LACTATION

A Comprehensive Treatise

VOLUME I

The Mammary Gland / Development and Maintenance

CONTRIBUTORS

R. R. ANDERSON

R. L. BALDWIN

R. DENAMUR

C. E. GROSVENOR

K. H. HOLLMANN

J. L. LINZELL

F. MENA

TAKAMI OKA

YALE J. TOPPER

H. ALLEN TUCKER

Y. T. YANG

LACTATION
A COMPREHENSIVE TREATISE

VOLUME I
The Mammary Gland / Development and Maintenance

Edited by

BRUCE L. LARSON / VEARL R. SMITH
Department of Dairy Science   *Department of Animal Science*
University of Illinois   *Colorado State University*
Urbana, Illinois   *Fort Collins, Colorado*

ACADEMIC PRESS New York and London   1974
A Subsidiary of Harcourt Brace Jovanovich, Publishers

ACADEMIC PRESS, INC.
111 Fifth Avenue, New York, New York 10003

United Kingdom Edition published by
ACADEMIC PRESS, INC. (LONDON) LTD.
24/28 Oval Road, London NW1

Library of Congress Cataloging in Publication Data

Larson, Bruce Linder, Date
 Lactation: a comprehensive treatise.

 Includes bibliographies.
  1. Lactation. 2. Milk. 3. Mammary glands.
I. Smith, Vearl Robert, Date joint author.
II. Title. [DNLM: 1. Lactation. 2. Lactation
disorders. WP825 L334L]
QP246.L38 599'.03 73-5298
ISBN 0−12−436701−1 (v. 1)

Contents

LIST OF CONTRIBUTORS viii

PREFACE ix

CONTENTS OF OTHER VOLUMES xi

PART I.   DEVELOPMENT AND STRUCTURE OF THE MAMMARY GLAND

Chapter One / **Cytology and Fine Structure of the Mammary Gland**

K. H. Hollmann

I. Uniformity of the Fine Structure of the Mammary Gland in Different Species 3

II. Light Microscopy of Half-Thin Sections of Mammary Tissues 5

III. Electron Microscopy of Mammary Tissues 14

IV. Virus Production in Normal Mammary Gland Cells 81

References 91

Chapter Two / **Endocrinological Control**

R. R. Anderson

I. Introduction 97

II. Measures of Mammary Gland Growth and Differentiation 99

III. Endocrine Regulation of Early Mammary Gland Differentiation and Growth 102

IV. Endocrine Changes during Puberty and Effects on Mammary Gland Growth 107

V. Normal Development of the Mammary Gland during Pregnancy and Pseudopregnancy 110

VI. Endocrine Control of Lactational Growth of the Mammary Gland 120

VII. Experimental Growth of the Mammary Gland 120

VIII. Nonhormonal Effects on the Mammary Gland 133

References 135

v

PART II. DEVELOPMENT AND MAINTENANCE OF LACTOGENESIS

Chapter Three / **Mammary Blood Flow and Methods of Identifying and Measuring Precursors of Milk**

J. L. Linzell

I.	Introduction	143
II.	Anatomy of Mammary Blood Vessels, Lymphatics, and Nerves	154
III.	Mammary Blood Flow	165
IV.	Mammary Lymph Flow	184
V.	Milk Precursors	186
VI.	Summary and Recommendations	219
	References	220

Chapter Four / **Neural and Hormonal Control of Milk Secretion and Milk Ejection**

C. E. Grosvenor and F. Mena

I.	Introduction	227
II.	Innervation of the Mammary Gland	228
III.	Removal of Milk from the Mammary Glands	236
IV.	Neuroendocrine Mechanisms in Milk Secretion	243
V.	Decline and Cessation of Lactation	266
	References	268

Chapter Five / **General Endocrinological Control of Lactation**

H. Allen Tucker

I.	Introduction	277
II.	Hormonal Control of Mammary Secretory Activity before Pregnancy	278
III.	Mammary Secretory Activity during Pregnancy	279
IV.	Hormonal Control of Lactogenesis	280
V.	The Lactation Curve	294
VI.	Hormonal Maintenance of Lactation	296
VII.	Effect of Nursing Intensity and Pregnancy on Lactation	315
VIII.	Conclusions	317
	References	318

Chapter Six / **Some Aspects of Mammary Gland Development in the Mature Mouse**

Yale J. Topper and Takami Oka

I.	Introduction	327
II.	Insulin and Serum Factor(s) Insensitivity	328
III.	Dynamics of Insulin Action	329
IV.	Cryptic Insulin Apparatus	330
V.	Insulin and Serum Factor(s) Sensitivity in Different States of Development	331
VI.	Sensitization by Prolactin	332
VII.	Protein Markers of Highly Developed Mammary Cells	334
VIII.	Requirement for Mitosis	335
IX.	Selection of a System for Further Study	336
X.	Developmental Status of Mammary Epithelial Cells in the Midpregnant Mouse	337
XI.	Synchronization of Midpregnancy Alveolar Cells	339
XII.	Additional Considerations	344
	References	346

Chapter Seven / **Enzymatic and Metabolic Changes in the Development of Lactation**

R. L. Baldwin and Y. T. Yang

I.	Introduction	349
II.	Mammary Enzyme Levels, Characteristics, and Relationships to Milk Synthesis	351
III.	Regulation of Mammary Enzyme Activities	389
IV.	Summary	406
	References	407

Chapter Eight / **Ribonucleic Acids and Ribonucleoprotein Particles of the Mammary Gland**

R. Denamur

I.	Introduction	414
II.	Ribonucleic Acids during Organogenesis and Secretory Differentiation of the Mammary Gland	415
III.	Nuclear RNA (nRNA) and Variations in DNA Transcription at the Moment of Functional Differentiation of the Mammary Gland	431
IV.	RNP (Ribonucleoprotein) Particles and Ribosomal RNA	438
V.	Transfer RNA of the Mammary Gland	447
	References	454
AUTHOR INDEX		467
SUBJECT INDEX		491

List of Contributors

Numbers in parentheses indicate the pages on which the authors' contributions begin.

R. R. ANDERSON (97), Department of Dairy Science, University of Missouri, Columbia, Missouri

R. L. BALDWIN (349), Department of Animal Science, University of California, Davis, California

R. DENAMUR* (413), Laboratoire de Physiologie de la Lactation, Institut National de Recherche Agronomique, C.N.R.S., Jouy-en-Josas, France

C. E. GROSVENOR (227), Departments of Physiology and Biophysics, University of Tennessee, Medical Units, Memphis, Tennessee

K. H. HOLLMANN (3), Department of Cancerology, Sarre University, and Collège de France, Laboratoire de Microscopie Électronique, Hôpital, Broussais, Paris, France.

J. L. LINZELL (143), Agricultural Research Council Institute of Animal Physiology, Babraham, Cambridge, England

F. MENA (227), Instituto de Investigaciones Biomédicas, UNAM, Ciudad Universitaria, Mexico

TAKAMI OKA (327), National Institute of Arthritis, Metabolism, and Digestive Diseases, National Ins 'utes of Health, Bethesda, Maryland

YALE J. TOPPER (327), National Institute of Arthritis, Metabolism, and Digestive Diseases, National Institutes of Health, Bethesda, Maryland

H. ALLEN TUCKER (277), Department of Dairy Science, Michigan State University, East Lansing, Michigan

Y. T. YANG (349), Department of Animal Science, University of California, Davis, California

* Deceased.

Preface

Only three decades ago, research on lactation was confined to relatively few land grant universities and occasional specialized research institutes around the world. Studies were limited to animals kept primarily for dairy purposes and augmented to a limited extent by the use of laboratory species. There was little relation between these studies and those on human lactation being performed in the medical profession.

However, all phases of lactation research have merged and expanded dramatically in the thirty years that have elapsed. With the development of more sophisticated equipment and techniques, scientists have searched for the elemental reactions involved in milk synthesis and for the ultrastructure of the organelles performing specific functions. The wide scope of subjects presented in this three-volume treatise, each by an eminent authority, indicates the breadth of research on lactation. The areas of interest represented are those oriented in the basic, health, medical, and agricultural sciences, all with specific interests in lactation.

Research during the past ten years has been especially active in the biological sciences. The accumulation of basic knowledge in the metabolism of tissues and cells has progressed rapidly, and advances in lactation have been no exception. Since the two volumes of "Milk: The Mammary Gland and Its Secretion" (edited by S. K. Kon and A. T. Cowie) were published in 1961 (Academic Press), no serious effort has been made to compile a comprehensive work on the subject of lactation. Such a compilation is the primary objective of this treatise. Some chapters in this work summarize developments of the past twelve years, while others cover areas that have grown in importance as more information has accumulated. For example, chapters on the fine structure of the mammary gland, the development and maintenance of lactation, and the biosynthesis of milk bring together a wide range of biochemical knowledge that has accumulated relative to the cellular mechanisms of hormones, structural elements, and the pathways in the synthesis of milk. Problems connected with consumption of milk that have become more apparent to the nutrition and medical specialists are treated in several chapters. Where applicable, through all the chapters, an attempt has been made to include information concerning a wide range of species, including man.

This treatise comprises three volumes containing a total of 28 chapters. The contents of this volume (I) are directed toward the structure and development of the mammary gland, leading to the maintenance of the gland in its specialized state of lactation. Emphasis has been placed on studies which have delineated the progression of these developmental changes at their most basic level. Electron microscopy, purified hormones, and techniques of molecular biology have been among the powerful tools used in this regard which have led to a rapidly increasing understanding of the changes that take place in cellular differentiation and their mediation by endocrinological factors. Volume II is concerned with the biosynthesis and secretion of milk and the diseases of lactation which affect the mammary gland. Volume III is concerned with the nutrition and biochemistry of milk, including the nutritional aspects of milk as a food and the maintenance of lactation in the whole animal of those species from which milk is utilized as a source of human food.

Our decision to undertake this project grew out of the feeling that an up-to-date summary of knowledge in the field was needed and that it would be of more use to compile a comprehensive treatise for the specialized scientist than to try to provide another textbook usable on the college level. We are pleased to have been able to obtain the contributions of so many outstanding scientists. We hope that this work achieves the desired synthesis of lactation research.

Note must be made of the untimely death in early 1973 of Dr. R. Denamur, author of Chapter 8. This article was originally written in French and translated into English. Dr. Denamur's death occurred before the galley proof was available which was subsequently corrected for errors by his former associates at Jouy-en-Josas. The final page proof was checked by the editors. Although we apologize for any errors that may be found in this article, we feel extremely fortunate that this monumental article by Dr. Denamur can be included in the treatise.

We wish to express our deepest appreciation to Corine R. Andersen and Helen J. Hegarty for their help in the editing of the manuscripts and in the preparation of the Subject Indexes.

BRUCE L. LARSON
VEARL R. SMITH

Contents of Other Volumes

VOLUME II: BIOSYNTHESIS AND SECRETION OF MILK / DISEASES

I. Biosynthesis of Milk

General Metabolism Associated with the Synthesis of Milk
C. L. Davis and D. E. Bauman

Biosynthesis of Milk Fat
D. E. Bauman and C. L. Davis

Biochemistry of Lactose and Related Carbohydrates
K. E. Ebner and F. S. Schanbacher

Biosynthesis of the Milk Proteins
B. L. Larson and G. N. Jorgensen

Cytological Aspects of Milk Formation and Secretion
R. G. Saacke and C. W. Heald

Membranes of the Mammary Gland
T. W. Keenan, D. James Morré, and C. M. Huang

II. Diseases of the Mammary Gland and Lactation

Pathophysiology of Prolactin Secretion in Man
Roger W. Turkington

Microbial Diseases of the Mammary Gland
F. H. S. Newbould

Ketosis
L. H. Schultz

Parturient Hypocalcemia, Hypomagnesemia, Mastitis-Metritis-Agalactia Complex of Swine
E. T. Littledike

Mammary Tumors in Mice
S. Nandi

AUTHOR INDEX–SUBJECT INDEX

**VOLUME III: NUTRITION AND BIOCHEMISTRY OF MILK /
MAINTENANCE**

I.   Biochemistry of Milk and Its Nutritive Quality

The Composition of Milk
   Robert Jenness

Genetic Variants of the Milk Proteins
   M. P. Thompson and H. M. Farrell, Jr.

General Environmental Contaminants Occurring in Milk
   Manfred Kroger

Physiological and Biochemical Aspects of the Accumulation of Contaminant Radionuclides in Milk
   F. W. Lengemann, R. A. Wentworth, and C. L. Comar

Immunoglobulins of the Mammary Secretions
   J. E. Butler

Immunological Problems of Milk Feeding
   Sidney Saperstein

Milk in Human Nutrition
   R. G. Hansen

II.   Maintenance of Lactation

Nutritional Requirements for Lactation
   W. P. Flatt and P. W. Moe

Environmental and Genetic Factors in the Development and Maintenance of Lactation
   R. W. Touchberry

AUTHOR INDEX–SUBJECT INDEX

PART I

DEVELOPMENT AND STRUCTURE OF THE MAMMARY GLAND

CHAPTER ONE

Cytology and Fine Structure of the Mammary Gland

K. H. Hollmann

I. Uniformity of the Fine Structure of the Mammary Gland in Different Species 3
II. Light Microscopy of Half-Thin Sections of Mammary Tissues 5
    A. The Mammary Gland at the Resting Stage (Mouse) .. 5
    B. The Mammary Gland during Pregnancy 6
    C. The Mammary Gland during Lactation 9
    D. Mitotic Activity in the Mammary Gland (Mouse) ... 9
    E. The Cytoplasmic–Nuclear Ratio in Different Stages of Mammary Activity 12
    F. The Mammary Gland during Milk Stasis 12
    G. The Regression of the Mammary Gland at the End of Lactation 13
III. Electron Microscopy of Mammary Tissues 14
    A. Structure of the Mammary Epithelium 14
    B. Fine Structure of the Glandular Cell 17
    C. Fine Structure of the Myoepithelial Cell 77
IV. Virus Production in Normal Mammary Gland Cells 81
    A. The Mammary Tumor Virus of the Mouse (MTV) .. 81
    B. Mammary Tumor Viruses in Other Species 85
    C. Leukemia Virus Transmitted through Milk 88
References 91

I. UNIFORMITY OF THE FINE STRUCTURE OF THE MAMMARY GLAND IN DIFFERENT SPECIES

Mammary gland cells from different species have an almost identical structure irrespective of the fact that the milk secreted by these cells varies widely in its chemical composition from one species to another. In all species the mammary cells accomplish their complex secretory function with the same cellular organelles, such as mitochondria, rough endoplasmic reticulum (or ergastoplasm), and Golgi apparatus. In the course of lactation the mammary gland cells modulate the composition and the yield of the milk to comply with the changing requirements of the young. They perform this by increasing the number, volume, or surface of the organelles whenever a higher synthetic activity is required.

Electron microscopic studies of more than 10 years deal with mammary tissues from humans (Waugh and Van der Hoeven, 1962; Bässler and Schäfer, 1969; Schäfer and Bässler, 1969; Hollmann and Verley, unpublished observations), cows (Feldman, 1961; Wooding, 1971a,b), goats (Wooding, 1971a,b; Hollmann, unpublished observations), sheep (Wooding, 1972; Hollmann, unpublished observations), pigs (Wooding, 1972), dogs (Hollmann and Verley, unpublished observations), cats (Hollmann and Verley, unpublished observations), rabbits (Hollmann, 1966; Hollmann and Verley, 1967; Girardie, 1967, 1968; Bousquet et al., 1969; Fiddler et al., 1971), hamsters (Bargmann et al., 1961; Ehrenbrand, 1964; Bargmann and Welsch, 1969), gerbils (Hollmann and Verley, unpublished observations), guinea pigs (Stockinger and Zarzicki, 1962; Girardie, 1967, 1968; Wooding, 1971a,b; Hollmann, unpublished observations), rats (Bargmann and Knoop, 1959; Bässler, 1961; Chentsou, 1964; Hollmann and Verley, 1967; Girardie, 1967, 1968; Helminen and Ericsson, 1968a,b,c; Helminen et al., 1968; Murad, 1970), and mice (Hollmann, 1959, 1960; Wellings et al., 1960a,b; Wellings and DeOme, 1961; Bargmann et al., 1961; Wellings and DeOme, 1963; Wellings and Philp, 1964; Girardie et al., 1964; Verley and Hollmann, 1966; Girardie et al., 1966; Hollmann and Verley, 1967; Rohr et al., 1968; Sekhri et al., 1967a,b; Girardie, 1968; Hollmann, 1968; Wellings and Nandi, 1968; Hollmann, 1969; Wellings, 1969; Hollmann and Verley, 1971). A uniform ground plan is shared by all mammary cells examined, and only insignificant differences have been observed, such as the size of the casein granules elaborated by mammary cells of different species (Table I).

TABLE I

DIAMETER OF PROTEIN GRANULES IN DIFFERENT SPECIES[a]

Species	Diameter (Å)
Human	300
Cow	800–1200
Rat	1500–3000
Mouse	3000

[a] Data from Bargmann (1962).

Other minor differences occur in the intensity of secretion during pregnancy. Girardie (1968), who examined mammary glands from mice, rats, guinea pigs, and rabbits, reported that the only difference observed in the four species concerns the moment when the first secretory granules become visible. Thus, at the end of the second third of pregnancy, "the milk secretion is considerable in the mouse, well under way in the rat, and only in its beginning in the guinea pig and the rabbit. The lipid synthesis appears in the prelactating mammary gland of the rabbit earlier than the protein synthesis" (Girardie, 1968). Such dissimilarities may rest on particular hormonal conditions or on the specific responsiveness of the mammary tissues, both proper to strains and species. Apparently, they have no major morphological substratum, although it cannot be ruled out that subtle quantitative differences in the cytoplasmic organelles (such as in the amount of ergastoplasm or mitochondria) occur at corresponding stages of pregnancy and parallel the functional divergencies reported. So far it appears justified to describe the fine structure of mammary cells in general without regard to the species.

II. LIGHT MICROSCOPY OF HALF-THIN SECTIONS OF MAMMARY TISSUES

The progress in tissue preservation and preparation achieved by techniques developed for electron microscopy improves notably the classic light microscopy. "Half-thin" (0.5–1.0 μm thick) araldite sections of osmium or glutaraldehyde fixed tissues stained with toluidine blue are a perfect material for high resolution photomicrographs. In half-thin sections of mammary gland cells, Golgi vacuoles, mitochondria, and ergastoplasmic arrangements are clearly distinguishable and casein granules of about 300 nm diameter can easily be detected within the vacuoles or outside the cells in the alveolar lumina (Figs. 4, 5, 7) (Hollmann and Verley, 1966). The following histocytological description is based on half-thin sections of mouse mammary glands and may serve as an outline of the general architecture of mammary tissues.

A. The Mammary Gland at the Resting Stage (Mouse)

The mammary gland of the newborn mouse consists of short primary ducts that begin at the nipple and branch into secondary and occasionally tertiary ducts terminating in end buds. The primary ducts are lined by a multilayered epithelium and have very narrow lumina (Sekhri *et al.*, 1967a). In the first 3 weeks of life end buds are rarely observed in the C57Bl/Crgl (Sekhri *et al.*, 1967a) or C3H mice (Nandi, 1959). From that time until puberty occurs, the ducts grow and pear-shaped end buds appear. After the mouse reaches puberty at the age of 8 weeks, the arborization of the ductal system and the formation of end buds progresses so that, in the 9-week-old mouse, the glandular tree occupies 90% of the fat pad (Sekhri *et al.*, 1967a). At the age of 3–4 months the mammary gland of virgin females consists of branching ducts lined by a single- or double-layered epithelium (Fig. 1), with interspersed myoepithelial cells. The ductal lumina are often filled with secretory material apparently rich in proteins. In the C57Bl mouse end buds are rare and true alveoli are absent at this stage (Sekhri *et al.*, 1967a), but strain differences exist (e.g., in C3H mice) as has been shown by Nandi (1958) and by Ranadive (1945).

B. The Mammary Gland during Pregnancy

During pregnancy the inactive mammary gland with its rudimentary parenchyma is transformed into a fully secreting tissue. This process re-

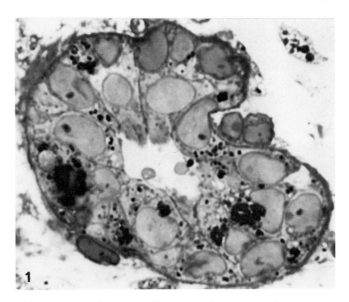

Fig. 1. Photomicrograph of a half-thin araldite section from a resting mouse mammary gland. The nuclei occupy a great part of the cells. The cytoplasm contains osmiophilic granules some of which coalesce and form irregular dark bulks. Toluidine blue; × 1700. (From Hollmann, 1969.)

quires growth of the grandular tree and differentiation of resting gland cells into functional cells. The sequence of events is quite similar in different species, and only their time course varies with the length of pregnancy.

1. First Half of Pregnancy

The mammary gland grows by dichotomous branching of the terminal portion of the duct system and by budding of alveoli. Thus the parenchyma successively replaces the fat pad (Fig. 2), which becomes more

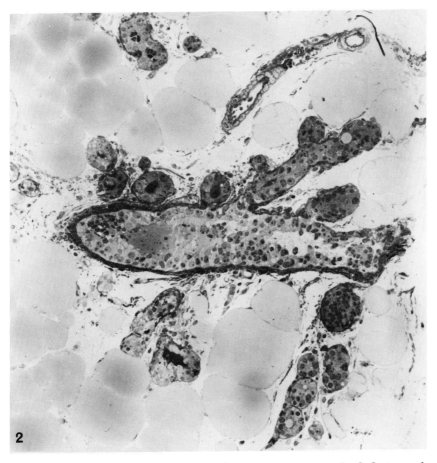

Fig. 2. Low-power light micrograph of a mouse mammary gland during early pregnancy. Ducts proliferate in the surrounding adipose tissue and give rise to alveoli. Araldite section, toluidine blue; × 225.

and more reduced and disappears completely at the end of pregnancy.

In the mouse, the first lobules are formed at the eighth or tenth day of pregnancy. The alveoli are rounder than before and have incipient or very narrow lumina generally devoid of secretory material. The glandular cells have become columnar, their infolded nuclei always occupying a great portion of the cell. The cytoplasm is more abundant, is denser, and contains numerous mitochondria and Golgi vacuoles. A few protein granules, enclosed in the vacuoles and lipid droplets of various size scattered through the cytoplasm, indicate the onset of secretory activity (Girardie, 1968). The lipid droplets are not extruded but are stored in the cytoplasm where they occupy about 20% of the volume (Fig. 3).

2. Second Half of Pregnancy

During the second half of pregnancy the growth of the gland continues and the secretory activity increases slowly. The lobulo-alveolar development becomes complete toward the last days of gestation, but the glandular lumina remains narrow until the time of parturition. At the third or second day ante partum the cytoplasm of the epithelial cells enlarges considerably and contains an increasing number of milk fat droplets, small at the cell basis but conspicuous in the apical region. Immediately before parturition they take up to 40% of the cytoplasmic volume (Fig.

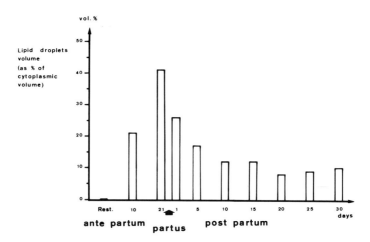

Fig. 3. The volume of milk fat droplets stored in mammary cells during pregnancy and lactation (mouse). The droplet volume is expressed as percentage of the cytoplasmic volume. A high storage takes place in the last few days before delivery. During lactation the milk fat droplets occupy about 10% of the cytoplasmic volume.

3). The Golgi vacuoles filled with protein granules also augment in size and number and accumulate under the apical plasma membrane. At the same time the nuclei of the epithelial cells take an ovoid shape with a smooth contour and have one, two, or even three large nucleoli. Although the glandular lumina are filled with protein granules, pictures evoking the release of secretory material are only rarely observed.

In the last hours before delivery the gland undergoes abrupt modifications. The secretory product, which takes up a great deal of the cytoplasm, is extruded and enters the alveolar cavities (Fig. 4). The lumina, overfilled with stagnating secretory material, become large and the outline of the alveoli becomes round. The glandular cells are cuboid or flat, their nuclei ovoid and turgescent, with conspicuous nucleoli. Their cytoplasm is abundant and contains numerous filamentous mitochondria and a clearly visible Golgi apparatus in the para- and supranuclear region, but there is almost no secretory material (Fig. 4).

C. The Mammary Gland during Lactation

The densely packed and fully distended alveoli give the lactating gland a spongy appearance. The structure of the alveoli is generally the same as observed immediately before delivery, except that the alveolar lumina are in some parts of the gland filled with fat droplets and protein granules, whereas in other parts they are almost empty. Correspondingly, the lining epithelium varies in different alveoli from high columnar to low cuboidal. Numerous filamentous mitochondria, large Golgi vacuoles, and an abundant ergastoplasm characterize the intensely secreting cells (Fig. 5). As a distinction from prelactating cells, which store most of the lipid droplets within the cytoplasm, the cells of the suckled gland contain rather few and small fat droplets (Figs. 3, 5). The myoepithelial cells with their extensions are embedded between the glandular cells so that the outline of the alveolus is round and smooth. In the course of lactation the gland preserves the same histocytological aspect.

D. Mitotic Activity in the Mammary Gland (Mouse)

In the mammary gland, as in other epithelia, new cells are needed in the course of cell renewal and in periods of growing. They are supplied by mitotic divisions. As far as the renewal of the mammary epithelium in a steady state is concerned, almost nothing is known about the turnover of resting or of functional cells. In periods of growing, mitotic figures are

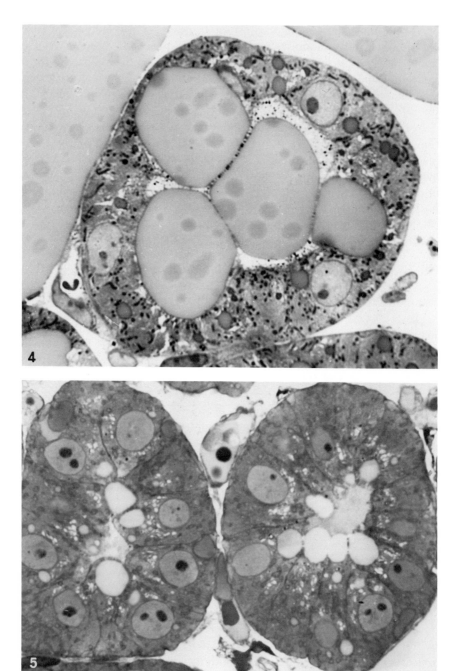

frequent in the end bud epithelium of prepubertal mice (Sekhri *et al.*, 1967a) and abundant in the developing gland of pregnant animals (Loeb and Hesselberg, 1917; Reece, 1956 quoted after Meites, 1961; Munford, 1964; Kriesten, 1965; Traurig, 1967a,b; and others).

In a quantitative study it has been shown (Kriesten, 1965) that the number of mitoses increases from about 1 per 1000 nuclei in the first days of pregnancy to a maximum of 10 per 1000 nuclei in the tenth day. Then the mitotic activity slopes down toward parturition. At the fifth day of lactation only 1 mitosis per 1000 nuclei was found, and later mitotic activity was almost nonexistent. Simultaneously with the decline of mitoses, the number of binucleated cells increases. According to Kriesten (1965), binucleated cells appear at the end of pregnancy and become more frequent with the beginning of lactation. Their number increases dramatically in the second half of lactation and attains more than 300 per 1000 epithelial cells at the twenty-first day. Kriesten believes that the binucleated cells originate from amitotic divisions and considers the doubling of the nuclei as a sign of an increased functional activity of the glandular epithelium.

Other investigators followed the cellular proliferation in the mouse mammary gland by means of radioautography after labeling with [³H]-thymidine (Traurig, 1967a,b) or by chemical determination of the DNA content (for review, Munford, 1964). Although for methodological reasons the different results are not easily superimposable, they suggest that there are two peaks of proliferative activity during pregnancy and a further new wave in the beginning of lactation. The latter observation raises the question whether lactating cells can enter mitosis. It seems that this indeed happens, since [³H]thymidine is incorporated in secreting cells (Traurig, 1967a), and mitotic figures are observed electron microscopically in lactating cells with a highly organized cytoplasm (Girardie, 1968; Hollmann, unpublished observation).

Fig. 4. Light micrograph of a bursting alveolus at the time of delivery (unsuckled gland, mouse). Note the large nuclei and prominent nucleoli and the numerous mitochondria in the cytoplasm (dark spots and filaments). Voluminous milk fat droplets fill the lumen or are retained in the cytoplasm. Araldite section, toluidine blue; × 1600.

Fig. 5. Two alveoli of a lactating gland, 24 hours postpartum (mouse). The glandular cells are columnar and have an abundant cytoplasm and large nuclei with prominent nucleoli. The Golgi field is clearly perceptible in the para- and supranuclear region. The alveolar lumina are smaller than in the cells just before delivery and do not contain stagnating secretory material. Araldite section, toluidine blue; × 1400. (From Hollmann, 1969.)

E. The Cytoplasmic–Nuclear Ratio in Different Stages of Mammary Activity

In the course of pregnancy and lactation, the cytoplasm of the mammary cells undergoes considerable modifications. Since the nucleus also changes in size or in number (binucleated cells, Section II,D) it is convenient to follow the cellular modifications by means of the cytoplasmic–nuclear ratio and to indicate the relative cytoplasmic volume as multiples of the nuclear volume. The changes occurring in the C/N ratio are represented in Fig. 6.

It is striking that the relative amount of cytoplasm increases considerably between parturition and the tenth day of lactation and that a further enlargement occurs between the fifteenth and the twentieth day. Since during the same period, particularly between the fifteenth and twentieth day of lactation, many cells become binucleated (Kriesten, 1965; Section II,D), the increase of the C/N ratio reflects a true enlargement of the cytoplasm. It seems that the functional activity of the mammary cells heightens immensely at this time (see also organelle development, Section III,B,4,b) and that the doubling of nuclei is necessitated to keep up with the cytoplasmic enlargement.

F. The Mammary Gland during Milk Stasis

During the first 24–48 hours after weaning, the mammary gland of the mouse remains unmodified (Verley and Hollmann, 1967). The alveoli,

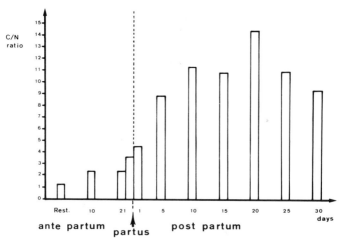

Fig. 6. Cytoplasmic–nuclear ratio (C/N) in mammary gland cells in successive stages of mammary activity. The relative amount of cytoplasm rises during pregnancy and reaches its maximum in the second half of lactation.

engorged with milk and distended, preserve their round outline. The epithelial cells are slightly flattened, but their nuclei are round or oval shaped as before, with large nucleoli. Their cytoplasm is abundant and contains dark blue stained clusters of irregular shape made up of coalesced protein granules.

It is difficult to determine on morphological grounds the precise onset of regression, i.e., the point of no return to the lactating stage. Apparently stasis can last for several days without inducing irreversible modifications. In the rat, lactation can set in again after 4 or 5 days of weaning, as reported by Silver (1956).

G. The Regression of the Mammary Gland at the End of Lactation

If the hormones required for maintaining lactation decrease, the histological and cytological organization of the mammary gland breaks down rapidly. The alveoli lose their round outline and their lumina, engorged with lipid droplets and protein granules, narrow (Fig. 7).

In the beginning of regression milk stasis still plays an important role and is accompanied by cellular modifications that lead the cells progressively to the resting stage (Fig. 8) or more abruptly to necrosis (Verley and Hollmann, 1967).

The cells devoted to necrosis lose their staining affinities and the cytoplasm becomes paler, somewhat granular or completely homogeneous. Other cells contain inclusions of different shape and size that consist of clumped protein granules or of autolysed cytoplasmic remnants (Fig. 9). The nuclei are preserved for a long time, but later undergo pyknosis. Finally, the cells shrink and disappear by lysis or by expulsion from the alveolus (Fig. 9). Degenerating cells are generally found either isolated or grouped as two or three adjacent cells, bordered on each side by surviving cells (Fig. 9). Such an arrangement allows the alveolar structure to be preserved when dying cells are eliminated.

In the course of this process, the myoepithelial cells apparently play a major role. Here and there they encompass completely the alveolar epithelium, thus constituting a second layer under the glandular cells (Figs. 7, 9). In other places they are contracted at the periphery of the alveolus. By their contractibility they probably facilitate the elimination of degenerated glandular cells and bridge the gap between the surviving cells.

Dying cells shed into the alveolar lumen have a vacuolated cytoplasm and are indistinguishable from bodies of Donné or colostrum corpuscles (Fig. 10; see also Section III,B,7) (Verley and Hollmann, 1967).

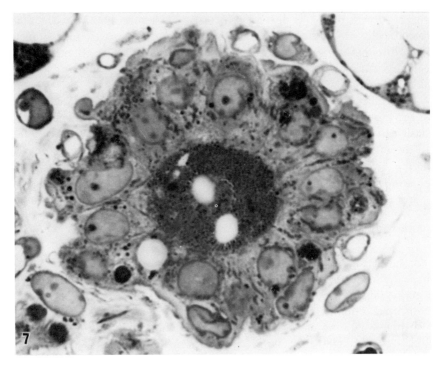

Fig. 7. Photomicrograph of an alveolus from a mouse mammary gland 2 days after weaning. The central cavity is filled with stagnating milk protein granules. The cytoplasm of the mammary cells is less abundant than during lactation. The nuclei are still large but the nucleoli are reduced in size. The myoepithelial cells protrude at the periphery of the alveolus and call forth an irregular contour. Araldite section, toluidine blue; × 1600. (From Verley and Hollmann, 1967.)

III.   ELECTRON MICROSCOPY OF MAMMARY TISSUES

A.   Structure of the Mammary Epithelium

Low power electron micrographs build the bridge between the histo-cytological aspects observed with the light microscope and the highly resolved morphology detectable with the electron microscope. Thus, low power views show nicely the structure of alveoli or ducts and rearrangements of tissue during pregnancy or at the end of lactation. They allow the identification of primary, secondary, and tertiary ducts under the electron microscope and the observation of marked differences in the three epithelia. Whereas the cells of primary ducts remain almost un-

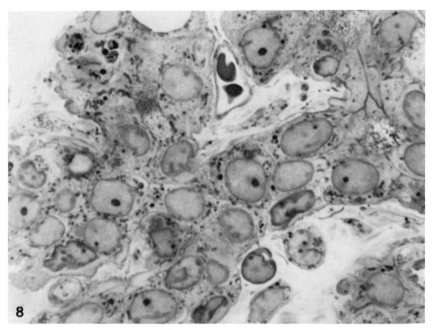

Fig. 8. Mouse mammary gland during regression. The glandular tree has a more solid structure and alveoli are reduced in size and number. The secretory activity has ceased and only a few protein granules are seen in the small lumina (on the right). Araldite section, toluidine blue; × 1500.

changed during lactation, the cells of secondary ducts are slightly stimulated and have a more abundant ergastoplasm and Golgi apparatus than they have in the resting stage. Tertiary duct cells differ noticeably from the preceding ones: they have parallel arrays of ergastoplasm, a pronounced Golgi complex, and are truly secreting (Sekhri *et al.*, 1967a). There seems to be an increasing sensitivity to lactogenic hormones from the primary duct to the peripheral structures, i.e., the alveoli.

The alveolus, which is indeed the most labile structure of the mammary gland, depends largely upon hormonal conditions and repeatedly undergoes profound rearrangements (Figs. 11–19). During pregnancy the alveolus is built up and consists of densely packed cells that accumulate large quantities of elaborated fat droplets in their cytoplasm. The alveolar lumen is very narrow or almost inexistent (Figs. 11, 12). At the point of delivery the alveolar structure becomes quite different (Fig. 13). There is now a large central cavity filled with voluminous fat droplets and small protein granules. The cells no longer store the synthesized secretory ma-

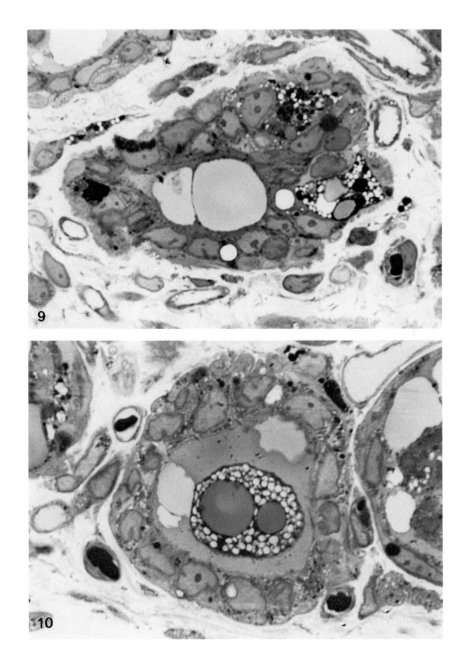

terial within their cytoplasm. The latter is moderately organized and the apical plasma membrane is covered with short microvilli. On the peripheral side of the alveolus, myoepithelial cells are disposed in a discontinuous second layer under the glandular cells (Fig. 13).

As lactation progresses and the gland is suckled, the alveolar lumen is less distended. The cells, in contrast, are turgescent and their lateral surfaces are stretched. The cytoplasm is packed with organelles and is more electron dense than in the preceding stages (Figs. 14, 15).

With the end of lactation a profound new rearrangement of the alveolar structure takes place (Figs. 16, 17). The cells become widely separated from one another and the intercellular spaces are congested by a flocculent material. The glandular cells are reduced markedly in number and size but the continuity of the alveolar structure is preserved as seen by the intact tight junctions (zonulae occludentes) on the luminal side and the unbroken basement membrane at the periphery of the alveolus.

At the end of regression the initial structure of a resting epithelium is regained (Figs. 18, 19).

B. Fine Structure of the Glandular Cell

Mammary cells are submitted to hormonal influences, which determine their functional activity. Under adequate stimulation resting gland cells develop into secreting cells and elaborate a complex secretory product containing proteins, fat, lactose, vitamins, minerals, and water.

In the course of lactation the cells vary the relative composition and the quantity of the secreted material. They accomplish this by continuously adjusting the development of the organelles, such as mitochondria, ergastoplasm, and Golgi apparatus, which together represent the synthetic apparatus of the cell (Fig. 46, p. 57).

Fig. 9. Regressing mammary gland of a rabbit, 8 days after weaning. The alveolus has an irregular contour and is bordered by contracted myoepithelial cells. Several cells are degenerating and contain numerous vacuoles and clusters of dark material. When they are shed in the alveolar lumen they take the aspect of Donné bodies (see Fig. 10). Araldite section, toluidine blue; × 1400. (From Verley and Hollmann, 1967.)

Fig. 10. Regressing mammary gland of a rabbit (same as Fig. 9). A corpuscle of Donné is seen in the alveolar cavity. Araldite section, toluidine blue; × 1550. (From Verley and Hollmann, 1967.)

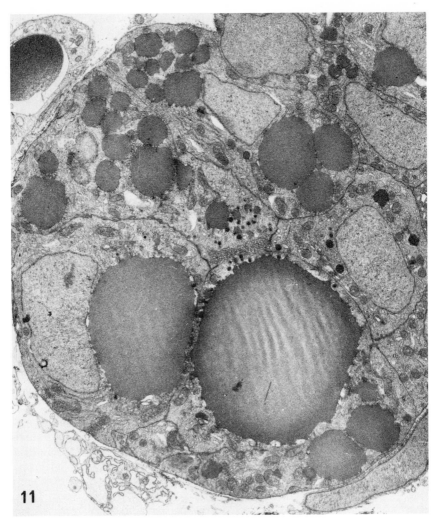

Fig. 11. Low-power electron micrograph of a developing alveolus from a mouse mammary gland at the fourteenth day of pregnancy. A central lumen is just incipient. The cytoplasm is still poor in organelles but contains numerous large fat droplets with dentate contours and a few (dark) protein granules. × 5000.

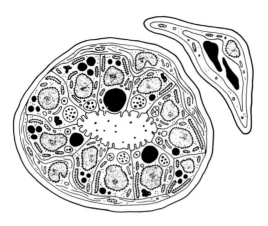

Fig. 12. Diagram of the structure of an alveolus in a prelactating gland (second half of pregnancy). The glandular cells have some ergastoplasm and Golgi elements and elaborate milk fat droplets and protein granules, but the secretory material is mostly stored within the cytoplasm and only rarely extruded into the lumen. Myoepithelial cells surround the glandular cells and the alveolus has a regular outline.

1. The Resting Cell

As already described (Section II,A) the resting gland is made of a branched duct system and end buds that represent the future alveoli. The ducts are divided into primary, secondary, and tertiary ducts according to the degree of branching (for the mouse see among others Nandi, 1958; Sekhri *et al.*, 1967a). On the ultrastructural level the epithelial cells of primary and secondary ducts have scalloped or lobated nuclei. Their cytoplasm, often limited to a small border around the nucleus, contains a few mitochondria, an inconspicuous Golgi apparatus, scattered ribosomes, and rarely some ergastoplasmic membranes (Figs. 20–22). The lateral surfaces of the cells are often intricate and show a well-developed junctional complex consisting of the three elements: zonula occludens, zonula adhaerens, and macula adhaerens (or desmosomes) (Farquhar and Palade, 1963; Figs. 20–23). In the zonula occludens the outer leaflets of the adjacent plasma membranes (plasmalemmata) are fused so that the intercellular space is obliterated in this region (Fig. 23). In the following zonula adhaerens the contiguous plasma membranes are not fused but separated by a 200 Å large intercellular space filled with a homogeneous material of low density (Figs. 20, 23).

In the desmosome (or macula adhaerens) the adjacent plasma membranes are also separated by an intercellular space, about 200 Å wide, which contains denser material than that in the zonula adhaerens. On the

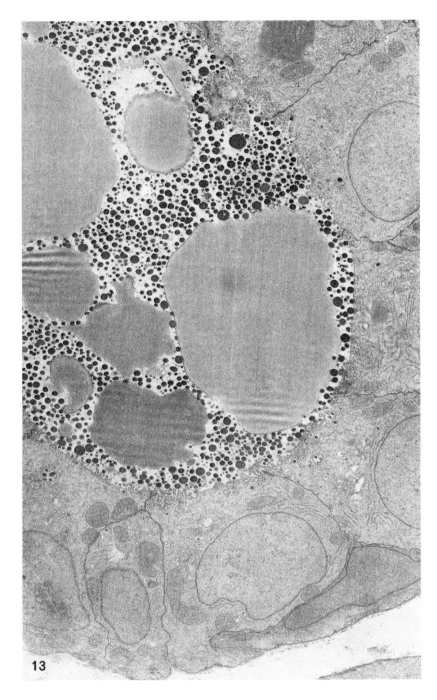

cytoplasmic side of each of the two membranes lies a dense plate on which bundles of fibrils converge from the cytoplasm (Figs. 21, 23).

A completely developed junctional complex is characteristic for ductal cells and therefore frequently observed in resting mammary epithelia. The alveolar cells, at least if they are functional, are held together by reduced junctional complexes consisting only of zonulae occludentes (and zonulae adhaerentes?).

According to Sekhri *et al.* (1967a) the cells of tertiary ducts have a somewhat more abundant cytoplasm but otherwise their structure is very similar to that of cells in the primary and secondary ducts.

The end buds are made of several cell layers bounding a small lumen. The end bud cells are different from duct cells and have a richer cytoplasm, a little more mitochondria, and a few ergastoplasmic cisternae (Fig. 24). Their Golgi apparatus is more developed than in ductal cells and consists of several lamellae and numerous vesicles. The apical surface of end bud cells is covered with short microvilli.

2. The Prelactating Cell

During pregnancy the resting cells progressively increase their organelle equipment so that, at the end of gestation, properly organized cells are ready for lactation (Hollmann, 1968, 1969; Hollmann and Verley, 1971).

a. THE BEGINNING OF PREGNANCY. In this stage the glandular cells have, like at the resting stage, a poor cytoplasmic organization, i.e., the different organelles are scanty. The mitochondria are few in number and small, with widely spaced internal cristae and minute mitochondrial granules. The ergastoplasm is sparse and the Golgi apparatus consists only of a few lamellae and vesicles. The nucleus is mostly lobated, has a scalloped contour, a fine granular and regularly dispersed chromatin, and small nucleoli. In the first stage of pregnancy no secretory product is visible in the cytoplasm, but some alveolar lumina contain a finely structured material suggesting degraded protein granules.

When pregnancy advances, the glandular cells undergo differentiation (Fig. 25). The mitochondria become more numerous with denser arranged internal cristae. The ergastoplasm develops, particularly in the

---

Fig. 13. Low-power electron micrograph of an alveolus from a mouse mammary gland immediately after delivery. The glandular cells are differentiated but have not yet reached the aspect of full lactating cells. The secretory product is released from the cells and stagnates in the central cavity. The cytoplasm contains a few protein granules and small fat droplets. × 6800.

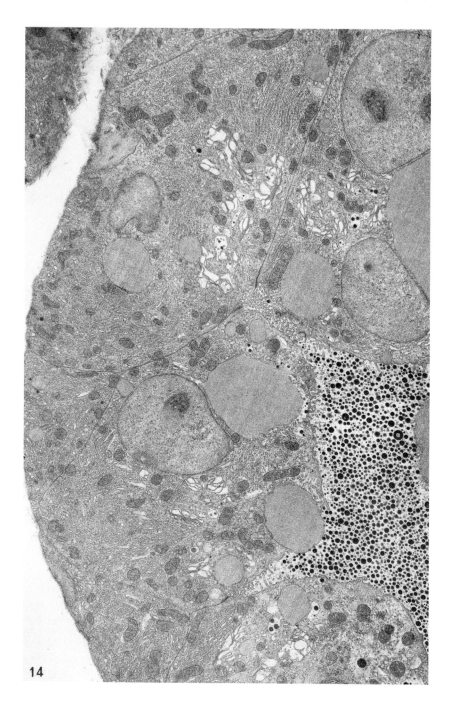

14

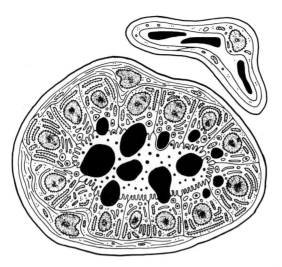

Fig. 15. Diagram depicting an alveolus from a lactating gland. The glandular cells are rich in organelles, and milk fat droplets and protein granules are released from the cells as soon as they are elaborated. The myoepithelial cells have a similar arrangement as that in the prelactating alveolus.

basal cytoplasm, and the Golgi apparatus increases in size and consists of flattened sacs, some vacuoles, and vesicles. This organelle is always located in the supra- and paranuclear region.

In the mouse the glandular cells begin to elaborate the first secretory products at about the eighth to tenth day of pregnancy (Girardie, 1968). At this time, milk fat droplets and protein granules appear in the cytoplasm, but the secretory activity is still moderate and only a part of the glandular cells is ready for secretion.

The first milk fat droplets become visible in the basal cytoplasm (Fig. 11). Their number and size vary from one cell to another. They are electron dense and have often an irregular or starlike contour. Most of them

Fig. 14. Portion of an alveolus from a mouse mammary gland at the fifth day of lactation. The alveolus has a smooth contour and the central cavity contains numerous protein granules. The cytoplasm of the mammary cells is abundant and completely occupied by the highly developed organelles. The ergastoplasmic cisternae are densely packed and predominate in the basal portion of the cytoplasm, whereas the Golgi elements are situated in the para- and supranuclear region. The mitochondria are scattered throughout the cell without preferential localization. Protein granules are seen in membrane bound vacuoles and large milk fat droplets are found at the apical pole of the cells. The cell in the upper right quadrant is binucleated. × 4800. (From Hollmann, 1969.)

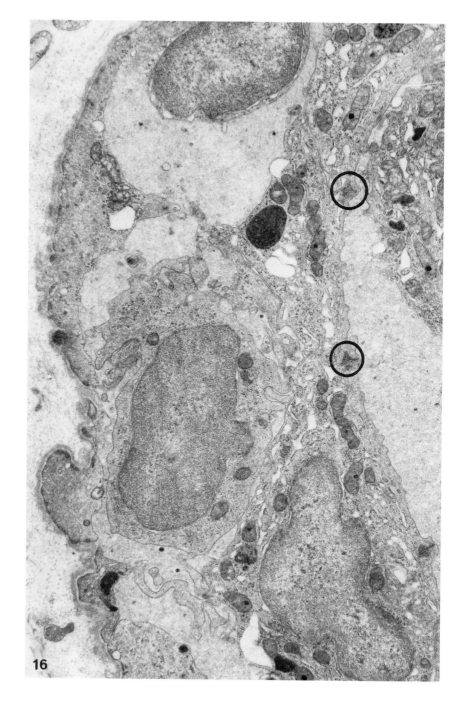

16

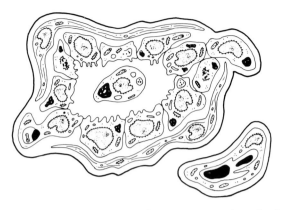

Fig. 17. Diagram of a collapsing alveolus in a regressing gland. The regular arrangement of the glandular cells is lost and the intercellular spaces are enlarged. Although the cells are at different stages of regression or on the way to necrosis, the wholeness of the alveolar structure is preserved by persistent juxtaluminal cell connections and by contracted myoepithelial cells at the base of the alveolus the contour of which thus becomes irregular. Necrotic cells are shed into the alveolar lumen or lysed and squeezed out toward the surrounding interstitial tissue.

are stored in the cytoplasm and the characteristic aspects of lipid extrusion are generally not observed.

The elaborated proteins appear as round granules of high electron density in vacuoles of the Golgi apparatus. At this stage of pregnancy they are not extruded into the alveolar lumen but remain in the cells. The first granules generally occur singly in small vacuoles, but later numerous granules accumulate and fuse within larger vacuoles and undergo a progressive degradation, as is the case at the end of lactation (see Section III,B,5 and 6). This process follows the same mechanism as that observed in other tissues such as the anterior pituitary (Smith and Farquhar, 1966; Fig. 26). It is accomplished with the aid of lysosomes (as dense bodies and multivesicular bodies), which are plentiful in the cytoplasm of early prelactating cells (Fig. 25). The secretory granules, enclosed in the vacuoles or liberated into the cytoplasm, are incorporated into dense bodies or into multivesicular bodies (Figs. 27–29) where they lose their

---

Fig. 16. Portion of a regressing alveolus from a rabbit mammary gland (8 days after weaning). The alveolar cells are separated by large intercellular spaces but are held together in the apical region by preserved junctional complexes (encircled) and at the periphery by myoepithelial cells and by a thickened basement membrane. In the alveolar lumen (on the right) a portion of a shed glandular cell can be recognized. × 8000. (From Hollmann and Verley, 1967.)

density and their characteristic fine structure. In subsequent steps the material is progressively degraded into vacuolated dense bodies that are eventually separated into free lipid droplets and dense bodies.

As already indicated by Smith and Farquhar (1966), dense bodies and multivesicular bodies are mainly involved in the degradation of secretory

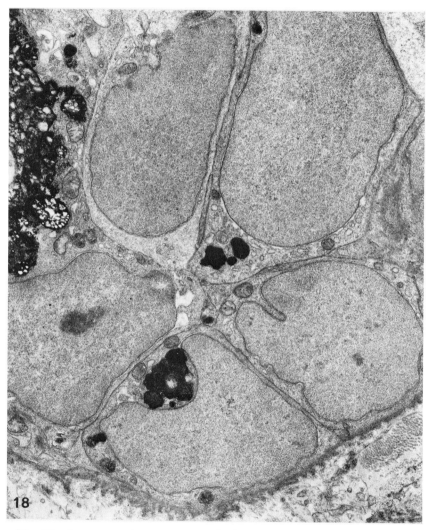

Fig. 18. Low-power electron micrograph of a resting acinus from a mouse mammary gland. The cytoplasm is reduced to a small border around the nucleus and contains only a few mitochondria, some lysosomes, and dark bulks of degradated material. × 7000. (From Hollmann, 1969.)

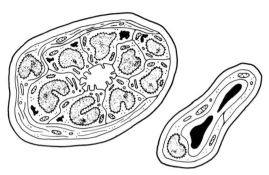

Fig. 19.   Diagram of a glandular structure at the resting stage. The central lumen is small or almost nonexistent, the nuclei are infolded, and the cytoplasm is reduced and contains few organelles. Secretory material is generally not produced, but lysosomes and bulks of electron-dense degradation products are often observed.

granules, whereas autophagic vacuoles (i.e., lysosomes containing sequestered cytoplasm and organelles) play an important part in the removal of degenerating cytoplasm. It is characteristic that autophagic vacuoles, abundant during regression, are almost absent in prelactating mammary cells. Obviously, the essential process in developing mammary cells is the permanent breakdown of the elaborated secretory material and not the degradation of cytoplasmic structures.

b. The Second Half of Pregnancy.   During this stage the cellular differentiation progresses, as can be seen by the further development of the cytoplasmic organelles. The mitochondria increase in size and number. The ergastoplasm continues to develop and consists of short and flattened cisternae predominantly at the base of the cell. The Golgi apparatus enlarges and attains at the end of pregnancy an almost identical aspect to that of lactating cells. It consists of flattened sacs, numerous vesicles, and vacuoles containing protein granules (Figs. 30, 31). The secretory activity intensifies and fat droplets and granule-laden vacuoles accumulate in the cytoplasm, particularly in the apical region (Figs. 27, 30). Some protein granules are extruded into the alveolar lumina (Fig. 30). Other granules are degraded, and multivesicular bodies and dense bodies are still numerous. However, free protein granules or proteinaceous bulks within the cytoplasm become rare and the process of intracellular degradation is apparently less important than in the preceding phase.

With the approach of delivery, milk fat droplets increase in number and size. The smaller droplets predominate in the basal cytoplasm, and the bigger ones occupy the apical region or bulge into the alveolar lumen. Although they take a great deal of the cytoplasm and compress the

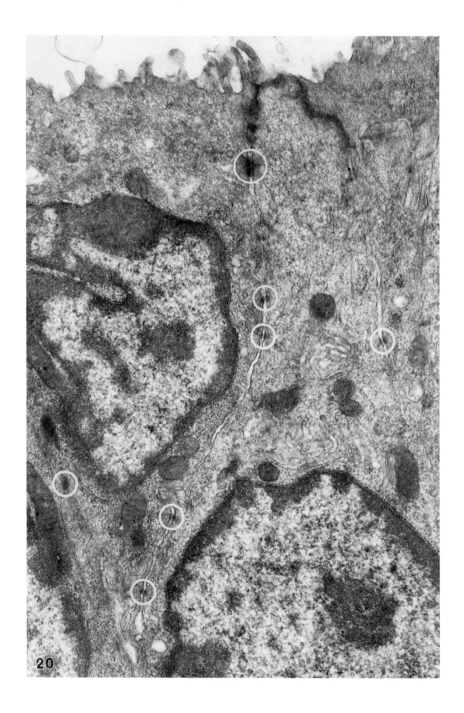

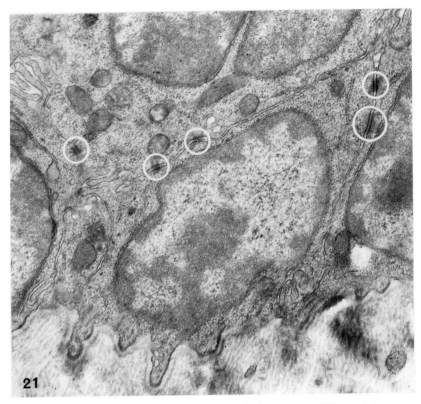

Fig. 21. Mammary cells from a resting gland of the mouse. The nuclei occupy a great part of the cells, and the organelles are poorly developed. Desmosomes (encircled) are numerous and the basal cytoplasm shows fingerlike projections surrounded by the basement membrane. × 26,000.

nucleus or push it toward the base, they are not released from the cell. The alveolar lumina are still narrow, filled with protein granules and only occasionally some lipid droplets and colostrum corpuscles (for the latter, see Section III,B,7).

In the last hours preceding delivery the structure of the glandular cell changes abruptly and nearly attains the aspect of the lactating cell (Figs. 13, 32). The mitochondria are dense and rich in cristae. The ergastoplasm

Fig. 20. Ductal cells from a resting mammary gland of the mouse. The cytoplasmic organelles are poorly developed. A small Golgi apparatus is seen above the nucleus. The lateral surfaces of the cells are connected by junctional complexes and numerous desmosomes (encircled). × 29,000.

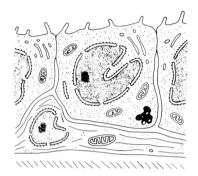

Fig. 22. Diagram depicting a resting mammary gland cell. The cell has a cubic shape and its apical surface has a few short microvilli. The nucleus is generally infolded and has a rather small nucleolus. The cytoplasm is reduced and poor in organelles, particularly in ergastoplasmic cisternae and Golgi elements.

is made of long cisternae arranged in parallel arrays at the base of the cell and in the paranuclear region. The Golgi apparatus is abundant, and most of the Golgi vacuoles contain well-defined protein granules.

The striking event at the end of pregnancy is the discharge of the secretory product into the alveolar lumina, which become distended. The cytoplasm of the glandular cells contains just a few newly formed lipid droplets, which now have round or ovoid contours. The multivesicular bodies have disappeared and pictures of intracytoplasmic degradation of secretory granules are no longer observed (Fig. 13).

3. The Lactating Cell

The fully lactating cell represents the summit of cytoplasmic organization (Figs. 33–40). The high development of the organelles indicates that the alveolar cells are now efficient metabolic factories for the production of casein, milk fat, β-lactoglobulin, lactose, and other components

The ergastoplasm, involved in the synthesis of proteins, consists of large groups of parallel cisternae that occupy a great portion of the cytoplasm (Fig. 39). Some cisternae are wide and contain a filamentous material (Fig. 39).

The Golgi apparatus, the site of formation of the definitive proteinaceous granules, comprises an assemblage of flattened sacs, large vacuoles and microvesicles (Fig. 40). The vacuoles originate from dilatations of the flattended sacs by pinching off. Most of them contain protein granules and are engaged in their transport to the apical cell surface.

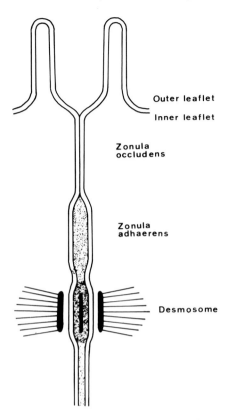

Outer leaflet

Inner leaflet

Zonula
occludens

Zonula
adhaerens

Desmosome

Fig. 23. Diagram of a completely developed junctional complex, consisting of three elements: zonula occludens (tight junction), zonula adhaerens (intermediate junction), and macula adhaerens (desmosome).

The mitochondria, scattered abundantly throughout the cytoplasm, have closely arranged cristae, a dense matrix, and several small intramitochondrial granules (Fig. 38).

The nucleus, large, round, or ovoid, has two or three prominent nucleoli. Two nuclei per cell may be observed (Fig. 14) although those pictures are less frequent in fine sections than they are in histological preparations (Section II,D).

The peculiar features of the lactating cells are best elucidated by quantitative description (Section III,B,4,b). Quantitative considerations also show that the organelle development does not reach a steady state but undergoes modifications in the course of lactation.

The "synthetic apparatus," i.e., the described organelles, elaborates the different milk constituents, two of which appear in a visible form

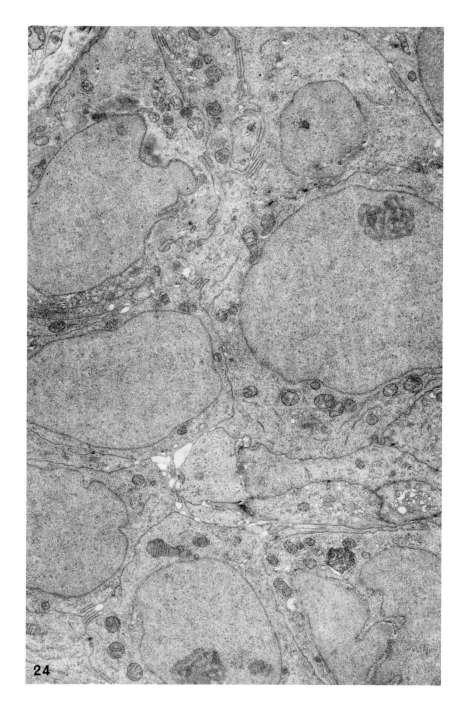

24

(Hollmann, 1959; Bargmann and Knoop, 1959): the protein granules (casein) and the milk fat droplets. The protein granules, enclosed in Golgi vacuoles, are round, electron dense, and have a subunit structure (Section III,B,4,a). Their diameter varies in different species and has been indicated from 300 Å (human) to 3000 Å (mouse) (see Table I). The milk fat droplets attain diameters of several microns. They are less electron dense than the protein granules and in contrast to the latter their density varies in different stages of lactation and depends widely on the procedure of fixation (Figs. 13, 14, 33, 34, 36). The smallest fat droplets occur in the basal cytoplasm, often between ergastoplasmic membranes (Bargmann and Knoop, 1959; Bargmann, 1962) or in contact with mitochondria.

Besides the organelles engaged in the synthetic process, other cytoplasmic differentiations are developed, although their role is not always obvious. Thus, microtubules with a diameter of about 220 Å have been described in lactating cells (Sandborn *et al.*, 1964). In the alveolar cells, they are arranged in horizontal and vertical directions, whereas in ductal cells they have only an apico-basal orientation. Their function as a conducting system or merely as a skeletal frame is still in question.

Other differentiations concern the plasma membranes. The luminal surface of the lactating cell is covered by microvilli that are up to 1 μm long. Bargmann (1962) counted 10–25 microvilli per μm^2 in the lactating gland of the hamster and assumes that they are involved in absorption of substances from the alveolar lumen. The microvilli shorten and disappear when fat droplets bulge in the alveolar cavity and tense the plasmalemma.

The basal side of lactating cells often has irregularly formed cytoplasmic processes (Bässler, 1961; Bargmann and Welsch, 1969). It seems that the basement membrane does not always follow the contour of these processes but bridges a few of them so that a complicated system of clefts is formed between the plasmalemma and the basement membrane (Bargmann and Welsch, 1969). According to Bargmann and Welsch (1969) the development of foot processes is particularly pronounced in mammary cells in the neighborhood of capillaries. That topographic relation and the observation of "coated vesicles" in the basal cytoplasm led Bargmann and Welsch (1969) to the opinion that the foot processes are involved in the uptake of substances from the extracellular space. In support of this hypothesis is the high enzyme activity, e.g., of alkaline

Fig. 24. Resting mammary cells from a human female 37 years old. The cells are poorly differentiated and show no signs of secretory activity.

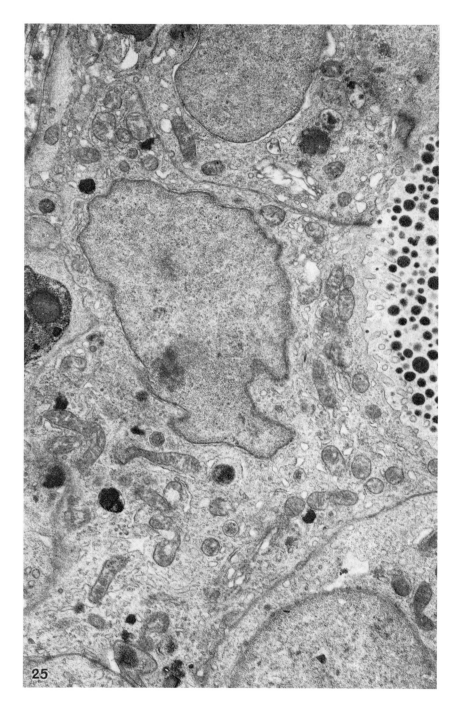

25

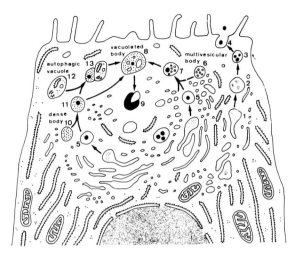

Fig. 26. Diagram illustrating some of the events occurring during milk stasis when a part of the elaborated secretory material is not released from the cell. The normal pathway of extrusion is indicated on the right of the diagram: flocculent material in dilated Golgi sacs (1) becomes condensed in Golgi vacuoles (2) and forms dense mature granules (3) which are released from the cell by fusion of the vacuoles with the surface membrane (4). When milk stasis occurs the elaborated material is degraded by the intervention of lysosomes: a protein-containing vacuole (5) fuses with a multivesicular body (6) or a dense body (10) forming complex structures (7 or 11) which develop into vacuolated bodies (8). The latter can undergo further modifications (9). When parallel cytoplasmic degradation takes place, as is the case during cellular involution, dense bodies (10 or 11) can merge with autophagic vacuoles (12) (i.e., lysosomes containing cytoplasmic constituents). These fused structures (13) are further degraded to yield a residual vacuolated body (8 and 9). The latter pathway is uncommon in prelactating cells but characteristic of involuting cells in the postlactating phase. (Adapted from Smith and Farquhar, 1966.)

phosphatase and glucose-6-phosphatase in the basal portion of lactating cells (Bässler and Paek, 1968).

Another characteristic aspect of the plasma membranes of lactating alveolar cells concerns the intercellular connections. The junctional complexes already described (Section III,B,1) are incomplete, and only the

Fig. 25. Portion of an alveolus from a mouse mammary gland at midpregnancy. The cytoplasm is much more abundant than in resting cells and contains numerous mitochondria, multivesicular bodies, lysosomes, and Golgi elements. The cells do not contain secretory material but the alveolar lumen (on the right) is filled with protein granules. The apical surface of the cells shows numerous microvilli. $\times$ 13,500.

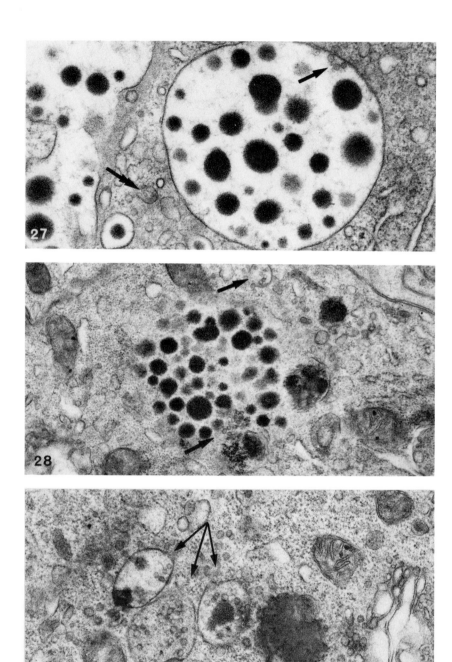

zonulae occludentes near the upper edges of the cells are regularly developed (Fig. 41). The zonulae adhaerentes can not be identified with certainty and desmosomes are generally absent (Hollmann, 1967). This particularity of the intercellular connection in lactating alveolar cells is probably of functional importance. The absence of desmosomes allows the intercellular spaces to become widely distended as is observed when milk stasis occurs (Hollmann, 1966; Hollmann and Verley, 1967).

4. Morphology of Milk Secretion

a. ELABORATION OF THE SECRETORY PRODUCT. i. *Elaboration of protein granules.* The milk proteins become at least partially visible as protein granules (about 300 nm diameter in the mouse) and their smaller components. They appear generally in the vacuoles of the Golgi apparatus (Bargmann and Knoop, 1959; Hollmann 1959; Wellings and DeOme, 1961; Wellings, 1969; and others), but occasionally, for instance in tumor cells, they occur in the ergastoplasmic cisternae (Hollmann, 1959). Several steps in the formation of the protein granule can be followed morphologically, and the time sequence of their elaboration can be established by high resolution autoradiography after injection of tritiated leucine.

(1) MORPHOLOGICAL STUDIES. It is clearly visible on electron micrographs that the protein granules have a distinct and regular substructure (Fig. 42). This characteristic pattern is observed in the granules contained in the Golgi vacuoles as well as in the granules released in the alveolar lumina.

According to Bargmann and Welsch (1969), who studied mammary tissues or milk from hamsters, rats, cows and humans, the larger protein granules are built up of chains of smaller particles with a diameter of

---

Figs. 27–29. Degradation of milk protein granules in prelactating mammary cells.

Fig. 27. Large vacuole from a prelactating cell containing numerous protein granules and some microvesicles (↑). A microvesicular body (⚡) is situated in the vicinity of the vacuole. Mouse mammary gland 24 hours antepartum; × 40,000.

Fig. 28. The secretory granules are liberated in the cytoplasm and in close relationship with microvesicular bodies (↑) and lysosomal structures. Mouse mammary gland, tenth day of pregnancy; × 27,000.

Fig. 29. Three microvesicular bodies (↑) one of which contains a dense granule which probably corresponds to an incorporated secretory granule. The dark mass with an irregular contour seems to be a residual body of degraded material. Mouse mammary gland, tenth day of pregnancy; × 37,000.

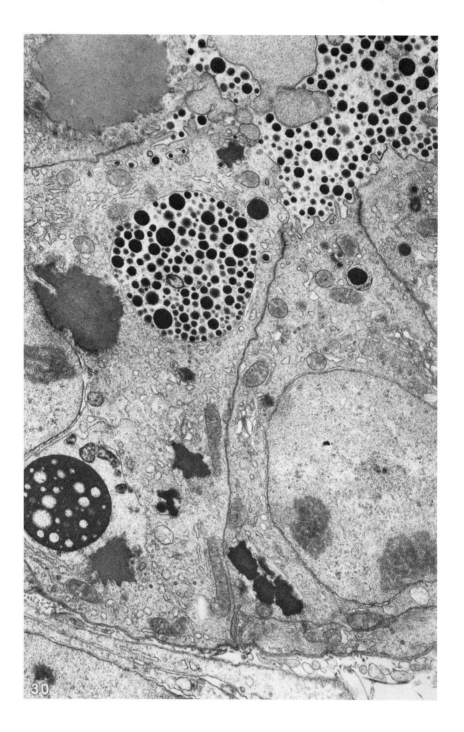

30

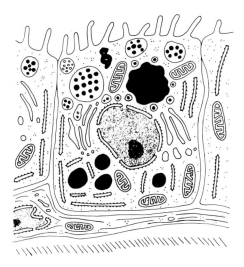

Fig. 31. Diagram illustrating the main features of a prelactating mammary cell (second half of pregnancy). The organelles involved in the secretory process are rather developed and the elaborated secretory product, protein granules, and milk fat droplets accumulate inside the cell. Pictures of extrusion are rare and a part of the stored secretory material is degraded by the lysosomal system (cf. Fig. 26).

150–200 Å. The latter structures seem to be composed of still smaller subunits that have a diameter of about 15–20 Å.

As Bargmann and Welsch (1969) emphasized, the last figures correspond to the size of casein molecules, which, according to the calculations of Waugh (1958), should have a diameter of 16 Å.

Besides these small structures observed in the Golgi compartment, other minute dense particles are found in the ergastoplasmic cisternae of lactating cells (Wellings and Philp, 1964; Helminen and Ericsson, 1968a; Hollmann and Verley, 1971) (Fig. 39). This material has a filamentous aspect, sometimes similar to that seen in the Golgi apparatus, and is loosely aggregated and in contact with the cisternal wall. After OsO_4 fixation for 48 hours, a dense deposit, which probably corresponds to the filamentous material (Hollmann and Verley, 1971) (Fig. 43), is found in the cisternae. The route by which the newly synthesized protein molecules get from the ergastoplasmic cisternae to the Golgi apparatus

Fig. 30. Mouse mammary gland cells at the fourteenth day of pregnancy. The cells contain numerous dark fat droplets of irregular shape, and vacuoles filled with protein granules. An unusual large vacuole at the upper pole of the cell on the left is a characteristic feature of milk stasis. × 13,500.

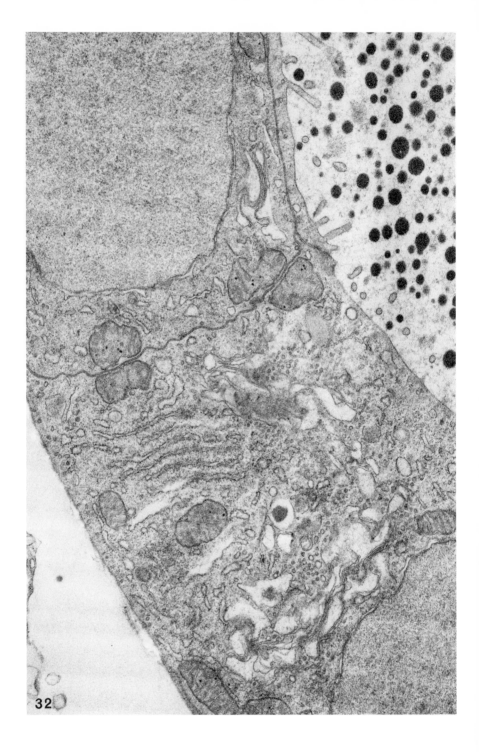

32

is not definitely elucidated. Earlier observations pointed out the existence of a continuity between ergastoplasm and smooth-surfaced Golgi lamellae (flattened sacs) (Palade, 1955; Haguenau and Bernhard, 1955). However, it is not established that such communications are widely distributed and really serve for the transfer of substances from one compartment to the other.

Studies on the intracellular transport of secretory proteins in pancreatic cells indicate that the material synthesized in the ergastoplasm is carried to the Golgi apparatus by means of small, smooth-surfaced vesicles that are usually located in the periphery of the Golgi complex (Jamieson and Palade, 1967). It is likely that a similar process takes place in the mammary gland, where microvesicles pinching off from the ergastoplasmic cisternae are frequently seen. After prolonged fixation in OsO_4 (Hollmann and Verley, 1971), numerous vesicles contain heavily stained material whereas others appear empty (Fig. 43). These morphological observations have to be interpreted with care, but they agree with the proposal that the microvesicles have a shuttle function and that the filled vesicles are on the way from the ergastoplasm to the Golgi apparatus whereas the empty ones are going from the Golgi to the cisternae (Figs. 43, 44).

Studies of the last years have shown that the Golgi apparatus has a much more complex function than was believed earlier. It was first suggested that it is devoid of synthetic activity and acts only through condensation of the proteinaceous substances elaborated elsewhere (Dalton and Felix, 1956). It is now recognized that the Golgi apparatus is involved in different functions: (1) in some final steps of the elaboration of protein secretion granules; (2) in the synthesis of some carbohydrate-containing substances (for instance mucoproteins in the goblet cell, Lane *et al.*, 1964, Hollmann, 1965; Neutra and LeBlond, 1966); and (3) in the process of membrane replenishment.

The precise way in which the organelle intervenes in the different processes still escapes our knowledge. As far as the synthesis of protein granules is concerned, it seems that a "condensation" of loose "precursor material" to densely packed protein granules takes place in the vacuoles (Fig. 42) since the definitive secretion granules preserve a characteristic

---

Fig. 32. Mouse mammary gland cells 3 hours before delivery (biopsy material). The cytoplasm is filled with organelles. The Golgi apparatus is developed and Golgi vacuoles contain protein granules. Several ergastoplasmic cisternae are arranged in parallel. The alveolar lumen on the upper right contain secretory granules. × 15,000. (From Hollmann, 1969.)

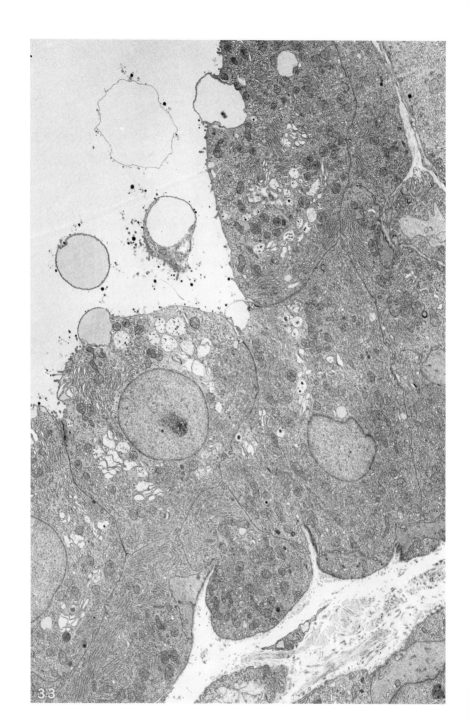

substructure (Bargmann and Welsch, 1969). Since the protein granules in the Golgi vacuoles react differently to prolonged OsO_4 fixation than the precursor material in the cisternae, it is quite possible that more complex chemical interactions occur in the Golgi compartment than just condensation (Hollmann and Verley, 1971).

(2) AUTORADIOGRAPHIC STUDIES. The sequential steps of protein synthesis in mouse mammary gland cells have been followed by high resolution autoradiography (Wellings and Philp, 1964; Verley and Hollmann, 1967; Stein and Stein, 1967; Rohr *et al.*, 1968). Tritiated leucine, one of the major amino acids of mouse milk protein (Wellings and Philp, 1964), is used as a tracer and its intracellular localization after different lapses of time determined by electron microscopy.

These studies reveal the following sequences of protein synthesis in lactating cells:

1. Twenty minutes after intravenous injection of tritiated leucine most of the radioactivity is detected over the ergastoplasm indicating that this is the primary site of protein synthesis.

2. Thirty minutes after injection the highest grain counts are observed over the Golgi apparatus.

3. Sixty minutes after injection the tracer is found both in the Golgi region and in the intraalveolar lumen.

The time sequence of radioactive tracing indicates that the ergastoplasm is the first site of protein synthesis and that the Golgi apparatus is involved in the further elaboration and transport of the proteinaceous secretory product.

A recent study of Rohr *et al.* (1968) completes the preceding results by semiquantitative data. These authors studied the incorporation of tritiated leucine between 5 and 240 minutes after intravenous injection and determined the percent distribution of silver grains over the different cellular compartments. They calculated the "relative specific localization" of the tracer by determining (a) the percentage of silver grains over a given compartment (e.g., Golgi apparatus) and (b) the relative surface of this compartment (as percent of the total cellular and luminar surface).

The relative specific localization is given by the quotient a/b. As represented in Fig. 45, the relative specific localization of [³H]leucine

Fig. 33. Full lactating mammary cells from a rat. Ergastoplasmic cisternae are abundant and densely packed, interspersed with numerous mitochondria. The Golgi elements are well developed and the vacuoles filled with protein granules. They occupy the para- and supranuclear region of the cells. × 4000.

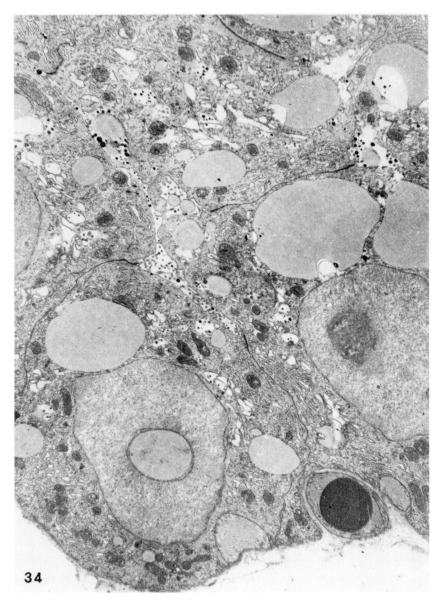

34

Fig. 34. Mammary gland cells from a gerbil at the second day of lactation. Besides the well-developed organelles, the cells contain numerous large fat droplets particularly in the apical cytoplasm. The cell at the lower left shows an "intranuclear" fat droplet which corresponds probably to a droplet situated in a nuclear invagination. × 6000.

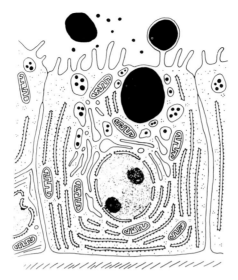

Fig. 35. Diagram of a fully lactating cell. The ergastoplasm is highly developed and oriented in parallel arrays in the para- and infranuclear region. Mitochondria are abundant and the large Golgi apparatus occupies the supranuclear portion of the cytoplasm. The secretory material is released from the cell as soon as it is elaborated: milk fat droplets are released by a pinching off mechanism and protein granules by fusing and opening of the transport vacuoles with the apical plasma membrane.

decreases steadily in the ergastoplasm and increases simultaneously in the Golgi compartment, where it attains a maximum at 30 minutes after injection. The half-life time of the labeled proteins in the ergastoplasm is about 22 minutes and in the Golgi field about 3 hours (Rohr *et al.*, 1968).

From the studies on mammary cells and from studies on other protein secreting glandular cells (see Jamieson and Palade, 1967) the intracellular pathway of milk proteins can be described as follows. The milk proteins are synthesized on the ribosomes, particularly on the membrane-bound ribosomes, i.e., the ergastoplasm (Gaye and Denamur, 1968, 1969). As is known from studies on isolated ribosomes, these structures are made of two subunits that generally escape observation in cell sections. However, occasionally they can be identified, and then it is seen that the larger subunit is attached to the cisternal membrane. It has been proposed that the newly synthesized polypeptide chains pass into the cisternal lumen through a channel in the larger subunit (Redman and Sabatini, 1966), but corresponding morphological observations are not yet available. In the next step the polypeptide chains seem to be trans-

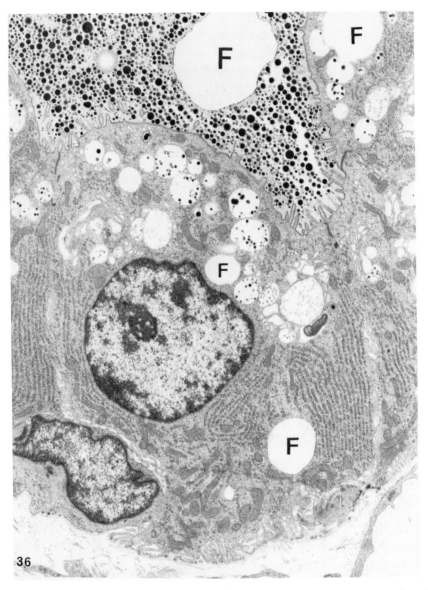

Fig. 36. Lactating mammary cells from a sheep showing well-developed and parallely oriented ergastoplasmic cisternae, particularly in the paranuclear region. The apical cytoplasm is occupied by Golgi vacuoles containing secretory granules. Note the numerous foot processes at the cell basis. F, Fat droplets. Glutaraldehyde perfusion; × 8600. (Courtesy of Dr. Linzell.)

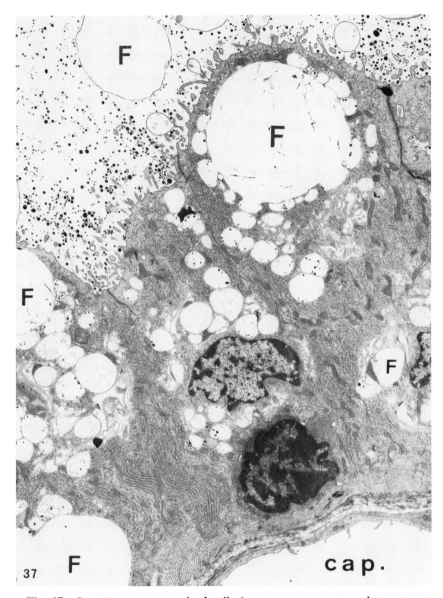

Fig. 37. Lactating mammary gland cells from a cow; same general structure as in other species. The differences in the preservation (for instance of the nuclei) are due to the fixation procedure (glutaraldehyde perfusion). The lipids of the milk fat droplets are completely extracted so that the droplets appear as empty vacuoles (F). Numerous smaller vacuoles containing protein granules are in close relationship with the milk fat droplets. On the lower right a capillary (cap.) is adjacent to the alveolar epithelium. × 7875. (Courtesy of Dr. Linzell.)

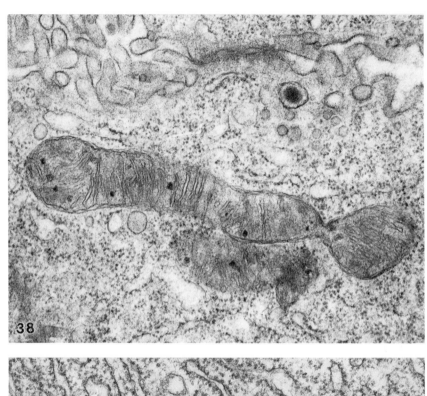

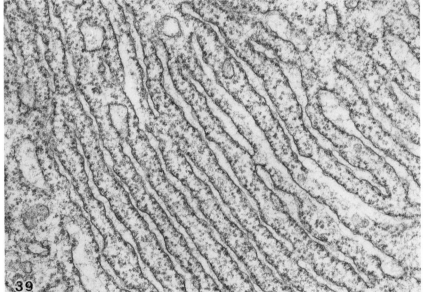

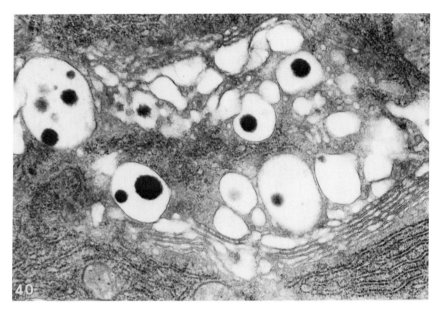

Fig. 40. Golgi apparatus of a mouse mammary gland cell at the ninth day of lactation. The three elements—flattened sacs, large vacuoles, and peripherally situated microvesicles—are clearly visible. Several vascuoles contain dense proteinaceous secretory granules. × 34,000.

ported in bulk materials from the ergastoplasm to the Golgi apparatus by means of smooth surfaced microvesicles, the peripheral elements of the Golgi complex (Jamieson and Palade, 1967).

Here occurs, within membrane-bound structures, the concentration of the primary secretory material and eventually further synthetic processes. The final milk protein granules are transported in membrane-bound vacuoles to the apical surface of the cell and released in the alveolar lumen.

ii. *Synthesis of milk fat and formation of droplets.* Ultrastructural studies of the mammary gland cells from different species have shown

---

Fig. 38. Mitochondrion from a mouse mammary gland at early lactation. Note the numerous internal cristae and the small mitochondrial granules. × 44,000.

Fig. 39. Detail of the ergastoplasm (or granular endoplasmic reticulum) of a lactating mammary gland of the mouse. The ergastoplasm consists of parallel arrays of cisternae. The cisternal membranes are studded on the outer surface with ribosomes of about 150 Å of diameter. Some of the cisternae contain a fine flocculent material. × 50,000.

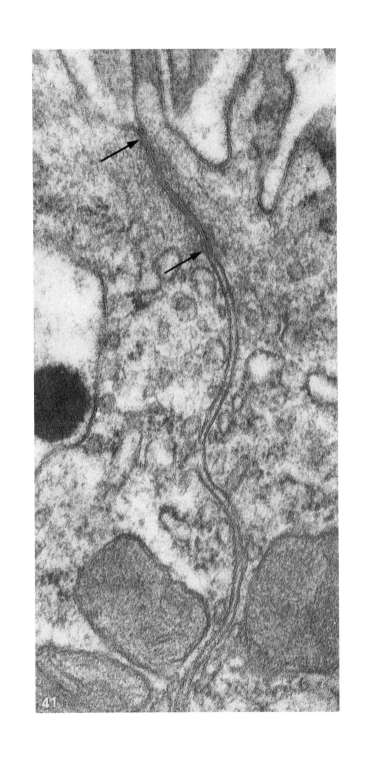

that in all cases the milk fat is produced by the cells as well-defined droplets (Figs. 14, 36) (Bargmann and Knoop, 1959; Hollmann, 1969; Wellings *et al.*, 1960a,b; Feldman, 1961; Sekhri *et al.*, 1967a; Wooding, 1971a,b; etc.). Small fat droplets generally appear in the basal cytoplasm, sometimes between ergastoplasmic cisternae. They are not bounded by a membrane.

In an autoradiographic study Stein and Stein (1966,1967) determined the different steps involved in the formation and the release of milk fat in the mammary gland of mice. At the sixth day of lactation the animals were injected intravenously with either [9,10-^{3}H]palmitic acid or [9,10-^{3}H]oleic acid.

After the usual exposure and development, silver grains were observed in succeeding lapses of time over the following cytoplasmic structures:

1. One minute after injection of labeled fatty acids the distribution of radioactivity varied among different cells. In some cells the grains were observed over the ergastoplasmic cisternae, in others over the intracellular lipid droplets. The labeled droplets were of all sizes and situated at the base of the cell as well as at the apex or even in the glandular lumen.

2. Ten minutes after the injection of oleic or palmitic acid silver grains were found over lipid droplets, mitochondria, and ergastoplasm.

3. At 30 and 60 minutes after injection the radioactivity was detected in lipid droplets in the apical region of the cell and in the lumina.

No silver grains were found over the protein granules in the Golgi apparatus, and the authors conclude that this organelle is not involved in the elaboration of milk fat droplets.

From this study it seems that the transfer of labeled fatty acids into the fat droplets is an extremely rapid process and that the first synthetic steps occur in the ergastoplasm. The finding that 95% of the fatty acids are esterified 1 minute after intravenous injection led Stein and Stein (1966, 1967) to the conclusion that the ergastoplasm is the site of fatty acid esterification. The lipids then aggregate *in situ* and acquire the droplet form.

Since silver grains are found over small as well as over large fat droplets, it is improbable that all droplets are freshly synthesized during the short time of 60 seconds after the injection of the labeled fatty acids. The growth of the droplets and their labeling seem to occur in two differ-

---

Fig. 41. Cellular contact between two lactating mammary gland cells. The zonula occludens in the juxtaluminal region is the main element of the junctional complex. Desmosomes are absent (mouse). × 90,000.

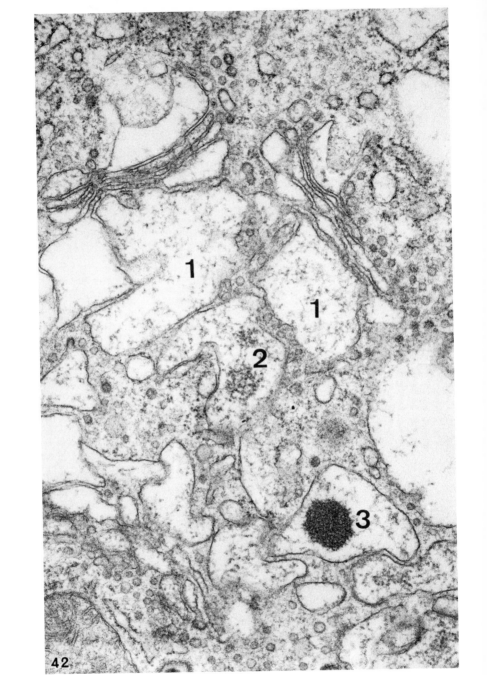

ent ways: (1) by new deposition of lipids in droplet form (small droplets at the base of the cell) and (2) by addition of newly synthesized lipids to preexisting droplets (peripheral growth of previously formed droplets). The result of this study, showing both small and large droplets labeled simultaneously, makes it unlikely that the lipid synthesis is limited to the basal portion of the cell as assumed earlier from descriptive studies.

iii. *Synthesis of lactose.* Little is known about the organelles involved in the synthesis of lactose, a process proper to mammary tissues.

In other than mammary cells, it has been shown that the Golgi apparatus plays an essential part in the uptake of sugars and in the synthesis of glycoproteins. There is accumulating evidence that this organelle is "the membrane–bounded compartment of the cell where enzymes involved in the synthesis of particular carbohydrate groups are present" (for review see Whaley *et al.*, 1972).

In mammary cells the enzyme lactose synthetase is said to be located on the Golgi lamellae (Coffey and Reithel, 1968, quoted by Kuhn, 1971) and Kuhn assumes that lactose is released in the lumen of the Golgi cavities. From the intracellular concentration of lactose (23 mM in the goat) and from the volume of the Golgi apparatus in lactating cells [7% of the cytoplasm in the mouse (Hollmann, 1968)], Kuhn estimated that the lactose concentration approaches 300 mM within the Golgi lumen. High-resolution autoradiography will be necessary to elucidate further the role of the Golgi apparatus in lactose synthesis during pregnancy and lactation.

b. THE DEVELOPMENT OF THE SYNTHETIC APPARATUS: QUANTITATIVE CONSIDERATIONS. Since the synthetic apparatus of the mammary cell develops gradually from the resting stage until full lactation it is interesting to find out whether a relationship exists between the amount of cytoplasmic organelles and the secretory activity of the cell. The development of organelles can be evaluated quantitatively from electron micrographs by volume or surface determinations (for review see Elias, 1951; Haug, 1955; Hennig, 1958; Sitte, 1965, 1967; Weibel *et al.*, 1966; and others).

Fig. 42. Golgi apparatus of a mouse mammary cell in the second half of lactation. Dilated sacs and vacuoles contain a fine granular material of about 150 Å, sometimes in a rosarylike arrangement (1) which aggregates (2), and forms the final secretory granules (3), which preserve the subunit structure. Numerous microvesicles are located at the periphery of the Golgi field. × 45,000.

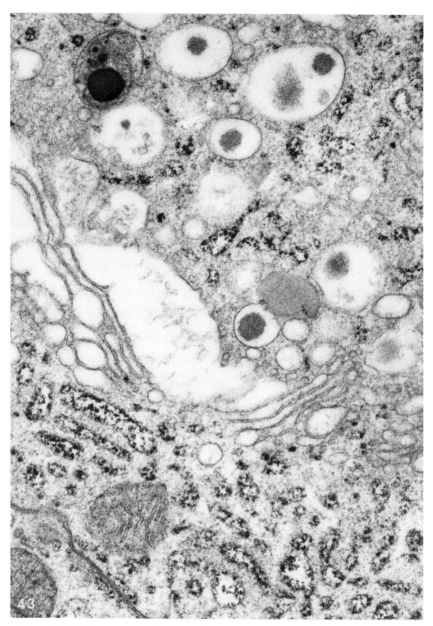

Fig. 43. Golgi region and surrounding ergastoplasm after OsO_4 fixation for 48 hours. Whereas the ergastoplasmic cisternae and some of the Golgi microvesicles are the site of osmium deposition the flattened Golgi sacs and "mature" vacuoles do not become impregnated by the osmium, no matter how prolonged the time of osmification. Although the chemical nature of this reaction is not clear, the staining differences between the two cellular compartments are noteworthy, and the observation that one

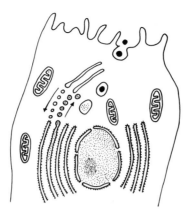

Fig. 44. The main organelles of the synthetic apparatus of the cell: the mitochondria as "powerhouses," the ergastoplasm (or rough-surfaced endoplasmic reticulum) engaged in the synthesis of secretory proteins, and the Golgi apparatus, a a complex system involved in the final steps of the secretory process, in the transport of the elaborated secretory granules to the apical surface of the cell, and in the supplying of new plasma membranes. The Golgi complex consists of three elements: smooth-surfaced flattened sacs, Golgi vacuoles, and small Golgi vesicles. The latter have a shuttle function between ergastoplasmic cisternae and Golgi apparatus and play a role in the transfer of the synthesized material from one compartment to the other.

The drawing of Fig. 46 indicates the cellular constituents analyzed morphometrically in mammary gland cells (Hollmann, 1967, 1968, 1969; Hollmann and Verley, 1971).

The results of these studies show that the quantitative development of mitochondria, ergastoplasm, and Golgi apparatus in mouse mammary cells shifts during pregnancy and lactation in a characteristic pattern.

i. *The mitochondria.* The mitochondria are the powerhouses of the cell and their number, size, and internal structure seem to be related to the intensity of cellular metabolism. The relative mitochondrial volume as percentage of the cytoplasmic volume is a useful value to describe the mitochondrial equipment of a cell and to compare it with that of other cells.

---

part of the microvesicles is heavily impregnated whereas the other part is not, agrees with the suggested shuttle function of the Golgi vesicles. The osmium-stained vesicles may be loaded vesicles on the way from the ergastoplasm to the Golgi apparatus whereas the "empty" ones are going from the Golgi to the cisternae. Note the presence of lysosomal structures. Mouse mammary gland at the end of lactation × 44,000. (From Hollmann and Verley, 1971.)

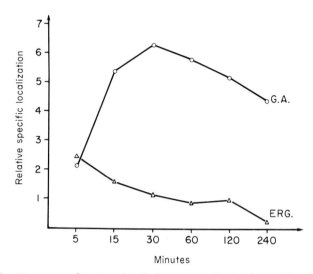

Fig. 45. Diagram indicating the "relative specific localization" of [³H]leucine in the ergastoplasm and in the Golgi field between 5 minutes and 4 hours after i.p. injection of the radioactive tracer. In the interval from 5 to 15 minutes the "leucine-activity" is located mainly in the ergastoplasm, in the following interval from 15 to 60 minutes, the main activity is found in the Golgi field (Adapted from the data of Rohr *et al.*, 1968).

During the different stages of mammary activity the mitochondrial volume varies in the following way (Fig. 47). From about 4.4% in the resting cell it increases rapidly during the first half of pregnancy and reaches a value of about 8% at the middle of pregnancy. Then a few days before parturition it increases again to about 10%. This value is maintained until the twentieth day of lactation, when a slow decrease begins.

ii. *The ergastoplasm.* The ergastoplasm, site of protein synthesis, consists of membranous sacs with attached ribosomes on its outer surface. Its development can be appreciated by the ergastoplasmic surface (μm^2) contained in a given volume of cytoplasm (μm^3).

In the first half of pregnancy the ergastoplasmic surface doubles (from 1.2 $\mu m^2/\mu m^3$ at the resting stage to 2.4 $\mu m^2/\mu m^3$ at the fourteenth day of pregnancy). Then it remains unchanged until 2 or 3 days before parturition (Fig. 48). At this time a new and rapid increase begins and continues until the fifth day of lactation when the highest value (about 5.3 $\mu m^2/\mu m^3$) is attained. Then there is a slope toward the tenth day and a further slight increase toward the twentieth day of lactation. Thereafter,

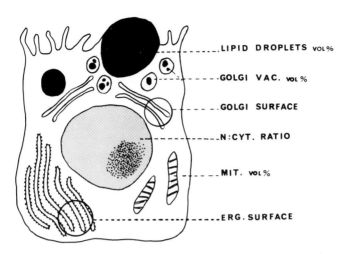

Fig. 46. Diagram of a mammary cell indicating the different cell constituents analyzed by morphometric methods. Mitochondria, Golgi vacuoles, and milk fat droplets have been characterized by their volume evaluated as percentage of the cytoplasmic volume (relative values). The development of ergastoplasmic cisternae and of flattened Golgi sacs has been determined by their surface, expressed as μm^2 per μm^3 of cytoplasm (absolute values). The proportion of cytoplasm to nucleus has also been evaluated. (From Hollmann, 1969; Hollmann and Verley, 1971.)

the ergastoplasmic development declines. Thus, two peaks are observed, one at the fifth day, the other at the twentieth day of lactation. It is interesting to note that during lactation the prolactin cells of the anterior pituitary show a similar ergastoplasmic development with maxima at the fifth and at the twentieth day (Verley and Hollmann, 1971) (Fig. 49). This suggests that the prolactin synthesis is particularly high at these periods and influences the amount of ergastoplasm in the mammary cells. The latter hypothesis seems to be supported by experimental data (see Denamur and Gaye, 1967). The high activity of the mammary cells at the twentieth day of lactation is further indicated by the ratio cytoplasm : nucleus, which attains at this time its maximum of 14 : 1 (Fig. 6) (Hollmann and Verley, 1971).

If the ergastoplasmic development in resting, prelactating, and lactating mammary cells is sufficiently characterized by the data obtained, it should be possible to test the influence of hormones on the development of this organelle. This has been tried with hydrocortisone (Hollmann and Verley, 1971), since *in vitro* experiments had indicated that this hormone favors the development of the ergastoplasmic cisternae (Mills and Topper, 1969). A mouse at the eighth day of lactation was injected with increas-

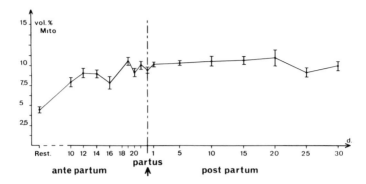

Fig. 47. Modification of the mitochondrial volume (evaluated as percentage of the cytoplasmic volume) in mammary gland cells of the mouse during pregnancy and lactation. The chondriome increases until parturition and then remains stable until the end of lactation (the standard deviation is indicated) (From Hollmann and Verley, 1971.)

ing doses of hydrocortisone and biopsies from mammary tissue were taken every day. The values obtained before hormonal treatment, after one injection (0.5 mg), and after five injections (0.5, 0.5, 1.0, 1.0, and 2.0 mg daily) are shown in Fig. 50. The data indicate some increase of the ergastoplasmic surface as compared with that of untreated animals. These results are of preliminary value, but they may illustrate the usefulness of morphometric methods for the evaluation of hormonal effects.

iii. *The Golgi apparatus.* The Golgi apparatus, which is closely involved in the final elaboration of proteins and probably in the synthesis of lactose,

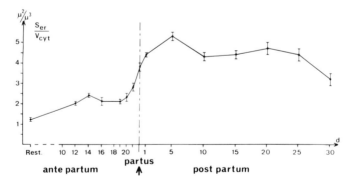

Fig. 48. Ergastoplasmic development [expressed in μm^2 of ergastoplasm per μm^3 of cytoplasm (μ^2/μ^3 in figure)] in mammary gland cells of the mouse during pregnancy and lactation (the curve represents a mean from several animals and different glands, thoracic and abdominal) (From Hollmann and Verley, 1971.)

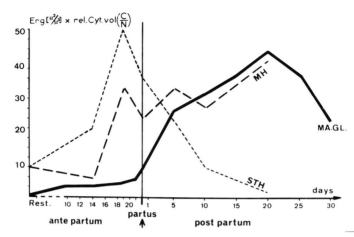

Fig. 49. Development of ergastoplasm in mammary gland cells (MA. GL.) and in mammotropic (MH) and somatotropic (STH) hypophyseal cells during pregnancy and lactation (mouse). In an attempt to approximate the ergastoplasmic surface *per cell* the relative cytoplasmic development (C/N) has been introduced and multiplied with the ergastoplasm (μm^2) per unit volume of cytoplasm (μm^3) (μ^2/μ^3 in figure). The diagram shows that both MH and STH cells have a high ergastoplasmic development in the last phase of pregnancy corresponding probably to a high functional activity during this time. Then the ergastoplasm decreases rapidly in STH cells, indicating that these cells are apparently not essential for the maintenance of lactation, whereas the ergastoplasm of MH cells remain abundant and goes parallel with the ergastoplasmic development in the mammary cells, suggesting an important role of this cell type for galactopoiesis, i.e., an enhancement of an already established milk secretion. (Data from Hollmann and Verley, 1971; Verley and Hollmann, 1971.)

is a complex system of three components: flattened sacs (seen as smooth lamellae on the electron micrographs), vacuoles, and microvesicles.

The development of the Golgi system can be appreciated by the determination of the surface of the sacs (μm^2 per μm^3 of cytoplasm) and the volume of the vacuoles (in percent of the cytoplasmic volume). The development of the two Golgi components follows closely the curve for that of the ergastoplasm (Figs. 51a,b). The volume of the Golgi vacuoles shows a steep increase with parturition and the onset of lactation (Fig. 51b).

The morphometric data available indicate a clear relationship between the build up of the synthetic apparatus, which attains a first level at the twelfth day of pregnancy and the appearance of the first secretory material at this time.

At parturition the mammary cell has not reached its full cytoplasmic

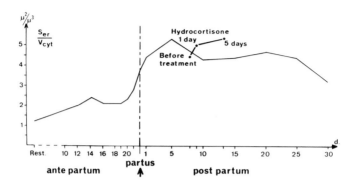

Fig. 50. Diagram to illustrate the application of morphometric methods for the evaluation of drug effects at the subcellular level. A lactating mouse is injected with hydrocortisone and biopsies of mammary tissue are taken the day before treatment, after 1 day (0.5 mg) of hydrocortisone, and after 5 days (0.5, 0.5, 1.0, 1.0, and 2.0 mg) of hydrocortisone treatment. The ergastoplasmic surface in the mammary cells of the treated animals is determined and compared with that of untreated animals at corresponding stages of lactation (From Hollmann and Verley, 1971.) ($\mu = \mu$m.)

organization and the initiation of milk secretion is not accompanied by a dramatic change in the organelle equipment of the cell (Hollmann, 1969). Mitochondria, ergastoplasm, and Golgi apparatus continue to augment in volume and surface until the fifth day of lactation, after which they increase only slightly (Hollmann and Verley, 1971).

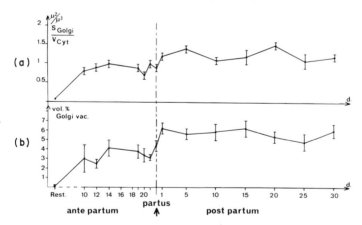

Fig. 51. Development of the Golgi apparatus in mammary cells during pregnancy and lactation (mouse). (a) Diagram indicating the membranous surface of flattened Golgi sacs and Golgi vacuoles [μm^2/μm^3 of cytoplasm (μ^2/μ^3 in figure)]. (b) Diagram showing the volume of the Golgi vacuoles (as a percentage of the cytoplasmic volume). (From Hollmann and Verley, 1971.)

c. RELEASE OF THE SECRETORY PRODUCT. i. *Release of fat droplets and formation of the milk fat globule membrane (MFGM).* Bargmann and Knoop (1959) first suggested that the extruded milk fat droplet is surrounded by a membrane that derives from the plasma membrane of the secretory cell. The authors described a mechanism by which the fat droplet becomes progressively enveloped by the luminal membrane and is ultimately pinched off into the alveolar cavity (Figs. 52, 53). This process, initially observed in the rat (Bargmann and Knoop, 1959), and then confirmed in the golden hamster and in the mouse (Bargmann *et al.*, 1961) is common to all species examined (Wooding, 1972).

Whereas Bargmann and Knoop (1959) and other authors believed that the apical membrane supplied the whole envelope of the fat droplet, Wooding (1971a; Wooding *et al.*, 1970) suggested that a part of the envelope originates from Golgi vacuoles. This proposal is founded on the current observation that Golgi vacuoles accumulate in the periphery of larger fat droplets and release their content concomitantly with the extrusion of the fat droplet. Wooding substantiated the close relationship of the two release mechanisms and traced the time course of the events, schematically represented in Fig. 54.

As the fat droplet approaches the apical pole of the cell, numerous Golgi vacuoles come up against its surface. Since membrane-bounded vacuoles fuse easily with the plasmalemma (see release of protein granules, Section III,B4,c,ii), they can intervene in the extrusion of fat droplets if they become stably linked with them. Such a closely associated Golgi vacuole then has a common contour with the fat droplet, and this common contour becomes the first part of the fat droplet membrane. In a following step the membrane of the Golgi vacuole fuses with the luminal plasma membrane, the vacuole opens and releases its content in the alveolar cavity. In this way the membrane of the vacuole becomes a part of the plasmalemma. The process continues with other fat-droplet-associated Golgi vacuoles and vesicles, and, by their successive fusion with the plasmalemma, the droplet emerges progressively from the cytoplasm. The definite membrane that surrounds the fat droplet is thus of two origins: one part is supplied by the plasmalemma whereas the other part comes from the membrane of Golgi vacuoles (Fig. 54).

As the fat droplet bulges in the alveolar lumen it does not fuse with the plasmalemma but remains separated from it by a layer of dense material 10–20 nm thick (Figs. 52, 53). This material, which often has localized thickenings, is of cytoplasmic origin (Bargmann *et al.*, 1961; Helminen and Ericsson, 1968a; Wooding, 1971a) and is still discernible after the release of the droplet from the cell. Thus the membrane of the

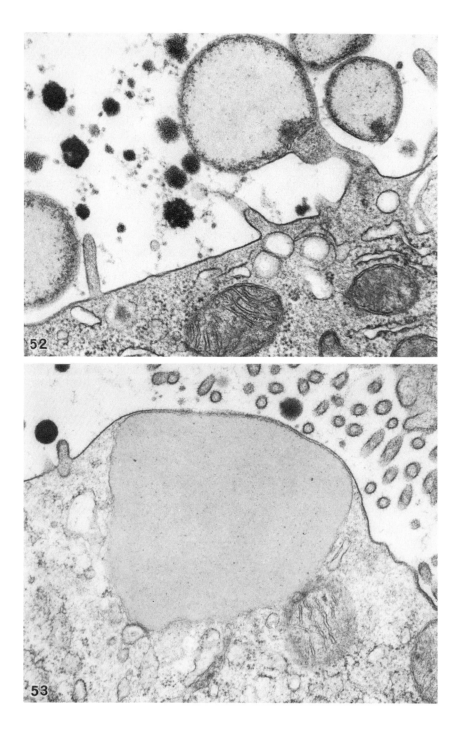

52

53

freshly secreted fat droplet consists, like that of the emerging droplet, of the plasmalemma and a thin electron-dense inner layer ("initial MFGM," Wooding, 1971b, 1972).

The initial MFGM is rapidly lost by blebbing off in small vesicles or by lifting off in sheets leaving a structureless "secondary MFGM" (Wooding, 1971b) proper to "older" fat droplets. The secondary membrane appears as a single contour that continuously surrounds the milk fat droplet.

The degradation of the initial MFGM into a secondary MFGM was observed on milk fat droplets from all the animals so far examined— human, horse, dog, wallaby, cow, goat, sheep, pig, mouse, rat, and guinea pig (Wooding, 1972).

The transformation of the initial MFGM into a secondary MFGM is in agreement with previously reported results, in particular with those of Keenan *et al.* (1970) who observed in high resolution electron micrographs that plasma membranes have a different structure than MFGM (corresponding probably to "secondary MFGM" of Wooding), although isolated fractions of the two types of membranes were chemically very similar. The reason the membranes of the fat droplets undergo structural rearrangements as soon as the free droplets are exposed to the milieu of the milk is still unknown.

ii. *Release of protein granules.* The release of the protein granules is effected by a process known as reverse pinocytosis or exopinocytosis. The protein granules are carried to the apical cytoplasm in membrane-bounded vacuoles originating from the Golgi apparatus. If the vacuole membrane comes in contact with the plasmalemma, the two membranes fuse and the vacuole opens and releases its content in the alveolar lumen (Fig. 54). That way the membrane around the vacuole becomes a part of the plasmalemma.

It is meaningful to see in this mechanism a source of replenishment for the plasma membranes lost during the extrusion of fat droplets (Patton and Fowkes, 1967). This again directs the attention to the role of the Golgi apparatus, which not only intervenes in the "maturing" of the protein granules and in their transport to the cell apex, but also acts as a generator for new membranes, as already suggested by Sjöstrand (1968).

iii. *The secretion modus in the mammary gland.* "Apocrine" or "mero-

---

Figs. 52 and 53. Extrusion of milk fat droplets.

Fig. 52. A fat droplet is completely enveloped by the plasmalemma and is on the point of pinching off. × 42,000.

Fig. 53. The large droplet has approached the apical plasma membrane and bulges in the alveolar lumen. Between the droplet and the plasmalemma a minute border of cytoplasm can be recognized. × 36,000.

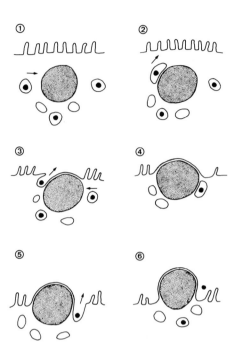

Fig. 54. Diagram of the release process of milk fat droplets reconstructed according to the proposition of Wooding (1971a). (1) When the fat droplet approaches the apical plasma membrane, "empty" or protein laden vacuoles accumulate at its periphery. (2) One or the other vacuole comes close to the fat droplet and becomes associated and shows a common contour with the droplet, separated only by a tiny rim of cytoplasm. If such a droplet-associated vacuole nears the apical plasma membrane, the two membranes fuse and the vacuole opens (3) and releases its content (milk serum or protein granules). (4) Then the recess in the plasma membrane disappears and by this way the fat droplet is drawn into the alveolar lumen. The process repeats with other vacuoles (4)–(6) until the droplet emerges almost completely from the cell and is pinched off.

crine"—this is the much debated question since the mammary gland is studied with the electron microscope and particularly since Bargmann *et al.* (1961) emphasized that the term "apocrine" is inappropriate for the milk secretion process and thus should be abandoned.

Following the first ultrastructural studies it appeared that the exteriorization of the secretory material was achieved without noticeable loss of cytoplasmic substance, but later it became evident that larger portions of cytoplasm, including organelles, may be pinched off with the fat droplets.

Although there is no doubt today that cytoplasmic substance is lost, the debate continues, mainly because the authors consider different points in the secretion process. Some of them lay stress on the mode of elaboration of the secretory material within the cytoplasm whereas others focus mainly on the mode of extrusion.

Bargmann *et al.* (1961) and Bargmann and Welsch (1969) underlined that the justification of the term "apocrine" depends on whether the detached cytoplasm is a true secretory material and thus an essential component of the milk or only an accidental by-product. They conclude that the term "apocrine secretion" should no longer be retained since it is associated with erroneous concepts that originated in the last century.

Girardie (1968), who observed rims of cytoplasm pinched off with the fat droplets, joins Bargmann's proposal and is of opinion that the quantity of cytoplasmic material lost is not significant and that the secretion type should be designated as "merocrine."

On the other side there are the authors who plead for the maintenance of the epithet "apocrine" as an adequate description for the release of secretory material in the mammary gland (Stockinger and Zarzicki, 1962; Kurosomi *et al.*, 1968; Helminen and Ericsson, 1968a; Wooding, 1971a; Wooding *et al.*, 1970; and others). They insist on the fact that "a part of the plasma membrane as well as a small amount of cytoplasm may be detached from the main cell body and released into the lumen along with the secretory substance proper" (Kurosomi *et al.*, 1968). Quite similarly Helminen and Ericsson (1968a) express their opinion when they state that the fat droplets "appeared to be pushed out of the cells together with a rim of cytoplasm, which later appeared to be detached. This kind of secretion evidently removed a part of the apical cytoplasm." They conclude, "Hence the findings seem to confirm the proposal that the term of "apocrine secretion" is justified . . . ." (p. 210). Herewith they meet the view of Stockinger and Zarzicki (1962) who believe that the cytoplasmic material lost in such a manner becomes an important constituent of the milk since they observed in the guinea pig that the cytoplasm pinched off with the fat droplets disintegrates immediately in the alveolar lumen thus supplying the milk with essential components such as enzymes and nucleic acids. From there, Stockinger and Zarzicki deduce that a true "apocrine" secretion as defined in the paper of Bargmann *et al.* (1961) indeed exists in the mammary gland.

Also Wooding (1971a) and Wooding *et al.* (1970) are convinced that appreciable fragments of the secretory cells are lost and that an "apocrine" type of secretion occurs in the mammary gland. To demonstrate that cytoplasmic materials do really enter the milk and that the crescents in contact with fat droplets in the alveolar lumen do not belong to neighboring cells situated out of the plane of section, Wooding *et al.* (1970) examined centrifuged milk from goats and guinea pigs. They found that about 1–5% of the fat droplets in the milk have crescents of cytoplasm (Fig. 55) containing ergastoplasm, free ribosomes, mitochondria, and vacuoles enclosing protein granules. The fat droplet and the cytoplasmic crescent are surrounded as a whole by a "unit membrane." Besides these "signets," cytoplasmic fragments devoid of nuclei were detected in centrifuged milk. The fragments contained organelles and occasionally secretory material, and the authors believe "that like the signets the fragments are part of the secretory cells lost in a classical apocrine manner."

Apart from the occasionally detached cytoplasmic crescents, there is a regular loss of a very small amount of cytoplasm that can be seen as a 10–20 nm thin layer of dense material at the inner surface of the fat droplet membrane (Wooding, 1971a,b). Based on these observations, Wooding (1971a) distinguishes, in agreement with Kurosomi (1961), two secretion mechanisms in the mammary gland. The extrusion of fat drop-

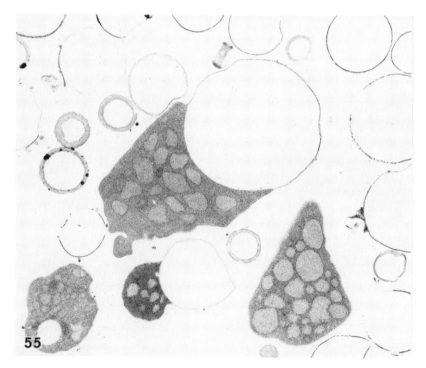

Fig. 55. Milk fat droplets from centrifuged goat milk with remnants of cytoplasm on one side ("signets" of Wooding *et al.*, 1970). × 8000. (Courtesy of Dr. Wooding.)

lets by pinching off from the plasma membrane including thereby cytoplasmic remnants is interpreted as an "apocrine" secretion, whereas the release of nonmembrane-bounded casein granules by exopinocytosis is considered as a "merocrine" secretion.

As seen from the preceding discussion, there is at the present time no more doubt that a constant loss of cytoplasmic substance occurs with the extrusion of the secretory material. This loss is called by most of the authors "apocrine secretion." It has to be asked if this is an adequate terminology for a phenomenon that is by definition *not* a secretion. Then, "secretion is the process by which cells absorb substances, transform them chemically or change their concentration and expel them" (de Robertis *et al.*, 1960). One has to be aware that it is a quite different thing if the cell loses parts of its own body or if the cell elaborates specific substances for exportation.

With this difference in mind, the term "apocrine" charged with an outdated conception would be better avoided for the description of the secretion modus in the mammary gland.

5. Cellular Aspects of Milk Stasis

As soon as the gland is no longer emptied by suckling or milking, the secretory material stagnates in the glandular lumina and within the glandular cells (Fig. 56). As the milk pressure increases in the gland, the elaboration of new secretory material diminishes (Peterson and Rigor, 1932; Smith, 1959; Zeilmaker, 1968).

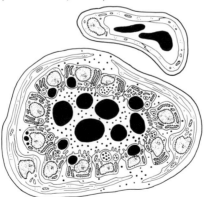

Fig. 56. Diagram depicting an alveolus during milk stasis. The central cavity is wide and filled with the stagnating secretory material. The glandular cells contain large amounts of elaborated protein granules and milk fat droplets. The spaces between the glandular cells and the glandular and myoepithelial cells are enlarged, but the structure of the cells and the architecture of the alveolus are almost intact.

In the early stage of milk stasis the mammary cell does not undergo ultrastructural modifications (Hollmann, 1966; Verley and Hollmann, 1966; Hollmann and Verley, 1967). Thus the morphology of the fully lactating cell is generally maintained. The nucleus is voluminous, oval shaped, and has a smooth contour and big nucleoli. The ergastoplasm is highly developed with parallel arrays, particularly in the basal cytoplasm. The mitochondria have the same shape and the same dense matrix with densely arranged cristae and small intramitochondrial granules. The aspect of the fat droplets and of the protein granules is unmodified.

If stasis progresses, the main feature observed is a disorder in the extrusion mechanism: fat droplets and protein granules are no longer released in the acinar cavity but are stored in the cell.

a. MODIFICATION OF THE PROTEIN GRANULES. The intravacuolar granules conglomerate into a bulky material (Wellings and DeOme, 1963; Hollmann, 1966; Helminen and Ericsson, 1968c). Then the vacuolar membranes break up and the proteinaceous material is released in the cytoplasm, where it is found as large masses with irregular outline and variable electron density (Figs. 57, 58). The subunits of the original granules are still recognizable but apparently have smaller dimensions than the subunits of freshly elaborated granules. Finally, the remnants of the vacuolar membrane disappear completely and the degradation of

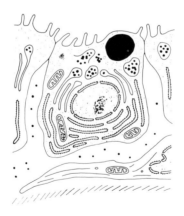

Fig. 57. Diagram showing the characteristic features of a mammary cell during milk stasis. The secretory products are stored in the cytoplasm. The protein granules accumulate within the Golgi vacuoles and merge together. If the overfilled Golgi vacuoles burst, the proteinaceous content enters the cytoplasm and undergoes degradation (see Fig. 26). The intercellular spaces are enlarged and sometimes contain protein granules. The juxtaluminal tight junctions (zonulae occludentes) are generally undamaged.

the proteinaceous material is completed within the cytoplasm following the mechanism already described (Section III,B,2,a).

b. Reflux of Secretory Material into the Intercellular Space. Besides the proteinaceous granules stored or degraded inside the glandular cell, other granules are found within the intercellular spaces or in the periaveolar tissue (Figs. 56, 57) (Bässler, 1961; Benedetti and Bartoszewicz, 1961; Hollmann, 1966; Verley and Hollmann, 1966; Sekhri *et al.*, 1967a; Girardie, 1968). It is not clear how the granules reach the extracellular spaces: by reflux from the alveolar lumen, by active transport to the intercellular boundaries, or merely by artificial rupturing of the bursting alveoli during tissue preparation. The absence of accompanying fat droplets may indicate that the liberation of protein granules in the extracellular space is due to a physiological process.

c. Autoradiographic Study. It seems that the occurence of milk stasis does not imply a breakdown of the synthetic activity of the cell. After injection of tritiated leucine the radioactive precursor is incorporated in newly formed protein granules as shown by high resolution autoradiography. The synthesis progresses in the same time sequence as during full lactation (Verley and Hollmann, 1966). It is noteworthy that the protein granules observed in the extracellular spaces also have the radioactive label and, therefore, represent freshly elaborated proteins (Verley and Hollmann, 1966).

6. Regression of the Mammary Gland at the End of Lactation

The regression of the mammary gland at the end of lactation is characterized by the disappearance of a bulk of parenchyma. Concomitantly the interlobar and interlobular connective and adipose tissues reappear. Thus, the loss of epithelial cells entails a rebuilding of the architecture of the gland.

a. Cellular Modifications. The cellular modifications observed in the course of regression reflect the interruption of the secretory activity, the return of one part of the cells to the resting stage, and the irreversible alteration and consecutive death of the other part of the cells.

A few days after the end of lactation the glandular cells undergo profound changes. Their shape becomes cubic, pearlike, or flat (Figs. 59, 60). The microvilli disappear so that the luminal surfaces have a smooth and often irregular contour (Figs. 16, 60).

The nuclei lose their round or slightly scalloped outline (Fig. 16) and become deeply infolded. Their chromatin remains finely dispersed, but the nucleoli reduce rapidly.

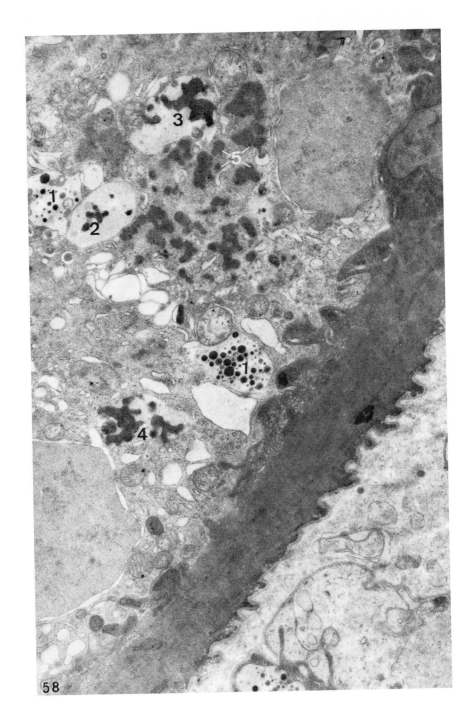

58

The ergastoplasm loses its parallel arrangement and breaks into smaller fragments and vesicles. Some cisternae persist in the basal portion of the cytoplasm but finally vanish almost completely while free ribosomes appear in increasing number.

The Golgi apparatus, situated as before in the supra- and paranuclear region, diminishes rapidly. The flattened sacs remain for some time, but the vacuoles diminish in size and number and no longer contain freshly elaborated protein granules.

The mitochondria of the regressing cells have a more translucent matrix, fewer and widely spaced cristae, and large intramitochondrial granules up to 200 nm in diameter (Fig. 61).

The milk fat droplets stored in the cytoplasm decrease in size. They are more electron dense than during lactation and have an irregular or star-shaped contour. Here and there they are in close contact with mitochondria (Fig. 61).

One of the most characteristic aspects of the regressing cell is the presence of a great number of lysosomes (Wellings and DeOme, 1963; Hollmann and Verley, 1967; Girardie, 1967; Helminen and Ericsson, 1968b; Sekhri *et al.*, 1967a), which appear as multivesicular bodies, dense bodies, and autophagic vacuoles (or autophagosomes). The latter are lysosomes containing remnants of cytoplasm or organelles (Figs. 62, 63).

The number of lysosomes varies from one cell to another and is apparently related to the intensity of the autophagocytic process engaged in the removal of the secretory material and in the reduction of the cytoplasm. The degradation of the cellular debris enclosed in the autophagosomes is accomplished by means of the lysosomal enzymes. The digested material appears as electron dense and often vacuolated masses (vacuolated bodies) that are released in the cytoplasm (Section III,B,2,a).

By way of autodigestion one part of the epithelial cells loses its cytoplasmic organization, diminishes in size, and returns gradually to the resting stage. Other glandular cells, particularly rich in autophagosomes, are more severly altered and degenerate (Fig. 63). They undergo similar cytoplasmic modifications as already described, but unlike the surviving cells they reveal nuclear changes. The chromatin conglomerates and the nucleus shrinks, breaks into fragments, and disappears. The dying cells

---

Fig. 58. Basal portion of an alveolus from a rabbit mammary gland during milk stasis. The Golgi vacuoles of the glandular cells contain protein granules (1) which fuse progressively (2, 3, and 4) and enter finally the cytoplasm where they are further degraded (5). The dark cell underlying the glandular cells is a myoepithelial cell. × 11,500. (From Hollmann, 1966.)

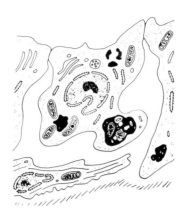

Fig. 59. Diagram illustrating the characteristic aspects of an involuting mammary gland cell at the end of lactation. The cell diminishes in size, the cytoplasmic organelles become reduced by a process of autodigestion in which lysosomes, the "suicide bags" (de Duve, 1963) of the cell play a major role. The bulks of dark material represent residual bodies resulting from the autophagic process.

are shed into the alveolar lumen where they are indistinguishable from colostrum bodies (Donné corpuscles) observed during pregnancy and early lactation (see Section III,B,7).

Other debris of necrotic cells are pushed into the connective tissue space where they are further degraded and disappear. Thus, there are two processes that lead to the reduction of the parenchyma: (1) the decrease of cell size and organelles in the surviving cell population and (2) the progressive degeneration and consecutive death of other cells. In both processes autodigestion of the cytoplasm with the intervening of lysosomes is an important mechanism.

Whereas most of the authors agree about the role of autophagocytosis in the reduction of the parenchyma, the opinions diverge about the part assumed by heterophagocytosis, i.e., the digestion of cells as a whole or as a portion of their cytoplasm by foreign cells such as macrophages (Helminen and Ericsson, 1968a,b,c; Helminen et al., 1968).

According to Wellings and DeOme (1963), Hollmann and Verley (1967), Sekhri et al. (1967b), who studied the morphology of regression in the mouse mammary gland, macrophages are scarce and apparently do not accomplish an important function in the reduction of epithelial cells. Wellings and DeOme (1963) stated: "Since phagocytes are not conspicuously abundant in the epithelial or stromal spaces during involution, morphological evidence does not suggest phagocytosis as a means of removal."

Helminen and Ericsson (1968a,b,c), who described the regression of the mammary gland in the rat, do not agree with this view and think that "macrophagelike cells" are involved in the uptake of epithelial cell cytoplasm and milk protein granules, particularly between the third and tenth day after weaning.

According to Helminen and Ericsson (1968b), the "macrophagelike cells" are interspersed among the epithelial cells and frequently situated on the basement membrane. They contain proteinaceous secretory granules and reveal the same enzyme activities as do the epithelial cells (Helminen *et al.,* 1968).

It is difficult to distinguish the "macrophagelike cells" described by Helminen and Ericsson in the alveolar epithelium of the rat from the degenerating epithelial cells observed in the mouse (Verley and Hollmann, 1967; Hollmann and Verley, 1967), since their fine structure is almost identical and both finally are shed into the alveolar lumen.

However, although the interpretations of Helminen and Ericsson do not overcome all doubts, it is likely that species differences exist in the process of tissue reduction and that macrophages play a more important role in other species than they do in the mouse.

b. Rebuilding of Architecture. The loss of epithelial cells entails a profound rebuilding of the architecture of the mammary gland. Whereas during milk stasis the structure of the alveolus is maintained, profound changes occur with the onset of regression.

The spaces between adjacent glandular cells and between glandular and myoepithelial cells become widely distended (Figs. 16, 59). As long as the glandular cells are held together in the apical region by persisting zonulae occludentes, a reflux of milk into the intercellular spaces is almost prevented. Nevertheless these spaces are filled with a slightly electron dense flocculent material, which results probably from degraded protein (Fig. 16). In the following steps, degenerating cells become detached and eliminated, whereas the remaining cells become dislodged mutually and here and there become arranged in multilayers.

In the course of regression the myoepithelial cells are longer and better preserved than the glandular cells. With their extensions they encircle like a hoop the vanishing alveolus. Their scalloped outline and their dense myofibrils strengthen the impression that the myoepithelial cells are firmly contracted and thus prevent the breakup of the alveolus (Figs. 16 and 58). The thickened basement membrane may also contribute to consolidate the remaining epithelium (Fig. 16).

Disappearance of the glandular cells and the shrinking of the glandular

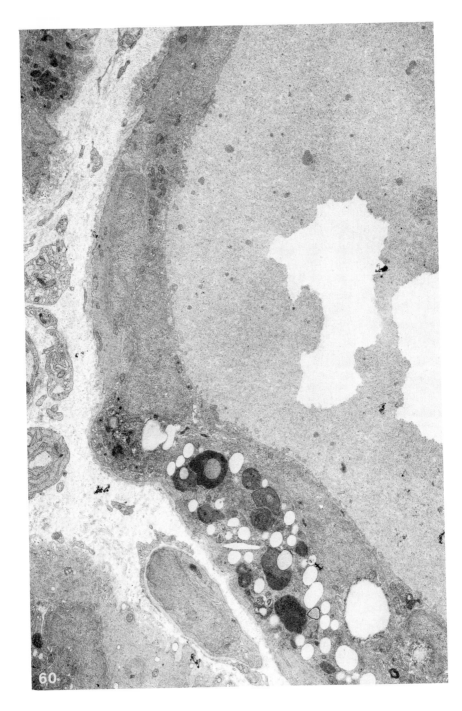

60

tree is accompanied by a new development of the mammary stroma. Fibroblasts are numerous and form bundles of collagen. Other connective tissue cells accumulate tiny fat droplets and develop into fat cells. The capillaries have smaller lumina and thickened basement membranes.

7. The So-Called Colostrum Cell or Corpuscle of Donné

The nature and significance of the so-called colostrum cell have been debated by light microscopists since the first description by Donné in 1844–1845 and have not been conclusively elucidated until today (for review Mayer and Klein, 1961).

The term "colostrum cell" is misleading in so far as this cell occurs not only during pregnancy and the beginning of lactation but also during other phases of glandular activity, especially during the regression of the gland after weaning (Girardie *et al.*, 1964; Hollmann and Verley, 1967; Sekhri *et al.*, 1967a; Wellings and DeOme, 1963). Sekhri *et al.* (1967a) observed "colostrum cells" as early as 12 hours after suspension of suckling and believe that their appearance is "the only evidence of the initiation of regression of the mammary gland at the light microscopic level" (Sekhri *et al.*, 1967a).

Among the classic researchers, one group considers the Donné bodies as modified leukocytes, lymphocytes, histiocytes, or other monocytic cells wandering through the alveolar epithelium and penetrating finally in the alveolar cavity. Another group believes that the corpuscle of Donné is of epithelial origin. The different opinions have been reviewed by Mayer and Klein (1961).

Recent studies with the electron microscope support the concept that at least in the mouse, the Donné bodies originate from the glandular cells of the alveolus since all kinds of transitional stages can be followed between the epithelial cells and the corpuscles of Donné (Girardie *et al.*, 1964,1966; Hollmann and Verley, 1967; Verley and Hollmann, 1967; Sekhri *et al.*, 1967a). This development is particularly clear during the regression of the gland after weaning (Hollmann and Verley, 1967; Sekhri *et al.*, 1967a; Girardie *et al.*, 1964; and others) but is the same during pregnancy (Girardie *et al.*, 1964; Murad, 1970; Hollmann and Verley, unpublished observation). It is closely related to a retention of

---

Fig. 60. Portion of an alveolus from a regressing mammary gland of the rabbit (eighth day after weaning). The cells are flattened and the reduction of cytoplasm and organelles is advanced. Some cells are filled with lysosomes. The alveolar lumen contains a rather homogeneous material but no protein granules or fat droplets. × 4500. (From Hollmann and Verley, 1967.)

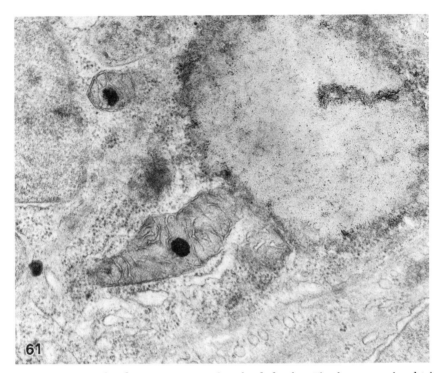

Fig. 61. Mitochondria in contact with a lipid droplet. The large mitochondrial granules are characteristic of involuting mammary cells. From a regressing mammary gland of a rabbit. × 40,000. (From Hollmann and Verley, 1967.)

secretory material within the cytoplasm, as soon as the equilibrium between the elaboration of this material and its extrusion is disturbed. Degenerative phenomena are associated. As described in Section III,B,6, the Golgi vacuoles become distended, the protein granules coalesce, and lysosomes and autophagic vacuoles that are involved in the removal of stored secretory material and superfluous organelles appear. The final stage of this process is a cell with a cytoplasm rich in vacuoles and lipid bodies. The degenerating cell then becomes detached from the alveolar epithelium and eliminated in the alveolar cavity. The desquamated cells, which look under the light microscope like the "corps granuleux" of Donné still have, under the electron microscope, characteristic features of epithelial cells.

In the mammary gland of mice, rats, and rabbits this is the course of events generally observed, whereas the passage of mesenchymal elements through the alveolar epithelium and their transformation in Donné bodies were not observed by Girardie *et al.* (1964), Hollmann and Verley (1967), and Sekhri *et al.* (1967a).

However, it should not be overlooked that the presently available ultrastructural observations on Donné bodies concern small laboratory animals and that differences may exist from species to species. As Lascelles (1969) reported in an immunological and light microscopic study, colostral cells from human and sheep mammary glands are monocytic cells that are "derived from the blood and enter the mammary gland in response to fat accumulation." The cells are said to be slowly motile under the phase microscope, sticking to glass, taking up cytophilic antibody, and phagocytizing carbon particles, properties that are highly specific for the monocytic macrophage series.

Thus, it is obvious that further electron microscopic observations from different species are needed before a general conclusion about the nature of Donné bodies can be drawn.

C. Fine Structure of the Myoepithelial Cell

The myoepithelial, or basket cells ("myothelia" of Hamperl, 1970), sometimes difficult to distinguish by light microscopy, have characteristic ultrastructural features that allow them to be identified easily under the electron microscope.

In the normal mammary gland they are widely spread contractile elements, which under pathological conditions can proliferate and participate in benign or malignant tumors. A review on the structure and histochemistry of "myothelia" in different tissues and particularly in the mammary gland has recently been written by Hamperl (1970).

1. Disposition

The myoepithelial cells are disposed longitudinally on the walls of the ducts and in a whorllike fashion on the alveoli. This disposition is easier to see in the light microscope than in the electron microscope (Richardson, 1949; Linzell, 1952). The body of the myoepithelial cell with the nucleus is arranged between the secretory cells and the tentaclelike prolongations are squeezed between or underlie the glandular epithelium. The myoepithelial cells with their branches are surrounded by the basement membrane (Figs. 58, 64, 66, 67).

According to Bargmann and Welsch (1969) the myoepithelial cells are situated preferentially near interalveolar blood capillaries (Fig. 66), and it is possible that their closeness to the vessels brings them under the

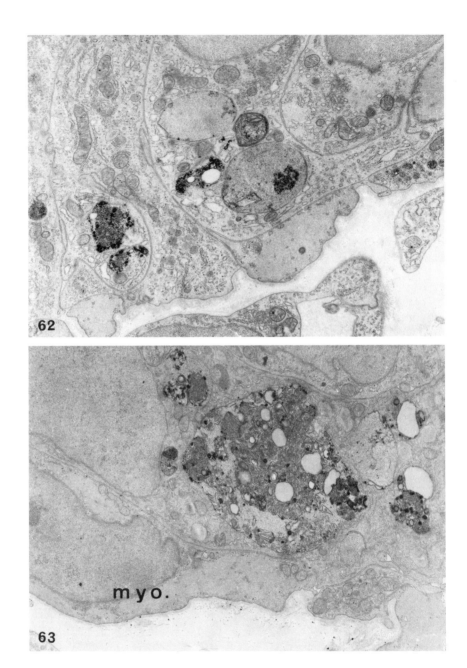

myo.

control of active substances passing through the capillary wall. Hamperl (1970) thinks, in agreement with Ellis (1965), that myothelia may fulfill some kind of transport function or control of the metabolism since they are sandwiched between the secretory epithelial cells and the stroma containing the nutrient vessels.

2. Ultrastructure

In the thin preparations for electron microscopy, the myoepithelial cells are almost never sectioned in their complete extension. Frequently, only one of their branches containing myofilaments or a portion of the clear cytoplasm with the indented nucleus is in the plane of cutting. In all cases, the myoepithelial cells (Fig. 64) can be easily distinguished from the glandular cells by: (1) the presence of myofilaments, (2) the tentaclelike prolongations at the base of the alveolus, (3) the clear cytoplasm with the poorly developed organelles, and (4) the indented nucleus.

The fine structure of the myoepithelial cell was first described in pathological material from mastopathia chronica cystica (Langer and Huhn, 1958) and in normal mammary glands of the rat and the mouse (Bargmann and Knoop, 1959; Hollmann, 1959).

These reports have since been confirmed by numerous authors (Waugh and Van der Hoeven, 1962; Bässler, 1961; Helminen and Ericsson, 1968a; Girardie, 1968; Wellings *et al.*, 1960a). As far as we know the structure of the myoepithelial cell is essentially the same in mammary glands of different species such as mouse, rat, hamster, gerbil, rabbit, cat, dog, goat, sheep, cow, and human.

The cytoplasm contains a characteristic fine felt of myofilaments mainly in the para- or infranuclear region (Figs. 64, 65).

Langer and Huhn (1958) already stated that the myofilaments are identical with those of smooth muscle cells and that they have a periodicity. The individual filament has a diameter of about 50 Å and a periodicity apparently similar to the I and Z stripes of skeletal muscle (Langer and Huhn, 1958; Haguenau, 1959; Ellis, 1965). The myofilaments of

Fig. 62. Basal portion of an alveolus from a mouse mammary gland during regression. The involuting cells contain numerous lysosomes (dense bodies, multivesicular bodies, autophagic vacuoles and residual bodies). × 12,000.

Fig. 63. A large lysosome containing remnants of cytoplasm and organelles in an involuting mammary cell from a mouse mammary gland during regression (same gland as Fig. 62). Myo, myoepithelial cell. × 10,000. (From Hollmann and Verley, 1967.)

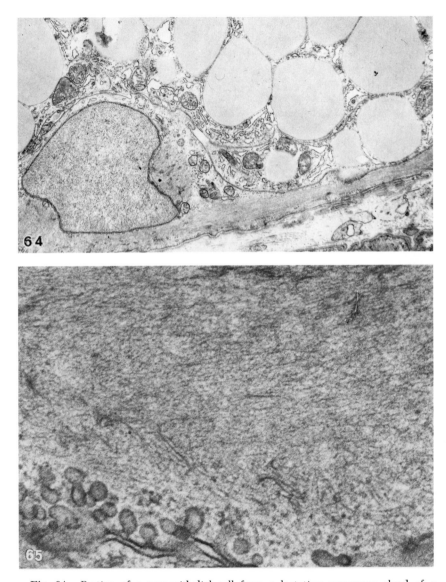

Fig. 64.   Portion of a myoepithelial cell from a lactating mammary gland of a
gerbil. The nucleus has an irregular shape and the cytoplasm contains few organelles.
The mitochondria are smaller than those of the adjacent glandular cell. The characteristic myofibrils are situated predominantly at the base of the cell and in the
tentaclelike processes. × 7500.

Fig. 65.   Fibrillar feltwork of a myoepithelial cell (mouse mammary gland, tenth
day of lactation). × 80,000.

myoepithelial cells contain actomyosin as Archer and Kao (1968) have shown in an immunofluorescence study using a fluorescein-labeled anti-actomyosin. Since myofilaments of smooth muscle cells also react positively with the same immunohistochemical stain, it can be concluded that both actomyosins are closely related or identical. According to Ellis (1965), who studied myoepithelial cells of human sweat glands, the myofilaments terminate near the basal site of the plasma membrane. There is indeed a zone of high electron density along the base of the cell that may be a site of attachment.

Besides the myofilaments, the myothelia have the common but poorly developed cytoplasmic organelles, i.e., a few mitochondria, a small Golgi apparatus, free ribosomes but almost no ergastoplasmic cisternae (Fig. 64). Glycogen granules are frequent. The nucleus has characteristic deep indentations. There is no indication for any secretory activity of the myoepithelial cell (Hollmann, 1959). However, numerous vesicles (Figs. 65, 66) arranged along the basal plasma membrane, and also often near the plasmalemma adjacent to the glandular cells, suggest an intense pinocytic activity, perhaps involved in the flow of metabolites to the secretory epithelium, as proposed by Ellis (1965).

IV. VIRUS PRODUCTION IN NORMAL MAMMARY GLAND CELLS

Milk is not only a beneficient substrate for nourishing the newborn but also in certain cases a dangerous vector for noxious substances and particularly for viruses that may cause infections, leukemia, or cancer. The transmission via the milk of the mammary tumor virus in the mouse is one of the best known examples.

A. The Mammary Tumor Virus of the Mouse (MTV)

Since Bittner (1936) discovered the so-called milk factor, which causes mammary cancer in many strains of mice, numerous studies have been devoted to this fascinating problem and have elucidated a good deal of the highly complex mammary carcinogenesis.

The responsible agent is a virus belonging to the paramyxoviruses. It has a diameter of 100–120 nm and a RNA-containing nucleoid of about 45 nm diameter (Figs. 68, 70). The viral envelope is covered by characteristic spikes 10 nm long, which are arranged in a hexagonal fashion (Figs. 68–70). The spikes have a typical structure consisting of a knob of 45 Å

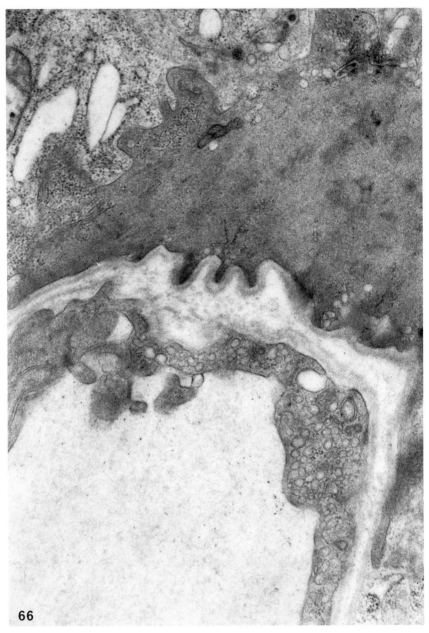

66

Fig. 66. Electron micrograph illustrating the frequently observed close topographic relation between a myoepithelial cell and a capillary. Both myoepithelial cell and capillary are surrounded by a basement membrane. From a lactating mammary gland of a rabbit. × 37,000.

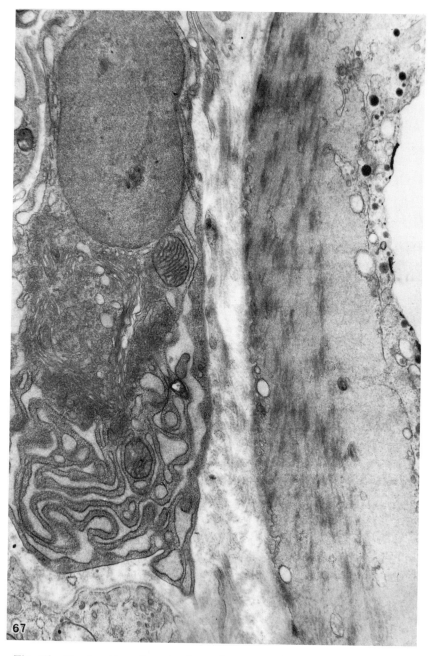

Fig. 67. Basal portion of an alveolus with a myoepithelial cell (right half of the figure) and adjacent stroma cells. From a mammary gland of a rabbit. × 21,500.

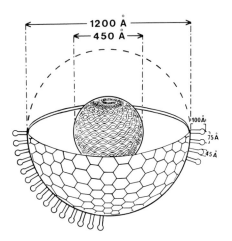

Fig. 68. Model of the mouse mammary tumor virus (MTV). The dimensions of the nucleoid and of the characteristic surface spikes are indicated. (From Hollmann, 1972a).

diameter and a stick anchored on the viral envelope (Fig. 69). The mammary tumor virus has been isolated from mouse milk and studied by physical, biochemical, and immunological means (see Sarkar and Moore, 1968, 1970; Sarkar *et al.*, 1969; Hollmann, 1972a,b; Hollmann and Verley, 1972a,b). If the virus is transmitted with the mother's milk, it is replicated electively in the mammary gland of the infected animal, particularly during pregnancy and lactation when the gland is stimulated by lactogenic hormones. Under these conditions, the MTV-virions (or B-particles, Bernhard *et al.*, 1955) can be detected at the apical surface of the glandular cells where they are elaborated by budding, often from the tip of a microvillus (Fig. 71). The mature and infectious particles are pinched off in the alveolar lumen.

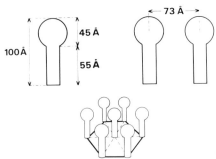

Fig. 69. Structure and dimensions of the spikes and their hexagonal disposition on the envelope of the mouse mammary tumor virus. (From Hollmann, 1972a.)

Other doughnut-shaped particles (A-particles) with an outer diameter of 70 nm, a concentric inner shell of 45 nm, and an electron-translucent center corresponding to the nascent nucleoid, are probably precursors of the B-particles (Bernhard *et al.*, 1955; Imai *et al.*, 1966; Smith, 1967). The A-particles are frequently situated in the Golgi region and often agglomerated in clusters that can be identified as inclusion bodies by light microscopy.

A- and B-particles are rare in unstimulated mammary cells (Feldman, 1963) but increase in number under the hormonal conditions that initiate lactation. In prelactating cells B-particles are found, intermingled with proteinaceous granules, within the distended Golgi vacuoles or in the alveolar lumina.

A peak of virus elaboration is attained with the onset of full lactation (Feldman, 1963; Miyawaki and Nishizuka, 1963; Girardie, 1968; Hollmann, unpublished observations).

In this connection, it is worthy to note that in the pregnant and lactating mouse, the secretory activity of somatotropic and mammotropic cells—as far as this can be concluded from their organelle development—coincides with the intensity of virus production. The development of ergastoplasm in MH and STH-cells (mouse) during pregnancy and lactation is indicated in Fig. 49.

The hormonal dependence of viral elaboration is further supported by the *in vitro* experiments of Lasfargues and Feldman (1963), who explanted mammary tissue from virus carrying pregnant R III female mice in organ culture. When such *in vitro* explants are treated with a combination of ovarian and hypophyseal hormones or with lactogenic hormones (MH), the production of B-particles is activated. Besides the hypophyseal hormones it seems that cortisol favors the replication of the mouse MTV. When cortisol is administered to C3H females, it stimulates virus proliferation and induces inclusion bodies consisting of A-particles in the cytoplasm of normal lactating mammary gland cells (Fig. 72) (Hollmann and Verley, unpublished observation) or of mammary tumor cells (Smoller *et al.*, 1961). As mentioned earlier (Section III,B,4,b) cortisol is likely to increase the amount of ergastoplasm in the mammary gland cell and may act in this way as a stimulus for protein synthesis and concomitantly for virus replication.

B. Mammary Tumor Viruses in Other Species

Viruslike particles have been described in mammary tumors of the rat (Hollmann and Riviere, 1959a,b; Engle *et al.*, 1969; Chopra *et al.*, 1970;

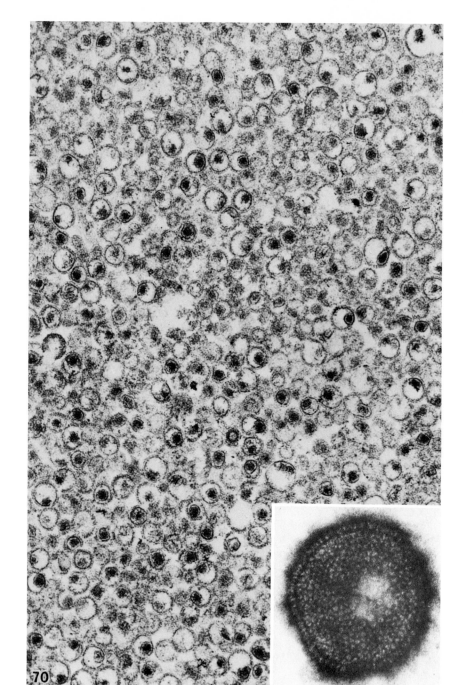

70

Fig. 70. Mammary tumor virus (B-particles) isolated by ultracentrifugation from mouse milk (high mammary cancer strain R III). Thin section of the pellet. The viral envelope and the nucleoid, often excentrically located, are clearly discernible. × 50,000. The inset at the lower right shows a high magnification of a negatively stained B-particle. The "spikes" on the envelope are easily recognized. × 300,000. (Courtesy Drs. D. H. Moore and N. Sarkar.)

Chopra and Taylor, 1970) and in human breast cancers (Dmochowski *et al.*, 1968a; Seman *et al.*, 1969) (for review see Hollmann and Verley, 1972).

Of great interest is the demonstration of viruslike particles, morphologically similar to or identical with the mouse MTV (Figs. 73, 74), in human milk (Moore *et al.*, 1971; Sarkar and Moore, 1972). Other findings such as the presence of 70 S RNA (Schlom *et al.*, 1972) and of RNA-dependent DNA polymerase (Schlom *et al.*, 1971; Dion and Moore, 1972; Das *et al.*, 1972) in human milk, and the possibility of hybridizing nucleic acids from murine mammary tumor viruses with nucleic acids from human breast cancer (Spiegelman *et al.*, 1972) support the hypothesis

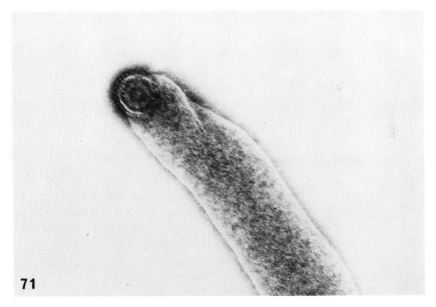

71

Fig. 71. Budding B-particle (mouse mammary tumor virus) from the tip of a microvillus. Negatively stained whole-mount preparation. × 120,000. (Courtesy of Dr. B. Kramarski.)

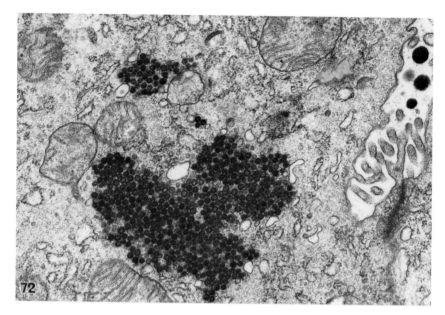

Fig. 72. Cluster of A-particles, the presumed precursors of the mature MTV-virions (B-particles), in the apical cytoplasm of a lactating mouse mammary gland cell. × 26,000.

that a human breast cancer virus related to the murine MTV may exist. This hypothesis will probably be under discussion during the coming years (for review see Hollmann, 1972a,b; Hollmann and Verley, 1972b).

C. Leukemia Virus Transmitted through Milk

Like the mammary tumor virus the leukemia virus (C-particle) can be found in the milk and in the mammary gland tissue. Dmochowski *et al.* (1963,1968b) observed leukemia virus particles in the milk of AKR mice and Hollmann *et al.* (1972) isolated an unusually high yield of C-particles from the milk of NZB mice (Figs. 75, 76). In the latter strain the lactating mammary cells elaborate, almost exclusively, C-particles, which are formed by budding from the plasma membranes (Hollmann *et al.*, 1972). Budding and mature C-particles were also observed in the mammary glands of pregnant C3H/f mice that had been injected intraperitoneally with the mouse leukemia virus (Feldman *et al.*, 1963).

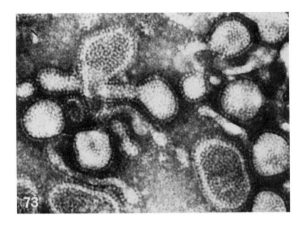

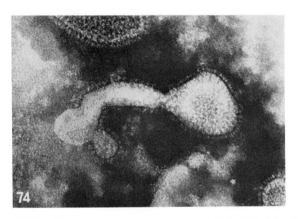

Figs. 73 and 74. Murine mammary tumor virus (M-MTV) (Fig. 73) compared with particles isolated from human milks (so-called H-MTV) (Fig. 74). The general structure and the arrangement and the length of the spikes are very similar. Negative staining. Fig. 73. M-MTV; × 125,000. Fig. 74. H-MTV; × 150,000. (Courtesy of Drs. D. H. Moore and N. Sarker.)

It is known that the mammary gland is not the only site for C-particle replication and that the leukemia virus is generally transmitted by other means than by the milk. However, under experimental conditions using highly potent mouse leukemia virus, transmission of the virus from one generation to another can take place through the milk. Gross (1962) reported that the mouse leukemia passage A virus was readily transmitted by the milk of nursing female mice provided that these mice had leukemia

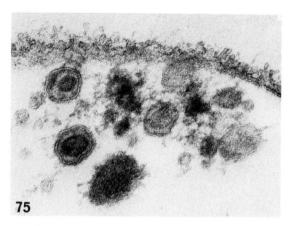

Fig. 75. C-particles in an alveolar lumen of a lactating mammary gland (NZB mouse). The dense nucleoid is generally situated in the center of the particle and the viral envelope has not the characteristic surface projections of the mammary tumor virus. × 110,000.

or were at the point of developing the disease at the time they were nursing. Thus, it appears that the quantity of virus transmitted by the milk is an essential factor for the induction of the disease.

Transmission of leukemia virus through the milk of nursing female mice was further reported by Law and Moloney (1961) and by Krischke and Graffi (1963). Although most of the present observations were made

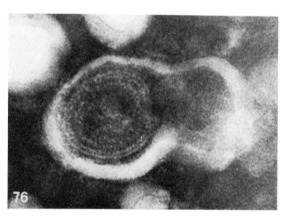

Fig. 76. Negatively stained C-particle isolated from the milk of NZB mice. The concentric rings made of a "macro-double helix" (not to be confused with the Watson-Crick double helix) show how the helical structures are coiled together to form the nucleocapsid. × 300,000.

on laboratory animals, the milk of other species should also be considered as a potential vector for the transmission of a leukemia agent.

ACKNOWLEDGMENTS

The author acknowledges gratefully the dedicated and skillful collaboration of Dr. J. M. Verley in the preparation of the manuscript and the technical assistance of J. Garaudel and P. Ferracci.

REFERENCES

Archer, F. L., and Kao, V. C. Y. (1968). *Lab. Invest.* **18**, 669.
Bargmann, W. (1962). *Z. Tierzüchtung Züchtungsbiol.* **76**, 416.
Bargmann, W., and Knoop, A. (1959). *Z. Zellforsch.* **49**, 344.
Bargmann, W., and Welsch, U. (1969). In "Lactogenesis" (M. Reynolds and S. J. Folley, eds.) pp. 43–52. Univ. of Pennsylvania Press, Philadelphia, Pennsylvania.
Bargmann, W., Fleischhauer, K., and Knoop, A. (1961). *Z. Zellforsch.* **53**, 545.
Bässler, R. (1961). *Frankfurt. Z. Pathol.* **71**, 398.
Bässler, R., and Paek, S. (1968). *Histochemie* **13**, 29.
Bässler, R., and Schäfer, A. (1969). *Z. Zellforsch* **101**, 355.
Benedetti, E. L., and Bartoszewicz, W. (1961). "Overdruk Elfde Jaarboek van Kankeronderzoek en Kankerbestrijding in Nederland," pp. 149–156.
Bernhard, W., Bauer, A., Guerin, M., and Oberling, C. (1955). *Bull. Cancer* **42**, 163.
Bittner, J. J. (1936). *Science* **84**, 162.
Bousquet, M., Fléchon, J. E., and Denamur, R. (1969). *Z. Zellforsch.* **96**, 418.
Chentsou, Y. S. (1964). *Acta Un. Int. Ca.* **20**, 1377.
Chopra, H. C., and Taylor, D. J. (1970). *J. Nat. Cancer Inst.* **44**, 1141.
Chopra, H. C., Bogden, A. E., Zelljadt, I., and Jensen, E. M. (1970). *Eur. J. Cancer* **6**, 287.
Coffey, R. G., and Reithel, F. J. (1968). Quoted by Kuhn, N. J. (1971). In "Lactation" (I. R. Falconer, ed.), pp. 161–176. Butterworth, London and Washington, D.C.
Dalton, A. J., and Felix, M. D. (1956). *J. Biophys. Biochem. Cytol. supp.* **2**, 79.
Das, M. R., Vaidya, A. B., Sirsat, S. M., and Moore, D. H. (1972). *J. Nat. Cancer Inst.* **48**, 1191.
de Duve, Ch. (1963). *Sci Amer.* **208**, 64.
Denamur, R., and Gaye, P. (1967). *Arch. Anat. Microsc. Morphol. Exp.* **56**, 596.
Dion, A. S., and Moore, D. H. (1972). Reverse transcriptase activity of murine mammary tumor virions (MuMTV): Analysis by polyacrylamide gel electrophoresis. To be published.
Dmochowski, L., Grey, C. E., Padgett, F., and Sykes, J. A. (1963). *17th Ann. Symp. Fundam. Cancer Res.*, p. 6 (Abstr.).
Dmochowski, L., Seman, G., Myers, B., and Gallager, H. S. (1968a). *Med. Record Ann.* **61**, 384.

Dmochowski, L., Langford, P. L., Williams, W. C., Liebelt, A. G., and Liebelt, R. A. (1968b). *J. Nat. Cancer Inst.* **40**, 1339.

Donné, A., (1844–45). "Cours de Microscopie," Bailliere, Paris.

Ehrenbrand, E. (1964). *Acta Histochem.* **18**, 1.

Elias, H. (1951). *Chicago Med. School Quart.* **12**, 98.

Ellis, R. A. (1965). *J. Cell Biol.* **27**, 551.

Engle, G. C., Shirhama, S., and Dutcher, R. M. (1969). *Cancer Res.* **29**, 603.

Farquhar, M. G., and Palade, G. E. (1963). *J. Cell. Biol.* **17**, 375.

Feldman, J. D. (1961). *Lab. Invest.* **10**, 238.

Feldman, D. G. (1963). *J. Nat. Cancer Inst.* **30**, 477.

Feldman, D. G., Gross, L., and Dreyfus, Y. (1963). *Cancer Res.* **23**, 1604.

Fiddler, T. J., Birkinshaw, M., and Falconer, I. R. (1971). *In* "Lactation" (I. R. Falconer ed.), pp. 147–160. Butterworth, London and Washington, D.C.

Gaye, P., and Denamur, R. (1968). *Bull. Soc. Chim. Biol.* **50**, 1273.

Gaye, P., and Denamur, R. (1969). *Biochim. Biophys. Acta* **186**, 99.

Girardie, J. (1967). "Histophysiologie de la grande mammaire. Etude histologique, histochimique, cytochimique et ultrastructurale." Ph.D. Thesis, Univ. of Strasbourg, Strasbourg, France.

Girardie, J. (1968). *Z. Zellforsch.* **87**, 478.

Girardie, J., Gros, C. M., Le Gal, Y., and Porte, A. (1964). *C. R. Soc. Biol.* **158**, 1940.

Girardie, J., Porte, A., Gros, C. M., and Le Gal, Y. (1966). *Laval Med.* (*Quebec*) **37**, 599.

Gross L. (1962). *Proc. Soc. Exp. Biol. Med.* **109**, 830.

Haguenau, F. (1959). *C. R. Acad. Sci. Paris* **249**, 182.

Haguenau, F., and Bernhard, W. (1955). *Arch. Anat. Microsc. Morphol. Exp.* **44**, 27.

Hamperl, H. (1970). *Current Topics Pathol.* **53**, 162.

Haug, H. (1955). *Z. Anat. Entwickl.-Gesch.* **118**, 302.

Helminen, H. J., and Ericsson, J. L. E. (1968a). *J. Ultrastruct. Res.* **25**, 193.

Helminen, H. J., and Ericsson, J. L. E. (1968b). *J. Ultrastruct. Res.* **25**, 214.

Helminen, H. J., and Ericsson, J. L. E. (1968c). *J. Ultrastruct. Res.* **25**, 228.

Helminen, H. J., Ericsson, J. L. E., and Orrenius, S. (1968). *J. Ultrastruct. Res.* **25**, 240.

Hennig, A. (1958). *Zeiss Werk-Z.* **30**, 78.

Hollmann, K. H. (1959). *J. Ultrastruct. Res.* **2**, 423.

Hollmann, K. H. (1960). *Bull. Soc. Roy. Belge Gynécol. Obstét.* **30**, 353.

Hollmann, K. H. (1965). *Z. Zellforsch.* **68**, 502.

Hollmann, K. H. (1966). *Z. Zellforsch.* **69**, 395.

Hollmann, K. H. (1967). *J. Microsc.* **6**, 61a.

Hollmann, K. H. (1968). *Z. Zellforsch.* **87**, 266.

Hollmann, K. H. (1969). *In* "Lactogenesis" (M. Reynolds and S. J. Folley, eds.), pp. 27–42. Univ. of Pennsylvania Press, Philadelphia, Pennsylvania.

Hollmann, K. H. (1972a). *Deutsch. Med. Woschr.* **97**, 620.

Hollmann, K. H. (1972b). *Annual Plenary Meeting of the European Organization for Research on the Treatment of Cancer* (*E.O.R.T.C.*), Semaine Cancérologique de Paris, June 19–23. *Biomedicine Rev. Eur. Clin. Biol.* (1973) **18**, 103–108.

Hollmann, K. H., and Riviere, M. R. (1959a). *C. R. Acad. Sci. Paris* **284**, 2917.

Hollmann, K. H., and Riviere, M. R. (1959b). *Bull. Cancer* **46**, 336.

Hollmann, K. H., and Verley, J. M. (1966). *Z. Zellforsch.* **75**, 601.

Hollmann, K. H., and Verley, J. M. (1967). Z. *Zellforsch.* **82**, 222.
Hollmann, K. H., and Verley, J. M. (1971). *In* "Lactation" (I. R. Falconer, ed.), pp. 31–45. Butterworth, London and Washington, D.C.
Hollmann, K. H., and Verley, J. M. (1972a). *Pathol. Biol.* **20**, 83.
Hollmann, K. H., and Verley, J. M. (1972b). *Symp. Thérapeut. non mutilantes des cancéreuses du sein* (in press).
Hollmann, K. H., and Verley, J. M., Sarkar, N. H., Charney, J., and Moore, D. H. (1972). *J. Nat. Cancer Inst.* **48**, 1243.
Imai, T., Hiromitsu, P., Matsumoto, A., and Horie, A. (1966). *Cancer Res.* **26**, 443.
Jamieson, J. D., and Palade, G. E. (1967). *J. Cell. Biol.* **34**, 577, and 597.
Keenan, T. W., Morre, D. J., Olson, D. E., Yunghans, W. N., and Patton, S. (1970). *J. Cell. Biol.* **44**, 80.
Kriesten, K. (1965). *Über den Funktionswandel des Milchdrüsenepithels bei der weissen Maus.* Inaugural-Dissertation (Dr. rer. nat.) Köln.
Krischke, W., and Graffi, A. (1963). *Acta. Int. Un. Cancer* **19**, 360.
Kuhn, N. J. (1971). *In* "Lactation" (I. R. Falconer, ed.), pp. 161–176. Butterworth, London and Washington, D.C.
Kurosomi, K. (1961). *Int. Rev. Cytol.* **11**, 1–124.
Kurosumi, K., Kobayashi, Y., and Baba, N. (1968). *Exp. Cell Res.* **50**, 177.
Lane, N., Caro, L., Otero-Vilardebo, L. R., and Godman, G. C. (1964). *J. Cell. Biol.* **21**, 339.
Langer, E., and Huhn, S. (1958). Z. *Zellforsch.* **47**, 507.
Lascelles, A. K. (1969). *In* "Lactogenesis" (M. Reynolds and S. J. Folley, eds.), pp. 138–139. Univ. of Pennsylvania Press, Philadelphia, Pennsylvania.
Lasfargues, E. Y., and Feldman, D. G. (1963). *Cancer Res.* **23**, 191.
Law, L. W., and Moloney, J. B. (1961). *Proc. Soc. Exp. Biol. Med.* **108**, 715.
Linzell, J. L. (1952). *J. Anat.* (*London*) **86**, 49.
Loeb, L., and Hesselberg, C. (1917). quoted by Meites, J. (1961). *In* "Milk: The Mammary Gland and Its Secretion" (S. K. Kon and A. T. Cowie, eds.), Vol. I, pp. 321–367. Academic Press, New York.
Mayer, G., and Klein, M. (1961). *In* "Milk: the Mammary Gland and Its Secretion" (S. K. Kon and A. T. Cowie, eds.), Vol. I, pp. 47–126. Academic Press, New York.
Meites, J. (1961). *In* "Milk: the Mammary Gland and Its Secretion" (S. K. Kon and A. T. Cowie, eds.), Vol. I, pp. 321–367. Academic Press, New York.
Mills, E. S., and Topper, Y. J. (1969). *Science* **165**, 1127.
Miyawaki, H., and Nishizuka, Y. (1963). *Gann* **54**, 391.
Moore, D. H., Charney, J., Kramarsky, B., Lasfargues, E. Y., and Sarkar, N. H., Brennan, M. J., and Burrows, J. H., Sirsat, S. M., Paymaster, J. C., and Vaidya, A. B. (1971). *Nature* (*London*) **229**, 611.
Munford, R. E. (1964). *Dairy Sci. Abstr.* **26**, 293.
Murad, T. M. (1970). *Anat. Rec.* **167**, 17.
Nandi, S. (1958). *J. Nat. Cancer Inst.* **21**, 1039.
Nandi, S. (1959). *Univ. Calif. Publ. Zool.* **65**, 1.
Neutra, M., and LeBlond, C. P. (1966). *J. Cell. Biol.* **30**, 119.
Palade, G. E. (1955). *J. Biophys. Biochem. Cytol.* **1**, 567.
Patton, S., and Fowkes, F. M. (1967). *J. Theoret. Biol.* **15**, 274.
Petersen, W. E., and Rigor, T. V. (1932). *Proc. Soc. Exp. Biol. Med.* **30**, 254.

Ranadive, K .(1945). *Proc. Indian Acad. Sci.* **22,** 18.

Redman, C. M., and Sabatini, D. D. (1966). *Proc. Nat. Acad. Sci.* (*Wash.*) **56,** 608.

Reece, R. P. (1956). quoted by Meites, J. (1961). *In* "Milk: The Mammary Gland and Its Secretion" (S. K. Kon and A. T. Cowie, eds.), Vol. I, pp. 321–367. Academic Press, New York.

Richardson, K. C. (1949). *Proc. Roy. Soc. London* **136,** 30.

Robertis, E. D. P. (De), Novinski, W. W., and Saez, F. A. (1960). "General Cytology," 3rd ed. Saunders, Philadelphia, Pennsylvania.

Rohr, H., Seitter, U., and Schmalbeck, J. (1968). *Z. Zellforsch.* **85,** 376.

Sandborn, E., Koen, P. F., McNabb, J. D., and Moore, G. (1964). *J. Ultrastruct. Res.* **11,** 123.

Sarkar, N. H., and Moore, D. H. (1968). *J. Microsc.* **7,** 539.

Sarkar, N. H., and Moore, D. H. (1970). *J. Virol.* **5,** 230.

Sarkar, N. H., and Moore, D. H. (1972). *Nature* (*London*) **236,** 103.

Sarkar, N. H., Charney, J., and Moore, D. H. (1969). *J. Nat. Cancer Inst.* **43,** 1275.

Schäfer, A., and Bässler, R. (1969). *Virchows Arch. Abt. A Pathol. Anat.* **346,** 269.

Schlom, J., Spiegelman, S., and Moore, D. H. (1971). *Nature* (*London*) **231,** 97.

Schlom, J., Spiegelman, S., and Moore, D. H. (1972). *J. Nat. Cancer Inst.* **48,** 1197.

Sekhri, K. K., Pitelka, D. R., and DeOme, K. B. (1967a). *J. Nat. Cancer Inst.* **39,** 459.

Sekhri, K. K., Pitelka, D. R., and DeOme, K. B. (1967b). *J. Nat. Cancer Inst.* **39,** 491.

Seman, G., Myers, B., Williams, W. C., Gallager, H. S., and Dmochowski, L. (1969). *Texas Rep. Biol. Med.* **27,** 839.

Silver, J. A. (1956). *J. Physiol.* (*London*) **133,** 65.

Sitte, H. (1965). *In* "Funktionelle und Morphologische Organisation der Zelle. 2. Wissensch. Konf. Ges. Dtsch. Naturforscher und Ärzte, Reinhardsbrunn, 1964. (K. E. Wollfarth-Bottermann, ed.), pp. 343–370. Springer, Heidelberg.

Sitte, H. (1967). *In* "Quantitative Methods in Morphology" (E. R. Weibel and H. Elias, eds.), pp. 167–198. Springer, Heidelberg.

Sjöstrand, F. S. (1968). *In* "The Membranes" (A. J. Dalton and F. Haguenau, eds.), pp. 151–210. Academic Press, New York.

Smith, V. R. (1959). "Physiology of Lactation," 5th ed., p. 93. Iowa State Univ. Press, Ames, Iowa.

Smith, G. H. (1967). *Cancer Res.* **27,** 2179.

Smith, R. E., and Farquhar, M. G. (1966). *J. Cell Biol.* **31,** 319.

Smoller, C. G., Pitelka, D. R., and Bern, H. A. (1961). *J. Biophys. Biochem. Cytol.* **9,** 915.

Spiegelman, S., Axel, R., and Schlom, J. (1972). *J. Nat. Cancer Inst.* **48,** 1205.

Stein, O., and Stein, Y. (1966). *Israel J. Med. Sci.* **6,** 773.

Stein, O., and Stein, Y. (1967). *J. Cell Biol.* **34,** 251.

Stockinger, L., and Zarzicki, J. (1962). *Z. Zellforsch.* **57,** 106.

Traurig, H. H. (1967a). *Anat. Rec.* **157,** 489.

Traurig, H. H. (1967b). *Anat. Rec.* **159,** 239.

Verley, J. M., and Hollmann, K. H. (1966). *Z. Zellforsch.* **75,** 605.

Verley, J. M., and Hollmann, K. H. (1967). *Z. Zellforsch.* **82,** 212.

Verley, J. M., and Hollmann, K. H. (1971). *In* "Lactation" (I. R. Falconer, ed.), pp. 93–103. Butterworth, London and Washington, D.C.

Waugh, D. F. (1958). *Disc. Faraday Soc.* **25,** 186.

Waugh, D., and Van Der Hoeven, E. (1962). *Lab. Invest.* **11,** 220.

Weibel, E. R., Kistler, G. S., and Scherle, W. F. (1966). *J. Cell. Biol.* **30,** 23.

Wellings, S. R. (1969). *In* "Lactogenesis" (M. Reynolds and S. J. Folley, eds.), pp. 5–26. Univ. Pennsylvania Press, Philadelphia, Pennsylvania.

Wellings, S. R., and DeOme, K. B. (1961). *J. Biophys. Biochem. Cytol.* **9**, 479.

Wellings, S. R., and DeOme, K. B. (1963). *J. Nat. Cancer Inst.* **30**, 241.

Wellings, S. R., and Philp, J. R. (1964). *Z. Zellforsch.* **61**, 871.

Wellings, S. R., and Nandi, S. (1968). *J. Nat. Cancer Inst.* **40**, 1245.

Wellings, S. R., DeOme, K. B., and Pitelka, D. R. (1960a). *J. Nat. Cancer Inst.* **25**, 393.

Wellings, S. R., Grunbaum, B. W., and DeOme, K. B. (1960b). *J. Nat. Cancer Inst.* **25**, 423.

Whaley, W. G., Dauwalder, M., and Kephart, J. E. (1972). *Science* **175**, 596.

Wooding, F. B. P. (1971a). *J. Cell. Sci.* **9**, 805.

Wooding, F. B. P. (1971b). *J. Ultrastruct. Res.* **37**, 388.

Wooding, F. B. P. (1972). *Experientia* **28**, 1077–1079.

Wooding, F. B. P., Peaker, M., and Linzell, J. L. (1970). *Nature* (*London*) **226**, 762.

Zeilmaker, G. H. (1968). *Int. J. Cancer* **3**, 291.

CHAPTER TWO

Endocrinological Control

R. R. Anderson

I.	Introduction	97
II.	Measures of Mammary Gland Growth and Differentiation ..	99
	A. Macroscopic Methods	99
	B. Microscopic Methods	100
	C. Biochemical Methods	101
	D. Evaluation of Various Methods	101
III.	Endocrine Regulation of Early Mammary Gland Differentiation and Growth	102
	A. Embryo	102
	B. Fetus	104
	C. Early Postnatal Life	107
IV.	Endocrine Changes during Puberty and Effects on Mammary Gland Growth	107
	A. Length of Estrous Cycles	107
	B. Recurrence of Estrous Cycles	109
V.	Normal Development of the Mammary Gland during Pregnancy and Pseudopregnancy	110
	A. Qualitative and Quantitative Studies	110
	B. Pseudopregnancy	113
	C. Contributions by Placenta and Fetus	118
VI.	Endocrine Control of Lactational Growth of the Mammary Gland	120
VII.	Experimental Growth of the Mammary Gland	120
	A. *In Vivo* Methods	120
	B. *In Vitro* Methods	131
VIII.	Nonhormonal Effects on the Mammary Gland	133
	A. Nutrition	133
	B. Mechanical Stimulation	134
	C. Drugs	134
	References	135

I. INTRODUCTION

Development of the mammary apparatus during intrauterine and extra-uterine stages was studied in a number of experimental animals by Turner and colleagues during the 1930's. Among the animals studied were the cow (Turner, 1930, 1931), rat (Turner and Schultze, 1931), mouse (Turner and Gomez, 1933a), guinea pig (Turner and Gomez, 1933b), rabbit (Rein, 1881; Balinsky, 1952), cat (Turner and deMoss, 1934), and dog (Turner and Gomez, 1934). The mammary gland begins to differentiate from the epithelium of the skin early in embryonic life. In both the male and female the primordial structures or anlagen of the mammary glands are the mammary lines. The lines are succeeded in rapid succession by structures indicative of ever-increasing growth and differentiation. These structures are the mammary streak, band, crest, hillock, and bud (Turner, 1952). The mammary bud gives rise to one or more primary sprouts, depending upon the mammalian species. While rats, mice, and cattle have a single primary sprout, primates have as many as 25.

Studies of mammary embryonic and fetal development have been done in perhaps no more than 30 of the estimated 19,000 species in the class Mammalia. It is unfortunate that a more concerted effort is not being made in this area. Based upon the evidence accumulated in relatively few species, the general concept of mammary development is that endocrine involvement in mammary gland growth and differentiation during embryonic and fetal life is relatively minor or even a nonentity. Growth of the gland in the male parallels that of the female in most species with the result that a teat develops, and it is associated with a cistern and rudimentary ducts. In a number of species studied, including the guinea pig, rabbit, and rat, the underdeveloped mammary gland of the male may be stimulated to a stage of considerable development by proper hormonal treatment.

Over the past several decades efforts have been made to determine the relationships between hormones and the mammary gland, both qualitatively and quantitatively. Since changes in development of the female mammary apparatus were particularly evident at puberty and during pregnancy, these conditions were studied much more than others. Hormones of the ovary were implicated very early as important stimulators of the mammary glands (Knauer, 1900; Loeb and Hesselberg, 1917). After the perfection of the hypophysectomy technique in the rat by P. E. Smith (1926), the stage was set for endocrinologists to demonstrate the importance of the pituitary gland to the mammary apparatus. The classic report of Ott and Scott (1910) demonstrated the need for the pituitary gland in milk removal, and the studies of Stricker and Grueter (1928) showed that the anterior pituitary elaborated a specific hormone involved in milk synthesis. These important findings concerning lactation served to generate interest by others in the aspect of mammary growth. During the 1930's, Turner and colleagues demonstrated that the ovarian steroid hormones were not effective in stimulating the mammary glands in the absence of the pituitary gland (Turner, 1939). By using replacement therapy in rats that had the pituitary, gonads, and adrenals removed, Lyons and co-workers were able to demonstrate the synergistic actions of hormones from the pituitary, ovaries, and adrenal glands (Lyons *et al.*, 1958). The introduction during the early 1950's of a chemical method based on DNA estimation to evaluate quantitatively growth of the mammary gland has lead to greatly increased knowledge of hormonal and mammary gland interaction *in vivo*. During the decade of the 1960's, the organ-culture, or *in vitro*, method has made possible a rapid increase in our understanding of the qualitative relationships between the endocrines and the mammary glands. Several excellent reviews concerning hormonal control of the mammary glands have appeared (Turner, 1939; Linzell, 1959; Jacobsohn, 1961). This chapter constitutes an effort to review selected investigations with emphasis on research conducted during the past decade.

II. MEASURES OF MAMMARY GLAND GROWTH AND DIFFERENTIATION

Progress in researching the actions of hormones on the mammary glands was not accelerated until several significant developments took place. Among these highlights were the ability to extirpate the pituitary gland of experimental animals, the purification of steroid hormones, and the development of morphological and chemical assays to qualify and quantify mammary gland proliferation. The assays may be divided into three general types: macroscopic, microscopic, and chemical methods.

A. Macroscopic Methods

Early measures of mammary gland growth included palpation to assess lactational potential of unbred heifers, outside measurements, visual observations, and weight of the mammary gland. Progress in the use of whole wet weights as a measure of mammary gland development was poor because of the high fatty tissue content of the gland which could not be separated from the parenchymal portion.

Weights of cows' udders were studied by Swett (1927), Gowen and Tobey (1927), Turner (1934), Emmerson (1941), and Matthews *et al.*

(1949). Gravimetric measurement of mammary glands in small laboratory mammals is not very successful when used as the only measurement, but it is often included in conjunction with other more reliable methods. Efforts to develop an objective and meaningful macroscopic method of mammary gland proliferation in laboratory animals was achieved using graph paper to measure areas of whole-mount preparations (Cowie and Folley, 1947; Flux, 1954) or by outlining the area and weighing the paper (Macdonald and Reece, 1960).

B. Microscopic Methods

Mammary glands have been observed microscopically for many years. Laboratory animals, such as rats which have thin sheets of glands, are readily used for the purpose of observing whole mounts. The glands are first fixed in Bouin's solution and stained with hematoxylin to emphasize outlines of epithelial cells. The thin sheets of mammary glands may be observed under a dissecting microscope for evidence of ducts, lobes, lobules, and alveoli (Wahl, 1915; Turner and Frank, 1930; Turner and Gardner, 1931). As such, they may serve effectively as a qualitative measure of mammary gland development. Attempts to quantify mammary gland whole mounts began with the mammogenic assay technique of Lewis et al. (1939) and Mixner et al. (1940). Recent investigations have been based upon this method as well (Singh and Bern, 1969; Singh et al., 1970).

Histological and cytological studies of the mammary gland have been numerous throughout the last two centuries. These have been reviewed by Turner (1952) and Mayer and Klein (1961). Although these procedures have been employed with success in elucidating the mechanisms involved in secretion of milk constituents, results obtained from using histological sections to quantify mammary development have not been reliable. For example, a complete cytological study of the mammary gland from the rat provided excellent information about cell constituents; but the constancy in cell numbers of cross sections of alveoli led the author to conclude that mammary gland growth was almost complete by the end of the first half of pregnancy (Weatherford, 1929). This conclusion was based on the fact that the numbers of nuclei per cross section of alveolus were 8.3 in the virgin, 9.3 on the fifth day, and 9.4 on the twenty-first day of pregnancy. The alveolar area index, which continues to be used as a supplement to other indices, was developed to measure mammary development (Richardson, 1953; Munford, 1963; Swanson et al., 1967). The method of serially sectioning mammary tissue for microscopic examination does have merit in qualifying the effects of various hormones on cytological and histological differentiation (Hardy, 1950; Lasfargues and Murray, 1959; Feldman, 1961; Rivera, 1964; Bern *et al.*, 1968). Ultra-structural changes of mammary epithelial cells during varying stages of development from the virgin to the lactating state have been studied. With the perfection of electron microscopy, increasing numbers of reports are appearing to relate intracellular structural changes to hormonal events (Ceriani *et al.*, 1970; Sekhri and Faulkin, 1970).

C. Biochemical Methods

After discoveries by Boivin *et al.* (1948) and Mirsky and Ris (1949) that deoxyribonucleic acid (DNA) is constant per somatic cell nucleus, it was suggested that DNA content of a particular tissue might serve as an estimate of cell numbers (Davidson and Leslie, 1950). This concept was applied to mammary gland tissue by Kirkham and Turner (1953, 1954), who pioneered the use of DNA measurement as a quantitative measure of mammary growth. Prior to this chemical method the procedures employed to measure growth of the mammary gland were not readily adaptable to rapid and reliable quantitative estimates. Other investigators quickly made use of the DNA procedure to test concepts concerning patterns and rates of mammary growth during estrous cycles, pregnancy, pseudopregnancy, and lactation (Shimizu, 1957; Greenbaum and Slater, 1957; Smith and Richterich, 1958; Nelson *et al.*, 1962; Tucker and Reece, 1963a).

D. Evaluation of Various Methods

Macroscopic measures of mammary gland development are subjective and lack both qualitative and quantitative properties. From the standpoint of practicality in evaluating dairy cattle and goats, these methods are the best that are available. Examples of attempts to quantitate macroscopic observations of the mammary glands include measurement of the angle of the floor of the udder (Turner, 1952), width and length of udder (Greenhalgh and Gardner, 1958), sonoray measurement of thickness of quarters to the median suspensory ligament (Caruolo and Mochrie, 1967), and water displacement and plaster casts (Linzell, 1966). Achievements in using these methods to evaluate mammary development have not been highly satisfactory. As a result little data have accumulated relating the effects of endocrines on mammary gland development based on these methods.

Semiquantitative methods for measuring mammary gland development have been based for the most part on the gross whole-mount observations of flat glands. These are limited to animals such as rats, mice, and rabbits. Kahn et al. (1965) developed a numerical scale for whole mounts from 0.5 to 4.0 to semiquantitate mammary growth and differentiation in rats so that statistical evaluation of the results was possible. Meites (1965) employed a scale from 1 to 5 using similar bases for arriving at a grade for a given whole mount, while Wrenn et al. (1966) graded ductal and lobule-alveolar development from 1 to 9.

Only the chemical determination of DNA has been a truly quantitative estimate of mammary gland growth (Turner, 1970). Several studies have been published to support the basic premise upon which this assay relies, namely, that the DNA is constant per somatic cell in the mammary gland (Griffith and Turner, 1957; Tucker and Reece, 1962). On the other hand, several other studies have suggested that DNA is not constant per cell in mammary gland tissue, and, therefore, DNA content is not a reliable estimate of mammary gland growth (Sod-Moriah and Schmidt, 1968; Simpson and Schmidt, 1970). Probably the best approach is to combine DNA measurements with whole-mount observations and/or histological sections of mammary tissue in order to obtain a reliable picture of mammary gland development (Munford, 1964; Sud et al., 1968). A comparison of the mammary gland area and DNA methods revealed that the two procedures correlate well, although it was pointed out that each has distinct advantages over the other (Munford, 1963; Nagasawa et al., 1966, 1967).

III. ENDOCRINE REGULATION OF EARLY MAMMARY GLAND DIFFERENTIATION AND GROWTH

A. Embryo

Information is becoming available concerning the hormonal control of the mammary gland in the embryo. We may consider the separation between embryonic and fetal development as that stage at which the primary sprout has reached full development. The mammary streak, band, line, crest, and hillock stages of growth and differentiation may or may not be under endocrine control. This is difficult to assess using in vivo experimental procedures because certain hormones of maternal source may cross the placenta to stimulate the embryo. Several in vitro studies of embryonic and fetal mouse mammary glands in organ culture have been conducted in an attempt to determine the effects of various hormones, separately and collectively, upon the mammary gland (Hardy, 1950; Lasfargues and Murray, 1959; Ceriani, 1970a,b).

Using 10- to 13-day mouse embryos, Hardy (1950) was able to cultivate the mammary apparatus for up to 25 days in a medium of chicken plasma and chick embryo extract. Although no hormones were added to the medium, growth of the mammary gland progressed through the mammary bud and primary sprout stages to the point where secondary ducts had grown into the fatty pad and a streakcanal formed at the end of the teat. Lasfargues and Murray (1959) found that mouse embryonic mammary tissue from 10- to 15-day embryos differentiated to that observed by Hardy when a biological medium was used, but not to as great an extent when Morgan's synthetic medium 199 was used. Addition of growth hormone or prolactin to the synthetic medium enhanced the ability of the mammary tissue to grow and differentiate. At the streak and band stage of mammary development some differentiation occurred in the absence of hormones. Of the five hormones tested in the organ-culture system, including estradiol, progesterone, growth hormone, prolactin, and cortisol, only growth hormone appeared to be concerned directly with growth of the mammary epithelium. Prolactin stimulated adipose tissue and the epithelium to prepare for lactation. Estradiol did not stimulate the epithelial tissue but did stimulate adipose tissue. Progesterone promoted the breakdown of ground substance and connective tissue, a function thought to be attributable to the mammary gland spreading factor (Elliott and Turner, 1954). Cortisol did not prevent differentiation but enhanced changes in the epithelium indicative of secretion. The action of cortisol seemed to override the growth hormone in that changes indicative of secretory function predominated over growth and differentiation of the epithelial cells attributable to growth hormone alone. Others have elaborated upon the findings of Lasfargues and Murray (1959) but with more mature mammary tissue than the embryonic anlage of the gland.

In the rat and mouse, mammary buds of the male separate from the Malpighian layer of the skin, the germinal layer from which the bud originated. The result of this separation is that there is no teat development in the male rat and mouse. However, the bud continues to exist and to differentiate into a primary sprout with secondary sprouts. This structure may be stimulated to develop into an elaborate network of ducts and lobule-alveoli under proper hormonal treatment. Indirect evidence that separation of the mammary bud from the epithelium in the 14-day embryo is hormonally controlled is based on the study by Raynaud

(1949) using testosterone. The separation in male embryo may be prevented by an antiandrogenic compound, cyproterone acetate (Elger and
Neumann, 1966; Neumann and Elger, 1966; Neumann *et al.*, 1966; Cupceancu *et al.*, 1969), or the separation may be encouraged in the female
embryo by norethisterone (Cupceancu and Neumann, 1969). Since the
action of cyproterone is to prevent separation of the mammary bud in the
male, it is assumed that in the normal male fetus the circulating level of
androgen, presumably testosterone, is sufficient to induce separation of
the mammary bud from the skin; thus, male rats and mice are characterized by the lack of nipples.

Stages of development of the mammary apparatus in relation to embryonic and fetal development may be confusing. Although the differentiation between embryo and fetus is at the end of 7 weeks in the human
(Thomas, 1968), it is approximately 90 days in the cow (Turner, 1952)
and 15 days in the rat.

B. Fetus

Endocrine control of mammary gland growth and differentiation in
fetal life is not well documented by *in vivo* work. The problems in experimental design and interpretation confronting the investigator in this
area of research endeavor seem almost insurmountable. However, some
experimental evidence, based on *in vitro* organ-culture work, does support
the concept that hormone control is important at this time. In most
mammalian species, with the exception of rats and mice, there is little
difference in the development of the mammary apparatus of males or
females to the secondary sprout stage. Beyond the stage of the secondary
sprouts, little more development than a primitive duct system takes place
in the male of most mammalian species having inguinal mammary glands.
The main reason for this is the lack of a fatty pad into which the ducts
may penetrate; a good example of this is the bovine (Turner, 1930).

Mammary gland development of the steer is very limited apparently.
One documented case may be cited. A Holstein steer was treated subcutaneously each day for 180 days with 200 mg progesterone and 200 μg
estradiol benzoate (EB). At the end of this period a daily injection of 0.3
mg EB per 45.4 kg body wt for 14 days was used to initiate lactation.
No more than 15 ml of milk per day was obtained from this animal,
indicating that the proliferation of mammary parenchyma was very
minimal indeed (Williams and Turner, 1961).

A second important reason for lack of growth and differentiation of
mammary glands in male fetuses is the production of androgens, which

are known to have an inhibitory action on development and differentiation of the gland of the female *in vivo* (Hoshino, 1965). However, the stage of development of the mammary apparatus and the sex of the individual is important, because testosterone propionate (TP) enhanced growth of the mammary gland in male mice whose mothers were treated with 5 mg TP on the fifteenth day of pregnancy. When the TP was given on the twelfth day of pregnancy, mammary development of both male and female fetuses was suppressed.

In vitro studies with androgens have been done on rat fetal tissue. Mammary glands obtained from the 17-day-old fetus (primary sprout stage) were cultured in a supporting medium and were stimulated to considerable growth and differentiation with insulin, prolactin, and aldosterone after 6 days. When testosterone was added at three different concentrations, the degree of inhibition in development was directly proportional to the level of testosterone (Ceriani, 1970a). In the case of midpregnancy mouse tissue, androgens, including testosterone, 17α-methyltestosterone, and 17α-ethynyl-19-nortestosterone, suppressed DNA synthesis in the presence of insulin, cortisol, and prolactin (Turkington and Topper, 1967).

Androgens secreted during uterine life of the bovine male fetus that is twin to a female may cause the female to be sterile. This animal is commonly referred to as a freemartin. The cause is commonly thought to be the passage of androgens produced by the male fetus into the female fetus's blood, suppressing the normal differentiation of the female reproductive organs. Alternative hypotheses have been discussed by van Tienhoven (1968). Little work has been done to determine the extent of mammary development in the freemartin, but one study reported in the literature concerned four Guernsey freemartins in which growth of the mammary gland was stimulated by injection of estradiol benzoate (EB) and progesterone for 180 days. This was followed by a high level of EB injection to stimulate lactation. Although 12 normal heifers responded well to the treatment, 3 of 4 freemartins were unable to lactate (Turner, 1959). Gross observation of the udders of the animals suggested that very little mammary growth occurred in the freemartins over the 180-day injection period.

Hormonal control of fetal mammary gland growth and differentiation in rats has been studied in organ cultures by Ceriani (1970a,b) and Ceriani *et al.* (1970). Mammary glands of 17-day fetuses were cultured in Waymouth's agar medium for 3, 6, or 9 days in the absence or presence of various combinations of hormones to determine the minimal hormonal requirements for mammary growth *in vitro*. Insulin was found to be a prime requirement for normal development of the mammary gland, verifying earlier findings by Elias (1959, 1962) and Ichinose and Nandi (1966) who used more mature sources of mouse mammary glands. However, it was pointed out that the primary sprout, called "the mammary gland anlage" by Ceriani, will survive and develop very slowly in the absence of any hormonal stimulus in the medium; this is in agreement with the findings of Voytovich and Topper (1967) that DNA replication will occur in the mammary bud of the mouse without the aid of insulin. Inasmuch as hormones are sometimes thought of as accelerators of autonomously occurring processes, especially in undifferentiated cells, these findings are not in conflict. It would seem that the schematic diagram presented by Ceriani to indicate the role of individual hormones in stimulating mammary gland growth and differentiation is a plausible one [Ceriani, 1970a (graph); Fig. 1]. Insulin accelerates growth of the primary sprout. It synergizes with prolactin in stimulating further growth and development. These two hormones plus aldosterone promote ductal differentiation and branching of the ducts. The stimulus to ductal differentiation is apparently initiated by aldosterone because this hormone alone in the medium will result in a miniature branched ductal gland. Prolactin in the medium stimulates growth and secretion, for there is no growth into the mesenchyme or secretion of the terminal cells when only insulin and aldosterone are in the medium.

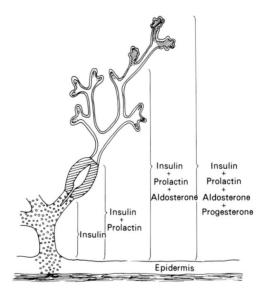

Fig. 1. Diagram indicating hormonal effects upon growth and differentiation of the mammary gland based on *in vitro* studies. (After Ceriani, 1970a.)

Addition of progesterone to the medium in the presence of insulin, prolactin, and aldosterone stimulated cell proliferation and granular secretion. 17β-Estradiol was not particularly effective nor was growth hormone. It was suggested that the optimal ratio of 1:1000 of estradiol to progesterone used *in vivo* is not the best ratio for *in vitro* studies.

C.   Early Postnatal Life

Growth of the mammary gland from birth to a period in advance of puberty is considered to be isometric, that is, it grows at the same rate as the rest of the body (Cowie, 1949). However, allometric growth commences much earlier than outward signs of puberty. This phenomenon has been documented in the rat (Cowie, 1949; Sinha and Tucker, 1966) and the bovine (Sinha and Tucker, 1969b). The accelerated rate of mammary growth maintains its high level until shortly after puberty when it again slows to an isometric rate or even less than general body growth. The slowdown in rate occurs in the rat at 60 days, which is about 20 days after the onset of puberty, and in the heifer at 9 months, which is about 3 months after the first sign of estrus.

Rapid prepubertal growth of the mammary gland may be caused by cyclic production of estrogens by the ovary (Sinha and Tucker, 1969a), which are released in response to gonadotropin cyclic activity that commences well in advance of puberty (Baker and Kragt, 1969). These phenomena have been documented in the rat and it is reasonable to assume that comparable conditions prevail in other mammalian species.

IV.   ENDOCRINE CHANGES DURING PUBERTY AND EFFECTS ON MAMMARY GLAND GROWTH

A.   Length of Estrous Cycles

Eutherian mammals generally have two types of estrus: continuous and cyclic. Several good examples of those showing continuous estrus or estrus for extended periods of time are the rabbit, ferret, and domestic cat. Ancel and Bouin (1911) described the rabbit mammary gland during continuous estrus as consisting of thickly branching mammary ducts. It has been observed that the duct system gradually develops after puberty in the domestic cat (Turner and deMoss, 1934), while there is apparently little or no duct proliferation of the mammary glands in ferrets during estrus (Hammond and Marshall, 1930).

Cyclic mammals are divided generally into those experiencing short estrous cycles of 4–6 days, such as the mouse, rat, and hamster, and those having longer cycles of 16–35 days, such as guinea pigs, sheep, swine, cattle, horses, and humans.

Several studies have detailed changes in the mammary glands of rats and mice during various stages of the estrous cycle. Since the luteal phase of the cycle is practically nonfunctional in these species, one would expect little additive growth of the gland with increasing cycles. Perhaps the first report to document changes in appearance of the mammary gland at different stages of the cycle in rats was that of Sutter (1921). He described a proliferation of the ducts into the fatty pad during proestrus and estrus. Others confirmed these observations and showed that the ducts involuted during metestrus and diestrus (Bradbury, 1932; Turner and Gomez, 1933a; Cole, 1933). By using the quantitative measure of DNA in the mammary gland, Sinha and Tucker (1969a) found that the mammary gland in the rat increased 8% from proestrus to estrus but was not significantly decreased through metestrus and diestrus. Of the five cycles studied in rats from 37 to 60 days old, there was a decline in mammary DNA between diestrus and the next proestrus. Growth during estrus was attributable to estrogens from the ovary and prolactin from the pituitary.

Animals displaying long estrous cycles from 15 to 35 days duration have a functional luteal phase that is usually associated with a predominance of progesterone secretion. It would be expected, therefore, that a more pronounced development of the mammary gland would occur in these animals compared to those having short 4- to 6-day cycles. Whole mounts and histological observations of mammary glands of guinea pigs revealed that the ducts proliferated during estrus (Loeb and Hesselberg, 1917; de Aberle, 1929; Turner and Gomez, 1933b). Mammary glands of virgin heifers were examined at various stages of the estrous cycle and ductal epithelial cells were found to develop just before estrus and to regress 8 days after estrus (Hammond, 1927). More recently, the histological observations have been augmented with biochemical data. Sinha and Tucker (1969b) sacrificed Holstein heifers on days 0 (estrus), 2, 4, 7, 11, 18, and 20 of the estrous cycle when the animals were approximately 17 months of age. The DNA of the glands increased by 118% from day 20 to the day of estrus and then declined through the cycle to the next estrus.

B. Recurrence of Estrous Cycles

Increased penetration of the mammary ducts into the fatty pad with each recurring estrous cycle has been indicated for many years. The rat was shown to have a rapid acceleration of ductal growth during the fourth and fifth weeks (just prior to vaginal opening which is during the sixth or seventh week) and again during the tenth week (Myers, 1917). In the mouse the duct system increases to approximately 70 days of age (Gardner and Strong, 1935) or even to as much as 90 days in the C57BL/6 strain of mice (Nagasawa *et al.*, 1967). Beyond 90 days there is a continuation of mammary growth in the virgin animal to the extent that some alveoli are differentiated. It should be pointed out, however, that female mice housed in colonies may experience spontaneous pseudopregnancy. The progesterone secretion by the corpus luteum of pseudopregnancy is significant in the rat (Fajer and Barraclough, 1967; Hashimoto *et al.*, 1968) and might explain the continued mammary proliferation and differentiation into alveoli in aged virgin mice.

Measuring gland growth in rats by specific mammary area or by chemical determination of DNA, Sinha and Tucker (1966) found that the most rapid proliferation of ducts into the fatty pad occurred between 23 and 40 days of age (prepuberal), while growth, measured by area, was significantly slower between 70 and 100 days. However, according to DNA measurements the rate of growth from 10 to 100 days was a straight line function between log of DNA and log of body surface, the exponential rate being greater than one (allometry).

In dairy heifers, weights and capacities of virgin animals increase gradually from 3 to 30 months (Matthews *et al.*, 1949). Capacities increase more rapidly than weight, suggesting that the ducts continue to proliferate into the fatty pad with each successive estrous cycle. A very thorough study by Sinha and Tucker (1969b), of mammary DNA, RNA, and hydroxyproline contents from Holstein heifers 0–12 months of age, showed that growth of the mammary gland began to accelerate at 3 months of age. This is several months in advance of puberty, which is 6 months of age in this breed. The rapid rate of mammary gland proliferation was 3.5 times as fast as body weight increase during the fifth to the ninth months of age. It then slowed to a rate of 1.5 times as fast as body growth from 10 to 12 months. From 12 to 16 months there was no additional growth on a unit body weight basis. This may be interpreted to mean that an isometric growth pattern of the mammary gland occurs from the first year onward. In absolute terms, the increase would be substantial because body weights of heifers at 2 years of age are about 60% greater than those at 1 year.

Based on the findings of Matthews *et al.* (1949), Turner reasoned that recurring estrous cycles are effective in enhancing mammary development to approximately 30 months of age. To test this hypothesis, virgin heifers were artificially induced to lactate at varying ages from 1 to 3 years of age, and milk production was used as an index of mammary development (Turner *et al.*, 1963). Maximum daily milk production in the yearlings was 2.4 kg; in the 2-year-olds, 3.5 kg; and in the 3-year-olds 6.8 kg. The evidence from this experiment, although indirect, tends to support the theory that growth of the mammary glands in cattle continues with successive estrous cycles to 30 months of age, even though the growth may be at an isometric rate with the body or even less than general body growth from 12 months to 3 years.

V. NORMAL DEVELOPMENT OF THE MAMMARY GLAND DURING PREGNANCY AND PSEUDOPREGNANCY

A. Qualitative and Quantitative Studies

Before the chemical measurement of mammary gland DNA to quantitate growth rate (Kirkham and Turner, 1953), virtually all studies concerning proliferation of the mammae during pregnancy were based on histological sections of alveoli and whole-mount observations of duct and lobule-alveolar extensions into the fatty pad. Quantitation of the whole-mount technique gained impetus with the publication by Cowie (1949) and is still recommended as a valuable supplement to chemical measurements (Munford, 1964; Nagasawa *et al.*, 1967; Sinha and Tucker, 1966, 1969b).

Early studies concerning the extent of mammary growth during pregnancy have been reviewed by Turner (1939, 1952) and Jacobsohn (1961). Generally, it may be said that primary ducts, emanating from the gland cistern, elongate and branch into the fatty pad in advance of and during recurring estrous or menstrual cycles. In most species, then, a fairly well-advanced duct system comprises the parenchymal portion of the mammary apparatus at the onset of the gestation period. During pregnancy the ducts proliferate further and further into the fatty pad until differentiation of the ductal end buds takes place. From this point the major type of architectural advance in mammary gland growth is that of grapelike clusters (lobules) of epithelial cells organized into a sphere (alveolus). Lobule-alveolar structures continue throughout pregnancy to proliferate into the farthest extremities of the fatty pad from the gland cistern. In some species the growth may continue into early lactation. The concept that proliferation of mammary parenchyma continues throughout pregnancy and into early lactation was a revolutionary concept developed as a result of using DNA as an index of mammary gland growth. Prior to that time, a commonly held concept of mammary growth during pregnancy held that virtually all growth of the duct and lobular-alveolar system occurred during the first two-thirds of pregnancy and that the last one-third of pregnancy was concerned with the initiation of mammary secretion (Turner, 1939). The earlier concept of mammary growth during pregnancy was based on histological, cytological, and whole-mount studies of mammary glands. Assumptions were based upon the observations available at the time and seemed quite reasonable, as evidenced by the series of whole mounts seen in Fig. 2.

Measurement of DNA in mammary gland tissue was first accomplished by Kirkham and Turner (1953, 1954) after Davidson and Leslie (1950) had suggested that DNA content of a tissue would be an excellent measure of cell numbers. An increase in cell numbers (hyperplasia) and in cell size (hypertrophy) could then be measured by this chemical determination. The RNA was measured by Kirkham and Turner (1953) to evaluate relative protein synthetic activity of the gland. Mammary gland proliferation is rapid during pregnancy in the rat as seen in Table I.

Chemical determination of DNA as a measure of mammary growth during pregnancy has been extended to other species, including the mouse (Nagasawa *et al.*, 1967; Brookreson and Turner, 1959; Wada and Turner, 1959a; Yanai and Nagasawa, 1971), guinea pig (Nelson *et al.*, 1962; Baldwin, 1966), rabbit (Denamur, 1961), hamster (Sinha *et al.*, 1970), and pig (Hacker, 1970). Quantitative studies of mammary gland growth during pregnancy in species other than the rat are summarized in Table II.

Earliest work in the rat by Kirkham and Turner (1953) and Shimizu (1957) suggested that total DNA in the mammary glands plateaued at midpregnancy, supporting the concepts presented prior to those studies. However, succeeding reports by Greenbaum and Slater (1957), Smith and Richterich (1958), Griffith and Turner (1961a), and Tucker and Reece (1963a,b) indicated that significant growth of the mammary glands of rats continued throughout all of pregnancy and, in fact, into early lactation. That mammary gland DNA continues to increase throughout pregnancy has been verified in other species studied to date, including guinea pigs (Nelson *et al.*, 1962), mice (Brookreson and Turner, 1959), hamsters (Sinha *et al.*, 1970), and pigs (Hacker, 1970).

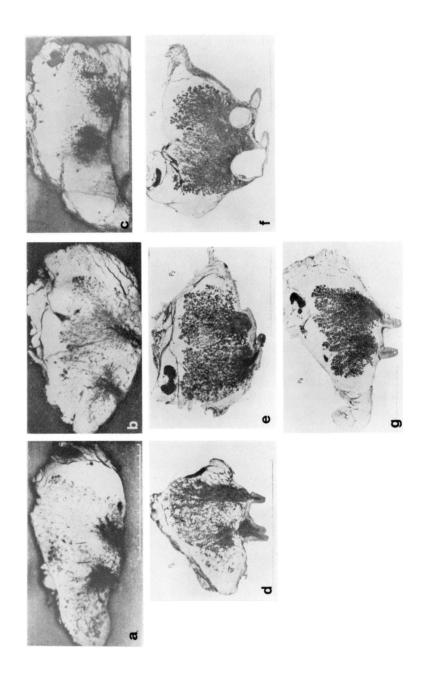

Evidence favoring the importance of hormones in controlling growth of the mammary glands during pregnancy is overwhelming. Early investigations centered around the concept that ovarian steroids, estrogens, and progesterone were responsible for growth and differentiation of the mammary gland during pregnancy. However, a number of studies with hypophysectomized animals revealed that pituitary hormones were intimately involved (Turner, 1939). The early studies led Turner to theorize the presence of and to search for an anterior pituitary hormone that synergized with estrogens to stimulate duct growth during estrous cycles and in early pregnancy. This was referred to as mammogen I (Lewis and Turner, 1939). A second anterior pituitary hormone, mammogen II, was thought to synergize with progesterone in midpregnancy to stimulate lobule-alveolar development (Mixner and Turner, 1943). The concept of pituitary involvement in mammary gland growth presently propounded by Turner considers a synergism with estrogens and progesterone of virtually all the adenohypophysial hormones to stimulate optimal mammary growth (Turner, 1970). Primary mammogenic activities appear to be intrinsic to prolactin and growth hormone with synergistic activities coming from adrenal corticoids via ACTH, thyroid hormones via TSH, and ovarian steroids via FSH and LH.

The interactions of hormones in stimulating proliferation of the mammary apparatus during pregnancy will be elaborated upon in the discussion concerning experimental growth of mammals.

B. Pseudopregnancy

A number of mammalian species experience a condition known as pseudopregnancy in which endocrine changes characteristic of pregnancy are brought about. The corpora lutea of the ovaries are maintained for a time and the mammary gland develops to variable degrees. Pseudopregnancy in the rat was described by Long and Evans (1922). Its length is approximately 13 days. Other small animals having pseudopregnancies running a duration of approximately one-half the normal length of gestation are the mouse (12 days), hamster (9 days), and rabbit (15 days). Turner (1939) reviewed the literature concerning the extent of mammary gland growth in various species during pseudopregnancy. It was con-

Fig. 2. Penetration of ducts and lobule-alveolar system into the fatty pad of cattle udder during successive months of pregnancy as follows: a, 1 month; b, 3 months; c, 4 months; d, 5 months; e, 6 months; f, 7 months; g, 8 months. Labels on udders refer to the number of the heifer. (After Hammond, 1927.)

TABLE I

DNA of the Six Abdominal–Inguinal Mammary Glands of the Rat during Pregnancy[a]

Day of pregnancy	No. of animals	Body weight (gm)	DFFT mean (mg)	DNA (μg/mg DFFT)[b]	Total DNA (mg/100 gm body weight)	Reference
5	21	253	288	25.2	2.83	Griffith and Turner, 1961a
10	21	255	363	33.0	4.52	Griffith and Turner, 1961a
15	19	264	422	43.0	6.76	Griffith and Turner, 1961a
18–20	19	324	749	33.2	7.63	Griffith and Turner, 1959
4	12	173	198	—	2.80	Tucker and Reece, 1963a
8	12	181	218	—	3.33	Tucker and Reece, 1963a
12	12	198	278	—	4.47	Tucker and Reece, 1963a
14	12	202	330	—	5.69	Tucker and Reece, 1963a
18	12	217	407	—	7.36	Tucker and Reece, 1963a
20	12	218	441	—	7.89	Tucker and Reece, 1963a
20	20	228	494	39.7	8.47	Kumaresan and Turner, 1965a
9	12	262	477	25.7	4.48	Anderson and Turner, 1968
12	12	262	426	28.9	4.70	Anderson and Turner, 1968
15	12	284	547	27.4	5.34	Anderson and Turner, 1968
18	12	271	578	33.9	7.27	Anderson and Turner, 1968
20	22	238	568	—	7.50	Kumaresan et al., 1967
14	10	257	512	—	5.68	Ferreri and Griffith, 1969
21	8	272	604	—	7.86	Ferreri and Griffith, 1969

[a] From Turner (1970).
[b] DFFT, dry fat-free tissue.

cluded that the growth of the mammary glands in rabbits, rats, and mice during pseudopregnancy was comparable to the growth during a similar period of pregnancy. It was suggested that pseudopregnancies could be classified as either the incomplete type or the complete type. Those animals demonstrating the incomplete type have been mentioned, while examples of the complete type have been observed in marsupials, domestic dogs, and foxes. Complete growth of the mammary glands and initiation of lactation have been observed in dogs and foxes.

With the development of the chemical measurement of DNA as a quantitative index of mammary growth, effects of pseudopregnancy on the glands have been studied. In the case of the mouse (Brookreson and Turner, 1959) and the rat (Anderson and Turner, 1968), growth of the mammary glands is minimal, being lower than at a comparable day of pregnancy. For instance, on day 12 of pseudopregnancy in the mouse the DNA of 7 mammary glands is 2.2 mg, while it is 4.2 mg on day 12 of pregnancy. In the rat, the six abdominal-inguinal glands contain 8.6 mg DNA on day 12 of pseudopregnancy and 12.2 on day 12 of pregnancy. Manipulation of the uterus to extend the length of pseudopregnancy by hysterectomy or growth of deciduomata resulted in a slight additional

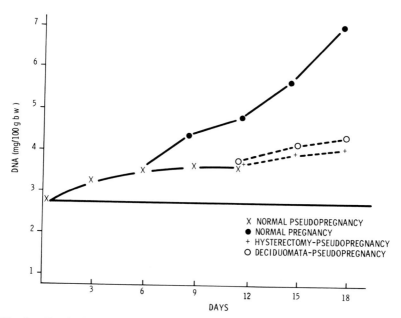

Fig. 3. Graph showing growth of six abdomino-inguinal mammary glands in rats during pseudopregnancy and pregnancy.

TABLE II

DNA of the Mammary Glands of Species Other than the Rat during Pregnancy

Species	Stage of pregnancy (days)	No. of animals	Body weight (gm)	DFFT (mg)	DNA (μg/mg of DFFT)	DNA Total (mg)	DNA Per 100 gm body weight (mg)	Reference
Swiss-Webster mouse (7 glands assayed)	(Virgin)	16	29.6	40.6	44.1	1.76	5.90	Brookreson and Turner, 1959
	12	14	36.9	95.3	46.9	4.34	11.71	Brookreson and Turner, 1959
	18	15	38.5	125.6	57.0	7.01	18.32	Brookreson and Turner, 1959
	(Virgin)	7	30.8	44.0	38.8	1.70	5.44	Wada and Turner, 1959a
	6	10	31.4	63.2	46.3	2.85	9.04	Wada and Turner, 1959a
	12	10	32.8	80.1	51.4	4.12	12.53	Wada and Turner, 1959a
	18	10	32.0	121.8	49.4	5.97	18.58	Wada and Turner, 1959a
C3H/He mouse (4 glands assayed)	(Virgin)	6–12	25.0	—	—	0.80	—	Nagasawa et al., 1967
	7	10	24.2	—	—	0.88	—	Yanai and Nagasawa, 1971
	14	8	28.7	—	—	1.83	—	Yanai and Nagasawa, 1971
	19	8	36.5	—	—	2.49	—	Yanai and Nagasawa, 1971
C57BL/6 mouse	(Virgin)	6–12	22.0	—	—	0.50	—	Nagasawa et al., 1967
	7	11	22.0	—	—	0.53	—	Yanai and Nagasawa, 1971

								Reference
	14	8	28.1	—	—	1.20	—	Yanai and Nagasawa, 1971
	19	8	32.9	—	—	1.75	—	Yanai and Nagasawa, 1971
Guinea pig (estimated values)	40	—	—	—	—	5.0	—	Nelson *et al.*, 1962
	55	—	—	—	—	10.0	—	Nelson *et al.*, 1962
	60	—	—	—	—	12.0	—	Nelson *et al.*, 1962
	68	—	—	—	—	20.0	—	Nelson *et al.*, 1962
(calculated values)	40	—	—	—	—	13.8	—	Baldwin, 1966
	60	—	—	—	—	18.3	—	Baldwin, 1966
Rabbit	1	—	—	—	—	15.0	—	Denamur, 1961
(estimated values, P × 10.1)	14	—	—	—	—	30.0	—	Denamur, 1961
	30	—	—	—	—	75.0	—	Denamur, 1961
Hamster	(Virgin)	22	108	204	19.2	3.9	3.6	Sinha *et al.*, 1970
	5	6	122	182	23.0	4.6	3.6	Sinha *et al.*, 1970
	10	13	128	256	43.3	11.1	8.7	Sinha *et al.*, 1970
	15	20	107	592	32.6	18.8	17.7	Sinha *et al.*, 1970
Domestic pig (values per gland)	(Virgin)	2	—	2.63[a]	46.5	121	—	Hacker, 1970
	25	1	—	2.48	45.1	108	—	Hacker, 1970
	50	1	—	2.24	50.9	115	—	Hacker, 1970
	100	2	—	14.38	39.9	580	—	Hacker, 1970
	110	4	—	34.90	36.0	1,218	—	Hacker, 1970
(values per gilt)	(Virgin)	2	—	36.8	—	1,700	—	Hacker, 1970
	25	1	—	33.5	—	1,400	—	Hacker, 1970
	50	1	—	28.9	—	1,400	—	Hacker, 1970
	100	2	—	201.3	—	8,100	—	Hacker, 1970
	110	4	—	458.5	—	15,850	—	Hacker, 1970

[a] All DFFT values for domestic pig are given in grams.

increase of mammary DNA (Fig. 3). Wrenn *et al.* (1966) measured mammary glands of rats by grading whole mounts arbitrarily from 1 to 9. At day 10 the pseudopregnant animals had 6.5 on the scale while pregnant rats had 7.0. At day 13 the pseudopregnant rats' mammary glands regressed to 5.0 while the glands of the pregnant rats attained a rating of 8.0.

C. Contributions by Placenta and Fetus

Well-known examples of placental contributions to mammary gland growth are human chorionic gonadotropin (HCG) and human placental lactogen (HPL). The former is produced by the chorionic tissue in specific Langhans cells. It is gonadotropic in action and thus stimulates secretion of estrogens and progesterone by the corpus luteum of the ovary. Its action may be considered as an indirect one. HPL probably provides the mammogenic hormonal stimulus required for mammary gland growth.

Other species that may be hypophysectomized during pregnancy with the conceptuses being carried to full term include the rat (Pencharz and Long, 1933) and mouse (Selye *et al.*, 1933). In these species the placental hormone appears to be luteotropic. It has also been shown to be mammogenic (Newton and Beck, 1939; Gardner and Allen, 1942). These findings are consistent with our present understanding that ovarian steroids require the presence of a synergistic hormone that normally comes from the anterior pituitary in order to promote the degree of mammary development that occurs in pregnancy. When the pituitary gland is removed, the placenta appears to be the source of the mammogenic hormone (mammotropin) required for gland growth. In addition to mammogenic and luteotropic properties, the placental factor of mice probably has lactogenic and somatotropic activities as well (Gardner and Allen, 1942). Rats hypophysectomized as early as day 6 of pregnancy were able to maintain pregnancy when injected with crude placentas from donors pregnant for 12 days. This demonstrated the luteotropic effect of the rat placenta (Averill *et al.*, 1950). A later study demonstrated the mammogenic, luteotropic and lactogenic properties of the placentae taken at day 12 of pregnancy (Ray *et al.*, 1955), while a study of day 12 placentas from mice show they had luteotropic and mammogenic activities (Cerruti and Lyons, 1960). A nearly normal amount of mammary growth from day 12 to day 20 of pregnancy in the hypophysectomized rat has been demonstrated using the DNA method for quantitation (Anderson and Turner, 1969). Kinzey (1968) reported that the mammogenic and luteotropic activities in placentas of protein-deficient rats were not impaired.

The source of rat placental mammogenic hormone was reported to be the trophoblastic elements (Matthies, 1967), which are fetal in origin. Minor mammogenic (or leuteotropic) activity has been ascribed to the deciduomata, which is maternal in origin (Wrenn et al., 1966; Anderson and Turner, 1968).

Placental mammogenic hormone (called "rat chorionic mammotropin," or "RCM," by Matthies, 1967) has been detected at day 12 of pregnancy in blood of hypophysectomized (Matthies, 1967; Linkie and Niswender, 1971) and intact rats (Cohen and Gala, 1969).

Content of placental mammogenic hormone in rats is high in day 11 and 12 placentas and drops off sharply in day 13 and 14 placentas (Linkie and Niswender, 1971). Two strains of mice having different levels of mammary gland development at comparable stages of pregnancy had no differences in placental mammogenic hormone content on days 14 and 19 of pregnancy (Yanai and Nagasawa, 1971). Perhaps the peak production had already occurred on day 12 of pregnancy.

A placental mammogenic hormone has been recovered from pig term placentas (McMurtry and Anderson, 1971, unpublished data). Whether or not other species have placental hormones that contribute to growth of the mammary apparatus is not known and must await future investigations. It will be interesting to determine if the placental hormone is similar to or different from the anterior pituitary hormone(s). The similarity between human pituitary growth hormone and human placental lactogen, a molecule having mammogenic and lactogenic properties, has been determined (Li et al., 1971). The two hormones are homologous in 96% of their respective molecules.

Contribution by the fetus to mammary proliferation is considered to be minimal or nonexistent, based on the studies of Leonard (1945), which showed that the placenta was able to remain viable and maintain mammary glands in hypophysectomized rats. Fetal contribution to mammary maintenance was examined by Desjardins et al. (1968), using DNA as a quantitative index of growth. When fetuses were removed on day 8 of pregnancy, the mammary glands on day 21 were found to have less DNA than normal pregnant animals on day 12. When fetuses were excised on day 12, the glands on day 21 had grown considerably, although not as much as those in normal pregnant animals or those having fetuses removed on day 16. These data suggest that viability of the placenta is dependent upon the fetus to day 12 of pregnancy. After that point, the placenta seems to be able to survive and produce placental mammogenic hormone in the absence of the fetus.

VI. ENDOCRINE CONTROL OF LACTATIONAL GROWTH OF THE MAMMARY GLAND

Continuation of mammary cell proliferation beyond parturition into early lactation has been demonstrated, using DNA as an index of growth, in rats (Griffith and Turner, 1961a; Tucker and Reece, 1963a,b), in mice (Brookreson and Turner, 1959), in rabbits (Denamur, 1961), in guinea pigs (Nelson et al., 1962), in hamsters (Sinha et al., 1970), and in pigs (Hacker, 1970). The relative contributions of growth during the postparturient lactation period in relation to total growth starting at conception are 54% in the domestic pig, 50% in the guinea pig, 40% in the rat, 22% in the mouse, 20% in the rabbit, and 6% in the hamster. Species variability in mammary cell multiplication during early lactation appears to be great. Data accumulated on the cow's mammary gland suggest that mammary growth following parturition is very minor if it occurs at all (Baldwin, 1966).

Hormones responsible for postparturient lactational mammary growth were studied by experimentally growing the mammary glands of rats with estradiol benzoate and progesterone for 19 or 24 days. Additional growth beyond the total mammary DNA at the end of pregnancy was accomplished with growth hormone and cortisol. Prolactin, alone or in combination with cortisol, did not increase DNA of the mammary glands significantly (Griffith and Turner, 1963). The ovaries were not required for the early lactational growth, suggesting that estrogens and progesterone were not involved in the process.

VII. EXPERIMENTAL GROWTH OF THE MAMMARY GLAND

A. In Vivo Methods

1. Endocrine Gland Extirpation and Replacement

a. ANIMAL MODELS. Early work on mammary gland growth showed that animals such as rats, mice, and rabbits with flat glands had a distinct advantage as experimental models because the glands could be peeled off the hide and prepared for histological and whole-mount observations. Furthermore, these animals could be kept under laboratory conditions very easily and the initiation of pregnancy could be timed. It was not surprising that the mouse served as the experimental model in the classic experiments of Allen and Doisy (1923) to extract the lipid soluble estrogenic hormone from the ovaries. The mouse and the rat served as good assay models because vaginal changes were observed without difficulty. These two species are still the most commonly used models for experimentation concerning the mammary gland, whether it is a study in developmental endocrinology, normal growth of the gland during pregnancy, or a study in mammary oncology. Other species have been used for comparative purposes, including guinea pigs, rabbits, hamsters, cats, and dogs. Experiments with cattle and goats have been important for reasons of improving productivity in farm animals. Monkeys have been used as experimental models because they are similar to humans.

b. Hormone Treatment. i. *Routes and vehicles of administration.* Hormones may be administered *in vivo* by several routes. These include intravenous, intraperitoneal, subcutaneous, intramuscular, intravaginal, sublingual, oral, buccal, ocular, and others. Most experimental procedures concerning growth of the mammary gland utilize the subcutaneous route. This is done because of ease and because a slow rate of absorption from the site of injection is generally desirable. Carriers for the ovarian steroids, estrogens and progesterone, are usually olive oil, sesame oil, corn oil, or propylene glycol because the steroids are soluble to some extent in these but to a very slight extent in an aqueous carrier. If an oil carrier is not desired, the steroid may be suspended in an aqueous medium with the aid of finely ground gum arabic. This is commonly used when adrenal corticoids are injected. Protein and polypeptide hormones are generally soluble in an aqueous medium if the pH is manipulated. A decided drawback to the injection into the subcutaneous area of a protein or polypeptide hormone in an aqueous medium is its rapid absorption into the blood from the site of injection. This results in the rapid metabolism of hormones that normally have a biological half-life of 20 to 30 minutes in the blood. If an injection regimen of once daily is used, the hormone is not present to fill the physiological need for the greater part of the day.

In the past 20 years many orally effective compounds have been synthesized. Much research has been done in experimental animals to test their effectiveness in stimulating mammary gland growth. The next decade will probably see many more compounds tested by routes of administration other than the common subcutaneous or oral routes.

2. Mammotropic Hormones

a. PITUITARY HORMONES. Experimental development of the mammary gland began in 1906, when Lane-Claypon and Starling attempted to stimulate mammary proliferation with aqueous extracts of placentas, fetuses, and ovaries. These experiments were not successful, but later studies with lipid extracts of the ovaries were successful (Frank and Rosenbloom, 1915). The discovery of estrogenic hormone by Allen and Doisy (1923) led to the observations that the hormone stimulated duct growth in the mammary glands of mice (Allen et al., 1924). Research efforts during the 1920's and 1930's centered around three themes: first, that estrogens stimulated duct growth for the most part and not lobule-alveolar growth; second, that progestin (progesterone) was responsible for lobule-alveolar development; and third, that in order for estrogens or progesterone to have an effect on the mammary gland, a hormone(s) from the pituitary gland was required (see review by Turner, 1939).

Full growth of the mammary apparatus in response to the anterior pituitary hormone having mammogenic activity, called "prolactin," or "mammotropin," was demonstrated by Clifton and Furth (1960). Pituitary tumors that produced large amounts of prolactin were grafted into recipient male rats previously adrenalectomized and gonadectomized to remove endogenous sources of steroid hormones. Whole mounts of the mammary gland clearly demonstrated the ability of the tumor-produced hormone to develop thickly populated lobule-alveolar mammary glands in male rats. This report aroused interest in the subject of hormonal control of mammary growth because previous research had suggested that ovarian steroids were able to synergize with insulin to stimulate mammary growth in hypophysectomized rats (Ahren and Jacobsohn, 1956) or that the anterior pituitary hormones synergized with estrogens and progesterone to allow the mammary gland to grow and differentiate (Lyons et al., 1958).

Additional evidence to support the findings that ovarian steroids were not required for full mammary gland development has been provided by Meites and co-workers using large doses of prolactin and growth hormone in triply operated rats (Talwalker and Meites, 1961), pituitary tumor transplants that produce abnormally high quantities of prolactin and growth hormone (Talwalker and Meites, 1964), implantation of normal rat adenohypophyses in close proximity to the mammary glands of immature, hypophysectomized female rats (Meites and Kragt, 1964), and injections four times daily for 10 days of physiological levels of prolactin and growth hormone to adrenalectomized-gonadectomized male rats (Meites, 1965). However, experimentation with mammary tumors suggested that ovarian hormones were required in synergism with pituitary hormone for growth of the tumors (MacLeod *et al.*, 1964).

It would be interesting to acquire data on DNA content of mammary glands developed by the stimulus of anterior pituitary hormones only and compare total DNA to glands from normal pregnant animals or ovariectomized animals in which mammary growth was induced with estrogen and progesterone. In our laboratory, mammary DNA in hypophysectomized rats was lower than virgin or ovariectomized rats. It was suggested that a hormone(s) from the anterior pituitary was required for maintenance of the duct system in the virgin animal, while in the absence of the pituitary gland, exogenously administered estrogen and progesterone slowed the rate of involution of the mammary ducts (Hahn and Turner, 1966).

b. STEROID HORMONES. Earlier reviews by Turner (1932, 1939) and Jacobsohn (1961) emphasized the significance of gonadal steroids in mammary gland development. Those which have received the most attention by investigators concerned with *in vivo* studies have been the estrogens, estrone and estradiol, and progesterone because these are the naturally secreted ovarian steroids. Turner (1939) introduced the concept that estrogens acted mainly upon the pituitary gland to stimulate secretion of mammogen I, while progesterone was effective in stimulating the release of mammogen II. The steroids then acted secondarily upon the mammary gland in a synergistic role to promote ductal growth in the case of estrogens and lobule-alveolar growth in the case of progesterone. Other concepts introduced into our thoughts concerning the role of ovarian steroids have been presented by Lyons *et al.* (1958) and Jacobsohn (1961). Some progress has been made by *in vitro* studies to clarify our understanding of the role of steroids in mammary gland growth. Further work in the area of molecular biology will be required before our full understanding of the role of steroids in mammary growth and differentiation is achieved.

Recent studies concerning the uptake of 17β-estradiol by rat mammary gland tissues have made use of autoradiography (Sander, 1968a). Radiolabeled estradiol was concentrated much more in epithelial cells than connective tissue or adipose tissue (Sander and Attramadal, 1968). Hypophysectomy performed 4 days prior to injection of estradiol did not influence the ability of rat mammary glands to take up estradiol (Sander, 1968b). Tritiated 17β-estradiol was concentrated in mammary tissue of the rat at one-third the amount in the uterus, two-thirds of the vagina, 11 times as much as omental adipose tissue, 17 times that of lung, and

42 times that of muscle, on a dry weight basis (Puca and Bresciani, 1969). It has also been found to concentrate in nuclei of epithelial cells of dimethylbenzanthracene-induced mammary tumors (Stumpf, 1969).

Progesterone uptake by mammary tissue has been studied in the rat (Lawson and Pearlman, 1964) and in the rabbit (Williams *et al.*, 1963; Chatterton *et al.*, 1969). It was suggested that progesterone is converted to 20α-hydroxypregn-4-en-3-one in the mammary gland of the rabbit and this metabolite of progesterone may have a stimulatory effect upon the mammary gland (Chatterton *et al.*, 1969).

Other studies of steroid uptake by the mammary gland include radio-labeled hexestrol, a synthetic estrogenic compound similar to diethylstilbestrol (Glascock and Hoeckstra, 1959) and testosterone by the mammary gland of the human (Deshpande *et al.*, 1963).

Investigations are continuing into the problem of determining optimal amounts and ratios of estrogens and progesterone required for maximum mammary growth. Variations in daily dosages of estrogens range from 1 to 500 μg and of progesterone from 1 to 200 mg. Ratios that are considered optimal range among species from 1 to 14 in goats to as high as 1 to 4000 in rats (Table III). Absolute amounts of estrogens and progesterone for optimal mammary growth may vary with other hormone secretion rates. For example, Moon and Turner (1960) found that

TABLE III

Ratios and Amounts of Estrogens and Progesterone for Mammary Gland
Growth *in Vivo*

Species	Estradiol benzoate (μg/day)	Ratio	Progesterone (mg/day)	Reference
Rat	1 (estrone)	1:4000	4	Lyons (1951)
Rat	1	1:3000	3	Moon *et al.* (1959)
Mouse	1	1:3000	3	Anderson *et al.* (1961)
Rabbit	24–96 (estrone)	1:42 to 1:104	1	Lyons and McGinty (1941)
Rabbit	15	1:67	1	Yamamoto and Turner (1956)
Guinea pig	15	1:67	1	Benson *et al.* (1957)
Cow	200	1:1000	200	Williams and Turner (1961)
Cow	343	1:250	86	Sud *et al.* (1968)
Goat	500	1:14	70	Schmidt *et al.* (1964)
Dog	10	1:1000	10	Trentin *et al.* (1952)

increases in thyroxine levels required increases in estrogen and progesterone for optimal mammary growth.

Attempts to develop the mammary gland of experimental animals to that found at the end of pregnancy have been relatively successful. Moon *et al.* (1959) used ratios of estrogen and progesterone from 1 to 1000 to as high as 1 to 10,000 injected for 19 days in rats. The experimentally developed mammary glands had DNA contents equal to rats pregnant 18–20 days. Further stimulation of the mammary glands of ovariectomized rats was achieved with addition of growth hormone and thyroxine (Kumaresan and Turner, 1965a), while pregnant rats responded with increased mammary DNA to growth hormone and insulin in one study (Kumaresan and Turner, 1966a) and to 0.75, 1.00, or 1.25 mg corticosterone per day in another (Kumaresan *et al.*, 1967). Postparturient lactational growth has been accomplished in part with growth hormone and cortisol after 19 days of estradiol benzoate (EB) and progesterone (Griffith and Turner, 1963). Using mammary area as a measure of gland growth, Macdonald and Reece (1962) found best results with 1 μg estradiol dipropionate every other day and 1 μg progesterone per day for 19 days in immature ovariectomized rats.

Experimental mammary growth in female and male mice revealed that 1 μg EB and 3 mg progesterone per day for 19 days were the best amounts (Anderson *et al.*, 1961). However, the level of DNA reached with these hormones was only 58% of the 18-day pregnant animals in the females and only 48% in the males. It was concluded that the placenta was an important contributor of hormonal stimuli to mammary growth in mice. Addition of cortisol and thyroxine improved growth and change of ratios of EB and progesterone improved the growth slightly, but it reached only 70% of the goal, which was the mammary DNA level at 18 days of pregnancy (Anderson and Turner, 1963).

Early studies on growth of the rabbit mammary gland in response to steroids have been reviewed (Turner, 1939). Experimentation with varying doses of estrone and progesterone showed that the best response was from 24 to 96 μg estrone and 1 mg progesterone per day for 25 days (Lyons and McGinty, 1941; Scharf and Lyons, 1941) or from 15 μg estradiol benzoate and 1 mg progesterone per day for 30 days (Yamamoto and Turner, 1956).

Studies in hypophysectomized rats and guinea pigs showed that estrogens and progesterone were not effective in stimulating mammary growth without the pituitary gland (Gomez and Turner, 1937). More recent experiments employing DNA as a quantitative measure of the mammary gland revealed that estrogen and progesterone in hypophysectomized rats slowed the rate of involution of the duct system from the normal estrous cycling virgin level to the lower level found after hypophysectomy (Hahn and Turner, 1966).

Immature male rats were treated with estradiol benzoate (EB) at a level of 1 μg per day for 20, 40, or 70 days starting at 20 days of age (Panda and Turner, 1966). The mammary glands were measured for DNA content with the result that EB stimulated rats had slightly lower DNA than controls after 20 or 40 days and slightly higher after 60 days. It was concluded that endogenous testosterone stimulated the controls better than EB stimulated the treated rats to 60 days of age (40 days injection), while at 80 days of age the testosterone in the controls was not effective in stimulating growth any further.

Growth of mammary glands of mature male gonadectomized rats in response to EB or to EB plus progesterone has been studied using DNA as an index (Srivastava and Turner, 1966a). Estrogen for 20 days had a very slight effect in increasing DNA while estrogen plus progesterone resulted in a significant increase in DNA. It was concluded that the mammary glands of male rats are able to respond to ovarian hormones almost as well as females.

The effect of testosterone propionate (TP) on the 2- to 5-day-old female rats is a sterile condition characterized by continuous vaginal cornification (Barraclough, 1961). To gain some insight into the effect of this treatment upon the mammary glands, neonates were treated with TP and after 120 days one group was sacrificed for DNA determination of the mammary glands. An 18% reduction in DNA below control animals was noted. A second group was ovariectomized at 120 days and treated daily with 2 μg EB and 6 mg progesterone for 19 days. When compared to a similarly treated control group, the DNA was 33% less (Kumaresan and Turner, 1966a). It was suggested that the lower level of growth in TP-sterilized rats was due to a decreased thyroid hormone secretion rate and less than normal secretion of anterior pituitary hormones, which may synergize with the ovarian steroids in stimulating lobule-alveolar growth.

Male rats were feminized in utero by the administration of cyproterone acetate from day 13 to day 22 of pregnancy. The teats were functional with openings to the outside, whereas normal male rats have no teats. The feminized males were gonadectomized at 300–350 gm body weight and injected subcutaneously with 2 μg EB and 6 mg progesterone per day for 19 days. After this, lactation was induced with 1 mg cortisol acetate, 1 μg EB, and 9 mg (3 × 3 mg/day) prolactin each day for 8 days. The mammary gland size was judged to be equal to a normal pregnant female and histology of the glands suggested that lactation was identical to similarly treated female control rats (Neumann *et al.*, 1966).

The role of androgens in mammary gland development has been studied (see Jacobsohn, 1961). An interaction of androgens with estrogens was suspected, and it was found that the male rat's mammary gland responded first to estrogens before androgens stimulated lobule-alveolar development (Jacobsohn, 1962a). This finding was confirmed and, in addition, it was found in a succeeding experiment that thyroxine enhanced the response of the mammary glands to ovarian hormones in male hypophysectomized rats treated with insulin and cortisone as well (Jacobsohn, 1962b).

More recently, Forsberg and Jacobsohn (1971) reported that male rats feminized with cyproterone acetate had mammary glands as well developed as control males of similar age. It was concluded that the feminized males were secreting sufficient androgen to develop their mammary glands similar to normal males.

A study concerning the mammogenic effects of androgens compared testosterone phenylpropionate with methandrostenolone, a synthetic steroid with low androgenic and high anabolic activity. This compound stimulated lobule-alveolar development and duct growth in gonadectomized male rats, whereas testosterone stimulated some lobule-alveolar development but no duct growth. It was suggested that the compound had estrogenic and androgenic effects (Ahren *et al.*, 1963).

Precursors and metabolites of progesterone have been tested for their ability to synergize with estrogen to grow the mammary gland in rats. Pregnenolone, 17α-hydroxyprogesterone, androstenedione, or testosterone propionate produced 29, 27, 36, and 33% of the mammary growth obtained by progesterone when combined with estradiol benzoate for a 19-day injection period (Damm *et al.*, 1961). The biological effectiveness of pregn-4-en-20β-ol-3-one was tested in rats and found to be about one-ninth as active as progesterone in synergizing with estrogen to stimulate increase of mammary DNA (Kumaresan and Turner, 1968). Orally effective progestagens from commercial sources were tried using mammary growth in rats as an index. Estradiol benzoate injected daily plus daily feeding of 1 mg/day of either Lutoral (6-chloro-6-dehydro-17-acetoxyprogesterone) or Provera (17α-hydroxy-6-methylpregn-4-en-3,20-dione-17-acetate) for 19 days stimulated mammary glands equal to estrogen and 3 mg progesterone treatment for 19 days of pregnancy (Griffith *et al.*, 1963). Norethynodrel, alone and combined with mestranol, was also shown to stimulate lobule-alveolar growth in rats equal to late pregnancy (Kahn and Baker, 1964).

c. PLACENTAL HORMONES. Because evidence is accumulating rapidly to show that the placenta is an important source of hormonal stimulant in maintenance of the corpus luteum and growth of the mammary gland, much work in this area is foreseen in the next decade. Recent investigations in this area have been mentioned in the section concerning growth of the mammary gland during pregnancy.

Luteotropic action of the placenta in the case of human chorionic gonadotropin is well known. The ability of the endometrial cups of the pregnant mare to elaborate a hormone that results in the formation and maintenance of a new set of corpora lutea is understood. However, these hormones are gonadotropic and not mammotropic. The finding that the human term placenta had hormonal activity that was lactogenic, somatotropic, and luteotropic (Josimovich and MacLaren, 1962; Josimovich et al., 1963; Kaplan and Grumback, 1964; Florini et al., 1966) served to provide an impetus for research on placentas of other mammals. Fortunately, the progress concerning characterization of biological and chemical properties of human placental lactogen has been rapid, with the result that its amino acid sequence is now known (Li et al., 1971). The mammogenic activity of this hormone has not been defined sufficiently well by in vivo assays, but growth and differentiation have been demonstrated in vitro (Turkington and Topper, 1966). It is 90% as potent as ovine prolactin in its mammogenic activity.

Jacobsohn (1961) reviewed the literature prior to that time concerning placental hormones. During the past decade interest has been renewed in the search for and identification of placental hormones in experimental animals, especially the rat. Matthies (1967) contributed greatly to knowledge concerning placental mammogenic hormone in the rat by identifying the source as being the trophoblastic elements in the fetal placenta and the time of maximum secretion as day 12 of pregnancy. The ability of the hormone elaborated by the rat placenta to stimulate mammary growth has been demonstrated directly (Lyons, 1944; Averill et al., 1950; Ray et al., 1955; Matthies, 1967; Cohen and Gala, 1969) and indirectly (Anderson and Turner, 1969). Direct evidence for the presence of prolactin in the mouse placenta from days 6 to 19 of pregnancy has been demonstrated (Kohmoto and Bern, 1970).

3. Metabolic Hormones

a. PANCREATIC HORMONES. The need for metabolic hormones such as insulin in experimental stimulation of mammary gland growth has been emphasized by Jacobsohn and colleagues (Donovan and Jacobsohn,

1960a,b; Jacobsohn, 1960, 1962b). Removal of the source of insulin from the rat is practically impossible, but treatment with alloxan destroys virtually all insulin-producing cells (β cells) of the pancreas. When rats were treated with alloxan and given estrogen plus progesterone for 19 days, mammary gland DNA was reduced 18% below control rats given the ovarian steroids. Rats given 3 units of insulin per day plus estrogen and progesterone after alloxan treatment had 66% more mammary DNA than similar controls (Kumaresan and Turner, 1965b). In pregnant rats, insulin at 3 units/day synergized with growth hormone (1–3 mg/day) to cause a 62% increase in mammary DNA over control animals (Kumaresan and Turner, 1966b). Studies using mammary tissue cultures have emphasized the need for insulin in the medium (Elias, 1959; Rivera, 1964; Ichinose and Nandi, 1966).

b. Thyroid Hormones. Thyroxine has been shown to stimulate the mammary gland when given in conjunction with insulin and cortisone to the hypophysectomized rat, but it has no effect alone (Etienne, 1960; Jacobsohn, 1960, 1962b). Thyroxine administered to pregnant rats at 2.5, 3.0, or 3.5 μg per 100 gm body weight per day had a slight beneficial effect on mammary gland DNA (Griffith and Turner, 1961b). Rats given estrogen and progesterone for 19 days were benefited significantly when the levels of estradiol benzoate and progesterone were doubled (Moon and Turner, 1960). A slight improvement in mammary gland growth was noted when 1, 2, or 3 μg thyroxine per 100 gm body weight was given per day to mice injected with ovarian steroids to stimulate mammary development (Anderson and Turner, 1963).

Others have observed detrimental effects on mammary development when excessive amounts of thyroxine were present (Meites and Kragt, 1965; Schmidt and Moger, 1967; Singh and Bern, 1969).

c. Adrenal Hormones. Hormones from the adrenal cortex include aldosterone, corticosterone, cortisone, and cortisol. All of these have been shown to be important in lactation. These corticoids have such profound effects upon general metabolic processes in the organism that they also influence mammary growth. Ahren and Jacobsohn (1957) presented histological evidence for the ability of corticoids to synergize with estrogens and progesterone to grow the mammary apparatus in the hypophysectomized rat and for that the corticoids act as the stimulus in thickening walls of ducts when insulin was given as well. A comparison of mammary DNA in ovariectomized-hypophysectomized rats versus virgin or ovariectomized rats revealed that the mammary gland had regressed. When the adrenals were removed as well as the hypophysis and ovaries, mammary

DNA was even lower (Hahn and Turner, 1967). This suggested that aldosterone might have a role in maintaining some integrity of previously developed mammary epithelium in the hypophysectomized rat, a concept that is supported by the *in vitro* studies of Ceriani (1970a). Adrenalectomized rats were treated with estrogens and progesterone to grow the mammary gland. The presence of glucocorticoid (prednisone or cortisol acetate) did not result in mammary growth, although the general health of the animals was excellent. Estrogen and progesterone in the absence of the adrenal glands did not grow the mammary glands as well as they did in animals having intact adrenal glands. Replacement with 100 μg prednisone or cortisol acetate per day in conjunction with the ovarian steroids resulted in mammary DNA equal to the respective control group. Deoxycorticosterone acetate was not sufficient replacement (Anderson and Turner, 1962). Corticosterone as additive therapy to ovariectomized rats given 2 μg estradiol benzoate and 6 mg progesterone per day for 19 days to grow the mammary glands was an effective synergist at levels of 0.75 and 1 mg/day (Hahn, 1967). Corticosterone at 1 mg synergized with thyroxine at 3 μg/100 gm body weight per day, bovine growth hormone at 1 mg and ovine lactogenic hormone to stimulate mammary growth in hypophysectomized rats to a level of DNA 97% above the control animals.

d. RELAXIN. Mammotropic activity of relaxin has been tested in mice by injecting it in combination with estradiol benzoate for 10 days. Mammary gland DNA reached a level equal to day 6 of pregnancy when 5 GPU per day of relaxin was used (Wada and Turner, 1959b). A similar experiment in rats resulted in a stimulation of mammary DNA equal to day 10 of pregnancy after 7 days injection of 1 μg estradiol benzoate and 15 or 45 GPU relaxin per day (Wada and Turner, 1959c). These experiments were designed to demonstrate the validity of a theory propounded by Turner stating that the estrogen and progesterone during pregnancy stimulate the release of relaxin, which in turn acts upon the mammary gland to aid in growth and differentiation. The theory has never been tested beyond the evidence in the two publications cited. Perhaps the future will see additional work accomplished concerning the relationship of relaxin to the mammary gland.

e. PARATHYROID HORMONE. Need for parathyroid hormone in mammary growth has not been very well documented. A study in rats of experimental growth with estrogens and progesterone in ovari-thyro-parathyroidectomized rats did not effectively show a need for parathyroid hormone in mammogenesis (von Berswordt-Wallrabe and Turner, 1960a). A second experiment using ovari-thyro-parathyroidectomized rats and dihydrotachysterol (AT 10) as a replacement for parathyroid hormone, indicated that AT 10 at a level of 20 μg/100 gm body weight per day for 19 days enhanced mammary growth significantly (von Berswordt-Wallrabe and Turner, 1960b).

f. PITUITARY HORMONES. Although it has been shown to have mammogenic properties (Lyons *et al.*, 1958), growth hormone may be considered to be a metabolic hormone. When DNA was used as a quantitative index of mammary growth, there was little increase in the hypophysectomized rat in response to 1 mg of bovine growth hormone per day for 19 days. On the other hand, growth hormone synergized with other hormones such as prolactin, corticosterone, thyroxine, and ovarian steroids (Hahn, 1967). Administration of 1 mg growth hormone for 19 days in ovariectomized rats was also ineffective in stimulating a significant increase in DNA (Moon, 1961). However, growth hormone was able to stimulate a significant increase when given with estradiol benzoate and progesterone. The synergistic action of growth hormone with the ovarian steroids in promoting an increase in mammary DNA was confirmed by Kumaresan and Turner (1965a). These experiments tend to support the findings of Lyons (1969) and Li *et al.* (1971), showing that the purest growth hormone preparations have both mammotropic and somatotropic activities intrinsic to the molecule.

B. *In Vitro* Methods

1. Evaluation of Responses

Since the successful experiments of Hardy (1950) in growing embryonic mouse mammary tissue in chicken plasma and chicken embryo extract, the organ culture method for evaluating mammary gland growth, differentiation, and secretion has been employed with great success. The response of the tissue to hormones in the medium may vary with time. The type of response may be a differentiation of the ducts into lobule-alveoli or an elongation of ducts without differentiation. In some studies, only histological observations of the cultural tissues have been made (Hardy, 1950; Lasfargues and Murray, 1959). In others, semiquantitative evaluation has been based on arbitrarily determined scores such as −, +, and + + (Rivera and Bern, 1961; Rivera, 1964; Ichinose and Nandi, 1966) or scoring 1 to 5 (Singh and Bern, 1969; Singh *et al.*, 1970). The latter are generally based on observations of stained whole mounts of the gland. Cell counting of clonally derived mammary tumor strains cultured *in vitro* has been used as a quantitative index (Posner *et al.*, 1970). Biochemical evaluation such as radioactive thymidine incorporation into DNA has been used (Stockdale and Topper, 1966a,b) as well as the time course of accumulation of the nonmetabolizable amino acid, α-aminoiso-butyric acid, by tissues *in vitro* (Topper *et al.*, 1970).

2. Hormones

a. MAMMOTROPIC HORMONES. Development of the embryonic mammary gland of mice *in vitro* progressed to some extent without hormonal stimulation (Hardy, 1950). In this study the mammary apparatus differentiated from a mammary bud to a primary duct and numerous secondary ducts and to a streakcanal in the teat without the aid of hormone stimulation in the medium. Later work by Lasfargues and Murray (1959) showed that prolactin and growth hormone had pronounced stimulatory effects on mammary growth and differentiation *in vitro*. The importance of insulin as a primary requirement for the maintenance of differential mammary tissue was demonstrated by Rivera and Bern (1961) and Rivera (1964). Differentiation of the mouse mammary gland from a duct to a lobule-alveolar type was found to occur only when aldosterone was available to synergize with the hormones that are generally considered mammotropic, namely, prolactin, growth hormone, estrogen, and progesterone (Ichinose and Nandi, 1966). Starting with fetal tissue, Ceriani (1970a) has found that insulin is required for prolactin to stimulate duct growth while aldosterone and progesterone enhance ductal branching and lobule-alveolar differentiation in the presence of insulin and prolactin.

Early *in vitro* work suggested that growth hormone was more effective as a stimulator of mammary epithelium growth and differentiation than was prolactin (Lasfargues and Murray, 1959). This was in the absence of insulin. When the importance of insulin to the integrity of tissue in cultured media was pointed out (Rivera and Bern, 1961; Rivera, 1964), the emphasis shifted in favor of prolactin as the more important hormonal determinant to mammary growth and differentiation (Ceriani, 1970a; Dilley, 1971). In some studies both prolactin and growth hormone are used (Ichinose and Nandi, 1966; Singh *et al.*, 1970), which lends support to the concept that the biological properties of these two anterior pituitary hormones overlap.

b. METABOLIC HORMONES. It is generally recognized as a result of *in vivo* studies that insulin, adrenal corticoids, and thyroxine are metabolic hormones; they have very little ability to stimulate mammary proliferation *in vivo* without the synergistic effects of the mammotropic hormones, prolactin and growth hormone. *In vitro* studies have demonstrated that some degree of growth and differentiation of mammary epithelium does occur under the stimulus of insulin or aldosterone. Therefore, it would appear that these hormones are mammotropic.

Thyroxine has been shown to have a synergistic effect at low concentrations *in vitro* while it is antagonistic to lobule-alveolar development of the mammary apparatus at high concentrations (Singh and Bern, 1969).

Organ-culture studies have shown that cortisol (Rivera and Bern, 1961), corticosterone (El-Darwish and Rivera, 1970), and aldosterone (Rivera, 1964; Ichinose and Nandi, 1966; Dilley, 1971) are synergistic with other hormones in stimulating mammary growth and differentiation. Adrenocortical steroids by themselves are ineffective in maintaining the alveolar structure of mammary glands from mice in late pregnancy (Rivera and Bern, 1961). Glands removed from animals pretreated *in vivo* with mammogenic hormones were maintained *in vitro* by aldosterone only when insulin was present as well (Ichinose and Nandi, 1966). Embryonic mammary tissue from mice was subjected to cortisol alone *in vitro* with the result that the epithelium differentiated abnormally and the surrounding adipose tissue replaced connective tissue (Lasfargues and Murray, 1959).

Requirements by mammary gland explants from midpregnant mice for various adrenal steroids were tested *in vitro*. All glucocorticoids were found to synergize with insulin and prolactin to stimulate epithelial cell differentiation (Turkington *et al.*, 1967).

Uptake of tritiated thymidine and grading alveolar development from 0 to 4 were used as indices of mitotic activity of immature rat mammary organ cultures. Explants cultured with insulin, prolactin, and aldosterone had significantly greater alveolar development and DNA synthetic activity than those receiving only insulin and prolactin. It was suggested that cell division in a proper hormonal environment precludes the differentiation of mammary epithelia from ducts to lobule-alveoli (Dilley, 1971) in a manner analogous to the cell division of alveolar cells prior to their differentiation into milk secretory cells (Stockdale and Topper, 1966a; Topper, 1968).

VIII. NONHORMONAL EFFECTS ON THE MAMMARY GLAND

A. Nutrition

Since growth of the mammary gland is dependent upon metabolic hormones, it would seem that factors related to changes in secretion rates of these hormones might also affect the mammary gland. Growth hormone has been shown to synergize with other hormones *in vivo* or *in vitro*. The growth hormone content of the pituitary gland of rats was progressively decreased by starvation for 24–96 hours (Friedman and Reichlin, 1965). Depriving rats of all food for 5–7 days resulted in a 40–50% reduction in the pituitary content of growth hormone and in a fivefold reduction in the amount of growth hormone releasing factor in the hypothalamus (Meites and Fiel, 1965). Rats given 75% or 50% of their normal food consumption reduced their thyroid hormone secretion rates by comparable amounts (Grossie and Turner, 1962). Sykes *et al.* (1948) maintained rats on a restricted diet from weaning to the end of pregnancy with a 30% reduction in food intake, body weight was reduced 23% and mammary gland weight 80%. The great reduction in weight of the glands was attributable mainly to a loss of the fatty pad and partly to reduction in parenchymal tissue. When ovariectomized rats were injected with 2 μg estradiol benzoate and 6 mg progesterone per day for 19 days and food was restricted to either 75% or 50% of normal, the DNA of the mammary glands was depressed only 4% and 18%, respectively (Srivastava and Turner, 1966b).

B. Mechanical Stimulation

Self-licking the mammary apparatus by the pregnant rat has been demonstrated to be a stimulus to growth of the mammary gland, using whole-mount observations (Roth and Roseblatt, 1967, 1968) and DNA determinations (McMurtry and Anderson, 1971). Pregnant rats were fitted with a collar to prevent self-licking; mammary glands were significantly less developed in these animals than in normal animals at the end of pregnancy. It was suggested that the afferent neural link between the mammary gland and hypothalamus was activated by licking with the result that prolactin secretion was increased. However, since mammary glands of hypophysectomized pregnant rats developed almost as well as normal pregnant rats (Anderson and Turner, 1969), it was concluded that the licking stimulus was a direct one. Perhaps it improved circulation of blood to the mammary apparatus and thereby enabled the hormones to stimulate greater growth of tissue.

C. Drugs

Little is known concerning the effect of drugs directly on mammary gland epithelia. Certain materials are used to suppress cellular actions in general. Colchicine and podophyllin are mitotic inhibitors and as such would be expected to slow the rate of mammary growth (Dilley, 1971).

Actinomycin D is used to block replication of messenger RNA at the DNA template. Puromycin suppresses protein synthesis at the ribosomal RNA level.

For the mammotropic effects of drugs such as phenothiazine derivatives, reserpine derivatives, and butyrophenones, which act primarily by affecting prolactin secretion via the hypothalamus, the reader is referred to Sulman (1970).

REFERENCES

Ahren, K., and Jacobsohn, D. (1956). *Acta Physiol. Scand.* **37**, 190.
Ahren, K., and Jacobsohn, D. (1957). *Acta Physiol. Scand.* **40**, 254.
Ahren, K., Arvill, A., and Hjalmarson, A. (1963). *Acta Endocrinol.* **42**, 601.
Allen, E., and Doisy, E. A. (1923). *J. Amer. Med. Ass.* **81**, 819.
Allen, E., Francis, B. F., Robertson, L. L., Colgate, C. E., Johnston, C. G., Doisy, E. A., Kountz, W. B., and Gibson, H. V. (1924). *Amer. J. Anat.* **34**, 133.
Ancel, P., and Bouin, P. (1911). *J. Physiol. Pathol. Gen.* **13**, 31.
Anderson, R. R., and Turner, C. W. (1962). *Proc. Soc. Exp. Biol. Med.* **109**, 85.
Anderson, R. R., and Turner, C. W. (1963). *Proc. Soc. Exp. Biol. Med.* **113**, 308.
Anderson, R. R., and Turner, C. W. (1968). *Proc. Soc. Exp. Biol. Med.* **128**, 210.
Anderson, R. R., and Turner, C. W. (1969). *J. Anim. Sci.* **29**, 183.
Anderson, R. R., Brookreson, A. D., and Turner, C. W. (1961). *Proc. Soc. Exp. Biol. Med.* **106**, 567.
Averill, S. C., Ray, E. W., and Lyons, W. R. (1950). *Proc. Soc. Exp. Biol. Med.* **75**, 3.
Baker, F. D., and Kragt, C. L. (1969). *Endocrinology* **85**, 522.
Baldwin, R. L. (1966). *J. Dairy Sci.* **49**, 1533.
Balinsky, B. I. (1952). *Trans. Roy. Soc. (Edinburgh)* **62**, 1.
Barraclough, C. A. (1961). *Endocrinology* **68**, 62.
Benson, G. K., Cowie, A. T., Cox, C. P., and Goldzveig, S. A. (1957). *J. Endocrinol.* **15**, 126.
Bern, H. A., Brown, D., and Ingraham, R. L. (1968). *J. Nat. Cancer Inst.* **40**, 1267.
Boivin, A., Vendrely, R., and Vendrely, C. (1948). *C. R. Acad. Sci. Paris* **226**, 1061.
Bradbury, J. T. (1932). *Proc. Soc. Exp. Biol. Med.* **30**, 212.
Brookreson, A. D., and Turner, C. W. (1959). *Proc. Soc. Exp. Biol. Med.* **102**, 744.
Caruolo, E. V., and Mochrie, R. D. (1967). *J. Dairy Sci.* **50**, 225.
Ceriani, R. L. (1970a). *Develop. Biol.* **21**, 506.
Ceriani, R. L. (1970b). *Develop. Biol.* **21**, 530.
Ceriani, R., Pitelka, D. R., Bern, H. A., and Colley, V. B. (1970). *J. Exp. Zool.* **174**, 79.
Cerruti, R. A., and Lyons, W. R. (1960). *Endocrinology* **67**, 884.
Chatterton, R. J., Jr., Chatterton, A. J., and Hellman, L. (1969). *Endocrinology* **85**, 16.
Clifton, K. H., and Furth, J. (1960). *Endocrinology* **66**, 893.
Cohen, R. M., and Gala, R. (1969). *Proc. Soc. Exp. Biol. Med.* **132**, 683.
Cole, H. A. (1933). *Proc. Roy. Soc. London B* **114**, 136.
Cowie, A. T. (1949). *J. Endocrinol.* **6**, 145.

Cowie, A. T., and Folley, S. J. (1947). *Endocrinology* **40**, 274.
Cupceancu, B., and Neumann, F. (1969). *Endokrinologie* **54**, 423.
Cupceancu, B., Neumann, F., and Ulloa, A. (1969). *J. Endocrinol.* **44**, 475.
Damm, H. C., Miller, W. R., and Turner, C. W. (1961). *Proc. Soc. Exp. Biol. Med.* **107**, 989.
Davidson, J. N., and Leslie, L. (1950). *Nature (London)* **165**, 49.
de Aberle, S. B. (1929). *Anat. Rec.* **42**, 1.
Denamur, R. (1961). *Ann. Endocrinol.* **22**, 768.
Deshpande, N., Bulbrook, R. D., and Ellis, F. G. (1963). *J. Endocrinol.* **25**, 555.
Desjardins, C., Paape, M. J., and Tucker, H. A. (1968). *Endocrinology* **83**, 907.
Dilley, W. G. (1971). *J. Endocrinol.* **50**, 501.
Donovan, B. T., and Jacobsohn, D. (1960a). *Acta Endocrinol.* **33**, 197.
Donovan, B. T., and Jacobsohn, D. (1960b). *Acta Endocrinol.* **33**, 214.
El-Darwish, I., and Rivera, E. M. (1970). *J. Exp. Zool.* **173**, 285.
Elger, W., and Neumann, F. (1966). *Proc. Soc. Exp. Biol. Med.* **123**, 637.
Elias, J. J. (1959). *Proc. Soc. Exp. Biol. Med.* **101**, 500.
Elias, J. J. (1962). *Exp. Cell Res.* **27**, 601.
Elliott, J. R., and Turner, C. W. (1954). *Endocrinology* **54**, 284.
Emmerson, M. A. (1941). *Vet. Ext. Quart. (School of Vet. Med., Univ. of Penn.)* **41**, 1.
Etienne, M. (1960). *Ann. Endocrinol.* **21**, 331.
Fajer, A. B., and Barraclough, C. A. (1967). *Endocrinology* **81**, 617.
Feldman, J. D. (1961). *Lab. Invest.* **10**, 238.
Ferreri, L. F., and Griffith, D. E. (1969). *Proc. Soc. Exp. Biol. Med.* **130**, 1216.
Florini, J. R., Tonelli, G., Breuer, C. B., Coppola, J., Ringler, I., and Bell, P. H. (1966). *Endocrinology* **79**, 692.
Flux, D. S. (1954). *J. Endocrinol.* **11**, 223.
Forsberg, J. G., and Jacobsohn, I. (1971). *Proc. Soc. Exp. Biol. Med.* **138**, 654.
Frank, R. T., and Rosenbloom, I. (1915). *Surg. Gynecol. Obstet.* **21**, 646.
Friedman, R. C., and Reichlin, S. (1965). *Endocrinology* **76**, 787.
Gardner, W. U., and Allen, E. (1942). *Anat. Rec.* **83**, 75.
Gardner, W. U., and Strong, L. C. (1935). *Amer. J. Cancer* **25**, 282.
Glascock, R. F., and Hoeckstra, W. G. (1959). *Biochem. J.* **72**, 673.
Gomez, E. T., and Turner, C. W. (1937). *Mo. Agr. Exp. Sta. Res. Bull.* **259**.
Gowen, J. W., and Tobey, E. R. (1927). *J. Gen. Physiol.* **10**, 949.
Greenbaum, A. L., and Slater, T. F. (1957). *Biochem. J.* **66**, 155.
Greenhalgh, J. F. D., and Gardner, K. E. (1958). *J. Dairy Sci.* **41**, 822.
Griffith, D. R., and Turner, C. W. (1957). *Proc. Soc. Exp. Biol. Med.* **95**, 347.
Griffith, D. R., and Turner, C. W. (1959). *Proc. Soc. Exp. Biol. Med.* **102**, 619.
Griffith, D. R., and Turner, C. W. (1961a). *Proc. Soc. Exp. Biol. Med.* **106**, 448.
Griffith, D. R., and Turner, C. W. (1961b). *Proc. Soc. Exp. Biol. Med.* **106**, 873.
Griffith, D. R., and Turner, C. W. (1963). *Proc. Soc. Exp. Biol. Med.* **112**, 424.
Griffith, D. R., Williams, R., and Turner, C. W. (1963). *Proc. Soc. Exp. Biol. Med.* **113**, 401.
Grossie, J., and Turner, C. W. (1962). *Proc. Soc. Exp. Biol. Med.* **110**, 631.
Hacker, R. R. (1970). Ph.D. dissertation, Purdue Univ., Lafayette, Indiana.
Hahn, D. W. (1967). Ph.D. thesis, Univ. of Missouri, Columbia, Missouri.
Hahn, D. W., and Turner, C. W. (1966). *Proc. Soc. Exp. Biol. Med.* **122**, 183.
Hahn, D. W., and Turner, C. W. (1967). *Proc. Soc. Exp. Biol. Med.* **126**, 476.

Hammond, J. (1927). "The Physiology of Reproduction in the Cow." Cambridge Univ. Press, London and New York.

Hammond, J., and Marshall, F. H. A. (1930). *Proc. Roy Soc. B* **105**, 607.

Hardy, M. H. (1950). *J. Anat.* **84**, 388.

Hashimoto, I., Henricks, D. M., Anderson, L. L., and Melampy, R. M. (1968). *Endocrinology* **82**, 333.

Hoshino, K. (1965). *Endocrinology* **76**, 789.

Ichinose, R. R., and Nandi, S. (1966). *J. Endocrinol.* **35**, 331.

Jacobsohn, D. (1960). *Acta Endocrinol.* **35**, 107.

Jacobsohn, D. (1961). In "Milk: The Mammary Gland and Its Secretion" (S. K. Kon and A. T. Cowie, eds.), Vol. I, pp. 127–160. Academic Press, New York.

Jacobsohn, D. (1962a). *Acta Endocrinol.* **41**, 88.

Jacobsohn, D. (1962b). *Acta Endocrinol.* **41**, 287.

Josimovich, J. B., and MacLaren, J. A. (1962). *Endocrinology* **71**, 209.

Josimovich, J. B., Atwood, B. L., and Goss, D. A. (1963). *Endocrinology* **73**, 410.

Kahn, R. H., and Baker, B. L. (1964). *Endocrinology* **75**, 818.

Kahn, R. H., Baker, B. L., and Zanotti, D. B. (1965). *Endocrinology* **77**, 162.

Kaplan, S. L., and Grumbach, M. M. (1964). *J. Clin. Endocrinol. Metab.* **24**, 80.

Kinzey, W. G. (1968). *Endocrinology* **82**, 266.

Kirkham, W. R., and Turner, C. W. (1953). *Proc. Soc. Exp. Biol. Med.* **83**, 123.

Kirkham, W. R., and Turner, C. W. (1954). *Proc. Soc. Exp. Biol. Med.* **87**, 139.

Knauer, E. (1900). *Arch. Gynäk* **60**, 322.

Kohmoto, K., and Bern, H. A. (1970). *J. Endocrinol.* **48**, 99.

Kumaresan, P., and Turner, C. W. (1965a). *J. Dairy Sci.* **48**, 592.

Kumaresan, P., and Turner, C. W. (1965b). *J. Dairy Sci.* **48**, 1378.

Kumaresan, P., and Turner, C. W. (1966a). *Endocrinology* **79**, 443.

Kumaresan, P., and Turner, C. W. (1966b). *Endocrinology* **78**, 396.

Kumaresan, P., and Turner, C. W. (1968). *Proc. Soc. Exp. Biol. Med.* **129**, 955.

Kumaresan, P., Anderson, R. R., and Turner, C. W. (1967). *Endocrinology* **81**, 658.

Lasfargues, E. Y., and Murray, M. R. (1959). *Develop. Biol.* **1**, 413.

Lawson, E. C. M., and Pearlman, W. H. (1964). *J. Biol. Chem.* **239**, 3226.

Leonard, S. L. (1945). *Anat. Rec.* **91**, 65.

Lewis, A. A., and Turner, C. W. (1939). *Mo. Agr. Sta. Res. Bull.* **310**.

Lewis, A. A., Turner, C. W., and Gomez, E. T. (1939). *Endocrinology* **24**, 157.

Li, C. H., Dixon, J. S., and Chung, D. (1971). *Science* **173**, 56.

Linkie, D. M., and Niswender, G. D. (1971). *Biol. Reprod.* **5**, 94.

Linzell, J. L. (1959). *Physiol. Rev.* **39**, 534.

Linzell, J. L. (1966). *J. Dairy Sci.* **49**, 307.

Loeb, L., and Hesselberg, C. (1917). *J. Exp. Med.* **25**, 285.

Loeb, L., and Hesselberg, C. (1917). *J. Exp. Med.* **25**, 305.

Long, J. A., and Evans, H. M. (1922). *Memoirs Univ. Calif.* **6**, 1.

Lyons, W. R. (1944). *Anat. Rec.* **88**, 446.

Lyons, W. R. (1951). *Colloq. Int. Cent. Nat. Rech. Sci.* **32**, 29.

Lyons, W. R. (1969). In "Lactogenesis: The Initiation of Milk Secretion at Parturition" (M. Reynolds and S. J. Folley, eds.), pp. 223–228. Univ. of Pennsylvania Press, Philadelphia, Pennsylvania.

Lyons, W. R., and McGinty, D. A. (1941). *Proc. Soc. Exp. Biol. Med.* **48**, 83.

Lyons, W. R., Li, C. H., and Johnson, R. E. (1958). *Recent Progr. Hormone Res.* **14**, 219.

Macdonald, G. J., and Reece, R. P. (1960). *J. Dairy Sci.* **43**, 1658.

Macdonald, G. J., and Reece, R. P. (1962). *Proc. Soc. Exp. Biol. Med.* **110**, 647.
MacLeod, R. M., Allen, M. S., and Hollander, V. P. (1964). *Endocrinology* **75**, 249.
Matthews, C. A., Swett, W. W., and Fohrman, M. H. (1949). *U.S.D.A. Tech. Bull.* **989**.
Matthies, D. L. (1967). *Anat. Rec.* **159**, 55.
Mayer, G., and Klein, M. (1961). In "Milk: The Mammary Gland and Its Secretion" (S.K. Kon and A. T. Cowie, eds.), Vol. I, pp. 47–126. Academic Press, New York.
McMurtry, J. P., and Anderson, R. R. (1971). *Proc. Soc. Exp. Biol. Med.* **137**, 354.
Meites, J. (1965). *Endocrinology* **76**, 1220.
Meites, J., and Fiel, N. J. (1965). *Endocrinology* **77**, 455.
Meites, J., and Kragt, C. L. (1964). *Endocrinology* **75**, 565.
Meites, J., and Kragt, C. L. (1965). *Endocrinology* **75**, 565.
Mirsky, A. E., and Ris, H. (1949). *Nature (London)* **163**, 666.
Mixner, J. P., and Turner, C. W. (1943). *Mo. Agr. Exp. Sta. Res. Bull.* **378**.
Mixner, J. P., Lewis, A. A., and Turner, C. W. (1940). *Endocrinology* **27**, 888.
Moon, R. C. (1961). *Amer. J. Physiol.* **201**, 259.
Moon, R. C., and Turner, C. W. (1960). *Proc. Soc. Exp. Biol. Med.* **103**, 149.
Moon, R. C., Griffith, D. R., and Turner, C. W. (1959). *Proc. Soc. Exp. Biol. Med.* **101**, 788.
Munford, R. E. (1963). *J. Endocrinol.* **28**, 35.
Munford, R. E. (1964). *Dairy Sci. Abstr.* **26**, 293.
Myers, J. A. (1917). *Anat. Rec.* **13**, 205.
Nagasawa, H., Iwahashi, H., Kuretani, K., and Fujimoto, M. (1966). *Endocrinol. Japon.* **13**, 344.
Nagasawa, H., Iwahashi, H., Kanzawa, F., Fujimoto, M., and Kuretani, K. (1967). *Endocrinol. Japon.* **14**, 23.
Nelson, W. L., Heytler, P. G., and Ciaccio, E. I. (1962). *Proc. Soc. Exp. Biol. Med.* **109**, 373.
Neumann, F., and Elger, W. (1966). *J. Endocrinol.* **36**, 347.
Neumann, F., Elger, W., and von Berswordt-Wallrabe, R. (1966). *J. Endocrinol.* **36**, 353.
Newton, W. H., and Beck, N. (1939). *J. Endocrinol.* **1**, 65.
Ott, I., and Scott, J. C. (1910). *Proc. Soc. Exp. Biol. Med.* **8**, 48.
Panda, J. N., and Turner, C. W. (1966). *Proc. Soc. Exp. Biol. Med.* **121**, 803.
Pencharz, R. I., and Long, J. A. (1933). *Amer. J. Anat.* **53**, 117.
Posner, M., Gartland, W. J., Clark, J. L., Sato, G., and Hirsch, C. A. (1970). *Develop. Biol. Suppl.* **4**, 114.
Puca, G. A., and Bresciani, F. (1969). *Endocrinology* **85**, 1.
Ray, E. W., Averill, S. C., Lyons, W. R., and Johnson, R. E. (1955). *Endocrinology* **56**, 359.
Raynaud, A. (1949). *Ann. Endocrinol.* **10**, 54.
Rein, G. (1881). *Arch. Milkr. Anat.* **20**, 431.
Richardson, K. C. (1953). *J. Endocrinol.* **9**, 170.
Rivera, E. M. (1964). *Endocrinology* **74**, 853.
Rivera, E. M., and Bern, H. A. (1961). *Endocrinology* **69**, 340.
Roth, L. L., and Rosenblatt, J. S. (1967). *J. Comp. Physiol. Psychol.* **63**, 397.
Roth, L. L., and Rosenblatt, J. S. (1968). *J. Endocrinol.* **42**, 363.
Sander, S. (1968a). *Acta Endocrinol.* **58**, 49.
Sander, S. (1968b). *Acta Endocrinol.* **59**, 235.

Sander, S., and Attramadal, A. (1968). *Acta Endocrinol.* **58**, 235.

Scharf, G., and Lyons, W. R. (1941). *Proc Soc. Exp. Biol. Med.* **48**, 86.

Schmidt, G. H., and Moger, W. H. (1967). *Endocrinology* **81**, 14.

Schmidt, G. H., Chatterton, R. T., Jr., and Hansel, W. (1964). *J. Dairy Sci.* **47**, 74.

Sekhri, K. K., and Faulkin, L. J., Jr. (1970). *In* "The Beagle as an Experimental Dog" (A. C. Andersen, ed.), pp. 327–349. Iowa State Univ. Press, Ames, Iowa.

Selye, H., Collip, J. B., and Thomson, D. L. (1933). *Proc. Soc. Exp. Biol. Med.* **31**, 82.

Shimizu, H. (1957). *Tohoku J. Agr. Res.* **7**, 339.

Singh, D. V., and Bern, H. A. (1969). *J. Endocrinol.* **45**, 579.

Singh, D. V., DeOme, K. B., and Bern, H. A. (1970). *J. Nat. Cancer Inst.* **45**, 657.

Sinha, Y. N., and Tucker, H. A. (1966). *Amer. J. Physiol.* **210**, 601.

Sinha, Y. N., and Tucker, H. A. (1969a). *Proc. Soc. Exp. Biol. Med.* **131**, 908.

Sinha, Y. N., and Tucker, H. A. (1969b). *J. Dairy Sci.* **52**, 507.

Sinha, Y. N., Anderson, R. R., and Turner, C. W. (1970). *Biol. Reprod.* **2**, 185.

Simpson, A. A., and Schmidt, G. H. (1970). *Proc. Soc. Exp. Biol. Med.* **133**, 897.

Smith, P. E. (1926). *Anat. Rec.* **32**, 221.

Smith, T. C., and Richterich, B. (1958). *Arch. Biochem. Biophys.* **74**, 398.

Sod-Moriah, U. A., and Schmidt, G. H. (1968). *Exp. Cell Res.* **49**, 584.

Srivastava, L. S., and Turner, C. W. (1966a). *Endocrinology* **79**, 650.

Srivastava, L. S., and Turner, C. W. (1966b). *J. Dairy Sci.* **49**, 1050.

Stockdale, F. E., and Topper, Y. J. (1966a). *Proc. Nat. Acad. Sci.* **56**, 1283.

Stockdale, F. E., and Topper, Y. J. (1966b). *Develop. Biol.* **13**, 266.

Stricker, P., and Grueter, F. (1928). *C. R. Soc. Biol.* **T99**, 1978.

Stumpf, W. E. (1969). *Endocrinology* **85**, 31.

Sud, S. C., Tucker, H. A., and Meites, J. (1968). *J. Dairy Sci.* **51**, 210.

Sulman, F. G. (1970). "Hypothalamic Control of Lactation." Springer-Verlag, New York.

Sutter, N. (1921). *Anat. Rec.* **21**, 59.

Swanson, E. W., Pardue, F. E., and Longmire, D. B. (1967). *J. Dairy Sci.* **50**, 1288.

Swett, W. W. (1927). *J. Dairy Sci.* **10**, 1.

Sykes, J. F., Wrenn, T. R., and Hall, S. R. (1948). *J. Nutr.* **35**, 467.

Talwalker, P. K., and Meites, J. (1961). *Proc. Soc. Exp. Biol. Med.* **107**, 880.

Talwalker, P. K., and Meites, J. (1964). *Proc. Soc. Exp. Biol. Med.* **117**, 121.

Thomas, J. B. (1968). "Introduction to Human Embryology." Lea and Febiger, Philadelphia, Pennsylvania.

Topper, Y. J. (1968). *Trans. N. Y. Acad. Sci.* **30**, 869.

Topper, Y. J., Friedberg, S. H., and Oka, T. (1970). *Develop. Biol. Suppl.* **4**, 101.

Trentin, J. J., Devita, J., and Gardner, W. U. (1952). *Anat. Rec.* **113**, 163.

Tucker, H. A., and Reece, R. P. (1962). *Proc. Soc. Exp. Biol. Med.* **111**, 639.

Tucker, H. A., and Reece, R. P. (1963a). *Proc. Soc. Exp. Biol. Med.* **112**, 370.

Tucker, H. A., and Reece, R. P. (1963b). *Proc. Soc. Exp. Biol. Med.* **112**, 409.

Turkington, R. W., and Topper, Y. J. (1966). *Endocrinology* **79**, 175.

Turkington, R. W., and Topper, Y. J. (1967). *Endocrinology* **80**, 329.

Turkington, R. W., Juergens, W. G., and Topper, Y. J. (1967). *Endocrinology* **80**, 1139.

Turner, C. W. (1930). *Mo. Agr. Exp. Sta. Res. Bull.* **140**.

Turner, C. W. (1931). *Mo. Agr. Exp. Sta. Res. Bull.* **160**.

Turner, C. W. (1932). *In* "Sex and Internal Secretion" (E. Allen, ed.), pp. 544–583. Williams and Wilkins, Baltimore, Maryland.

Turner, C. W. (1934). *Mo. Agr. Exp. Sta. Res. Bull.* **211.**

Turner, C. W. (1939). *In* "Sex and Internal Secretions" (E. Allen, ed.), 2nd Ed., pp. 740–803. Williams and Wilkins, Baltimore, Maryland.

Turner, C. W. (1952). "The Mammary Gland. I. The Anatomy of the Udder of Cattle and Domestic Animals." Lucas Bros. Publ., Columbia, Missouri.

Turner, C. W. (1959). *Mo. Agr. Exp. Sta. Res. Bull.* **697.**

Turner, C. W. (1970). *Mo. Agr. Exp. Sta. Res. Bull.* **977.**

Turner, C. W., and deMoss, W. R. (1934). *Mo. Agr. Exp. Sta. Res. Bull.* **207.**

Turner, C. W., and Frank, A. H. (1930). *Mo. Agr. Exp. Sta. Res. Bull.* **145.**

Turner, C. W., and Gardner, W. U. (1931). *Mo. Agr. Exp. Sta. Res. Bull.* **158.**

Turner, C. W., and Gomez, E. T. (1933a). *Mo. Agr. Exp. Sta. Res. Bull.* **182.**

Turner, C. W., and Gomez, E. T. (1933b). *Mo. Agr. Exp. Sta. Res. Bull.* **194.**

Turner, C. W., and Gomez, E. T. (1934). *Mo. Agr. Exp. Sta. Res. Bull.* **207.**

Turner, C. W., and Schultze, A. B. (1931). *Mo. Agr. Exp. Sta. Res. Bull.* **157.**

Turner, C. W., Williams, R., and Hindery, G. A. (1963). *J. Dairy Sci.* **46,** 1390.

van Tienhoven, A. (1968). *In* "Reproductive Physiology of Vertebrates," pp. 12–14. Saunders, Philadelphia, Pennsylvania.

von Berswordt-Wallrabe, R., and Turner, C. W. (1960a). *Proc. Soc. Exp. Biol. Med.* **103,** 536.

von Berswordt-Wallrabe, R., and Turner, C. W. (1960b). *Proc. Soc. Exp. Biol. Med.* **104,** 599.

Voytovich, A. E., and Topper, Y. J. (1967). *Science* **158,** 1326.

Wada, H., and Turner, C. W. (1959a). *J. Dairy Sci.* **42,** 1198.

Wada, H., and Turner, C. W. (1959b). *Proc. Soc. Exp. Biol. Med.* **101,** 707.

Wada, H., and Turner, C. W. (1959c). *Proc. Soc. Exp. Biol. Med.* **102,** 568.

Wahl, H. M. (1915). *Amer. J. Anat.* **18,** 515.

Weatherford, H. L. (1929). *Amer. J. Anat.* **44,** 199.

Williams, R., and Turner, C. W. (1961). *J. Dairy Sci.* **44,** 524.

Williams, W. F., Turner, G. D., and Lynch, J. (1963). *J. Dairy Sci.* **46,** 642.

Wrenn, T. R., Bitman, J., de Lauder, W. R., and Mench, M. L. (1966). *J. Dairy Sci.* **49,** 183–187.

Yamamoto, H., and Turner, C. W. (1956). *Proc. Soc. Exp. Biol. Med.* **92,** 130.

Yanai, R., and Nagasawa, H. (1971). *J. Dairy Sci.* **54,** 906.

PART II

DEVELOPMENT AND MAINTENANCE OF LACTOGENESIS

CHAPTER THREE

Mammary Blood Flow and Methods of Identifying and Measuring Precursors of Milk

J. L. Linzell

I. Introduction 143
 A. Principles 144
 B. History of Attempts to Measure Mammary Substrate
   Uptake 146
II. Anatomy of Mammary Blood Vessels, Lymphatics, and
   Nerves 154
 A. Large Blood Vessels 155
 B. Small Blood Vessels 155
 C. Vascular Shunts 158
 D. Teat Blood Vessels 161
 E. Mammary Lymphatics 161
 F. Mammary Vasomotor Nerves 163
III. Mammary Blood Flow 165
 A. Methods of Measuring Mammary Blood Flow 165
 B. Rate of Mammary Blood Flow 174
 C. Factors Controlling Mammary Blood Flow 181
IV. Mammary Lymph Flow 184
V. Milk Precursors 186
 A. Methods of Identification 186
 B. Identified Precursors 204
 C. Mechanism of Mammary Uptake 218
 D. Fasting Metabolism 219
VI. Summary and Recommendations 219
 References 220

I. INTRODUCTION

A major reason for being interested in the mammary glands is the wish to know how milk is made, and the starting point in that investigation is

143

to ask, From what is it made? At present three methods are available. First, a labeled compound may be given, and it is determined whether a labeled product is found in milk. Second, the requirements of mammary tissue are studied *in vitro* using homogenates, isolated cells, slices, organ culture or perfusion of whole glands. Third, arterial and mammary venous samples are taken from intact animals to see whether significant quantities of the possible precursor are in fact taken up by the normal mammary tissue.

Ideally, all methods should be used for alone each can give misleading data. This chapter tries to summarize the advantages and disadvantages of each method of approach and will try to indicate where technical errors have led to inadequate or misleading data. Many previous studies, ostensibly quantitative in nature, have done little more than show whether a particular substance should or should not be considered as a possible milk precursor. Thus, only the major precursors are identified, and much more remains to be learned about the uptake of minor components and hormones and the variability in time in the uptake of all substances. I will try to explain and excuse past failures and inadequacies and, if I am thorough, should indicate to the reader where, if she or he is interested, new attempts may be made. This may be worthwhile because two observations make me think that there may still be unrecognized milk precursors: (1) Isolated perfused glands of goats, given all the known substrates and hormones believed to be necessary for lactation, produce about half the quantity of milk that they were making in the animal (Hardwick and Linzell, 1960; Linzell *et al.*, 1972b). (2) It is not possible to fully restore to normal the halved milk yield produced by fasting goats for 24 hours, when the same substrates are infused intravenously (Linzell, 1967b).

A. Principles

The majority of attempts to measure the uptake of milk precursors have been made in intact, usually conscious animals (cows and goats). Most of the difficulties and errors of this method will be appreciated by recounting the history of the attempts, but first the principles involved must be clearly understood. The earliest investigators appreciated that all the precursors used by the tissue to synthesize milk must come ultimately from the blood and it is easy to work out the following simple equations.

Organ uptake = quantity arriving in arterial blood − quantity leaving in
venous blood   (1)

Organ uptake = organ blood flow × blood arteriovenous difference in concentration (2)
Organ uptake = milk output − (lymph output and tissue storage) (3)

If (2) and (3) are measured simultaneously for as many different substances as possible we should be in a fair position to reason from what
milk is made. These considerations were understood 60 years ago and
yet we still do not have all the information to answer the question, From
what is milk made? Why not? Not, I think, because no one was interested, but because these basic things are so difficult to measure and
study. In spite of warnings from previous reviewers it is still not always
appreciated that this often is a sphere of study where a casual pass at the
subject with inadequate methods is not good enough; it must be done
properly or not at all and to do it properly one must pay great attention
to detail, because there are traps for the unwary.

Equations (1), (2), and (3) are a statement of the principle of Fick
(1870), who realized that you could calculate the output of blood from
the heart from a knowledge of the total O_2 consumption or CO_2 output
of an animal, and the simultaneously measured arteriovenous difference
(a − v) of O_2 and CO_2 across the lungs, through which all the blood from
the heart passes. Knowing a − v you can easily calculate how much
blood has to pass through the lungs to account for the total gas absorbed
or given up. Actual measurements were not made until many years later,
but in several forms the Fick principle is widely used, not only for cardiac
output, but to measure blood flow through organs and tissues, and, as in
the present case, to measure their metabolism. It is of great importance
in physiology, but unfortunately the principle, which is so simple to state,
bristles with difficulties to apply. Several authors have given warnings of
the snags but Zierler (1961) has treated the subject mathematically and
shown that the Fick principle can only be applied to measure tissue
metabolism when: (1) the blood flow is constant, (2) the tissue metabolism is constant, (3) the arterial concentration of substrates is constant,
and (4) the venous blood sample is representative of that of the whole
tissue.

He also showed that if the flow changes, then the status quo is reestablished as soon as it has remained constant for a time equal to the longest
transit time of a particle through the organ. He recommended taking two
pairs of a − v samples at an interval not longer than the mean transit
time (volume of distribution divided by the blood flow). Furthermore,
he stated that to compare the a − v of two substances in a single pair of
samples it is necessary to know that the distribution of their transit times
is the same.

A consideration sometimes overlooked is that the flow and arterio-venous measurements must correspond, i.e., if blood flow is measured, a − v determinations must be made on blood, not on plasma. If the volume of distribution in blood of the substance under consideration is known, a correction may be applied from measurement of the hematocrit. Unless a substance is only distributed in plasma, it is usually best to analyze whole blood.

A further potential complication in the case of the lactating mammary gland is that water is withdrawn from the blood to be transferred into milk, and this will raise slightly the concentration of substances in the venous blood and lead to an underestimate of uptake.

B. History of Attempts to Measure Mammary Substrate Uptake

Kaufmann and Magne (1906) in France were the first to measure the uptake of a precursor by the mammary glands. This was done in the conscious cow and was highly successful. They reported that blood taken from the mammary vein (milk vein) had significantly less glucose than jugular blood, but only during lactation, and that the jugular-mammary vein difference was related to the level of milk production. Their value of 14–18 mg/100 ml plasma for cows giving 12 liters of milk per day is remarkably accurate and they correctly deduced that glucose is the precursor of lactose. They also appreciated that these two veins can be punctured without anesthesia and without grossly disturbing the animal, and must have appreciated that stress can vitiate measurements, due to disturbing the steady-state conditions demanded for the Fick principle.

At this early date the importance of glucose for lactose synthesis and the nature of milk precursors were demonstrated in heroic experiments by Foa. First he showed that two glands removed from a lactating goat gave, over 7 hours, similar quantities of milk of identical composition, when one gland was joined by its main artery and vein to the carotid artery and jugular vein of another lactating goat and the other gland was similarly joined to a virgin goat (Foa, 1908a). This important experiment was not repeated until Linzell (1963b) transplanted two lactating glands by vascular anastomosis to the necks of two other goats, one a lactating female and the other a castrated male goat and got similar yields of milk from the two glands, which were 80% of previous over the first 24 hours. This suggests that there is nothing special circulating in the blood during lactation, and foreshadowed the much later discovery that only very simple precursors are required by the mammary glands to make milk

Foa (1908b) also showed that glucose is the main sugar in the blood of lactating, as well as in nonlactating, rabbits and dogs and demonstrated that in a lactating goat there was less glucose in mammary venous blood than in carotid blood. Then Foa (1912) perfused in isolation sheep and goat glands with Ringer solution and made further important discoveries. Glucose was found to be essential in the perfusate for lactose formation but galactose had no effect. In the most successful perfusions where defibrinated blood was included in the perfusate to prevent edema, the milk formed contained lactose, casein, and fat; glucose was removed from the perfusate by the tissue and when more was added, lactose concentration in the milk rose. He also observed fat in the watery "milk" produced when olive oil, triolein, oleic, and linoleic acids were added to the Ringer-only perfusate, and the iodine number was lower than that in the perfusate, suggesting alteration in lipid composition by the tissue. A few years later Cary (1920) reported that α-amino-N concentration was similar in mammary vein and jugular vein blood of nonlactating cows, but 16–34% lower in mammary vein blood of lactating cows. He estimated that amino acid uptake was sufficient to account for the milk protein secreted.

Thus, 50 years ago there was good evidence that glucose is the precursor of lactose and suggestive evidence that plasma fatty acids and amino acids form milk fat and protein respectively and that glucose could support the secretion of "normal" milk. Precursor uptake had been measured in conscious animals, udders had been perfused, and within a few years mammary glands had been successfully grown in organ culture (Maximow, 1925).

After this excellent start, the Kaufmann-Magne technique was enthusiastically used by Meigs and his colleagues in America, with disastrous results. Kaufmann and Magne carefully said that their results showed that the udder removed more glucose from arterial blood than the head did, but Meigs assumed that they had shown that jugular blood is identical to arterial blood as far as the udder is concerned and, unfortunately, this is not true for all substrates. Meigs et al. (1919) reported that mammary vein blood in cows had less phospholipid than jugular blood and incorrectly deduced that phospholipid is the main precursor of milk fat (Meigs, 1922). How did this error arise?

Blackwood and Stirling (1932) reported that jugular blood is not equivalent to arterial blood in cows. They obtained arterial blood from the radial artery and compared its composition with that of jugular and mammary vein blood and found that the hematocrit and the iron concentration were significantly higher in jugular blood. Therefore, they concluded that the jugular — mammary vein difference of phospholipid detected by Meigs *et al.* was due not to mammary uptake, but due to removal of water by the salivary glands during passage through the head. They pointed out that cows can produce 60 liters of saliva a day and thought that this would lead to the 3–10% increase in hematocrit they measured in jugular blood as compared with arterial blood. However, I think that this is wrong! Sixty liters/day is 42 ml/minute, and to raise the hematocrit 3–10% would imply a head blood flow of only 420–1400 ml/minute, an unlikely range, because head blood flow in goats is at least 400 ml/minute (Baldwin and Bell, 1963; Linzell, 1965), and in cows would be expected to be 5–10 times this. Later Folley and Peskett (1934) showed that marked hemo-concentration occurs in the jugular vein just after releasing the choke rope that is frequently used to raise the vein to facilitate venepuncture in cows. However, the important point is that Blackwood (1934) showed that when arterial blood is compared with mammary blood there is no a — v of phospholipids, which cannot therefore be a significant precursor of milk fat. This is now believed to be correct. Also, Blackwood (1932) reported an a — v of amino acids and correctly concluded that these are precursors of milk protein.

As with arteriovenous measurements and udder perfusion the first use of tissue slices was quite successful. Grant (1935) demonstrated that lactating guinea pig tissue could form lactose from glucose but not from galactose, mannose, and fructose, and that no more lactose was formed from glucose + galactose than from glucose alone (Grant, 1936). However, this useful technique was not exploited until nearly 10 years later (Folley and French, 1948) when a whole series of productive investigations ensued (see Folley, 1956).

At this stage a more thorough study of the technique of arteriovenous sampling in cows was made by Graham *et al.* (1936a), who devised the technique of puncturing the internal iliac artery per rectum. They then made the important observation that stress and excitement could vitiate the results, leading to temporary cessation of uptake (no a — v) and/or to large differences in hematocrit between arterial and mammary venous blood that is not seen in undisturbed animals. This was amply confirmed by Shaw and Petersen (1939). Methods of detecting and avoiding stress are dealt with later, but, in spite of the care of early workers, following severe criticism of several reviewers (e.g., Folley, 1949) the method fell into disrepute.

Note that, up to this time, no one had attempted to measure blood flow through the mammary glands while taking a — v samples. Jung (1932a,b), who took no blood samples, measured mammary blood flow in conscious goats, but I believe his figures are too low. He inserted, under local anesthesia (ethyl chloride spray), a Ludwig stromuhr into the mammary artery of goats, held on their sides, and obtained figures of 60 and 62 ml/minute in two lactating goats giving 2.4 liters of milk per day. The mean figure from current work is 800 ml/minute (see later). Jung (1933) then wrote a theoretical paper explaining why mammary blood flow was so unexpectedly low, but later it was found that holding the goat on its side and inserting a flow cannula into the mammary vessel, under local anesthesia, lowered the blood flow (to 40% of previous in Linzell's 1960b experiments). I also suspect that the stromuhr further lowered flow in Jung's experiments, due to arterial spasm and/or release of serotonin (5-hydroxytryptamine), which is at a very high concentration in goat platelets and is released when blood comes into contact with the foreign surfaces. Serotonin is a powerful vasoconstrictor in the mammary gland (Hardwick and Linzell, 1960). Jung admitted that his blood flow figures might be lowered by stress but clearly did not think this would be lowered by twelvefold. It may be mentioned in passing that although mammary arterioles have very well-developed sympathetic constrictor nerve fibers (Linzell, 1950; Hebb and Linzell, 1970), and are very sensitive to adrenaline and noradrenaline (Hebb and Linzell, 1951), (Fig. 1) the mechanism by which mammary blood flow falls in response to stress has not been determined and this needs doing. However, it is known that both adrenaline (Ely and Petersen, 1941) and sympathetic nerve stimulation (Linzell, 1955) can so lower mammary flow as to partially block milk ejection by preventing oxytocin from reaching the mammary myoepithelial cells.

The work of Lintzel (1934) is important because, in addition to measuring a − v, he was the first to try to measure udder blood flow simultaneously in conscious lactating goats. He does not say so, but he employed the Fick principle to estimate blood flow, by dividing the measured output of products in milk by the a − v of the blood precursor, and he was remarkably successful. He found that milk fat output divided by a − v for plasma neutral lipid, gave a figure of 540 liters of blood passing through the udder for each liter of milk formed; milk protein output divided by a − v amino acid N gave 450, and milk phosphate output divided by a − v inorganic P gave 476. This is excellent, because the mean figure for blood flow and milk yield measured directly many years later is 493 ± 15 (Linzell, 1968) (Table I). Lintzel got a figure of only 256 for lactose output divided by glucose a − v but realized that this must be wrong because some glucose is oxidized, which at that time could not be allowed for quantitatively. In fact, Annison and Linzell

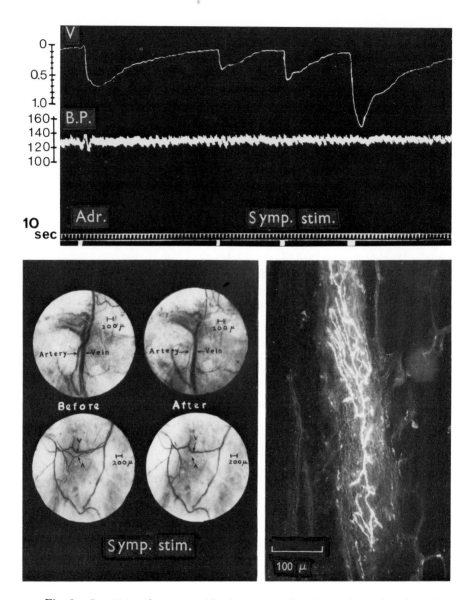

Fig. 1.   Sensitivity of mammary blood vessels to adrenaline and noradrenaline. *Top,*
Anesthetized dog. Volume record (V) of one mammary gland in a plethysmograph.
Adrenaline, 2 μg intravenously (A) causes vasoconstriction but has a negligible effect
on the blood pressure. Stimulation of the sympathetic nerves for 5, 10, and 15 seconds
has a similar effect. (From Linzell, 1950.) *Bottom, left,* Anesthetized cat. Effect of
stimulating the sympathetic nerves on the surface mammary blood vessels. Note

(1964) found that 16–34% of glucose taken up is oxidized, but this correction only brings Lintzel's figure to 383 and his a − v of glucose is still rather large. His arterial level of glucose was abnormally high at 71 mg/100 ml, possibly due to the stress of obtaining arterial blood by cardiac puncture. Nevertheless, Lintzel's work is a milestone in that he established a sound method of measuring mammary blood flow, which still has its uses.

Lintzel's work was soon repeated in the cow by Graham *et al.* (1936b) with similar results, and the Fick method became the established method of studying milk secretion in cows and was widely used for a decade. Workers using the method realized the importance of avoiding stress; this they did by speed and skill in sampling, by taking the venous sample first, and by measuring the Hb or hematocrit of their arterial and mammary venous samples to check that the animal was undisturbed. They also estimated blood flow, usually by measuring milk Ca, plasma Ca a − v, and applying the Fick principle; Ca, being a mineral, must be entirely passed from blood to milk.

However, progress was unimpressive and wrong data were obtained, which have been cataloged and critically reviewed by Barry (1964). The main difficulty was in measuring the small a − v of minor components. Far from being low as Jung claimed, mammary blood flow is relatively high during lactation, about 3–6 times that of the average of all tissues in goats. This meant that often workers were looking for small a − v on top of a high plasma level (e.g., in the case of Ca a fall from 10 to 9.73 mg/100 ml of plasma), often outside the accuracy of the analytic methods.

Graham (1937) made a valiant attempt to measure a − v and blood flow simultaneously in the goat using a direct method of flow estimation, a thermostromuhr on the milk vein. He removed one gland and tied off all veins except the milk vein and even exteriorized the carotid artery to be able to take arterial samples without stress. However, he found that the glucose uptake was only sufficient to account for half the lactose formed, whereas we now believe that enough glucose is taken up to account for all the lactose and glycerol in milk and for about half the CO_2 produced by the gland as well (Annison and Linzell, 1964). Since Graham's a − v was somewhat high, his blood flow must have been a serious underestimate. The reason, I think, is that he overlooked the fact

---

that the arterioles constrict completely but the venules are unaffected. (From Linzell, 1950.) *Bottom; right,* Arteriole in a rabbit mammary gland showing the rich innervation with fluorescent sympathetic fibers containing noradrenaline. (From Hebb and Linzell, unpublished.) Note: $1\mu = 1\mu m$.

TABLE I

<small>Comparison of Mammary Blood Flow Calculated on the Fick Principle with Direct Measurement by Thermodilution[a]</small>

Component measured	Thermodilution measurement	
Blood flow (ml/min per 100 gm-tissue)	43.5 ± 1.7	
Milk yield (ml/min per 100 gm-tissue)	0.09 ± 0.004	
Ratio (milk yield/ blood flow)	$\therefore 43.5/0.09 = 483$	(Mean: 483 ± 15)

	Fick calculations		
	Precursor [a − v (mg/100 ml blood)]	Product [milk concentration (mg/100 ml)]	Ratio (product/ precursor)
Amino acid N versus milk protein N	1.04 ± 0.08	460 ± 90	$460/1.04 = 442$
Glucose versus lactose and glycerol	14.4 ± 0.9 (% oxidized: $25 \pm 3\% = 3.6$)	Lactose: 4600 ± 400 Glucose equivalent: 4840 ½ Glycerol: 270	$4840 + 270/$ $14.4 - 3.6$ $= 474$
Triglyceride (TG) and acetate versus fatty acids	TG: 6.7 ± 0.3 = 6.0 fatty acids Acetate: 5.7 ± 0.4 (% oxidized: $47 \pm 6 = 2.7$ mg) 3.0 mg acetate yields 1.77 mg fatty acid	Fat: 4300 ± 700 (contains 3760 fatty acids)	$3760/6.0 + 1.77$ $= 483$

[a] Linzell (1966a). Data from six goats giving 1–5 liters of milk daily.

that, having tied off all the mammary veins except the one his flowmeter was applied to (the milk vein), once the animal lies down and occludes this vein, the blood has no escape route. Under these circumstances, the numerous small veins connecting the gland to the surrounding skin and muscle quickly enlarge, and only a proportion of the blood must have been flowing through his flowmeter. I can make this criticism because I later and independently made the same error myself (Linzell, 1960a).

This brings us to the final error that trapped early workers: often the venous blood they took was not solely representative of the blood draining the whole udder. This arose from an incorrect account of the venous drainage of the cow's udder that had persisted since the first description by Fürstenburg (1868).

Fürstenburg described the anatomy of the main blood vessels of the cow's udder and noted that, when detached from the animal, from both the left and right halves, two large and one medium sized veins apparently emerge. Unfortunately, he evidently did not look inside them because he would have found that they all contained valves, whose direction clearly indicate that on each side only one of these veins carries blood away from it. Becker (1937) discovered the valves in the medium sized vein (the perineal), showing that this vessel carries blood from the vulva toward the udder and not from the udder to the vulva and this is correct. It was not until 1955 that the venous drainage of the udder was determined in conscious animals (Linzell and Mount, 1955; Linzell, 1960a). The important point is that this work showed that in some animals there is the possibility of variable quantities of nonmammary blood entering the milk vein. Thus, one cannot select cows, goats, or sheep at random for this type of work, but must carefully examine each animal for the degree of incompetence of the valves in the mammary veins (see Section V, A, 3, d for methods). An additional advantage of this careful selection is that it is possible to pick animals where the total flow from one-half of the udder leaves in the milk vein.

Application of this knowledge enabled me (Linzell, 1957, 1960b, 1960a) to devise a method of measuring udder blood flow easily and repeatedly for long periods in conscious undisturbed goats and, in addition, ensured that venous samples fully representative of the tissue were obtained. The methods require prior surgical preparation of the animal, but these do not interfere with lactation and, once complete, the animals can be used repeatedly for years. Thus, the first extensive measurements were made of mammary substrate uptake and product output according to Eqs. (2) and (3), which because of the generally good agreement were probably essentially correct (see Linzell, 1968).

It was not until later that all the necessary measurements were made simultaneously in the cow (Kronfeld *et al.*, 1968). Although they used a method of blood flow measurement which tends to overestimate (see Section III, A, 5, a) nevertheless, an impressive amount of information was obtained and clear quantitative differences in udder and general metabolism were detected between normal, fasting, and ketotic cows. This is an excellent example of benefits to be derived from painstaking work.

Annison and Linzell (1964) and Annison *et al.* (1968) made an advance by combining mammary uptake experiments with turnover measurements and significantly increased the amount of information that can be obtained from an experiment. By taking mammary blood samples and measuring mammary blood flow and milk yield during isotope dilution studies, one can make reasonable estimates simultaneously in conscious undisturbed animals of total body turnover of two substrates (^{14}C- and ^{3}H-labeled), the contribution of the ^{14}C-labeled compound to total CO_2 output, the proportion of each milk component derived from the labeled compounds, the mammary uptake of these and other components, in quantitative terms, which can be related to the output in the milk of products derived from them, the mammary uptake in relation to total body turnover, the contribution of ^{14}C-labeled compounds to mammary CO_2, and the proportion of the precursor oxidized by the mammary gland.

II. ANATOMY OF MAMMARY BLOOD VESSELS, LYMPHATICS, AND NERVES

In placental mammals, mammary glands are found in different regions of the body and they partake of the blood, lymph, and nerve supply of the area in which they happen to be located, so one may deduce that there is nothing very specific or unusual about mammary blood vessels, lymphatics, and nerves. Failure to remember this led to the erroneous account of the venous drainage of the cow's udder by the first investigators.

Humans, monkeys, elephants, and bats have pectoral mammary glands deriving their blood supply from intercostal, lateral thoracic, and internal mammary (internal thoracic) blood vessels. Cows, sheep, goats, horses, and guinea pigs have inguinal mammary glands and share the blood and nerve supply of the skin of the inguinum. Whales and dolphins have glands beside the vulva. Rats and mice have mammary glands widely spread in the inguinal to pectoral regions, and in cats, dogs, and rabbits the glands extend from the axilla to the groin and in pigs from the xiphisternum to the groin, so that, as might be expected, mammary blood and nerve supply in these animals is multiple. Some aquatic rodents (e.g., coypu, *Myocastor coypus*) even have mammary glands on the back or dorsal thorax. The important point is that mammary glands in all species are entirely skin structures and therefore, not unexpectedly, their gross blood and nerve supply is basically similar to that of skin.

A. Large Blood Vessels

The major vessels to mammary glands are described and illustrated in some textbooks of anatomy. Linzell (1953a) deals with the cat, dog, rabbit, rat, mouse, and guinea pig; Puget and Toty (1956) with the dog; Linzell (1960a) with the goat, sheep, and cow; Barone and Monnet (1955) with the horse; Palic (1954) with the sheep; Vladimirova (1958) and Srukov (1962) with the goat; Zietzschmann (1917), Becker and Arnold (1942), and El Hagri (1945) deal with the cow; Nishinakagawa (1970) deals with all these species plus the hamster, and gives useful diagrams and the common variations noted in individuals of the various species.

B. Small Blood Vessels

If it is agreed that there is nothing particular about the large mammary vessels, there are reasons for imagining there may be something special about the smallest ones. First, because mammary blood flow is so extremely labile and thus warrants consideration, and second, because it is particularly difficult to obtain a complete injection of all mammary arterioles and capillaries with injection masses, particularly with rubber latex, due to mammary vasoconstriction occurring at death or during preparation of the tissue in anesthetized animals. Furthermore, several monographs and reviews give grotesquely oversimplified or distorted diagrams of the relation of the small blood vessels to the secretory cells.

Wahl (1915) was the first to study the smallest mammary blood vessels. He examined whole mounts of mammary glands of rabbits after injection with India ink. He reported that the concentration of capillaries around the mammary ducts and end buds of virgin animals was higher than in the surrounding fatty connective tissue and that, as the glands grow during pregnancy, the vascularity around the mammary tissue increases. The arterioles and venules supplying the capillary network come from surrounding cutaneous and muscular vessels, but new ones are formed from capillaries and, as the mammary tissue expands outwards, new vessels extend and tend to follow the ducts into new lobules. However, arterioles, and less frequently, venules, do approach from other directions.

Dabelow (1933, 1934) extended Wahl's account to the rat, mouse, and guinea pig and reported three further findings: (1) that the mammary lobules, as they grow and displace adipose tissue cells, also take over the existing adipose tissue capillaries so that few new capillaries are formed, although some are transformed into arterioles and venules by acquiring a smooth muscle sheath; (2) the arteriole and venules supplying fat and mammary lobules approach in one of three ways: (a) intralobular, (b) extralobular, but from the same direction, (c) extralobular from any direction; (3) that, like the fat lobules, neighboring mammary lobules are joined by common capillaries bridging the connective tissue sheath between them. This he believed allowed blood to be shunted from an inactive lobule to an active one.

Soemarwoto and Bern (1958) and Nishinakagawa (1970) studied, in whole mounts, the distribution of blood vessels to the mammary glands of mice at different stages of the reproductive cycle, and animals endocrinectomized and/or treated with hormones. They confirm Dabelow's report that the mammary tissue grows into and takes over the blood supply to the fat in which it lies. Nishinakagawa (1970) surprisingly states that (a) in the nonlactating animal capillary plexuses are only found around the fat cells and end buds of the mammary ducts, (b) only the main ducts have a sheath of small blood vessels, (c) capillary plexuses are only seen around small ducts during development, (d) alveoli form in small fat lobules, already possessing a capillary network, (e) only during lactation when all the adipose tissue has been displaced by secreting mammary tissue are there well-developed capillary networks seen closely surrounding the alveoli and ducts. He concludes that vascular development precedes growth of new ducts and alveoli and was able to mimic the increase in vascularity with injections of progesterone or estrogen plus progesterone.

The technique used by these two authors to delineate the blood vessels was to inject a large volume of India ink in saline intravenously into the anesthetized animals so it would be seen only in those vessels that were patent at the time of death. Thus, there is the possibility that not all capillaries would be filled. Nevertheless, this method might be expected to give a valid assessment of the functional vascularity at different stages of the reproductive cycle.

The distribution of small blood vessels to the actively secreting glands of dogs, cats, and goats was studied by Linzell (1971a) using postmortem specimens injected with India ink, dyes, dyed gelatin, and rubber latex, or with the blood vessels distended with blood by tying the veins in life. They were examined with a binocular dissecting microscope either during dissection of the whole cleared specimen or in thick sections (50–250 μm) (Fig. 2). In these species the richness of the mammary blood supply was confirmed. Each alveolus is surrounded by a network of 5–10 capillaries, each section approximately 50 μm long and 10–15 μm apart.

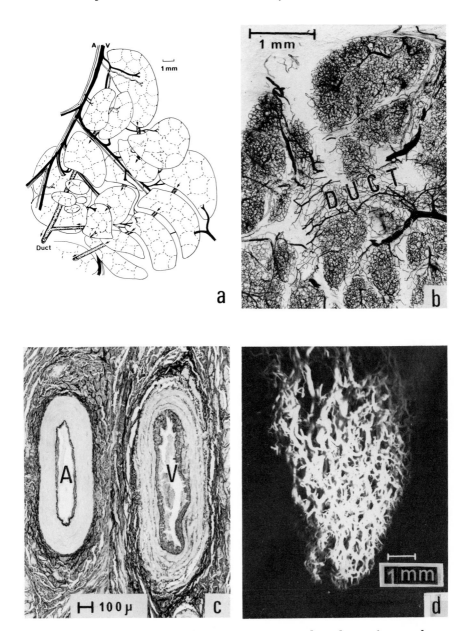

Fig. 2. Mammary blood vessels. a, Lactating cat. Independence of major ducts and blood vessels. b, Thick section (100 μm) of lactating cat mammary gland injected with red and blue gelatin: arteries, pale gray; veins, black. c, Artery and vein in a goat's teat. Elastic stain. d, Latex cast of veins in cat's teat.

As observed by Dabelow (1933, 1934), each lobule made up of alveoli draining into a small duct had its own capillary network supplied by one to three arterioles and drained by one to three venules. Both the afferent and efferent vessels approached from all directions in an apparently random fashion (Fig. 2a,b). The ductule draining the lobule also has a surrounding capillary network derived from the same supply (Fig. 2b). In these specimens capillaries bridging neighboring lobules were not seen. Furthermore, it is difficult to believe that no new capillaries are formed during mammary development in animals such as guinea pigs, cows, and goats, where the volume of the functional glands so exceeds that of the nonlactating animal. As the gland grows all available space is quickly filled by newly formed ducts and alveoli and the overall size of the gland increases exponentially, about eightfold in goats (Linzell, 1966b). The exact way in which the mammary tree grows, particularly in late pregnancy, has not been described (Dabelow says that duct branching is dichotomous). However, in general it involves upward and outward growth away from the teat. This must involve a considerable growth of new blood vessels of all types, at a rate equal to that of the mammary tissue, and specifically for the mammary tissue.

It should be noted that mammary ducts do not have a specialized blood supply as salivary gland ducts do (Fig. 2b). The structure of mammary ducts is very similar at all levels (Linzell and Peaker, 1971a) and the capillary network surrounding them is supplied by arterioles and venules at intervals from the surrounding lobular supply (Linzell, 1971a). Gostev (1968) noted that the capillaries in folds of the ducts in goat glands were well-developed and suggested that these are the regions where reabsorption of ions takes place. However, there is nothing in mammary tissue resembling the striated duct region of the salivary gland, where active ionic exchange takes place and there is a much denser network of capillaries than around the alveoli. Indeed recent work shows that mammary ducts are impermeable to the main constituents of milk (Linzell and Peaker, 1971a).

C. Vascular Shunts

In many tissues arteries and veins are capable of being joined directly, thus shunting blood away from the capillaries, so that, while the overall blood flow through the tissue may remain constant, the proportion flowing through capillaries, where effective exchange of gases and nutrients takes place, can vary widely. Two structures have been described that accomplish this shunting.

1. Arteriovenous Anastomoses

Discovered by Hoyer (1877) and seen and understood best in the rabbit's ear, they are present in many tissues. These classical A-V shunts are short, twisted, thick-walled vessels, with an irregular lumen of 60–100 μm in diameter, which directly connect a small artery to its neighboring vein, draining the same capillary bed. In the conscious rabbit with a glass observation chamber in the ear these shunts can be seen to open and close randomly at different frequencies but all are open when the rate of blood flow through the ear is high and it is very warm (Clark, 1938). Indeed, this is a means of preserving exposed tissues from frostbite. A-V shunts are abundant in the tips of the fingers, the nose and ear and particularly in the feet of arctic birds. Not surprisingly, they are also found at the tip of the teat (Moriconi, 1953; Manente, 1954; Nisbet, 1956; Linzell, 1971a) and doubtless help to maintain its blood flow in cold conditions (Fig 3a). They could also help to maintain flow during suckling and milking. These A-V shunts are structures capable of passing particles of up to 60–100 μm. In goats they are only found in the teat and mammary skin and thus could hardly shunt blood effectively away from mammary secretory tissue, since the teats and skin form only 10–20% of the udder.

In a goat's udder, in which the blood vessels appeared to be completely injected with monastral fast blue dye, Linzell (1971a) observed small, dye-filled vessels in the walls of the cistern that at first appeared to be small arteries but which lacked the internal elastic lamina characteristic of arteries (Fig. 3b). Classical A-V shunts also have no elastic coat but have thick walls of modified muscle cells, which the cisternal vessels lacked. If these vessels are a modified type of A-V shunt, then they could shunt blood away from secretory tissue and could be functionally important.

2. Arteriovenular Bridges or Thoroughfare Channels

These structures, first recognized by Zweifach (1939) in the mesentery, are vessels, somewhat larger than capillaries, that join the end of an arteriole directly to its venule. Off this channel the true capillaries branch, the entrance to each being controlled by a sphincter. The opening and closing of these capillary sphincters effectively control flow through the capillary bed and was observed in the living mesentery. In the mammary gland very occasionally similar vessels were seen by Linzell (1971a) in injected specimens, but the living tissue would need to be studied to verify their existence and their mode of functioning.

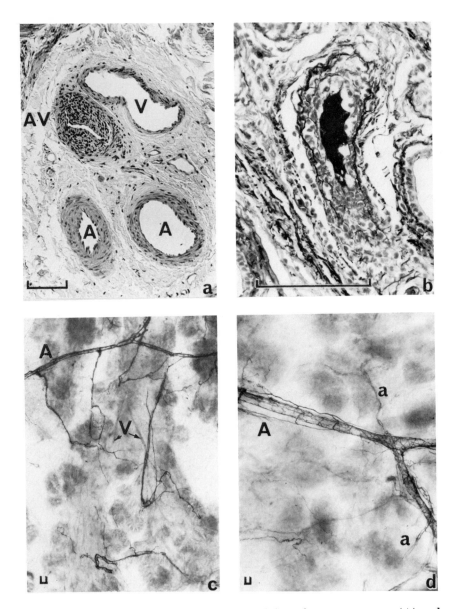

Fig. 3. a, Classical arteriovenous shunt (A-V) lying between its artery (A) and vein (V). Tip of goat's teat. Hematoxylin and eosin. b, Possible small A-V shunt in the cistern of a goat's udder. Lumen contains blue dye injected into main artery. Elastic stain. c, Nerves in involuting rabbit mammary gland which follow arteries (A) closely, veins (V) not innervated. (From Hebb and Linzell, unpublished.) d, Nerves in

D. Teat Blood Vessels

Apart from the high concentration of A-V shunts the other blood vessels to the teat are specialized. The arteries tend to run straight along the length of the teat but the veins form an extensive network throughout the structure (Fig. 2d). Furthermore, at first sight they resemble arteries, having a thick muscular wall. They can be distinguished by the thicker intima and by elastic tissue distributed throughout the muscle (Fig. 2c). These veins would be better suited to maintain blood flow during suckling, when the teat is subjected to large positive and negative pressures.

E. Mammary Lymphatics

The arrangement and structure of lymphatics are of some interest. This was studied mostly in the last century when a controversy arose that has been settled only recently, the subject having been neglected for over 60 years. According to one school of thought the finest mammary lymphatics resemble those illustrated in textbooks of histology, and start in among the alveoli, but others thought that this was an artifact due to injecting masses into the tissue when the fluid forces channels for itself that do not exist in life. Such workers believed that there are no lymphatics inside the lobules and that excess tissue fluid enters the finest lymphatics which surround the lobules, but do not enter them. Recent work supports this view.

If it is agreed that the technique of injecting colored fluids into the tissue is liable to produce artifacts, there is also the difficulty of distinguishing empty blood capillaries from lymph capillaries in sections of uninjected tissue. Therefore, it is preferable to inject the blood capillaries with a colored substance so that they can be distinguished from the lymphatic capillaries but it is difficult to be certain that every blood capillary is filled. However, in specimens where all blood capillaries appear to be injected, all the smallest vessels inside lobules have dye in them. Furthermore, in specimens where the blood capillaries were filled with blood by tying off the veins in life (Linzell, 1971a) or injecting blood into the arteries postmortem (Lee and Lascelles, 1969) and in cases of staphylococcal mastitis where there is intense vascular congestion, in all these specimens very few lymph capillaries are seen inside lobules.

---

lactating rabbit, all following arteries (A) and arterioles (a). Secretory alveoli not innervated. Whole mount. Butyrylcholinesterase. (From Hebb and Linzell, unpublished.)

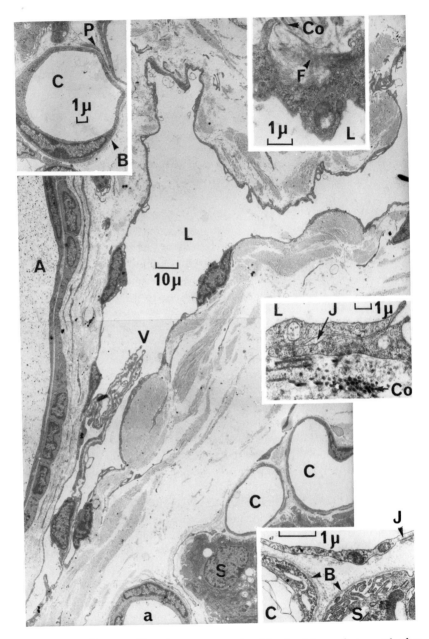

Fig. 4. Capillaries and lymphatics in a goat's udder fixed by perfusion with gluta-raldehyde. Lymphatic with a valve (V), lies in the interlobular connective tissue, next to an artery (A): C, blood capillary; S, secretory cells; J, junction of lymphatic

Finally electron microscopy confirms this view (Fig. 4), because blood and lymphatic capillaries can be distinguished at the ultrastructural level. I have studied this in goat mammary glands fixed by perfusion with warm glutaraldehyde. This not only preserves fine structure but prevents the collapse and distortion of the tissue which tends to occur when fresh tissue is cut. Electron micrographs show the following features:

Capillaries. These are usually circular in cross section. The endothelial cells are of uniform thickness (0.2–2.0 μm) and are joined by tight junctions. There is a well developed basement membrane and pericytes, which are rather sparce and therefore not seen in every section (Fig. 4).

Lymphatics. These are much larger than blood capillaries but irregular in profile. The walls are thin (0.1–0.5 μm) and sometimes valves can be seen (Fig. 4); veins with valves can be distinguished because they have smooth muscle in the wall. The endothelial cells of lymphatics are not joined by tight junctions (Fig. 4), the nuclei tend to bulge into the lumen; there are no pericytes and only a very poorly developed basement membrane (Fig. 4). However, there are characteristic fine anchoring filaments passing from the wall in places into the surrounding collagen fibers (Fig. 4), and long projections of cytoplasm pass into the surrounding collagen.

F. Mammary Vasomotor Nerves

These must be mentioned in this chapter because they can readily reduce mammary blood flow in stress. Being a skin structure, the mammary glands share its innervation, which is sensory, and adrenergic sympathetic. This has been established in dogs, cats, goat, sheep, and cows. In the goat and sheep the data is the most complete (Linzell, 1959). The udder is mainly innervated by the external spermatic and perineal nerves, which carry sensory fibers from the gland (the dermatomes overlap) and carry to it vasomotor fibers from the lumbar and sacral sympathetic chains. These fibers innervate the smooth muscle in the teat and the gland's arteries and arterioles and originate in the thoracic and lumbar ganglia of the sympathetic chain. The preganglionic fibers to these postganglionic

---

endothelial cells. Note the absence of tight junction and basement membrane. B, Basement membrane of blood capillary and secretory cells; Co, collagen; F, anchoring filaments; a, arteriole; P, pericyte; L, lumen. Note: $1\mu = 1\mu$m. Micrographs by courtesy of R. D. Burton, and Dr. F. B. P. Wooding.

nerves enter the chain in white rami communicantes between thoracic 8 and lumbar 5 (Fig. 5).

Recent examination of mammary innervation by histochemical techniques reveals the very rich network of sympathetic nerves, which accompany all arteries and arterioles (Hebb and Linzell, 1970; Lukáš et al., 1971), down to the smallest. Indeed all the nerves, sensory and sympathetic, follow the arteries closely (Figs. 1,3; Hebb and Linzell, 1970). Since the mammary glands are very sensitive to injected adrenaline and noradrenaline (Hebb and Linzell, 1951; Fig. 1), it is not surprising that in anesthetized animals stimulation of the sympathetic nerves which act by releasing noradrenaline severely reduces mammary blood flow. The significance of these findings is that in the conscious animal, very mild stress or disturbance can reduce mammary blood flow, e.g., venipuncture in the goat (Linzell, 1971b), and in the rat lifting the animal from the nest (Hanwell and Linzell, 1972). Whether this is due to reflex vasomotor activity and to release of adrenaline has not been established but this is immaterial to the investigator who wishes to measure mammary arteriovenous differences, who clearly must take careful steps to avoid even

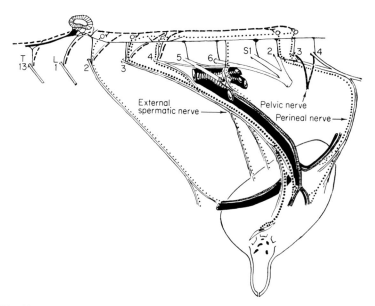

Fig. 5. Sympathetic innervation of the udder of the goat. The sheep and cow are similar. Note that vasodilator parasympathetic fibers in the pelvic nerves do not reach the udder. Sympathetic preganglionic (— — —); sympathetic postganglionic (. . . . . .); parasympathetic (————). (From Linzell, 1959.)

mild stress in taking the blood samples. There are several instances where the data obtained were wrong because this advice was ignored.

III. MAMMARY BLOOD FLOW

A. Methods of Measuring Mammary Blood Flow

In anesthetized animals all methods can be used, although this may be of little interest because blood flow and milk yield tend to fall under anesthesia. A simple and accurate method in a heparinized animal is to cannulate one mammary vein (tying off all the others) and to arrange for the blood to flow into a funnel and thence back into the animal via any other vein. Flow is then measured with a drop recorder, stop watch and cylinder, orifice meter, bubble flowmeter or several other types (see Green, 1948). A Gaddum (1929) flowmeter is excellent in this situation. Mammary glands can be circumcised, leaving the main vessels intact, and then placed in a plethysmograph so that the flow can be measured by venous occlusion with a volume recorder (Linzell, 1950; Vladimirova, 1954). It is better to insert a cannula or flowmeter into a vein because the serotonin released from platelets goes away from the tissue and is removed by the lungs. In an artery serotonin release can cause a fall in mammary blood flow, unless an antagonist is used (bromo-LSD or methysergide) and these may have other effects. The following methods of measuring blood flow have been used in conscious animals.

1. Electromagnetic Flowmeter

This was applied aseptically around the main artery in goats (Reynolds *et al.*, 1968), and the leads were brought out through the skin of the flank so that the animal could be attached to the recording apparatus at intervals. This is excellent for short-term experiments and for studying factors that influence udder blood flow. Its limitations are (a) its life is limited because it causes gradual closure of the artery due to fibrosis and even erosion; (b) it can only be calibrated by opening the vessel and making a timed collection of the blood distal to the instrument; (c) to get a true zero on the recorder the artery needs to be clamped distally during recording; fortunately in many goats this can be accomplished manually, although several implantable occludes have been described (e.g., Jagenau *et al.*, 1969; Sham *et al.*, 1970). Recently, Houvenaghel *et al.* (1972) and Dhondt *et al.* (1973), using an electromagnetic flowmeter in the conscious cow, were able to produce zero flow by occluding the external iliac artery manually per rectum.

2. Thermodilution

Linzell (1957, 1960b, 1966a) adapted Fegler's (1954, 1957) thermo-dilution method to measure udder blood flow in goats and later in cows. The principle of the method is that saline cooler than the blood is in-jected at known temperature and constant rate (Linzell, 1966a) into the milk vein near the udder in the standing animal. A thermocouple or thermistor, lying in the vein 10–25 cm downstream measures the fall in temperature of the blood and saline mixture. Knowing the temperature of the blood upstream, the rate of blood flow can be calculated (Fig. 6).

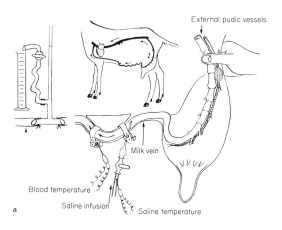

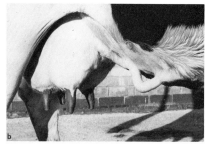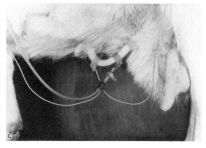

Fig. 6.   a, Measurement of udder blood flow by thermodilution, in a milk vein loop. At the time of exteriorizing the vein, the vessels crossing between the two halves of the udder and minor veins in front of it are removed. (From Linzell, 1966a, by per-mission of the American Heart Association, Inc.) Milk vein loop in a cow (b) and goat (c).

Fegler (1957) showed that his technique could be used to measure flow in the abdominal and thoracic vena cavae. Later Fronek and Ganz (1960) showed that it also worked in arteries. These results are somewhat surprising because it might be thought that in deeply buried vessels error would arise due to heat exchange with the vessel wall and its surrounding tissues. Fegler (1957) showed that what happens is that the vessel wall is cooled but that it quickly rewarms as fresh warm blood flows past it (i.e., gives up its "coolth") so that indicator is not lost from the bloodstream. The shape of the concentration time curve is flattened and lengthened, but the area under it is little altered. In spite of these facts, a reason thermodilution is particularly suitable for estimating udder blood flow is that the vein is superficial. Indeed, to be able to use the method repeatedly, many times a day, the milk vein is exteriorized as a long, skin-covered loop (Fig. 6). This facilitates repeated puncture for the insertion of the injection needle and thermistor probe and, since the vein is surrounded by air of much lower thermal conductivity than that of tissues, there is even less chance of the method overestimating true flow due to loss of indicator.

As currently used in my laboratory, the cool saline is injected at very constant rate using a piston and velodyne motor. This fluid passes into a thin-walled rubber bag in a 3-liter reservoir of sterile pyrogen-free saline, which is thus displaced into the vein; a thermistor monitors the temperature just before it enters the vein. The saline enters the vein via a hypodermic needle with the end blocked and with three small radially placed holes near the tip. These three fine jets facilitate mixing with the blood, which is the essence of the method. To assess the proportion of the total mammary flow that is measured during the saline injection the external pudic vein is manually occluded (Fig. 6) (see Section V,A,3).

3. Thermostromuhr

This instrument had a vogue in the 1930's and was used by Graham (1937) in the goat's milk vein. It heats the blood and measures the rise in temperature downstream. The rise in temperature varies with the log of velocity. Because of technical difficulties in measuring the exact amount of heat transferred to the blood, the instrument was calibrated empirically.

4. Indicator Dilution

A simple method is to inject an indicator that remains intravascular, e.g., Evans blue dye (T 1824), into the mammary artery to measure the concentration–time curve in the veins. I have used either single rapid injections or a continuous infusion, although for this it is necessary to know the concentration of recirculated dye upstream of the injection site. In normal animals this method is limited in that catheterization of the artery must be done under anesthesia. However, in goats bearing one gland transplanted to the neck and supplied by an exteriorized carotid artery, arterial injection is easy (Linzell 1963b, 1971b), and the other carotid, also exteriorized, can be used to obtain the "upstream" concentration of the recirculated dye.

5. Fick Methods

Several methods are based on the Fick principle.

a. NITROUS OXIDE. Kety and Schmidt (1945) devised this method for measuring brain blood flow in man, and Reynolds (1964) has applied it to the goat's udder. N_2O is freely diffusable in blood and tissues and during a period of breathing a gas mixture containing it (15%), the time taken for an organ to become saturated with the gas is proportional to the rate it is delivered to the organ, i.e., to its blood flow. If the total gas (Q) in the organ and the mean arteriovenous difference during uptake [$\int(a - v)\, dt$] are known, then the rate of blood flow (F) can be calculated by dividing the former by the latter.

$$F = Q/\int(a - v)dt \qquad (4)$$

The partition coefficient between blood and tissue must be known and a correction applied if this is not unity. It is difficult to measure the total gas taken up, but its concentration is easier to estimate, being equal at saturation to the concentration in the venous blood. Therefore, if both sides of Eq. (4) are divided by the weight of the organ, flow is obtained per unit weight of tissue. This is a limitation of the method for most organs but, fortunately, it is possible to measure udder volume in goats and even cows during life (Linzell, 1960b, 1966b; Kjaersgaard, 1968a).

For this method it is necessary to take frequent samples of arterial and mammary venous blood for 15–30 minutes and the animal must be trained to breathe through a mask, without disturbance. It tends to underestimate flow by 19%, probably partly because N_2O is lost through the skin of the udder (Reynolds et al., 1968).

Other diffusible substances can replace N_2O. I have found that ^3HOH suffers from the same disadvantage as N_2O, but urea is not lost through the skin and is a better indicator, if anything slightly overestimating flow. Ethanol or aminoantipyrine could also be used. Another fact that is usually not allowed for is that blood water is 85% whereas tissue water is only 70%. This would result in an overestimate by the factor of 85/70, i.e., 1.09 for substances distributed in water.

b. ANTIPYRINE. Rasmussen (1963) proposed a simple method of estimating mammary blood flow, when he was studying the excretion of drugs into milk. He pointed out that the Fick principle can be invoked when a diffusible substance is passing from milk to blood as well as from blood to milk. He injected a known quantity of antipyrine solution into the teat and found that it was absorbed exponentially, as would be expected if the process is passive. In this case he knew the quantity absorbed by measuring the amount left in the milk after a given period (about 40 minutes). During the absorption period he took 4–5 pairs of arterial and mammary venous blood samples and, knowing the rate of absorption at the time of sampling, could calculate the blood flow. Rasmussen allowed a period of 10 minutes for the antipyrine solution to distribute itself in the milk ducts before he started sampling, but Kronfeld (1969) improved the method by taking more frequent samples and integrating the area inscribed by the arterial and venous curves as in Kety and Schmidt's N_2O method.

When compared with the electromagnetic and thermodilution methods, Rasmussen's original method tended to overestimate for reasons that were unknown (Rasmussen and Linzell, 1964; Reynolds et al., 1968). The improved method has not been checked, nevertheless in cows a plot of milk yield versus bood flow measured with antipyrine (Kronfeld et al., 1968) falls substantially above a similar plot of milk yield versus blood flow measured in this laboratory by thermodilution (Fig. 10). Moreover, Kronfeld et al. (1968) comments that in their experiments the udder uptake of glucose was sometimes equal to the total entry rate of glucose into the circulation of the cow, which is impossible. Since it is unlikely that the entry rate and mammary a − v of glucose were seriously in error, this must indicate an overestimation of udder blood flow. This is a great pity because the method is so simple.

c. CLEARANCE METHODS. An estimate of the blood flow per unit volume of tissue can be made from the rate at which a freely diffusible indicator is cleared from the tissue; the faster the flow the quicker the elimination (Kety, 1949). First the tissue is loaded with the indicator, and, after loading, the rate of disappearance is measured after the input has ceased. A neat twist to this method is to use hydrogen gas (Aukland et al., 1964) or radioactive xenon and krypton (Holzman et al., 1964). because these are almost completely eliminated from the venous blood in one passage through the lungs and, thus, it is not always necessary to measure the arterial concentration, because this is virtually zero. Hydrogen can be measured with a hydrogen electrode, as used for pH measurement, except that it is not kept saturated with hydrogen gas. The radioactive gases can be detected outside tissue because they are γ-ray emitters.

Since diffusible substances are cleared, exponentially, it is only necessary to measure the $t_{\frac{1}{2}}$ and to estimate the flow (F).

$$F = \lambda(\ln 2/t_{\frac{1}{2}}) \tag{5}$$

where λ is the partition coefficient between blood and tissue of the indicator.

d. METABOLIC FICK METHODS. The method, introduced by Lintzel (1934), estimates mean mammary blood flow from the mean a − v of a precursor and the measured quantity of the product transferred to the milk in a given time. Some of its advantages in studies of mammary metabolism are that this method integrates flow over the period, during which milk yield is measured and that the measurements may be made on the same samples that are taken for a − v analysis. The method was widely used in the late 1930's and early 1940's using Ca as the precursor and product.

Linzell (1960b) compared this method with flow measured by thermodilution in goats. The mean data were in agreement, but there was great variation, chiefly due to the difficulty of measuring accurately the a − v of Ca, which is only of the order of 0.2 mg/100 ml. This could be much less of a problem using atomic absorption spectrometry. However, other substances can be used that have a much larger a − v. For example, in experiments where the turnover of glucose is being measured by the injection of tracer amounts of [^{14}C]glucose, the proportion of the a − v of glucose oxidized can be measured from the increase in specific radioactivity of CO_2 across the gland (Annison and Linzell, 1964). The only remaining major products of glucose are milk lactose, triglyceride glycerol, and citrate. In the goat and cow such experiments show that at least 85% of milk lactose is derived from plasma glucose, and about half the citrate and glycerol. Thus the error is not too great if it is assumed that all the lactose comes from glucose and the contributions to glycerol and citrate are ignored, and the blood flow is calculated from the a − v glucose and the output of lactose and CO_2. Since the proportion of glucose oxidized is reasonably constant in fed undisturbed goats (25 ± 3%, Annison and Linzell, 1964, and unpublished observations), a rough estimate may be made by measuring only a − v glucose and milk lactose.

Other candidates for accurate measurement of blood flow by the Fick principle are some of the essential amino acids, which are entirely transferred to the synthesized milk proteins and have a large extraction (a − v is 40–70% of the arterial concentration). Lysine, leucine, and threonine look the most useful. Since the amino acid composition of milk protein is unlikely to vary, it should be only necessary to determine the proportion of the chosen amino acid in synthesized protein and thereafter to measure only total milk protein output, because the quantity of plasma protein transferred to the milk is normally negligible.

It must be emphasized that this method demands that during the period of the measurements the rate of milk secretion must be stable (see Section I,A). However, comparison of mean data shows that there is good agreement between blood flow calculated by the Fick method and blood flow directly measured by thermodilution (Table I).

6. Ultrasonic Methods

These are relatively new but are of great promise. As originally used, two crystals were placed diagonally across the bloodstream and first one transmitted and the other received and then the functions were reversed. This involved measuring very tiny differences in time between receiving the signal, depending on whether the sound was traveling with or against the stream, and this was difficult. However, later the method was simplified electronically by employing the Doppler-Shift principle (Franklin *et al.*, 1961). Both crystals face the same way but each is at about 45° to the direction of flow. The waves of ultrasound are transmitted by one crystal and the reflected waves received by the other. If the objects reflecting the waves are moving, the frequency of the reflected signal is altered slightly (increased or decreased depending on whether the particles are approaching or receding), and electronically it is relatively easy to compare the received frequency with that emitted, and to filter out the changed (Doppler) frequency, which is directly proportional to the velocity of the moving reflectors. In blood the red blood corpuscles readily reflect ultrasound, and the big advantage of this technique in physiology is that the method can be applied across unopened undamaged vessels, indeed, even if they are covered by other tissues, including skin (Stegall *et al.*, 1966). For example, I have successfully applied this method to measure the velocity of blood flow in a "milk vein" loop (Fig. 6) or a carotid loop supplying a transplanted mammary gland. The method is simple, bloodless, and effective. Unfortunately, the main snag is that it measures blood velocity and not flow, so that it is necessary to know the diameter of the blood vessel to be able to calculate flow, and to be sure that it does not vary during an experiment. However, even here ultrasonics promises to be of help. It is possible to fire a pulse of ultrasound straight across the vessel and to pick up and display on an oscilloscope the various objects in its path that reflect the sound waves (Arndt and Klauske, 1971). The walls of the vessel can be identified because they pulsate in unison with the heart beat. Knowing the velocity of sound in the tissue and the time taken to receive the reflected wave, it is possible to calculate the distance of the reflecting surface. Thus the possibility exists of a double ultrasonic probe, for application around a vessel (either buried aseptically in the body or applied percutaneously), which will monitor continuously both the blood velocity and the diameter of the vessel.

7. Indicator Fractionation

Sapirstein (1956) developed a method of estimating blood flow simultaneously to all organs. He pointed out that if a freely diffusible substance is injected rapidly into the right atrium it is thoroughly mixed in the heart and lungs and passes to all organs in equal concentration. If the circulation is stopped as soon as the blood has passed through an organ, the quantity of the indicator in it is determined by the blood flow, i.e., the proportion of the cardiac output received by it. If the cardiac output is known, the blood flow to any organ can be measured. The method is limited because the animal must be killed, but it has proved valuable in this laboratory in studying cardiovascular phenomena in the lactating rat.

Sapirstein (1956), originally used ^{42}KCl as the indicator and thought, that, since K would be actively pumped into cells as soon as it diffused into the extracellular space, extraction would be almost 100%, the first time round the circulation. Thus, there would be a brief period when the isotope was mostly entering the tissues with very little in the veins. However, in a later paper using ^{42}KCl, $^{86}RbCl$ or [^{131}I]iodoantipyrine (Sapirstein, 1958) he found in fact 40% of the indicator returned to the right heart after the first circulation. Nevertheless, in rats the distribution in many different organs was stable between 6 and 64 seconds, suggesting that the extraction of the isotope by each of them did not vary markedly. Thus, he stated that an essential criterion of the method is that the extraction of the indicator by an organ to be studied must be equal to that of the body as a whole and that this can be determined by showing that the isotope content remains constant during a time equal to several circulation times. The method will underestimate total flow in organs with a large number of A-V shunts, with a low extraction of indicator, but it will indicate capillary flow which may be useful to know. In general the values obtained by Sapirstein's technique for many organs are in good agreement with those obtained by other methods.

Chatwin *et al.* (1969) successfully applied Sapirstein's method to the mammary glands in the rat, using ^{3}HOH as the indicator, and they extended its usefulness by simultaneously estimating the cardiac output by Fegler's thermodilution technique. They demonstrated a large increase in both mammary blood flow per gram of tissue and in the proportion of the cardiac output taken by the mammary glands during lactation. Later, Linzell (1969), using [^{125}I]iodoantipyrine, investigated the cardiovascular changes occurring at parturition in rats. Hanwell and Linzell (1973) more thoroughly explored the mammary extraction of ^{86}RbCl, which is probably the ideal indicator for mammary work. Mammary isotope content rises to a peak at 10 seconds and remains stable for 5 minutes or even longer, but usually the animals are killed at 45 seconds. It is not essential to stop the circulation by guillotining the animal as Sapirstein did, an overdose of pentobarbitone is satisfactory, and this means that the method can be used in the conscious animal on its nest with the young, injecting the indicator and the anesthetic via a plastic catheter chronically implanted into the right atrium via a jugular vein (Hanwell *et al.*, 1972).

8. Semiquantitative Methods

Linzell (1953b) tested heated thermocouples thrust into the tissue to record local blood flow. These give satisfactory records in the liver but, in mammary glands, were insensitive, and sometimes local flow increased when total flow decreased. In humans (Pickles, 1953; Abolins, 1954) and goats (Vladimirova, 1955) a thermal index based on the observation that mammary skin is hotter than neighboring skin has been used. The differential temperature between the two sites can be recorded painlessly with thermocouples or thermistors and certainly varies with the stage of lactation, estrous cycle, etc. It would seem to be more an indicator of mammary skin blood flow, and it is not known how this correlates with mammary blood flow. Thermography has also been used to detect the raised skin temperature during lactation in women (Vuorenkoski *et al.*, 1969). Pickles (1949, 1952) applied a fluctuating pressure to the breast in a plethysmograph applied to the chest wall and showed that the amplitude of the resultant air pressure wave was related to the blood flow. The method gave similar qualitative changes during the cycle as the thermal index (Pickles, 1953). Berkow and Jacobson (1940) trans-illuminated the breast and showed that the pulsations recorded by a photocell were larger when the blood flow increased. Gostev (1967) used a novel means of getting biopsy samples quickly in conscious goats for the histological determination of the number of capillaries containing blood cells. He fired a circular punch into the udder from a shotgun!

9. Comments

It should be noted that several methods of measuring mammary blood flow depend on obtaining a valid venous sample. Thus, for measuring flow it is as important to understand the complexities of mammary venous drainage, as it is for obtaining valid arteriovenous difference measurements.

The following section shows that the main factor influencing mammary blood flow is the rate of milk secretion. Thus, if an experimenter not in a position to measure blood flow can obtain valid arterial and mammary venous blood samples from conscious undisturbed animals and knows the mean milk yield, then Figs. 7–9 may be used to estimate mean blood flow and its likely upper and lower limit, with an accuracy that may well be sufficient to decide if a substance is removed from the blood in significant quantities. The mean data can also be used to compare with blood flow calculated from the metabolic Fick principle on the same blood and milk samples.

B. Rate of Mammary Blood Flow

1. Goat

Most is known about blood flow in conscious trained goats as measured by the thermodilution method (Linzell 1960b; 1966b), and there is a close correlation over the course of a lactation between the rate of udder blood flow and milk yield. There is an abrupt rise at parturition (Reynolds, 1970, Fig. 7), but during established lactation the variation in blood flow from hour to hour and day to day is of the order of 10% of the mean, occasionally as high as 30%. This is consistent with the rate of milk secretion also being remarkably stable in undisturbed animals. Mild stress (Linzell, 1960b; Linzell, 1971b) and fasting (Linzell, 1967a; Annison *et al.*, 1968) lower udder blood flow.

In Fig. 7 are scatter plots of 100 estimations of udder blood flow made in the course of other work at all stages of the reproductive cycle in 20 animals, by the continuous thermodilution method (Linzell, 1966a).

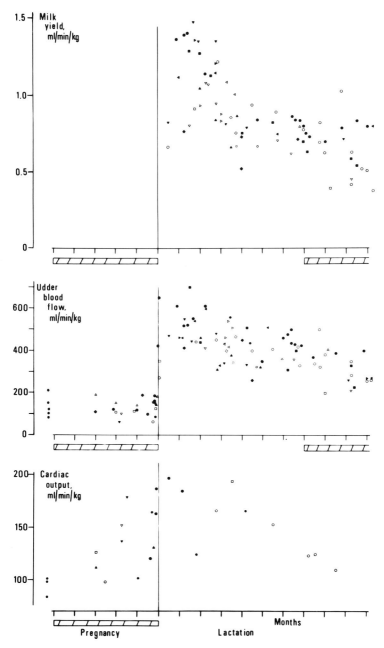

Fig. 7. Scatter plot of values of udder blood flow and cardiac output measured by thermodilution in 20 goats during 5 lactations and the milk yield on the same day. Cardiac output rises during pregnancy but mammary blood flow only in the last day.

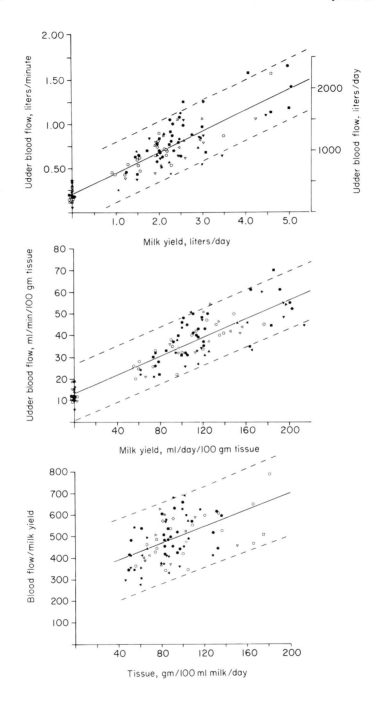

Some animals were studied during five lactations. They supplement the earlier data of Linzell (1960b), who systematically studied udder blood flow over the whole reproductive cycle in a smaller number of animals, with similar results. Analyses of variance show that age, lactation, and stage of lactation have no influence on udder blood flow under normal conditions in established lactation, which is solely related to milk yield. During established lactation, the peak blood flow (about 1.5 liters/minute) coincides with the peak milk yield and is equivalent to 60 ml/minute per 100 gm of udder tissue, which is at least 3 times the average for all organs (i.e., cardiac output divided by the body weight) (Figs. 7, 8). After the peak of lactation there is a steady decline in udder blood flow, but at a rate slower than the rate of decline in milk yield. In advanced lactation the efficiency of the udder is less than it is at peak yield in that more blood passes through the udder for each gram of milk formed (Figs. 8, 9). Thus, the blood flow:milk yield ratio, first calculated by Lintzel (also in goats) and much quoted and used since, of about 500:1 is only an approximation and does not apply when the milk yield is very low, when the ratio is over 1000:1 and rapidly becomes infinite as lactation ceases. Figures 8 and 9 show that at maximum milk yield the ratio is about 400:1 rising to 500:1 over the main part of the lactation curve, which lasts 6–9 months in dairy goats. At low yields (natural or due to fasting) it is 700 to 1000:1. In Saanen goats this is when the daily yield is 0.5–1 liter; in relation to the size of the udder, the yield is then only 25–50 ml/day per 100 gm of udder tissue.

These data are from the A.R.C. Institute of Animal Physiology herd of dairy goats, which are mostly pure bred Saanen, British Saanen, and a few British Alpine. However, very similar data were obtained by me in the Unilever Laboratory at Bedford and by Reynolds *et al.* (1968) in Philadelphia using Saanen, Nubian, French Alpine, and other crossbred dairy breeds. Furthermore, this Institute has a herd of Welsh goats, which give less than half the yield of the Saanens and have commensurately smaller udders (Linzell, 1966b). Extensive use of these animals in udder perfusion experiments, where milk yield before perfusion and blood flow and udder weight during it are accurately known, show that milk yield/blood flow data are not significantly different. Thus, these data may be used to predict udder blood flow from the easily measured milk yield, with an accuracy of about ±30%.

Fig. 8. Data from Fig. 7 replotted to show the relation between milk yield and blood flow. Efficiency decreases at low milk yield, because blood flow for the formation of a given quantity of milk increases.

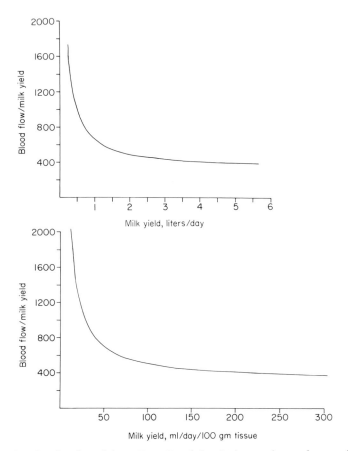

Fig. 9. Graphs plotted from Figs. 7 and 8, which may be used to predict blood flow from the milk yield in goats.

The close association between blood flow and milk yield is also maintained on fasting, both falling to about half by 16 hours (Linzell, 1967a; Annison *et al.*, 1968) (Table IV). However, it is not known which is cause and which is effect.

These figures are for total udder blood flow, but the secretory tissue forms only a part of it, 80–90% in full lactation. The blood flow in the various tissues forming the udder has been determined by Hanwell and Linzell (unpublished) using [86]RbCl or radioactive microspheres injected into the mammary artery *in vivo* (conscious or anesthetized) or *in vitro* (perfused). Before recirculating occurred, the blood flow was stopped (after 45 seconds), and the distribution of the isotope in the tissue was determined. It was found that the blood flow through the skin, teat capsule, and fat were similar, but that during lactation only blood flow through secretory tissue was 2–3.5 times higher. Mammary lymph node blood flow was also higher. Within the secretory tissue itself there was some variation in flow of the order of 70–200% of the mean.

2. Cow

A number of measurements are now available using the antipyrine and the continuous thermodilution methods. Rasmussen (1965) showed that his antipyrine method worked in the cow, giving figures of 1–22 liters/ minute, 22–101 ml/minute per 100 gm tissue. Following injection of the antipyrine into the two glands on one side it was detected in the opposite milk vein confirming the existence of venous anastomoses between left and right halves of the udder. Therefore antipyrine should be injected into all four glands. Kjaersgaard (1968b) used the method to demonstrate the dramatic rise in udder blood flow at calving and Kronfel et al. (1968) used the method and reported figures of 3.3–9.3 liters/ minute, but more important they reported that, as in the goat, there was a significant correlation with milk yield. Kronfeld (1969) improved the method of calculation, studied the rise in udder blood flow at calving, and summarized data of his own and from Rasmussen's laboratory, on fed, fasting, and ketotic cows in established lactation, which again demonstrates an excellent correlation between udder blood flow and milk yield. On the average, a cow with a yield of 20 liters/day had an estimated udder blood flow of just over 10 liters/minute, i.e., BF/MY 750:1. This is higher than the average for goats and does suggest that, as in goats, the antipyrine method overestimates blood flow. Indeed, Kronfeld et al. (1968) pointed out that using this data at high yield, udder glucose uptake, equaled the total entry rate of glucose into the circulation, an unlikely finding.

Measurements of udder blood flow by thermodilution made in this laboratory are lower than the antipyrine data (Annison, 1971; Linzell and Crowe-Swords, unpublished). The mean is about 6 liters/minute for a yield of 20 liters/day, BF/MY 430:1, which is in reasonable agreement with the goat data (Fig. 10). As in the goat, one milk vein was exteriorized as a skin covered loop and minor veins were removed (Fig. 6). Nevertheless, some evidence was obtained that overestimation occurred (udder glucose uptake equal to or greater than entry rate) due to veins crossing between the two halves of the udder, which, as in the goat, should be removed. This is most easily done in dry animals.

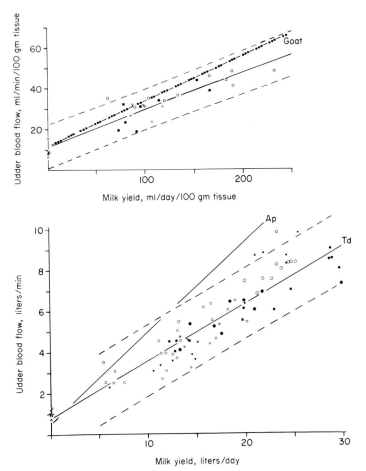

Fig. 10. Relation between milk yield and blood flow, measured by continuous thermodilution in seven cows. Also shown are similar data for the cow using the antipyrine method (Kronfeld, 1969) and for the goat, using thermodilution.

3. Other Species

Since the metabolic rate of small animals is greater than that of large ones, it is not surprising that mammary blood flow per 100 gm of tissue is greater for goats than for cows (Figs. 8 and 10), and one would expect it to be still higher for smaller species. In lactating cats and dogs plethysmography gave figures of only 21 ± 5 ml/minute per 100 gm (Linzell, 1950 and unpublished), but this was probably lowered due to anesthesia and surgery. Isolated glands perfused with perfused lungs in circuit to remove serotonin showed maximum flows of 30 for the cat and 55 for the dog (Hebb and Linzell, 1951), but the rate of milk secretion was not known. The Sapirstein–Fegler techniques give more reliable estimates, and in a guinea pig on day 3 of lactation a figure of 133 was obtained (Linzell and Setchell, unpublished). Recently, using the Sapirstein–Fegler techniques, mammary blood flow has been measured in five conscious rats suckling litters of twelve and was found to be 101 ± 5 ml/minute per 100 gm. (Hanwell and Linzell, 1972).

C. Factors Controlling Mammary Blood Flow

So far two facts have been emphasized. Firstly, in conscious undisturbed animals mammary gland blood flow is relatively stable from hour to hour and day to day, and, secondly, that mild stress readily lowers it. In spite of the fact that both these findings are important aspects of mammary physiology, no one has investigated how they are brought about, neither the cause of the dramatic rise in blood flow at parturition nor the mechanism by which stress and fasting lower it. Both are fruitful fields for further study.

Reynolds (1969), who demonstrated that mammary blood flow in goats begins to rise 2–3 days before parturition, nevertheless suggested that the cause of the increase in udder blood flow at term is that uterine blood is diverted to the mammary glands. However, this cannot be the whole story because, in rats, Linzell (1969) found that although uterine blood flow fell from 10% of the cardiac output (17.2 ± 1.8 ml/minute) to less than 1% within an hour of parturition (1.6 ± 0.13 ml/minute) the mammary gland contribution rose from 4.5% (5.1 ± 0.5 ml/minute) to only 7% (7.91 ± 0.6 ml/minute) during the first day of lactation, and to 8% (9.4 ± 0.5 ml/minute) on day 2.

Most of the substances known to affect the microcirculation in other organs have been tested on the mammary glands, mostly in the isolated perfused preparation or in anesthetized animals.

1. Vasoconstrictors

Mammary blood vessels are exquisitely sensitive to adrenaline and noradrenaline. Doses of 1–10 μg injected or infused IV which have no effect on general blood pressure reduce mammary blood flow in the anesthetized dog (Linzell, 1950; Fig. 1), and in the conscious goat (Linzell, 1971b). Hebb and Linzell (1951) found that when perfused lungs were included in a perfused mammary gland circuit, mammary blood flow increased and the sensitivity to adrenaline increased 100- to 1000-fold; in dogs, cats, and goats the threshold reached was 10^{-8} $\mu g/gm$ of tissue. In Linzell's experiments in which microgram doses IV caused mammary vasoconstriction in dogs and goats (confirmed by Houvenaghel, 1970, in sheep and goats, and Dhondt et al., 1973, in cows), it may be estimated from cardiac output data (Fig. 7) that the concentration of adrenaline reaching the mammary gland is of the order of 10^{-6} $\mu g/ml$ of blood. Since mammary blood flow is about 0.5 ml/gm tissue per minute, the quantity of adrenaline delivered to the tissue is well above the threshold dose. Thus, if it can be established that the adrenal gland in conscious dogs and goats is capable of releasing microgram quantities per minute, then adrenaline is a serious contender as a regulator of mammary blood flow. Measurements are not available, but in anesthetized (Crone, 1965) and conscious sheep (Setchell and Waites, 1962) insulin hypoglycemia causes the continual release for long periods of 0.1–0.5 $\mu g/minute$ per kg body weight, i.e., about 5–10 $\mu g/minute$, which is well within the range that would seriously reduce mammary blood flow. In lactating goats Linzell (1967b) found that insulin hypoglycemia could lower milk yield without altering glucose a — v, which suggests that the udder blood flow fell due to adrenaline release.

In large doses the antidiuretic hormone (ADH vasopressin) is well known to cause vasoconstriction in many organs, and it does also in perfused cows' udders (1000 mU, Petersen, 1942) and in conscious goats 10 mU/minute, Peaker and Linzell, (1973). However, it is very doubtful if the very much smaller quantities that are released in conscious animals in the course of water balance regulation have this vascular response on the mammary glands. Oxytocin in large doses can also cause vasoconstriction in the perfused udder of cows (Petersen, 1942) and goat (Hardwick and Linzell, 1960). However, Reynolds et al. (1968) found in conscious goats that 1000 mU (about 10 times the quantity believed to be released in response to milking) had negligible effects on mammary blood flow and in the work of Linzell and Peaker (1971b) a goat that was very sensitive to oxytocin showed an increase in flow to 20 mU injected ia. Houvenaghel et al. (1972) also found that small doses (100–500 mU) increased udder blood flow in the conscious cow.

Serotonin (5-hydroxytryptamine) is a mammary vasoconstrictor in microgram quantities and is an infernal nuisance in perfusion and other experiments when it is released from platelets as they come in contact with foreign surfaces (see Linzell, 1954; Hardwick and Linzell, 1960; Linzell et al., 1972b). In udder perfusion experiments using whole blood, there is often a fall in blood flow to very low levels over 3–4 hours. This is undoubtedly partly due to serotonin but also to the platelets themselves, which aggregate and progressively block small blood vessels. It is not known whether serotonin release or platelet clumping have these effects in conscious animals under physiological conditions.

Some prostaglandins are pharmacologically vasoactive compounds formed by and released from many organs (Ramwell and Shaw, 1969). Since they are derived from fatty acids, it would not be surprising if the mammary glands that are synthesizing large quantities of fatty acids did not also produce prostaglandins. Pickles (1953), measured changes in mammary blood flow in the human using his baroplethysmograph method (Pickles, 1949, 1952) and his thermal circulation index (Pickles, 1953). He found mammary flow to be lowest during menstruation. Later he pointed out that prostaglandin F_{2a}, which is released from the uterus at this time is a potent constrictor of veins, and suggested that it might reduce mammary blood flow. Linzell (quoted by Pickles, 1967) found that 10 μg had no effect on flow in an isolated perfused goat udder but later found that 28 μg/minute infused into the mammary artery of a conscious goat caused a marked fall in blood flow.

The pCO_2 of mammary venous blood in goats is 50 mm Hg and in perfused glands both a high pO_2 and a low pCO_2 reduce mammary blood flow (Hebb and Linzell, 1951; Kumar *et al.*, 1953; Hardwick and Linzell, 1960; Linzell *et al.*, 1972b). These conditions are produced by equilibrating the blood in the artificial lung with gas mixtures different to those occurring *in vivo* (i.e., higher in O_2 and lower in CO_2 content). It is unlikely that a raised pO_2 ever occurs under physiological conditions, but a fall in pCO_2 could occur in animals that are panting in very hot humid climates and might be related to the poor milk production under such conditions.

Linzell (1950) found that lowering the temperature of the blood in perfusion experiments to 25°C caused a marked but reversible fall in blood flow. However, Hardwick and Linzell (1960) found that goat udders perfused at 34°–36°C gave as much milk as those perfused at 39°C (the normal udder temperature). It seems unlikely that changes in blood temperature would cause changes in mammary blood flow under *in vivo* conditions, but, since the organ is exposed to the atmosphere, this should be borne in mind. Tsakhaev (1959) found that at very low environmental temperatures denervated glands showed a fall in milk yield.

2. Vasodilators

In dogs and cats acetylcholine and histamine in doses of 0.1–1.0 μg both cause vasodilatation (Linzell, 1950); acetylcholine in very small doses and histamine both also cause milk ejection. This was taken by Petersen (1942) to indicate that the mammary glands have a parasympathetic as well as a sympathetic innervation. In detailed anatomic and physiological experiments in goats and sheep, Linzell (1959) could find no evidence for this.

Two substances that also cause mammary vasodilatation in conscious goats are adenosine and bradykinin. Adenosine can also be very useful in perfusion experiments in reversing vasoconstriction due to unknown causes. The adenosine phosphates are also dilator compounds and have been proposed as being concerned in the control of the microcirculation (Holton and Holton, 1954), while recently Hilton and Vrbová (1970) have suggested that phosphate, released during activity, is a dilator in muscle. NaH_2PO_4 is also a dilator in the mammary glands of conscious goats.

Bradykinin is remarkable in that it causes mammary vasodilatation *in vivo* (Reynaert *et al.*, 1968; Linzell *et al.*, 1972) but vasoconstriction *in vitro* (Linzell *et al.*, 1972). Possibly related to this is the fact that reactive hyperemia *in vivo* is reversed to reactive constriction *in vitro*. Thus, in conscious or anesthetized goats following complete cessation of blood flow due to arterial occlusion, when the clamp is removed, the initial blood flow is much raised (Linzell, 1953b; Linzell *et al.*, 1972), suggesting that a vasodilator, produced by the tissue, has accumulated during the period of zero flow. By contrast, when the blood flow is stopped to perfused glands, upon resumption the initial flow is low and only regains its initial value over 2–3 minutes (Linzell *et al.*, 1972), suggesting the production of a vasoconstrictor substance during the period of ischemia.

3. Comment

At present it is not possible to say with certainty whether any of the substances known to alter mammary blood flow are in fact involved in controlling it *in vivo*. This is partly because it is only recently that mammary blood flow can be measured in conscious animals; anesthetized animals are possibly not suitable because flow is already greatly lowered (Linzell, 1971b). Secondly, we have no accurate knowledge of whether any of these substances appear in the circulation of the mammary glands in conscious animals.

IV. MAMMARY LYMPH FLOW

Several reviewers of studies of mammary metabolism by the arteriovenous difference technique have pointed out the potential error of

ignoring lymph flow (e.g., Kay, 1947; Folley, 1949). However, the measurement of this by cannulating lymphatic draining mammary tissue only
became simple when fine plastic tubing became available (Linzell, 1960c).

Most workers who have collected mammary lymph have cannulated
one or more of the main trunks draining a whole gland, but these are
usually most easily found distal to a lymph node, e.g., the superficial
inguinal node. One must be cautious in accepting that this is in fact
mammary lymph because the node has a rich blood supply (see Section
III,B), and Rasmussen and Linzell (1964) showed that antipyrine in
lymph was partially reabsorbed into the bloodstream in the node, raising
the possibility of alteration of lymph quantitatively and qualitatively as it
traverses the node. Lymph ducts afferent to the node are more numerous
but smaller and harder to find, but of course they do carry real mammary
lymph, although no one duct carries lymph from the whole gland; indeed,
some drain mainly the skin and teat (El Hagri, 1945; Ziegler, 1959), and,
since lymph has the same osmotic pressure as plasma, it seems probable
that this equilibrium may be achieved in the node, where there is ample
.opportunity for osmotic equilibration to occur between adjacent lymphatic
sinuses and blood capillaries. However, in some of their experiments on
mammary uptake and release of triglycerides, glycerol, and fatty acids in
the goat, West *et al.* (1972) found that the concentration and specific
radioactivities of these compounds were very similar in lymph collected
from ducts afferent and efferent to the node. An unexpected finding was
that when glycerol and fatty acids were released during the hydrolysis of
doubly labeled triglyceride in the capillary endothelial cells, both passed
extensively across the extracellular space into the secretory cells and then
into milk, but only glycerol appeared in lymph in the expected concentration. Very little labeled fatty acids were found in lymph either afferent
or efferent to the lymph node, although it is known that they crossed the
extracellular space between the blood capillaries and the secretory cells
because they appeared in milk fat in large quantities. These findings are
of general interest in the question of whether lymph is identical to extracellular fluid. In the mammary gland it is not, because it is clear that the
extracellular fluid inside lobules has a different composition (in this case
more fatty acids) than outside where the fluid is first collected to become
lymph.

It must be remembered that lymph nodes also receive lymph from all
other structures in the area: skin, muscle, and connective tissue. In cows,
goats, and sheep this includes the lymphatics of the vulva, and, in these
species, the lymph flow from this organ is very high at parturition and for
a while falsely led me to believe that red blood cells enter mammary
lymph at term (Linzell, 1960c). I was collecting lymph from the efferent

duct of the superficial inguinal lymph node (often called the "mammary node") in a goat in late pregnancy, and just before parturition, blood appeared in the lymph and clotted in the cannula. Later I found that Evans blue dye (T 1824) injected into the tissue around the vulva appeared in the lymph emerging from the superficial inguinal lymph node, so that it was clear that the lymph duct carries lymph from the whole inguinal area, although of course this mostly comes from the mammary glands, the largest organ in the region.

Mammary lymph flow has now been measured often for several weeks continuously, in conscious goats (Linzell, 1960c; Reynolds, 1962), sheep (Lascelles and Morris, 1961), and cows (Peeters et al., 1963; Lascelles et al., 1964), as well as in anesthetized animals (Linzell, 1960c) and in isolated perfused udders (Hardwick and Linzell, 1960; Linzell et al., 1972b).

Mammary lymph flow is higher than from most organs. It is related to the rate of milk secretion and at maximum, over 2 ml/hour per 100 gm of tissue, which is about equal to that from the liver. Nevertheless, the error of ignoring lymph flow in arteriovenous difference work is very small, because mammary blood flow during full lactation is at least 1000 times the rate of flow of lymph flow so that the quantities of substates likely to leave in lymph are much less than the error of measuring mammary uptake from a − v times blood flow.

V. MILK PRECURSORS

A. Methods of Identification

1. Isotopes

The increasing availability of labeled biochemical compounds have added greatly to our knowledge of milk synthesis. However, there are snags. A labeled substance may be transformed into another compound elsewhere in the body, which is in turn taken up by the mammary gland and used to synthesize some milk component. For example, labeled lactate is readily transformed into glucose in the liver, and the labeled glucose is converted to lactose in the mammary gland. Thus, the results of such an experiment do not show that the mammary glands take up lactate and make lactose from it. Nevertheless, there is a net uptake of lactate by the mammary glands (Linzell, 1968) so there is the possibility of incorporation of its carbon into milk compounds. A way around this problem is either to use the isolated perfused gland or to give the labeled lactate to one gland and to compare the specific activities of lactose and other milk components in the milk of this gland (*I*) with those of the other glands (*C*); if the *I/C* ratio is significantly greater than 1.0 this will demonstrate local incorporation by the injected gland. Kleiber and Luick (1956) injected their isotope into the teat canal, but this does not yield quantitative data. Wood *et al.* (1957) infused into the artery of one side of the udder, even diverting the venous blood for a period to increase the chance of detecting a raised *I/C* ratio. However, the surgery involved lowered the milk yield and partly vitiated the quantitative results. To simplify arterial catheterization previous exteriorization of the vessel as a skin covered loop gives the greatest chance of causing minimal disturbance of the animal. This is difficult *in situ* (Linzell, 1963a), and in the goat and sheep, in particular, it is necessary to divide the vessels crossing between the two glands. In goats, the most effective solution is to transplant one gland to the neck, where the artery is anastomosed to one carotid artery, which is exteriorized as a skin covered loop (Linzell, 1963b). These preparations lactate excellently and can be used in such studies for years (see Linzell, 1971b). Since the mammary vein is joined to the jugular, arteriovenous measurements are also easily made and now blood flow can be continually monitored at any time by the application of an ultrasonic flowmeter to the exteriorized artery percutaneously (see Section III,A,6).

A further difficulty in interpreting isotopic data is that, within the mammary tissue itself, labeled atoms may be transferred to other compounds by exchange reactions due to the overlap of metabolic pathways, so that the label ends up in several different products in the milk. Some biochemists have considered that this is an insuperable bar to the interpretation of isotopic data. However, it is to be hoped that, as we get more complete data of the total throughput of all compounds, it will be possible to give a complete description of the movement of atoms from plasma into milk (see Fig. 21). Clearly, a computer will be necessary but I suspect that the definition of precursors and products will be then a question of semantics.

2. *In Vitro* Techniques

These all give clear answers and tell one what the tissue can do, but not necessarily what it does do *in vivo*.

a. HOMOGENATES AND TISSUE SLICES. These have been used mainly for fundamental biochemical studies, which have considerably assisted in the identification of milk precursors. Modern ancillary aids such as ^{14}C- and

[3]H-labeled compounds, liquid scintillation counting, chromatography, etc., have considerably increased the usefulness of these simple techniques so that, doubtless, they will continue to be used. Usually the normality of slices is assumed rather than assessed. However, the O_2 uptake of goat udder slices (Folley and French, 1949) is the same as that measured *in vivo* (Linzell, 1960b) and, as might be expected, O_2 uptake per gram of tissue was much higher for small animals. Linzell and Peaker (1971c) noted that intracellular [K] was higher in slices of mammary tissue incubated in nutrient media than in fresh tissue. In fact "fresh tissue" has suffered anoxia following the killing of the animal, which allows K to leak from the cells.

For incubations lasting longer than 3 hours it is essential to avoid contamination with microorganisms because their rate of multiplication is such that their metabolism could become a substantial fraction of the total at and after this time.

b. Isolated Mammary Cells.   Unfortunately these lose the ability to synthesize lactose in 16–18 hours even though they survive for long periods (Ebner and Larson, 1959). Nevertheless, bovine cells separated from fat cells aseptically by treatment with collagenase (Ebner *et al.*, 1961) and subsequent centrifugation in 0.33 M sucrose are very useful in short experiments, and, recently, Kinsella and McCarthy (1968) have shown that fat synthesis and secretion goes on for 3 days at a rate similar to that *in vivo*. They were even able to watch by phase contrast microscopy the slow expulsion of lipid droplets from the cells. Pitelka *et al.* (1969) found that although the cells' ultrastructure showed abnormalities during preparation they quickly reverted to normal once they were incubated in nutrient media, and Abraham *et al.* (1972) showed that such cells synthesize fat, lactose, and protein, at greater rates than slices. Twarog and Larson (1964) showed that the later loss of the ability to synthesize lactose was accompanied by a loss of UDPG pyrophosphorylase activity. If the cause of this can be discovered and remedied, the usefulness of *in vitro* preparations might be considerably enhanced.

c. Organ Culture.   The technique, in which little pieces of mammary tissue rather than separated cells of pregnant mice are cultured, is now being used extensively in endocrinological studies (see Forsyth, 1971). Great emphasis has been laid on the response of the tissue to hormones, with evidence of synthesis of casein (Turkington and Topper, 1966) and ultrastructural signs of secretion, but a serious fact is that lactose synthesis has been reported to be very low (Forsyth *et al.*, 1969). This may be because the hormonal treatment is not optimal. Normal lactating tissue has not been cultured and this might synthesize more lactose in organ culture. Clearly a more detailed assessment of this potentially valuable technique is needed.

d. Perfusion. Whole mammary glands maintained in isolation are the easiest *in vitro* preparation to assess, because milk yield can be measured directly and compared with the previous yield *in vivo*. This was not reported by early workers (Foa, 1912; Petersen *et al.*, 1941; Peeters and Massart, 1947), but it later became clear that the yield is only about half or less of what it had been on the animal before perfusion in cows (Tindal, 1957) and goats (Hardwick and Linzell, 1960; Linzell *et al.*, 1972b). The most detailed studies are of those in the goat (Hardwick and Linzell, 1960; Linzell *et al.*, 1972b). The strange thing is that the yield does not behave as early workers assumed, i.e., normal at first and then falling steadily as the preparation fails. The yield falls immediately when perfusion starts but is maintained at 50% of previous for 6–8 hours and then starts to decline. The preparation is satisfactory in that milk is only produced if substrates are given, and the composition of the minimum requirements of glucose, fatty acids, amino acids, and minerals is very similar in its properties to what is removed by the goats udder *in vivo* (Table III). The addition of minor components and hormones brings about no improvement in milk yield, and β-hydroxybutyrate, lactate, and chylomicra, which are taken up from the plasma *in vivo* can be omitted from the substrates without producing a further fall in yield. The perfused gland is also a little different in its amino acid requirements (Mepham, 1971; Linzell *et al.*, 1972b).

In spite of deficiencies, perfused mammary glands have provided important data. Petersen and Ludwick (1942) showed that blood taken from a cow just after milk ejection, caused ejection when given to a perfused udder. Hardwick *et al.* (1961) discovered that glucose is essential for milk secretion by showing that without it the yield is negligible and that as soon as it is given secretion starts within an hour. Other sugars cannot substitute for glucose (Linzell *et al.*, 1972b), and it is difficult to see how this work could have been done without the perfused gland. Later Hardwick *et al.* (1963) showed that glucose was a more important source of energy than acetate. Uptake of chylomicra and their use to form milk fat was first conclusively shown in perfused glands (Lascelles *et al.*, 1964).

Thus in all *in vitro* techniques quantitative data must be treated with reserve, and data can even be different qualitatively from that obtained *in vivo*. The onus is on the experimenter to ascertain how normal his preparation is and to assess the significance of his data.

3. Measurement of Arteriovenous Differences *in Vivo*

As emphasized in the introduction, these must be made by simultaneously taking samples of arterial and mammary venous blood under stable conditions. Thus, the main emphasis of this section is on efficient sampling of arterial and venous blood in conscious calm animals.

However, successful measurement of a − v can give misleading data. For example, in the case of plasma free fatty acids (FFA), there is no significant a − v, but they are in fact taken up and used to synthesize milk fatty acids. The reason is that the uptake is masked by the simultaneous release of fatty acids into the venous blood. In this case it was only when labeled FFA were infused and were found to be transferred to milk in quantity that the true mechanism came to light (see Section V, B,3).

a. Avoidance of Stress. Early workers in the field appreciated that stress can vitiate arteriovenous measurements, and several studies were made on methods of detecting and avoiding it (see Folley, 1949). Graham *et al.* (1936a), who devised the technique of taking arterial blood from cows from the iliac arteries per rectum, recommended using three operators, taking the venous blood first (as this causes less distress) and that, if more than 4 minutes was taken in all, the attempt should be abandoned as the results would be worthless. They also stressed that the hematocrit of the arterial and venous samples should be almost identical, and they routinely measured this as a check. Graham *et al.* (1936a) did this because they thought that blood can become markedly concentrated or diluted in its passage through the udder in stress, but this seems improbable. Barcroft *et al.* (1925) showed that the spleen in dogs acts as a reservoir of red blood cells, which are rapidly injected into the circulation when it contracts in response to exercise and stress. In the goat and horse this can raise the hematocrit up to 25% in a short time (Anderson and Rogers, 1957; Tarten and Schalm, 1964), and this seems to be the most likely cause of rapid changes in hematocrit in disturbed conscious animals. Thus, it is equally as important to take notice of the arterial level as it is to ascertain that arterial and venous values are identical. In this laboratory in lactating animals the arterial hematocrit of samples taken via indwelling catheters is $27 \pm 1.7\%$ in goats, $28 \pm 0.3\%$ in cows, $26 \pm 2\%$ in horses, and $31.5 \pm 1.3\%$ in pigs.

It is possible to detect distress by careful observation of the animal. Dilatation of the pupil is a sensitive indicator, but a rise in blood pressure and tachycardia can also occur. Linzell (1971b), found that in the presence of such signs in the goat there is a fall in mammary blood flow, and that even simple venipuncture can initiate these reactions. Since the blood flow in transplanted (i.e., denervated) glands also falls, this is probably due to circulating adrenaline. Adrenaline also releases glucose from liver glycogen so a raised blood glucose may also be evidence of stress. In this laboratory measurements of arterial blood glucose concentrations in conscious undisturbed catheterized lactating animals give values of 45.5 ± 1.5 mg/100 ml blood in goats, 52 ± 2 in cows, 52.5 ± 2.8 in pigs, and 59.5 ± 4.5 in horses. Therefore, in the experiments of Foa (1908b), Lintzel (1934) on goats, where arterial glucose was 97.6 and 71.3 mg/100 ml, respectively, in those of Shaw *et al.* (1938) on cows and Charton *et al.* (1965) on sheep, where arterial glucose rose as high as 82 and 130 mg/100 ml and in those of Spincer *et al.* (1969) on pigs, where arterial plasma glucose was 122 ± 4 mg/100 ml, it seems possible that the animals were stressed, so that there is some doubt about the accuracy of these measurements. Arterial lactate may be also raised in excitement from less than 10 mg/100 ml in cows (Powell and Shaw, 1942; Hartmann, 1966) and goats (Linzell, 1968) to over 60 mg/100 ml (Shaw *et al.*, 1938) and at the higher levels there is an increased mammary a − v.

Reineke *et al.* (1941a,b) in goats and Shaw (1946) in cows used general anesthesia as a means of avoiding stress because it reduced variability in arteriovenous differences. However, Linzell (1960b, 1971b) found that general anesthesia in goats can markedly reduce mammary blood flow and milk yield, particularly if combined with surgery. This is partly due to abnormal posture because holding a goat on its side reduces mammary blood flow, whereas cyclopropane anesthesia (after pentobarbitone induction) for 2.5–5 hours in sitting goats, had very little effect on milk yield. Pentobarbitone anesthesia in lactating prone rats did not reduce cardiac output, mammary blood flow, or milk yield (Hanwell and Linzell, 1972) and in pigs a − v of many substrates were not significantly different from values obtained in conscious animals (Spincer *et al.*, 1969), although Linzell *et al.* (1969) did note a fall in a − v of glucose and amino acids and a rise in FFA levels. Linzell *et al.* (1969) found that the tranquilizer Spiperone immobilized lactating sows for catheterization of blood vessels under local anesthesia and did not appear to influence a − v, mammary blood flow, or milk yield. In goats it is difficult to immobilize the animal and leave it standing, which is necessary for sampling mammary venous blood. A further snag in using anesthesia or tranquilizers in goats is that if mammary blood flow does fall (e.g., from change of posture) its recovery is very slow, often taking an hour or more (Linzell, 1960b). Clearly, a − v measurements would be meaningless during this period.

Thus sedation and tranquilization can be used to obtain arterial and mammary venous samples from fractious, dangerous, or timid animals, but it must be borne in mind that defense reactions can be induced that could give misleading data and, if possible, one should monitor mammary blood flow and milk yield. It seems preferable to familiarize the animal to the experimental set up and to take samples from previously catheterized vessels particularly in ruminants. The development of a more efficient tranquilizer would be a boon.

b. SAMPLING ARTERIAL BLOOD IN CONSCIOUS UNDISTURBED ANIMALS. It is generally recognized that blood is so thoroughly mixed in the heart and lungs that blood in all the arteries is identical in composition. Therefore, it is not necessary to obtain blood from the mammary arteries themselves, and this is very fortunate because they are often rather small and/or inaccessible: of course, it is also important that mammary blood flow should not be reduced, as it easily can be, by spasm, due to needle puncture or due to the presence of a catheter reducing the cross-sectional area of the mammary artery.

Another important fact is that puncture of an arterial wall is painful when done with anything but a very fine sharp needle (Linzell, 1963a). Even where local anesthesia is used, the amount of restraint needed can be sufficient to induce mild stress responses, and as Zierler (1961) has clearly shown these must be avoided in arteriovenous difference work. In some very docile animals with a carotid loop the artery can be punctured with a fine sharp needle, but it is far safer to be certain of obtaining stable conditions to insert a catheter under local anesthesia and to wait for at least an hour before sampling.

Following Kaufmann and Magne (1906), early workers regarded jugular blood as "arterial" as far as the udder is concerned in cows. Blackwood and Stirling (1932) found that jugular hematocrit is raised, which they wrongly thought is because the head of ruminants removes much water during salivation. Later Folley and Peskett (1934) found that compressing the jugular veins with a tourniquet raises the hematocrit (see also Section V,A,3,a). If properly taken from undisturbed animals, there is little difference in hematocrit between carotid and jugular blood (Table II). However, since the head and neck in farm animals is largely bone, skin, and muscle, it is not surprizing that jugular blood has significantly less acetate, and more lactate and amino acids than the carotid blood. Human muscles also release amino acids (Felig *et al.*, 1970). It is clearly unwise to regard jugular blood as arterial as far as the mammary glands are concerned. Indeed, one should be cautious in regarding jugular blood as typical of general circulating blood in ruminants; this advice is almost universally ignored, even though it is easy to catheterize the right ventricle and pulmonary artery via the jugular vein without the use of X-rays in the standing horse (Chauveau and Marey, 1861), goat (Linzell, 1966c), and cow (Kronfeld *et al.*, 1968). Various arteries have been used to collect blood in conscious animals.

i. *Cow.* Blackwood and Stirling (1932) punctured the radial artery and Graham *et al.* (1936a) used the external iliac artery approached per rectum or per vaginam (Maynard *et al.*, 1938). However, the latter and subsequent workers (Shaw and Petersen, 1939) found that this is apt to distress the animal. Fisher (1956) described a technique of puncturing the brachial artery where it crosses the first rib with a 10-cm 18 gauge needle inserted just medial to the point of the shoulder 15° below horizontal; of course local anesthesia must be used. It is not known if catheters can be inserted into the artery through the needle or over a wire by Seldinger's (1953) technique at such a depth.

TABLE II

COMPOSITION OF BLOOD TAKEN FROM THE CAROTID ARTERY (A), PULMONARY ARTERY (PA), AND JUGULAR VEIN (JV) IN RUMINANTS[a]

Sample	A	PA	JV
Hematocrit (%)	25 ± 0.6	24.8 ± 0.72	26 ± 0.93
Blood glucose (mg/100 ml)	41.0 ± 1.9	40.3 ± 2.0	40.0 ± 1.95
Blood lactate (mg/100 ml)	4.6 ± 0.38	5.08 ± 0.52	5.83 ± 0.55[b]
Plasma *a*-amino N (mg/100 ml)	5.01 ± 0.57	4.97 ± 0.69	6.41 ± 0.75[b]
Plasma free fatty acids (mEq/liter)	0.32 ± 0.01	0.39 ± 0.03	0.34 ± 0.03
Plasma acetate (mEq/liter)	1.37 ± 0.16	1.30 ± 0.15	0.92 ± 0.18[c]

[a] The samples were taken simultaneously from unrestrained fed animals (three lactating and two dry goats and two lactating cows) via indwelling catheters. Paired t tests showed that A and PA were not significantly different but that JV was for lactate, amino acids, and acetate. Mean ± S.E. of mean.

[b] $p < 0.05$.

[c] $p < 0.001$.

Emery *et al.* (1965) reported in several papers using "tail" blood as arterial. It is apparent that some times they hit the coccygeal artery and sometimes the coccygeal vein, but they argue that this is immaterial since the tail is mostly skin, bone, and tendon, which remove very small quantities of substrates so that tail venous blood is almost identical in composition to arterial blood This they found to be true for glucose and acetate, but it would have to be demonstrated for other compounds. In cows I have catheterized the coccygeal artery, and one advantage is that the tail can be easily anesthetized by epidural injection of local anesthetic into the sacrococcygeal space. Thus, one can take a little time to find the artery without stressing the animal. Using epidural anesthesia, I have also catheterized the perineal artery below the vulva. An incision is needed because the vessel is 2–5 cm deep. However, once found in the fat it is easy to cannulate.

In my opinion, the most satisfactory way of obtaining arterial blood in cows is to catherize the carotid artery a few hours before the experiment. I have done this by making conventional loops of Van Leersum (1911) (see Linzell, 1963a) or by bringing the artery under the skin just lateral to the jugular vein where it can be catheterized percutaneously. As pointed out by Kronfeld *et al.* (1968), it is not necessary to implant a plastic plate beneath the artery as recommended by Hartmann and Lascelles (1964); if the muscle is carefully sewn beneath it, the artery remains subcutaneous indefinitely.

ii. *Sheep and goat.* In goats Lintzel (1934) employed cardiac puncture, and much earlier Barcroft *et al.* (1919) were able to puncture the left ventricle from the fourth intercostal space on the left and the right ventricle from the third space, and thus to measure cardiac output. However, their animals were held on their right sides, and, even with training, some struggled.

Many workers have inserted catheters under anesthesia into various arteries of sheep and goats and brought the end of the catheter out of the back; these catheters have remained patent for days or even weeks. For long experiments it is best if the end of the catheter lies in a fast flowing stream (e.g., the aorta) as this decreases the chance of thrombi forming on the end of the catheter.

For longer term and for the greatest certainty and facility most workers agree that a carotid loop is best (Graham *et al.*, 1937). Later, Bone *et al.* (1962) and Jha *et al.* (1961) reported that carotid loops have a limited life in sheep and goats, but I have exteriorized the carotid, often both left and right, by Van Leersum's (1911) technique in 60 goats. With care these remain patent and useful for the remainder of the animal's life (up to 8 years in my laboratory).

iii. *Pig.* To collect arterial blood without disturbance in lactating sows, it is necessary to cannulate the vessel beforehand under local or general anesthesia. Pig arteries are relatively difficult to catheterize because they readily go into intense spasm, and rigid catheters, as they are advanced into the vessel, can easily separate the intima from the media causing blockage. However, once successfully cannulated it is easy to bring the catheter out through the skin of the back or flank, and this is tolerated remarkably well by the sow. However, the piglets, which are very inquisitive and very efficient at rooting with their snouts, very quickly damage interesting objects projecting from their mother. Quite elaborate metal covers are necessary to protect the catheters between sampling periods (Linzell *et al.*, 1969, Fig. 11). Arteries that have been

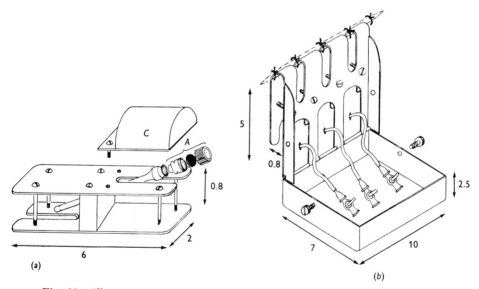

Fig. 11. Illustration of two methods used of bringing catheters through the skin of sows, which allowed easy sampling and prevented damage when not in use. a, Luer-lok hypodermic needle fixed to a block, which is sandwiched between two plates fixed to the skin, one inside and the other outside. The catheter can be flushed through by injecting through the rubber diaphragm of the male adaptor (A), which is removed for sampling. A cover (C) protects the assembly from investigation by the piglets. b, Metal box fixed to the skin, which can be closed over catheter holes and also contains the light plastic tap closing the catheters. Both devices were made of stainless steel, dimensions in centimeters; the only critical dimension is 0.8 cm, the thickness of the skin. Not drawn to scale. (From Linzell *et al.*, 1969.)

successfully used in sows are the carotid, internal saphenous, external pudic, and superficial mammary branches of the internal thoracic (Linzell *et al.*, 1969; Weirich *et al.*, 1970). The auricular artery can also be cannulated (Anderson and Elsley, 1969), but it is rather too small to obtain reasonably sized blood samples quickly for mammary work.

iv. *Horse.* It is possible to puncture the external maxillary and even the carotid artery (lateral to the jugular, 15–25 cm in front of the shoulder, Gabel *et al.*, 1964) but whether the needle can be left in long enough or a catheter can be inserted through it over the wire by Seldinger's technique is not known. Tavenor (1969) says that there is not enough skin to make carotid loops in horses, but I have found that this is not true. However, as in the cow a simpler technique is to relocate the artery subcutaneously by stitching muscle beneath it lateral to the jugular. It is not necessary to support the artery by a plastic plate as recommended by Tavenor (1969).

c. Sampling Mammary Venous Blood in Conscious Animals. Theoretically this should present no difficulties if the location of the mammary veins is known. However, there is a danger of obtaining nonmammary blood, particularly in ruminants and horses, so the subject warrants discussion because, as mentioned in the history of the subject, interesting and important changes occur in mammary venous drainage, with age and parity.

d. Variations in Venous Drainage of Mammary Glands. In all animals the skin of the ventral abdomen is principally supplied by two arteries and their accompanying veins. The first emerges through the muscle beside the xiphisternum and originates from the internal thoracic vessels (called "internal mammary," for obvious reasons, in man). These vessels pass backwards beneath the skin and anastomose with the second pair of main vessels, which pass through the inguinal canal and mainly supply the groin. These vessels are most correctly called the "cranial" and "caudal superficial epigastric," but the posterior vessels are often called the "subcutaneous abdominal," and the vein is, of course, the milk vein of cows, sheep, and goats. It is often forgotten that the milk vein is accompanied by an artery.

In pigs, dogs, cats, and rabbits the mammary glands lie all along the abdomen and are supplied by the cranial and caudal superficial epigastric vessels, which enlarge to form a single pair of large vessels running dorsal to and often through mammary tissue (see Section II). A catheter passed well into this vein, almost anywhere along the abdomen, will mainly sample mammary venous blood in these lactating animals, i.e., the proportion of blood from skin and subcutaneous tissue will be small providing, of course, that the tip of the catheter does not lie near any gland that has involuted due to not being suckled. After a few days of lactation involution is easily detected because such a gland is smaller than the rest.

In ruminants, horses, and guinea pigs, the mammary glands are inguinal and so only the caudal superficial epigastric vessels drain the mammary tissue (Linzell, 1960a, Figs. 12, 13). However, as is well known, the cranial superficial epigastric vein is also enlarged in ruminants in lactation and forms the front part of the milk vein. It remains small in virgin females and males. The reason for the enlargement of this vein in breeding females is that valves become incompetent as the posterior vein enlarges to carry away the large amount of blood entering the inguinal area as the mammary glands begin to function. The functional valves normally ensure that blood drains forwards into the cranial vein at the front of the abdomen and backward into the caudal vein at the back, but this is only true in males and virgin females (Fig. 13).

The situation has been most extensively studied in goats. In young animals and in males, the valves were found to be competent, and the vein in front of the udder contained no mammary blood. However, as the udder grows, the great increase in blood flow into the inguinal area dilates

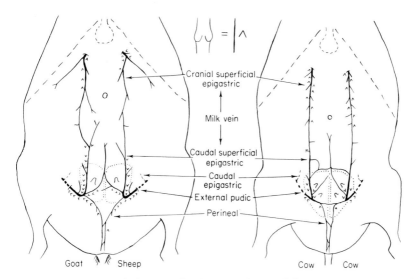

Fig. 12. Diagram of the superficial veins of the abdomen in ruminants. The angles of branching and position of the valves clearly indicate the direction of blood flow. All the veins are accompanied by arteries. (From Linzell, 1960a.)

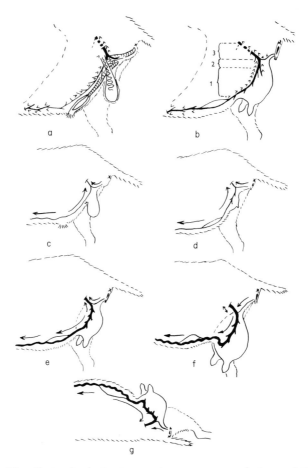

Fig. 13. The effects of valvular incompetence on venous drainage of the udder in goats. a and b, Position of valves in the male and female. (1) Valves always incompetent in breeding females; (2) valves usually incompetent in older females; (3) valves sometimes incompetent in old females. c–g, Usual direction of venous blood flow in standing animals. c, All males; d, virgin females; e, primiparous females; f, multiparous females; g, direction of flow in all females, when held supine. (From Linzell, 1960a.)

the vein, and some of the forward valves become incompetent, so that when the animal stands some mammary blood flows forward into the milk vein as was always thought. In some older animals, and in most parous goats in very late pregnancy, the rise in intraabdominal pressure causes incompetency of valves in the external pudic vein as well and forces some blood from the abdomen into the milk vein. In that case only a proportion of blood carried in the milk vein is of mammary origin, sometimes less than half (Fig. 14; Linzell, 1960a, 1966a).

In the standing animal the veins of the abdominal wall form an alternate route to the vena cava for the return of udder blood to the heart, but they empty into the anterior (cranial) and not posterior (caudal) vena cava. Since these two venous channels also meet in the inguinal region (Fig. 6), a complete circle is formed so that there must be some point at which the flow divides to enter either the cranial or caudal vena cava. In virgin females and males, the "watershed" point is near the umbilicus for the superficial veins, but in older females, owing to the valvular incompetence, it moves further backward and small variations in the position of this critical point have a great influence on mammary venous drainage. In goats four alternative conditions may exist in standing animals (Fig. 13):

1. The milk vein contains no mammary venous blood, because all the valves are competent. This obtains in males and virgin females and changes during the first pregnancy to condition (2).

2. The milk vein has mammary venous blood, but it originates from the front of the udder only, because the front valves only are competent.

3. The milk vein carries the total venous outflow, because all the valves in the milk vein are incompetent but those in the external pudic are competent. This occurs in a proportion of animals in the second lactation and beyond.

4. The milk vein contains all the mammary venous blood plus a variable amount from the abdomen due to incompetence of valves in the external pudic vein as well (Figs. 14, 15). This occurs in about 30% of mature lactating goats, and probably in all in late pregnancy, except the first.

As Becker and Arnold (1942) first demonstrated, in cows the perineal vein never carries mammary blood away from the udder but takes vulval blood into the external pudic veins (Figs. 13, 14). In conditions (1) and (2) this blood returns to the heart via the external pudic veins, but in conditions (3) and (4) it enters the milk vein in standing animals. This, is then a source of error, but fortunately in all goats, except virgins, it is too small a proportion of the total flow to be of consequence.

When animals are lying down all are in condition (1), because the milk vein is compressed. They are also in condition (1) when lying on their backs (Linzell, 1960a).

Fewer cows have been studied physiologically, but the situation is basically the same as in goats, although somewhat more in the experimenter's favor. Twenty-five udders have been dissected, and in ten cases

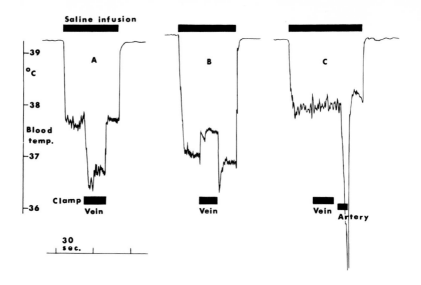

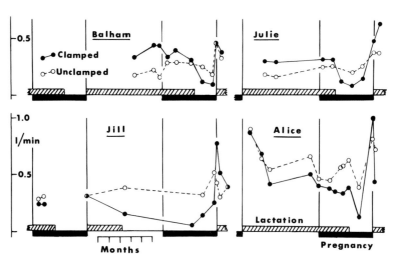

Fig. 14. *Top,* Effects in goats of manual compression of external pudic vein on flow in the "milk vein" loop. A, Flow decreases. B, Flow increases. C, No effect, but occluding artery just behind the vein reduced the flow. *Bottom,* Measurements of flow in the milk vein of goats with and without manual clamping of the external pudic vein, at different stages of the reproductive cycle. See Figs. 6 and 13 for anatomy. In all four animals when they were not lactating, if clamping was omitted, udder blood flow would be seriously overestimated, but during lactation the results are consistent and characteristic of the animal. (From Linzell, 1966a by permission of the American Heart Association Inc.)

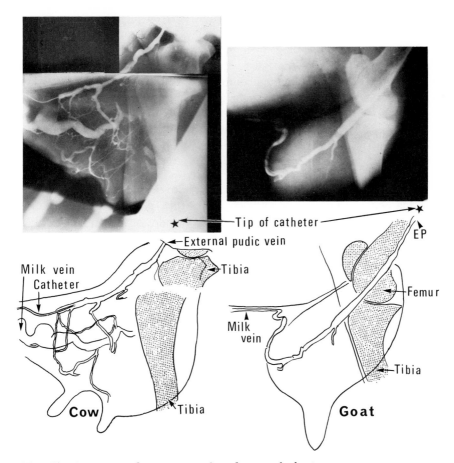

Fig. 15. Angiograms demonstrating that, due to valvular incompetence, nonmammary venous blood can enter the milk vein from the external pudic vein in a Jersey cow and a Saanen goat. Catheters were passed from the milk vein back into the external pudic vein in the standing animal. Note the S-shaped bend within the udder of the goat. See Fig. 13.

angiography of the mammary veins was carried out in the living animal beforehand. There are fewer backwardly pointing valves in the milk vein of cows than in sheep and goats and these are well within the udder (Fig. 12) so that by 1 year of age (before puberty) the milk vein just in front of the udder contains blood from the front glands, in standing animals (Linzell, 1960a). In three cows injection of contrast medium into the external pudic vein showed that the valves there were incompetent,

and, because the radio-opaque medium was detected in the milk vein
(Fig. 15) and in two others, the valves were partially incompetent.
Further quantitative studies were made on seven surgically prepared cows
(five Jerseys and two Friesians), with a milk vein loop and minor veins
removed. The effect of manual compression of the external pudic vein was
tested as in the goat (Fig. 13) for its effect on the rate of blood flow in
the milk vein. In three late pregnant animals this usually caused a fall in
flow, but during lactation this occurred only 9 times out of twenty-nine
trials, and the maximum dilution with nonmammary blood was 60%,
mean 26%, on these occasions.

   i. *Ruminants.*   We are now in a position to decide how to get a sample
of mammary venous blood from any animal. It is essential to try to obtain
venous blood that is representative of the whole organ. Under anesthesia
it is safest to sample from the external pudic vein after having tied off
all other veins. In conscious animals, one has two choices, either to sample
from the external pudic, or from the more accessible milk vein. To sample
from the external pudic vein catheters can be passed into it via the
perineal vein, via a branch supplying lateral udder skin and inside of the
thigh, or via one of the venous branches crossing the midline. However,
surgery is required to cannulate all these vessels. In some conscious
animals catheters can be passed easily backwards along the milk vein
into the external pudic, but in most this is difficult because of its great
tortuosity (Fig. 15). To sample from the milk vein is easy, but it must
be remembered that it only carries mammary venous blood in standing
animals over a certain age, which is 1 year in cattle and after the first
half of pregnancy in goats, and in such animals the proportion of blood
from surrounding tissue may form a sizeable proportion of the total.
Animals in condition (3) may be sought, but they must be studied carefully to ascertain this (Linzell, 1960a, 1966a), and there is the risk that
they will pass to condition (4) where nonmammary blood passes, in
standing animals, from the abdomen to the milk vein. Ligation of the
external pudic vein to prevent this (Graham, 1937) is unsatisfactory because when the animal lies down the milk vein is occluded and, with
both major exits closed, many small collaterals open up (Linzell, 1960a).
Temporary occlusion with plastic snares and inflatable cuffs were satisfactory for a few days, but ultimately all foreign substances tied around
vessels surgically cause thrombosis and then blood leaves via the collateral
veins (Linzell, 1960a). Eventually the simple and effective method was
devised of manually compressing the external pudic between the udder
and the abdomen at the time of sampling or flow measurement when the

animal is standing (Fig. 6). In a goat one gently grips the base of the udder high in the groin. The paired external pudic veins lie immediately in front of the arteries, which pass vertically into the udder, and certainly will be squeezed if the arteries are felt pulsating just behind the fingers and thumb. This has been confirmed by observing the effect of this compression on blood flow recorded continuously in the milk vein (Linzell, 1966a), using the continuous thermodilution method or ultrasonic flowmeter (Fig. 14).

Manual compression of the external pudic vein is not so easy in cows, because the lateral suspensory ligament of the udder is thicker than in the goat. This makes it less easy to palpate the artery, which is the landmark, and less easy to decide whether one is occluding the vein. In the goat there is often a brief surge in flow as the vein is released, which is characteristic of successful compression, irrespective of whether the mean flow is raised or lowered during occlusion. This is a useful sign in the cow also.

ii. *Pig.* The abdominal skin is drained by the same veins as in ruminants, but glands lie all along the abdomen. The homologous vein to the "milk vein" of ruminants lies just lateral to the abdominal mammary glands and is visible through the skin in many animals (Fig. 16). This can then be punctured with a needle or a catheter can be inserted percutaneously. Care should be taken to see that the glands immediately adjacent to the sampling site are being suckled so that true mammary venous blood is obtained.

However, usually the animal will be anesthetized to insert an arterial catheter as well. Thus, it is just as well to simultaneously insert a venous catheter into the vein in a region draining a fully functional gland. Usually this can be done via a skin side-branch (Fig. 16) so that flow is not reduced (Linzell *et al.*, 1969). The catheter is brought out of the skin of the flank beside the arterial catheter (Fig. 11).

iii. *Horse.* The venous drainage of the horse udder is basically similar to that in cows, goats, and sheep except that there is on each side an additional large vein (not accompanied by an artery) that drains into the femoral vein (Barone and Monnet, 1955). This vein usually joins the external pudic vein and Nishinakagawa (1970) calls it the principal mammary vein. However, my dissections show that this vein also receives several large branches draining the perineum, the inside of the thigh, and the skin lateral to the udder, which can be used to catheterize it. The vein in front of the udder, at first glance, appears to be the "milk vein" (Fig. 17). However, it does not carry mammary venous blood because the

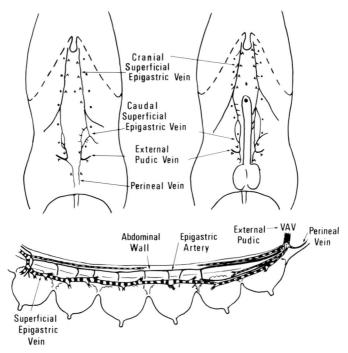

Fig. 16. Veins of pig mammary glands. *Top*, Dissections of female and male piglets, showing the superficial abdominal veins (and their valves), which drain the mammary glands in adults. *Bottom*, Dissection of mammary glands of a lactating sow. The mammary arteries are chiefly derived from the epigastric artery whilst the veins drain into the superficial epigastric veins.

valves remain competent. It may be a tributory of either the external pudic or the principal vein, and it is often difficult, without surgery, to pass catheters back along into either of the main veins. A further difficulty is that there is very great individual variation. I have dissected six lactating udders and no two are the same in their venous drainage (Fig. 17).

B. Identified Precursors

Arteriovenous differences have been successfully measured in conscious undisturbed cows, goats, and pigs and are very similar in each species (Table III). The most data available are for the goat, and this is plotted in Fig. 18 to illustrate the magnitude of the extraction of various blood constituents and also to show that the main precursors of milk are

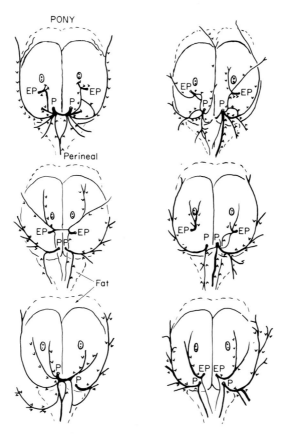

Fig. 17. Variations in venous drainage of the udder in the lactating horse. One pony (*top, left*) and five thoroughbreds. EP, External pudic vein; this is accompanied by the main artery (not shown); P, principal vein, which empties into the femoral, and frequently joins the EP and the opposite P. This vein mainly drains the skin of the thigh and perineum.

glucose, fatty acids, amino acids, and minerals, a very simple mixture, which also proves to be very similar to that required by isolated perfused glands to maintain milk secretion (Hardwick and Linzell, 1960; Linzell *et al.*, 1972b). The mammary metabolism of the major milk precursors are reviewed by Annison (1971), Mepham (1971), and Bickerstaffe (1971).

Barry (1964), in a critical review of the identification of milk precursors by arteriovenous measurements, commented increduously on the variability of a − v quoted in the literature and somewhat reluctantly concluded that to demonstrate uptake, extraction must be more than 20%. However, two factors are concerned, analytic error and biological variation. Not

TABLE III

Arteriovenous Differences across the Mammary Glands of Conscious Lactating Animals[a]

	Goat A	Goat E	Cow A	Cow E	Pig A	Pig E
Blood						
O_2, vols/100 ml	11.85 ± 0.8 (38)	45 ± 1.3 (38)	14.37 ± 0.24 (19)	29 ± 1.3 (19)	12.9 ± 0.6 (6)	33 ± 6 (6)
Glucose (mg/100 ml)	45.5 ± 1.5 (34)	33 ± 1.4 (34)	49.5 ± 1.3 (29)	25 ± 1.3 (29)	6.6 ± 1.3 (13)	30 ± 1.2 (13)
Acetate (mg/100 ml)	8.9 ± 0.6 (34)	63 ± 2 (34)	9.07 ± 0.56 (28)	56 ± 2 (28)	1.90 ± 0.02 (11)	45 ± 1.5 (11)
Lactate (mg/100 ml)	7.13 ± 0.3 (11)	28 ± 3 (11)	8.2 ± 0.61 (30)	10 ± 3 (30)	12.5 ± 0.75 (11)	15 ± 2 (11)
Plasma, (mg/100 ml)						
β-Hydroxybutyrate	5.8 ± 0.47 (9)	57 ± 3 (9)	5.3 ± 0.62 (23)	40 ± 4 (23)	1.24 ± 0.04 (11)	15 ± 1.2 (11)
Acetoacetate	0.25 ± 0.05 (4)	8 ± 8 (4)	0.55 ± 0.011 (8)	34 ± 13 (8)	0.58 ± 0.03 (7)	2 ± 4 (7)
Triglycerides	21.9 ± 2.5 (10)	40 ± 5 (10)	9.04 ± 0.69 (20)	58 ± 2 (20)	31.9 (11)	22 (11)
Free fatty acids	8.7 ± 0.4 (18)	3 ± 4 (18)	7.98 ± 0.75 (25)	4 ± 5 (25)	0.42 ± 0.1 (6)	−2 ± 10 (6)
Phospholipids	160 ± 19 (8)	4 ± 3 (8)	80 ± 19 (11)	0 ± 5 (11)	55.3 ± 0.6 (10)	5.5 ± 1 (10)
Cholesterol	37 ± 4 (7)	−5 ± 6 (7)	23 ± 4 (5)	0 ± 1 (5)	17.2 ± 0.65 (10)	1 ± 1.6 (10)
Cholesterol esters	100 ± 17 (7)	2 ± 4 (7)	183 ± 17 (11)	1 ± 3 (11)	24.0 ± 2.3 (3)	15 ± 7.5 (3)
Free glycerol	0.34 ± 0.06 (6)	7 ± 4.5 (6)				

	A	E	A	E	E	A	E
Methionine	0.27 ± 0.02 (10)	72 ± 9 (10)	0.25 ± 0.02 (10)	57 ± 5 (4)	33	0.81 ± 0.07 (10)	37 ± 1 (10)
Phenylalanine	0.70 ± 0.05 (10)	63 ± 5 (10)	0.72 ± 0.02 (11)	43 ± 3 (4)	38	2.11 ± 0.08 (12)	32 ± 0.7 (12)
Leucine	2.07 ± 0.08 (10)	63 ± 5 (10)	2.18 ± 0.11 (11)	44 ± 1 (4)	49	4.28 ± 0.16 (12)	33 ± 1.6 (12)
Threonine	0.96 ± 0.06 (10)	60 ± 2 (10)	0.98 ± 0.05 (11)	34 ± 1 (4)	34	2.69 ± 0.09 (12)	23 ± 1.2 (12)
Lysine	2.13 ± 0.19 (10)	49 ± 6 (10)	1.24 ± 0.05 (11)	59 ± 1 (4)	56	4.22 ± 0.20 (12)	26 ± 0.7 (12)
Arginine	2.53 ± 0.11 (10)	48 ± 7 (10)	1.29 ± 0.07 (11)	47 ± 4 (4)	46	4.08 ± 0.18 (12)	27 ± 1.4 (12)
Isoleucine	1.79 ± 0.08 (10)	47 ± 5 (10)	1.73 ± 0.06 (11)	45 ± 1 (4)	38	3.01 ± 0.08 (12)	31 ± 1 (12)
Histidine	1.04 ± 0.12 (10)	42 ± 5 (10)	0.98 ± 0.03 (11)	27 ± 2 (4)	28	2.41 ± 0.014 (12)	25 ± 0.7 (12)
Valine	2.79 ± 0.11 (10)	37 ± 5 (10)	3.07 ± 0.14 (11)	27 ± 2 (4)	27	4.90 ± 0.20 (12)	26 ± 1.3 (12)
Glutamate	1.93 ± 0.11 (10)	58 ± 4 (10)	0.94 ± 0.03 (11)	56 ± 5 (4)	55	6.24 ± 0.22 (12)	39 ± 1.6 (12)
Tyrosine	0.95 ± 0.07 (10)	39 ± 5 (10)	0.72 ± 0.03 (11)	45 ± 5 (4)	50	2.58 ± 0.09 (12)	25 ± 2 (12)
Asparagine	0.89 ± 0.07 (10)	37 ± 7 (10)	0.42 ± 0.05 (7)		31	0.62 ± 0.08 (5)	1 ± 9 (5)
Proline	2.59 ± 0.19 (10)	36 ± 6 (10)	0.81 ± 0.11 (7)		26	4.46 ± 0.19 (10)	31 ± 2.5 (9)
Ornithine	1.11 ± 0.14 (10)	36 ± 7 (10)	0.93 ± 0.04 (10)	42 ± 4 (4)	52	1.90 ± 0.23 (5)	16 ± 8 (5)
Aspartate	0.28 ± 0.03 (10)	33 ± 7 (10)	0.15 ± 0.01 (11)	50 ± 9 (4)	23	0.44 ± 0.03 (11)	13 ± 2 (11)
Alanine	1.66 ± 0.1 (10)	25 ± 4 (10)	1.61 ± 0.06 (11)	19 ± 4 (4)	5	3.65 ± 0.21 (11)	9 ± 1 (12)
Glutamine	3.74 ± 0.27 (10)	23 ± 5 (10)	2.63 ± 0.23 (7)		23	6.40 ± 1.21 (4)	9 ± 4 (4)
Glycine	6.85 ± 0.78 (10)	5 ± 2 (10)	1.79 ± 0.07 (11)	10 ± 2 (4)	8	5.14 ± 0.21 (12)	−0.3 ± 0.7 (12)
Citrulline	1.93 ± 0.18 (10)	3 ± 6 (10)	1.24 ± 0.07 (11)	12 ± 3 (4)	7	—	
Serine	1.41 ± 0.12 (10)	0 ± 7 (10)	0.89 ± 0.07 (11)	31 ± 4 (4)	20	1.66 ± 0.12 (4)	22 ± 3 (4)

a The extraction (E) is the a − v expressed as a percentage of arterial concentration (A). Data for the goat is taken from animals in the author's laboratory, much of it published in papers mentioned in the text. For the cow, the details taken from Hartmann and Lascelles (1964), Verbeke and Peeters (1964), Hartmann (1966), Kronfeld et al. (1968), and Bickerstaffe et al. (1974), and for the pig, from Spincer et al. (1969), and Linzell et al. (1969). The second value for E for amino acids in the cow is from Verbeke and Peeters (1964), who give only mean a and a − v values. Numbers in parentheses are number of observations.

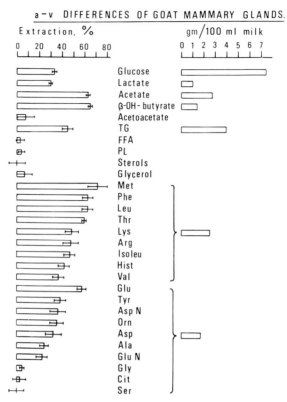

Fig. 18. Summary of the main precursors of milk in the goat. On the left the extraction $(a - v)/A$; on the right the uptake.

many workers have published their errors. Heap and Linzell (1966) showed that $a - v$ of progesterone was greater than the error of their assay determined from duplicates by the method of Snedecor (1950). In goats and pigs Linzell *et al.* (1969) reported that the same method gave the following coefficients of variation: free and bound fatty acids 1%; CO_2 1.5%; O_2 2%; amino acids 4%; acetate, glucose, and phospholipids 6%; lactate 7%; methionine and proline 10%; cholesterol 11%; and cholesterol esters 12%. In the cow Kronfeld *et al.* (1968) found it to be 1.9–4.0% for glucose and 1.9–13.6% for acetate. Thus, for all these methods $a - v$ of more than 13.6% would be unlikely to occur by chance in more than 1 in 20 trials, and in many a much smaller $a - v$ would be significant. Kronfeld *et al.* (1968) correctly points out that it depends on the method and the analyst. A further consideration is consistency; if it is found that there is a small but consistent $a - v$, which is less than the error in the method, this suggests a genuine uptake, but other methods are necessary to prove it, e.g., measurement of a − v and transfer to milk of the labeled compound either *in vivo* or *in vitro*.

1. Glucose

Glucose was the first milk precursor identified in the cow (Kaufmann and Magne, 1906) and goat (Foa, 1908b), and it is probably the most important, because without it milk secretion almost ceases in isolated perfused goat glands (Hardwick *et al.*, 1961). The reason is now clear. Glucose is essential for the final stage of lactose formation, for the reaction with UDPgalactose (Watkins and Hassid, 1962), and there are now several reasons for thinking that lactose, after it is secreted, draws water from the cell osmotically, thus accounting for the very small volume of milk, very rich in fat and protein, formed by perfused goat glands deprived of glucose (see Linzell and Peaker, 1971c).

In conscious animals there are also good reasons for accepting the importance of glucose as a key milk precursor. Upon fasting, the milk yield in goats sinks, between the eighth and sixteenth hour, to about half the fed level, and the mammary glucose uptake falls to 31% (Linzell, 1967a; Table IV). This can be restored to about 85% by an intravenous infusion of glucose (Linzell, 1967b), and in some fed animals the milk yield also can be increased by glucose infusion (Linzell, 1967b).

Annison and Linzell (1964) were the first to determine the fate of glucose taken up by the udder of the fed goat. They found that 25% was oxidized and that the remainder was quite sufficient to account for all the lactose and glycerol found in milk. Barry (1952) had shown that glucose was the main precursor of lactose. In the work of Annison and Linzell (1964) at least 85% of lactose and 50% of glycerol were derived from glucose (Annison, 1971). This would almost account for the glucose uptake, after that oxidized has been subtracted (Fig. 19).

Other experiments suggest that glucose may be used to form some other components. Mepham and Linzell (1968) infused [^{14}C]glucose into the mammary artery in lactating goats and detected radioactivity in serine, alanine, glutamate, and aspartate of the synthesized milk protein of the infused gland. According to the views of Black (1970) much of this labeling could be due to exchange reactions, whereby ^{14}C entering the Krebs citric acid cycle is randomized as the cycle turns and thus is transferred to compounds in equilibrium with compounds in the main metabolic pathways. However, as the earlier arteriovenous difference data of Mepham and Linzell (1966) showed, the uptakes of serine, aspartate,

TABLE IV

Effects on Whole Body and Mammary Metabolism of a
24-Hour Fast in Lactating Goats[a]

	Fed	Fasted
Nutrient yield		
Milk[b]	100	40 ± 3.4
Lactose[b]	100	31 ± 3.4
Fat[b]	100	81 ± 6.7
Protein[b]	100	81 ± 4.9
Whole body		
Glucose entry rate[c]	3.6 ± 0.43	1.3 ± 0.42
Acetate entry rate[c]	5.2 ± 0.3	1.16 ± 0.25
FFA entry rate[c]	0.3 ± 0.12	4.0 ± 1.3
CO_2 derived from glucose[b]	9 ± 0.7	4 ± 1.0
CO_2 derived from acetate[b]	27 ± 3.0	9.5 ± 0.5
CO_2 derived from FFA[b]	0.3 ± 0.15	23
Udder		
Volume of empty tissue[b]	100	83 ± 3.2
Glucose uptake[c]	62.9 ± 11.5	13.1 ± 2.5
Acetate uptake[c]	26.4 ± 5.0	1.6 ± 0.8
FFA uptake[c]	0	13.0
CO_2 derived from glucose[b]	38.8 ± 4.2	9 ± 1.0
CO_2 derived from acetate[b]	26.0 ± 2	11 ± 2
CO_2 derived from FFA[b]	0	17.5
Glucose oxidized[b]	25.4 ± 3.3	7.5 ± 2.5
Acetate oxidized[b]	44	62.5 ± 17.5
FFA oxidized[b]	0	13 ± 6
Blood flow[c]	43.5 ± 1.7	23 ± 3
O_2 uptake[c]	2.34	1.05 ± 0.1
R.Q.	1.4 ± 0.04	0.85 ± 0.045
Glucose uptake[d]	73	39 ± 4
Acetate uptake[d]	20	4 ± 2
FFA uptake[d]	0	40

[a] From Annison and Linzell (1964), Linzell (1967a), Annison *et al.* (1967),
(1968), and unpublished data.
[b] Results given as percent.
[c] Results given as milligrams per minute per kilogram of body or tissue.
[d] Results given as percent of entry rate.

glutamate, and alanine are seriously short of that expected if the source
of these amino acids in synthesized milk protein is the free amino acid in
the plasma. Thus, we must admit that the glucose carbon could be considered as a possible source of the carbon in these amino acids in milk.
Nevertheless, comparison of specific activities of the amino acids and of
plasma glucose showed that amino acid synthesis cannot be a major

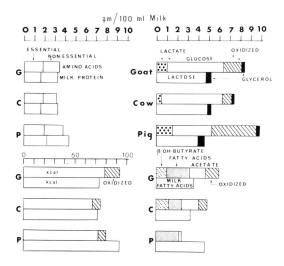

Fig. 19. Summary of uptake, output data for lactating goats, cows, and pigs.

use of glucose. This probably is an example of a situation where all three methods of identifying precursors will be needed to reveal the truth.

Folley and his colleague (see Folley, 1956) discovered an important difference in mammary metabolism between ruminants (sheep, goats, and cows) and other animals (rats, mice, and rabbits); only in the latter can the mammary tissue synthesize fatty acids from glucose. The pig, which like the rat, is an omnivore, also can form short-chain and some long-chain fatty acids from glucose (Linzell *et al.*, 1969), but the horse cannot (Linzell *et al.*, 1972a).

2. Amino Acids

Early workers considered that the mammary uptake of amino acid N was sufficient to account for all the milk N and that most of the milk protein must be synthesized in the tissue. This is most probably correct, but there was a period when amino acid uptake was reported to be significantly less than protein output, and it was then that claims were made for a significant a − v of a glycoprotein (see Barry, 1964). When labeled amino acids became available it soon became apparent that in the case of lysine, tryosine, methionine, glutamate, glutamine, glycine, threonine, and serine, the plasma free amino acids are the main source of the same residues in the milk protein (see Barry, 1964; Mepham, 1971), but the overall picture was not resolved until all the necessary measurements were made simultaneously in the goat, i.e., a − v of all the amino acids, udder blood flood, and milk protein synthesis (Mepham and

Linzell, 1966). This revealed that all the essential amino acids are removed from the plasma in quantities sufficient to account for the corresponding synthesized milk protein. This was also true for many nonessential amino acids, although there was more variability between animals; the uptake of serine was consistently less than output, there was an uptake of ornithine, and amino acid not present in milk protein, and the uptake of arginine was 3–4 times output.

Recently a few measurements have been made of a − v of all the amino acids and the blood flow and milk yield in cows (Bikerstaffe et al., 1973). As in the goat, uptake of all essential and some nonessential amino acids is sufficient to account for all the amino acid residues in the milk protein and again arginine uptake is excessive, 1.5–2 times that necessary.

In the pig (Linzell et al., 1969; Spincer et al., 1969) there is also reasonable evidence that essential amino acids are removed from the plasma at the rate expected from quantities of protein being synthesized and again a − v of nonessential acids are variable. Unlike the goat and cow, arginine uptake is not excessive and serine uptake is large. However, there are low a − v of other nonessential amino acids and pig as well as goat mammary tissue has the ability to synthesize some amino acids, since ^{14}C is transferred from glucose to casein in perfused pig glands.

The significance of the excessive arginine uptake in cows and goats is unknown but Mepham and Linzell (1967) were able to show that there is an accumulation of urea in the perfusate during perfusion of goat glands and, when [^{14}C]arginine was included in the substrates, radioactivity was detected in ornithine, proline, and urea. Thus, part of the labeled arginine, which is also transferred to protein, seems to be deaminated. Labeled ornithine also gives rise to proline in the perfused sheep udder (Verbeke et al., 1965).

3. Fatty Acids

Fatty acid uptake varies with the species, the main difference of course, being that herbivores that ferment cellulose through microbial action in the stomach or hind gut, have raised blood levels of volatile fatty acids, mainly acetate, which are absorbed by the mammary glands and used partly for energy and partly for the synthesis of the longer chained fatty acids of milk fat. This is most clearly worked out in ruminants (Folley, 1956; Bickerstaffe, 1971), but in rabbits (Popjak et al., 1949) and horses (Linzell et al., 1972a) the mammary utilization of acetate is highly significant.

Even in the pig, there is a small uptake of acetate (Linzell et al., 1969).

In fact acetate uptake by the mammary gland in all species is greater than is apparent, because the tissue also produces acetate in fed and fasting animals (Annison and Linzell, 1964; Annison *et al.*, 1968). This is revealed when [14C]acetate is infused, because the specific activity of acetate in mammary venous blood is less than in arterial blood, indicating the release of unlabeled acetate by the tissue.

Following the discovery in ruminants of the importance of volatile fatty acid formation by microbial fermentation in the rumen, and of the mammary uptake of acetate (McClymont, 1951) as well as utilization of acetate for the synthesis of short-chain fatty acids of milk fat (Folley, 1956), the earlier reports of a substantial uptake of triglyceride (then called neutral lipid) in the goat (Lintzel, 1934) and cow (Maynard *et al.*, 1938) were forgotten. However, in fact, they are equally as important as acetate, and in the last decade this has been well documented.

In cows, Riis *et al.* (1960) showed that when a labeled colloidal lipid fraction of plasma was harvested from one animal and injected into another, label was transferred to milk fat. Later in goats Barry *et al.* (1963) confirmed the large extraction of lipid, but reported that it was confined to the triglyceride fraction and within that class to the chylomicra and the low density lipoproteins. About the same time Lascelles *et al.* (1964) prepared labeled chylomicra by infusing [3H]stearate into the duodenum of a goat, collecting the chyle, and confirmed the ability of mammary tissue to extract these very large particles from the plasma. Radioactivity was rapidly transferred from the labeled chylomicra to milk fat, in isolated perfused goat glands and in conscious goats. In fact, in the latter about half the total radioactivity was trapped in the udder within 16 minutes, and, when a gland was then removed and perfused in isolation without further label, radioactivity was still transferred to synthesized milk fat (Lascelles *et al.*, 1964). Also, at this time, the importance of acetate as a precursor of milk fat was downgraded when Annison and Linzell (1964) found, in goats infused with [14C]acetate, that about half the acetate taken up by the udder was oxidized and that the remainder was not sufficient to form more than 45% of the total milk fatty acids (Fig. 19). However, this is counterbalanced by the discovery that there is a substantial extraction 65 ±2% of β-hydroxybutyrate in goats (Barry *et al.*, 1963) and cows (Shaw, 1942; Kronfeld *et al.*, 1968) and by the later demonstration that the labeled natural isomer is taken up and handled by isolated perfused glands very much like acetate (Linzell *et al.*, 1967).

The magnitude of the extraction of chylomicra and low-density lipoproteins was surprising, but independent work by two groups on the mouse and goat revealed the mechanism that turns out to be important for understanding the uptake of fat by all tissue, including adipose tissue. The explanation was anticipated by D. S. Robinson, because in his collaboration with Barry *et al.* (1963), he reported that the goat's udder releases lipoprotein lipase into the venous blood. This is the clearing factor lipase released by heparin. This enzyme was also detected in the perfusate when goat's udders were perfused in isolation, even when no heparin was used (Lascelles *et al.*, 1964). Its importance became clear when Annison *et al.* (1967) infused labeled free fatty acids into lactating goats. Although there was no net a — v of this fraction across the udder, (confirming the same finding of Barry *et al.* 1963), nevertheless, large amounts of the radioactive acids were transferred to milk fat. More significantly there was a substantial fall in specific activity across the udder showing that unlabeled fatty acids had been released by the tissue into the venous plasma. The story for the goat was completed when chylomicra, labeled both in the glycerol and fatty acid parts of the molecule, were infused. Both glycerol and fatty acids were transferred to milk fat in quantity, but, more importantly, free labeled glycerol and fatty acids appeared in the venous blood (West *et al.*, 1972). Clearly, the chylomicra had been hydrolyzed before uptake by the secretory cells. The fact that the released glycerol and very little of the fatty acids were also detected in mammary lymph, strongly suggested that hydrolysis occurred on or in the endothelial cells (Fig. 20). This would account for the lipase released into mammary venous plasma.

The independent work of Schoefl and French (1968) beautifully confirmed the goat work. These workers also injected chylomicra into lactating animals (mice) but examined the mammary tissue with the electron microscope and by histochemistry. They clearly showed lipase activity to be confined to the capillaries and that, at the ultrastructural level, the endothelial cells engulf the large fat particles into intracellular vesicles, where hydrolysis must occur, because no fat particles were seen outside the capillaries in the extracellular space, where we had detected free glycerol and fatty acids in the goat (West *et al.*, 1972). Blanchette-Mackie and Scow (1971) have confirmed the intracellular location of hydrolysis in vesicles in the endothelial cells in adipose tissue of rats; in the goat, Annison and his colleagues (Bickerstaffe *et al.*, 1970) have presented chemical evidence from experiments using doubly labeled chylomicra and fat emulsions and chemical analogues of triglycerides (glycerol ethers) that hydrolysis is almost complete, although a little may be absorbed as the monoglyceride, with the fatty acid on the 2 position of glycerol.

Support for the importance of FFA for milk fat synthesis comes from the study of fasting lactating animals, in which it has long been known

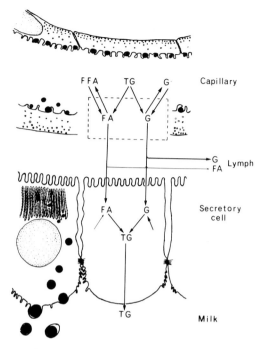

Fig. 20. Summary of mechanism of transfer of long-chain fatty acids and glycerol to milk fat in the goat. TG, Triglyceride; FA, free fatty acids; G, glycerol.

that, in spite of the fall in milk yield, the milk fat concentration rises. As in all fasting animals, there is a large rise in plasma FFA due to mobilization of fat stores, and in the cow (Kronfeld, 1965) and goat (Linzell, 1967a) there is then a consistent mammary a − v, not seen in fed animals that have a low plasma FFA. In fact, since uptake of acetate and triglycerides (TG) fall on fasting, FFA are the main precursors of milk fat. Infusion of labeled palmitate, stearate, or oleate in 24-hour fasting goats (Annison *et al.*, 1968) confirmed that they were transferred to milk fat, and showed that FFA accounted for 61% of the fat precursors and for 46% of the milk fatty acids. The uptake of hydroxybutyrate falls slightly, but the tissue uses some of its own large store of fat (Linzell *et al.*, 1967), because empty udder volume shrinks by 17% within 24 hours and milk fatty acid output is higher than uptake (Annison *et al.*, 1968). By measuring a − v of all components and using isotopes, it is possible to trace the movements of the precursors through the tissue in a comprehensive manner (Fig. 21).

It must be emphasized that the uptake of triglycerides by hydrolysis in

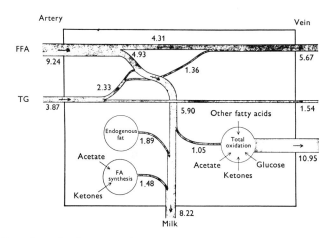

Fig. 21. Flow of palmitate carbon through the udder of a fasting (24-hour) goat, calculated from simultaneous measurements of a − v, blood flow, milk yield, and composition and changes in specific radioactivities. All values in milligrams C per minute. In the first 24 hours of fasting the empty udder volume shrinks by 17%. (From Annison *et al.*, 1968).

mammary capillaries has been demonstrated in both ruminants and non-ruminants, and, since there is an a − v of TG in the cow (Graham *et al.*, 1936b; Hartmann and Lascelles, 1964), pig (Linzell *et al.*, 1969), and horse (Linzell *et al.*, 1972a), this mechanism is probably universal, as is also the uptake of long-chain free fatty acids. The main difference between the species is that ruminants have lost the ability to synthesize fatty acids from glucose but use acetate and hydroxybutyrate instead. It also appears that acetate and β-hydroxybutyrate are as important to the ruminant udder as a source of energy as they are as a source of carbon for short-chain fatty acid synthesis.

4. Minor Components

Milk is a complicated fluid containing many minor components, which must all originate from the plasma, directly or following chemical alteration in the tissue of another precursor. All minerals must pass from plasma to milk, so it is pointless to measure their a − v, except as a means of assessing blood flow by the Fick principle (see Section III,A,5,c). In this connection K, Ca, PO_4 and I_2 may be recommended because they are concentrated in milk, compared to plasma. Nevertheless, because mammary blood flow is relatively high, their a − v may be difficult to measure accurately. Other minor components may be of interest because they may help us to understand the secretory mechanism and to identify rate limiting steps. It is worth emphasizing that the mixture of glucose, fatty acids, and amino acids is only capable of sustaining half the expected milk yield in the isolated perfused goat's udder (Linzell *et al.*, 1972) and cannot fully restore the reduced yield of the fasted animal (Linzell, 1967b). In the perfused gland many other substances (including hormones) have been added to this substrate mixture, without significantly increasing the milk yield (Linzell *et al.*, 1972) so that we still do not know what is lacking.

The concentrations of vitamins A, C, and D in milk appear to reflect their corresponding plasma concentrations, but most of the B vitamins except B_{12} are more concentrated in milk than in plasma.

In conscious lactating goats the ratio of the concentrations in milk and plasma range from 82 for biotin to 2 for folic acid. Mammary uptake equalled or exceeded output in the milk for biotin, pantothenic acid, riboflavin, nicotinic acid, and vitamin B_{12}, and the results were variable for thiamine, pyridoxine, and folic acid. In isolated perfused glands the concentration of all vitamins in milk fell (except nicotinic acid) and panthenate and riboflavin added to the blood raised their concentrations in milk (with riboflavin the milk became yellow). However, there was no increase in milk yield. (Ford and Linzell, unpublished).

Measurements are also in progress with carnitine, which is involved in fatty acid metabolism. It is particularly high in ruminant tissues and present in milk, being raised in ketosis. Snoswell and Linzell (unpublished) found that there is a twenty- to thirtyfold concentration of carnitine in milk and that mammary tissue has an even higher concentration (127–161 nmoles/gm). Nevertheless, the loss of milk would deplete the tissue in 3 days and in two out of three goats there was an extraction of 50–100%.

These results illustrate both the difficulties of detecting mammary uptake of minor components and also that the method is not completely discredited as a means of identifying minor but possibly important milk precursors.

Hormones are dispersed in the plasma and are usually considered to affect the target tissues by virtue of their concentration. The idea of the target organ responding as it takes up the hormone is seldom considered, but this occurs in the case of the mammary gland with progesterone (Heap and Linzell, 1966), and to a small extent in the case of cortisol (Paterson and Linzell, 1971) and estrone (Challis and Linzell, 1973).

C. Mechanism of Mammary Uptake

This is clearly important but has been little studied. It has been noted that, in the cow and goat, in the case of glucose (Graham *et al.*, 1936b; Linzell, 1960b), acetate (McClymont, 1951; Linzell, 1960b), and many nonessential amino acids (Mepham, 1971), the a − v is proportional to the arterial concentration. This implies that extraction is a passive process but this may not be true. The observations were made in the normal range of blood concentrations; outside this the results are different. I have records over a wider range for glucose and these show that, down to very low arterial levels, the mammary glands can still extract the necessary quantities of glucose, while at very high concentrations the a − v does not increase. Furthermore, in the case of essential amino acids there is no relation between a − v and arterial concentration (Mepham, 1971).

These data are incomplete and, therefore, possibly misleading because extraction would be expected to be influenced by blood flow, which must be known also, in order to calculate uptake or flux. Only in the goat was blood flow also measured, and these data suggest that, in late lactation, blood glucose concentration and a − v rise, without a commensurate fall in udder blood flow and milk yield. This shows that in late lactation the mammary glands are less efficient in that they appear to require more glucose to form a given quantity of milk.

To decipher the mechanism by which the mammary glands remove precursors, it is more informative to consider individual animals over short time intervals. In the work of Linzell (1967b) it may be noted that in fasting animals and in those given insulin, a − v was unaffected, while blood flow fell, to account for the fall in glucose uptake. This shows that under these circumstances the mammary glands can remove a constant quantity of glucose, quite independent of the arterial glucose level. Perfused glands show similar properties (Linzell *et al.*, 1972b). In addition, if the arterial concentration is raised by infusing glucose and there is an increased synthesis of milk or lactose, sometimes the a − v is not raised, the increased uptake of glucose being accompanied by a rise in mammary blood flow. In many organs the uptake of diffusible substances is flow limited. When glucose is absent, mannose and fructose can enter the cell because they sustain the same O_2 uptake as glucose, but experiments should be done to test whether other sugars and glucose analogues compete with glucose, by infusing two together. However, it seems probable that, once a substance reaches a capillary, the rate limiting step will be the entrance into the cells, which is likely to be by facilitated diffusion with a carrier in the cell membrane.

D. Fasting Metabolism

Caution must be exercised in the timing of arteriovenous measurements because striking changes in mammary metabolism occur within a relatively few hours after the last meal, even in ruminants. In the goat, if feed is withdrawn after morning milking, by evening milking the yield is reduced only slightly to 90% of expected, but by next morning it is only about half previous (Linzell, 1967a). The large quantitative differences in whole animal and udder metabolism occurring at this time are summarized in Table IV. Hartmann and Lascelles (1965) and Kronfeld *et al.* (1968) encountered similar changes in cows fasted 2–4 days, and there was an increased mammary uptake of β-hydroxybutyrate. Kronfeld (1965) showed that in cows plasma FFA levels started to rise 8–12 hours after a feed, so the timing is similar to the goat. In monogastric animals changes would probably be quicker. Further work is needed on the fluctuations in mammary metabolism in relation to feeding.

VI. SUMMARY AND RECOMMENDATIONS

The rate of mammary blood flow is of interest because· it is closely related to the rate of milk secretion, although it seems that milk yield controls blood flow and not vice versa. Factors affecting both are mentioned. A fall in mammary blood flow is one of the sensitive indicators of stress. To accurately identify and measure the uptake of milk precursors it is necessary to use three techniques:

1. The employment of labeled compounds (usually isotopically) *in vivo* and *in vitro*. Proviso: in whole animals incorporation of the label into milk does not necessarily mean uptake of the compound because of the possibility of transformation into other precursors elsewhere in the body. Infusion into only one gland overcomes this and is excellent when combined with method 3.

2. Use of *in vitro* techniques. Substances suspected of being milk precursors must be given in normal or tracer amounts to mammary gland homogenates, isolated mammary secretory cells, mammary tissue growing in organ culture, and/or isolated perfused whole glands and the uptake

and metabolism of the compound measured. If possible, the output of products derived from the substance should also be measured.

3. Simultaneous measurements should be made *in vivo* of the arterio-venous difference of the substance as well as the mammary blood flow and the output of possible production in the milk. Generally this means using trained, conscious, surgically prepared animals.

REFERENCES

Abolins, J. A. (1954). *Acta Obstet. Gynecol. Scand.* 33, 60.
Abraham, S., Kerkof, P. R., and Smith, S. (1972). *Biochim. Biophys. Acta* 261, 205.
Anderson, D. M., and Elsley, F. W. H. (1969). *J. Agr. Sci. Cambridge* 72, 475.
Anderson, R. S., and Rogers, E. B. (1957). *Amer. J. Physiol.* 188, 178.
Annison, E. F. (1971). *In* "Lactation" (I. R. Falconer, ed.), p. 281. Butterworths, London and Washington, D. C.
Annison, E. F., and Linzell, J. L. (1964). *J. Physiol. London* 175, 372.
Annison, E. F., Linzell, J. L., Fazakerley, S., and Nichols, B. W. (1967). *Biochem. J.* 102, 637.
Annison, E. F., Linzell, J. L., and West, C. E. (1968). *J. Physiol. London* 197, 445.
Arndt, J. O., and Klauske, J. (1971). *Proc. Int. Symp. Mod. Tech. Physiol. Sci., Munich.* p. 2.
Aukland, K., Bower, B. F., and Berliner, R. W. (1964). *Circ. Res.* 44, 164.
Baldwin, B. A., and Bell, F. R. (1963). *J. Physiol. London* 167, 448.
Barcroft, J., Boycott, A. E., Dunn, J. S., and Peters, R. A. (1919). *Quart. J. Med.* 13, 35.
Barcroft, J., Harrison, H. A., Orahovats, D., and Weiss, R. (1925). *J. Physiol. London* 50, 443.
Barone, R., and Monnet, C. (1955). *Bull. Soc. Sci. Vet. Lyon* 57, 73.
Barry, J. M. (1952). *Nature (London)* 169, 878.
Barry, J. M. (1964). *Biol. Rev.* 39, 194.
Barry, J. M., Bartley, W., Linzell, J. L., and Robinson, D. S. (1963). *Biochem. J.* 89, 6.
Becker, R. B. (1937). *J. Dairy Sci.* 20, 408.
Becker, R. B., and Arnold, P. T. D. (1942). *Fl. Agr. Exp. Sta. Tech. Bull.* p. 379.
Berkow, S. G., and Jacobson, M. B. (1940). *Endocrinology* 26, 986.
Bickerstaffe, R. (1971). *In* "Lactation" (I. R. Falconer, ed.), p. 317. Butterworths, London and Washington, D. C.
Bickerstaffe, R., Annison, E. F., and Linzell, J. L. (1974). *J. Agr. Sci.* (In press).
Bickerstaffe, R., Linzell, J. L., Morris, L. J., and Annison, E. F. (1970). *Biochem. J.* 117, 39P.
Black, A. L. (1970). *In* "Physiology of Digestion and Metabolism in the Ruminant" (A. T. Phillipson, ed.), p. 452. Oriel Press, Newcastle.
Blackwood, J. H. (1932). *Biochem. J.* 6, 772.
Blackwood, J. H. (1934). *Biochem. J.* 28, 1346.
Blackwood, J. H., and Stirling, J. D. (1932). *Biochem. J.* 26, 357.
Blanchette-Mackie, E. J., and Scow, R. O. (1971). *J. Cell. Biol.* 51, 1.

Bone, J. F., Metcalfe, J., and Parer, J. T. (1962). *Amer. J. Vet. Res.* **23,** 1113.

Cary, C. A. (1920). *J. Biol. Chem.* **43,** 477.

Challis, J. R. G., and Linzell, J. L. (1973). *J. Endocrinol.* **57,** 451.

Charton, A., Faye, P., Hervy, R., Bernard, C., and Gueslin, M. (1965). *C.R. Seances Soc. Biol.* **159,** 1509.

Chatwin, A. L., Linzell, J. L., and Setchell, B. P. (1969). *J. Endocrinol.* **44,** 247.

Chauveau, J. P. A., and Marey, E. J. (1861). *C.R. Hebd. Seances Acad. Sci.* **53,** 622.

Clark, E. R. (1938). *Physiol. Rev.* **18,** 229.

Crone, C. (1965). *Acta Physiol. Scand.* **63,** 213.

Dabelow, A. (1933). *Gegenbauer. Morphol. Jb.* **73,** 69.

Dabelow, A. (1934). *Anat. Anz.* **78,** Verh. Anat. Ges. 165.

Dhondt, G., Houvenaghel, A., Peeters, G., and Verschooten, F. (1973). *Arch. Int. Pharmacodyn.* **201,** 195.

Ebner, K. E., Hoover, C. R., Hageman, E. C., and Larson, B. L. (1961). *Exp. Cell Res.* **23,** 373.

Ebner, K. E., and Larson, B. L. (1959). *J. Dairy Sci.* **42,** 916.

El Hagri, M. A. A. M. (1945). *Brit. Vet. J.* **101,** 27, 51, 75.

Ely, F., and Petersen, W. E. (1941). *J. Dairy Sci.* **24,** 211.

Emery, E. S., Brown, L. D., and Bell, J. W. (1965). *J. Dairy Sci.* **48,** 1647.

Fegler, G. (1954). *Quart. J. Exp. Physiol.* **39,** 153.

Fegler, G. (1957). *Quart. J. Exp. Physiol.* **42,** 254.

Felig, P., Pozefsky, T., Marliss, E., and Cahill, G. F. (1970). *Science* **167,** 1003.

Fick, A. (1870). *Verhandl. Phys.-Med. Ges. Würzb.* **2,** 16.

Fisher, E. W. (1956). *Vet. Rec.* **68,** 691.

Foa, C. (1908a). *Arch. Fisiol.* **5,** 520.

Foa, C. (1908b). *Arch. Fisiol.* **5,** 533.

Foa, C. (1912). *Arch. Fisiol.* **10,** 402.

Folley, S. J. (1949). *Biol. Rev.* **24,** 316.

Folley, S. J. (1956). "The Physiology and Biochemistry of Lactation." Oliver and Boyd, Edinburgh.

Folley, S. J., and Peskett, G. L. (1934). *J. Physiol. London* **82,** 486.

Folley, S. J., and French, T. H. (1948). *Nature (London)* **161,** 933.

Folley, S. J., and French, T. H. (1949). *Biochem. J.* **45,** 117.

Forsyth, I. A. (1971). *J. Dairy Res.* **3,** 419.

Forsyth, I. A., Jones, E. A., and Barrett, M. A. (1969). *Rep. Nat. Inst. Res. Dairy, Shinfield* 112.

Franklin, D. L., Schlegel, W., and Rushmer, R. D. (1961). *Science* **134,** 564.

Fronek, A., and Ganz, V. (1960). *Circ. Res.* **8,** 175.

Fürstenburg, M. H. F. (1868). "Die Milchdrusen der Kuh." Engelmann, Leipzig.

Gabel, A. A., Hamlin, R., and Smith, C. R. (1964). *Amer. J. Vet. Res.* **25,** 1151.

Gaddum, J. H. (1929). *J. Physiol. London* **67,** 16P.

Gostev, A. V. (1967). *Bull. Exp. Biol. Med.* **63,** 103.

Gostev, A .V. (1968). *Nerv. Sist.* **9,** 71.

Graham, W. R. (1937). *J. Biol. Chem.* **122,** 1.

Graham, W. R., Kay, H. D., and McIntosh, R. A. (1936a). *Proc. Roy. Soc. London B* **120,** 319.

Graham, W. R., Jones, T. S. G., and Kay, H. D. (1936b). *Proc. Roy. Soc. London B* **120,** 330.

Graham, W. R., Turner, C. W., and Gomez, E. T. (1937). *Mon. Agr. Exp. Station Res. Bull.* **260,** 3.

Green, H. D. (1948). *Methods Med. Res.* **1,** 66.

Grant, G. A. (1935). *Biochem. J.* **29,** 1905.

Grant, G. A. (1936). *Biochem. J.* **30,** 2027.

Hanwell, A., Fleet, I. R., and Linzell, J. L. (1972). *Comp. Biochem. Physiol.* **41A,** 659.

Hanwell, A., and Linzell, J. L. (1972). *J. Physiol. London* **226,** 24P.

Hanwell, A., and Linzell, J. L. (1973). *J. Physiol. London* **233,** 93.

Hardwick, D. C., and Linzell, J. L. (1960). *J. Physiol. London* **154,** 547.

Hardwick, D. C., Linzell, J. L., and Mepham, T. B. (1963). *Biochem. J.* **88,** 213.

Hardwick, D. C., Linzell, J. L., and Price, S. M. (1961). *Biochem. J.* **80,** 37.

Hartmann, P. E. (1966). *Aust. J. Biol. Sci.* **19,** 495.

Hartmann, P. E., and Lascelles, A. K. (1964). *Aust. J. Biol. Sci.* **17,** 935.

Hartmann, P. E., and Lascelles, A. K. (1965). *Aust. J. Biol. Sci.* **18,** 1025.

Heap, R. B., and Linzell, J. L. (1966). *J. Endocrinol.* **36,** 389.

Hebb, C. O., and Linzell, J. L. (1951). *Quart. J. Exp. Physiol.* **36,** 159.

Hebb, C. O., and Linzell, J. L. (1970). *Histochem. J.* **2,** 491.

Hilton, S. M., and Vrbová, G. (1970). *J. Physiol. London* **206,** 29P.

Holton, F. A., and Holton, P. (1954). *J. Physiol. London* **126,** 124.

Holzman, G. B., Wagner, H. N., Iio, M., Rabinowitz, D., and Zierler, K. L. (1964). *Circulation* **30,** 27.

Houvenaghel, A. (1970). *Arch. Int. Pharmacodyn.* **186,** 190.

Houvenaghel, A., Peeters, G., and Verschooten, F. (1972). *Arch. Int. Pharmacodyn.* Suppl. 182, **196.**

Hoyer, H. (1877). *Arch. Mikrosk. Anat.* **13,** 603.

Jagenau, A. H. M., Schaper, A., and Rens, W. (1969). *Pflügers Arch.* **310,** 182.

Jha, S. K., Lumb, W. V., and Johnston, R. F. (1961). *Amer. J. Vet. Res.* **22,** 948.

Jung, L. (1932a). *C.R. Soc. Biol.* **109,** 737.

Jung, L. (1932b). *C.R. Soc. Biol.* **109,** 1052.

Jung, L. (1933). *Lait* **13,** 307.

Kaufmann, M., and Magne, H. (1906). *C.R. Hebd. Seances Acad. Sci.* **143,** 779.

Kay, H. D. (1947). *Brit. Med. Bull.* **5,** 149.

Kety, S. S. (1949). *Amer. Heart J.* **38,** 321.

Kety, S. S., and Schmidt, C. F. (1945). *Amer. J. Physiol.* **143,** 53.

Kinsella, J. E., and McCarthy, R. D. (1968). *Biochim. Biophys. Acta* **164,** 53.

Kjaersgaard, P. (1968a). *Acta Vet. Scand.* **9,** 177.

Kjaersgaard, P. (1968b). *Acta Vet. Scand.* **9,** 180.

Kleiber, M., and Luick, J. R. (1956). *Ann. N. Y. Acad. Sci.* **64,** 299.

Kronfeld, D. S. (1965). *Vet. Rec.* **77,** 30.

Kronfeld, D. S. (1969). *In* "Lactogenesis" (M. Reynolds, and S. J. Folley, eds.). Univ. Pennsylvania Press, Philadelphia, Pennsylvania.

Kronfeld, D. S., Raggi, F., and Ramberg, C. F. (1968). *Amer. J. Physiol.* **215,** 218.

Kumar, S., Lakshmanan, S., Corbin, E. A., and Shaw, J. C. (1953). *Amer. J. Physiol.* **173,** 82.

Lascelles, A. K., Cowie, A. T., Hartmann, P. E., and Edwards, M. J. (1964). *Res. Vet. Sci.* **5,** 190.

Lascelles, A. K., Hardwick, D. C., Linzell, J. L., and Mepham, T. B. (1964). *Biochem. J.* **92,** 36.

Lascelles, A. K., and Morris, B. (1961). *Quart. J. Exp. Physiol.* **46**, 206.
Lee, C. S., and Lascelles, A. K. (1969). *Amer. J. Anat.* **126**, 489.
Lintzel, W. (1934). *Lait* **14**, 1125.
Linzell, J. L. (1950). *Quart. J. Exp. Physiol.* **35**, 295.
Linzell, J. L. (1953a). *Brit. Vet. J.* **109**, 427.
Linzell, J. L. (1953b). *J. Physiol. London* **121**, 390.
Linzell, J. L. (1954). *Rev. Can. Biol.* **13**, 291.
Linzell, J. L. (1955). *J. Physiol. London* **130**, 257.
Linzell, J. L. (1957). *J. Physiol. London* **137**, 75P.
Linzell, J. L. (1959). *Quart. J. Exp. Physiol.* **44**, 160.
Linzell, J. L. (1960a). *J. Physiol. London* **153**, 481.
Linzell, J. L. (1960b). *J. Physiol. London* **153**, 492.
Linzell, J. L. (1960c). *J. Physiol. London* **153**, 510.
Linzell, J. L. (1963a). *Amer. J. Vet. Res.* **24**, 223.
Linzell, J. L. (1963b). *Quart. J. Exp. Physiol.* **48**, 34.
Linzell, J. L. (1965). Quoted by Folley, and Knaggs (1965). *J. Endocrinol.* **33**, 301.
Linzell, J. L. (1966a). *Circ. Res.* **18**, 745.
Linzell, J. L. (1966b). *J. Dairy Sci.* **49**, 307.
Linzell, J. L. (1966c). *J. Physiol. London* **186**, 79P.
Linzell, J. L. (1967a). *J. Physiol. London* **190**, 333.
Linzell, J. L. (1967b). *J. Physiol. London* **190**, 347.
Linzell, J. L. (1968). *Proc. Nutr. Soc.* **27**, 44.
Linzell, J. L. (1969). *In* "Lactogenesis" (M. Reynolds, and S. J. Folley, eds.), p. 153. Univ. Pennsylvania Press, Philadelphia, Pennsylvania.
Linzell, J. L. (1971a). *In* "Lactation." (I. R. Falconer, ed.), p. 41. Butterworths, London and Washington, D.C.
Linzell, J. L. (1971b). *In* "Lactation." (I. R. Falconer, ed.), p. 261. Butterworths, London and Washington, D.C.
Linzell, J. L., Annison, E. F., Bickerstaffe, R., and Jeffcott, L. B. (1972a). *Proc. Nutr. Soc.* **31**, 72A.
Linzell, J. L., Annison, E. F., Fazakerley, S., and Leng, R. A. (1967). *Biochem. J.* **104**, 34.
Linzell, J. L., Fleet, I. R., Mepham, T. B., and Peaker, M. (1972b). *Quart. J. Exp. Physiol.* **57**, 139.
Linzell, J. L., Mepham, T. B., Annison, E. F., and West, C. E. (1969). *Brit. J. Nutr.* **23**, 319.
Linzell, J. L., and Mount, L. E. (1955). *Nature (London)* **176**, 37.
Linzell, J. L., and Peaker, M. (1971a). *J. Physiol. London* **216**, 701.
Linzell, J. L., and Peaker, M. (1971b). *J. Physiol. London* **216**, 717.
Linzell, J. L., and Peaker, M. (1971c). *J. Physiol. London* **216**, 683.
Linzell, J. L., and Peaker, M. (1971c). *Physiol. Rev.* **51**, 564.
Lukáš, Z., Lukášová, J., and Ryšánek, D. (1971). *Z. Mikrosk-Anat. Forsch.* **84**, 219.
Manente, B. A. (1954). II. *Pan-Am. Congr. Vet. Med. S. Paulo.* D.6.
Maynard, L. A., McCay, C. M., Ellis, G. H., Hodson, A. Z., and Davis, G. K. (1938). *Cornell Univ. Agr. Exp. Station Memoir* 211.
Maximow, A. (1925). *Virchows. Arch. Pathol. Anat. Physiol.* **256**, 813.
McClymont, G. L. (1951). *Aust. J. Agr. Res.* **2**, 158.
Meigs, E. B. (1922). *Physiol. Rev.* **2**, 204.
Meigs, E. B., Blatherwick, N. H., and Cary, C. A. (1919). *J. Biol. Chem.* **37**, 1.

Mepham, T. B. (1971). *In* "Lactation" (I. R. Falconer, ed.), p. 297. Butterworths, London.

Mepham, T. B., and Linzell, J. L. (1966). *Biochem. J.* **101**, 76.

Mepham, T. B., and Linzell, J. L. (1967). *Nature (London)* **214**, 507.

Mepham, T. B., and Linzell, J. L. (1968). *Biochem. J.* **107**, 18P.

Moriconi, A. (1953). *Atti. Soc. Ital. Sci. Vet.* **7**, 358.

Nisbet, A. M. (1956). *Nature (London)* **178**, 1477.

Nishinakagawa, H. (1970). *Bull. Fac. Agr. Kagoshima Univ.* **20**, 1.

Palic, D. (1954). *Acta Vet. Belgrade* **4**, 85.

Paterson, J. Y. F., and Linzell, J. L. (1971). *J. Endocrinol.* **50**, 493.

Peaker, M., and Linzell, J. L. (1973). *J. Endocrinol.* **57**, 87.

Peeters, G., Cocquyt, G., and de Moor, A. (1963). *Ann. Endocrinol.* **24**, 717.

Peeters, G., and Massart, L. (1947). *Arch. Int. Pharmacodyn.* **74**, 83.

Petersen, W. E. (1942). *Proc. Soc. Exp. Biol. Med.* **50**, 298.

Petersen, W. E., and Ludwick, T. M. (1942). *Fed. Proc. Fed. Amer. Soc. Exp. Biol.* **1**, 66.

Petersen, W. E., Shaw, J. C., and Visscher, M. B. (1941). *J. Dairy Sci.* **24**, 139.

Pickles, V. R. (1949). *Quart. J. Exp. Physiol.* **35**, 219.

Pickles, V. R. (1952). *Quart. J. Exp. Physiol.* **37**, 175.

Pickles, V. R. (1953). *J. Obstet. Gynaecol. Brit. Emp.* **60**, 301.

Pickles, V. R. (1967). *Biol. Rev.* **42**, 614.

Pitelka, D. R., Kerkof, P. R., Gagné, H. T., Smith, S., and Abraham, S. (1969). *Exp. Cell. Res.* **57**, 43.

Popjak, G., Folley, S. J., and French, T. H. (1949). *Arch. Biochem.* **23**, 509.

Powell, R. C., and Shaw, J. C. (1942). *J. Biol. Chem.* **146**, 207.

Puget, E., and Toty, M. (1956). *Rev. Méd. Vét.* **107**, 84.

Ramwell, P. W., and Shaw, J. E. (1969). *Recent Progr. Horm. Res.* **26**, 139.

Rasmussen, F. (1963). *Acta Vet. Scand.* **4**, 271.

Rasmussen, F. (1965). *Acta Vet. Scand.* **6**, 135.

Rasmussen, F., and Linzell, J. L. (1964). *Quart. J. Exp. Physiol.* **49**, 219.

Reineke, E. P., Stonecipher, W. D., and Turner, C. W. (1941a). *Amer. J. Physiol.* **132**, 535.

Reineke, E. P., Williamson, M. B., and Turner, C. W. (1941b). *J. Dairy Sci.* **24**, 317.

Reynaert, H., Peeters, G., Verbeke, R., and Houvenaghel, A. (1968). *Arch. Int. Pharmacodyn. Therap.* **176**, 473.

Reynolds, M. (1962). *J. Dairy Sci.* **45**, 742.

Reynolds, M. (1964). *Amer. J. Physiol.* **206**, 183.

Reynolds, M. (1969). *In* "Lactogenesis." (M. Reynolds, and S. J. Folley, eds.), p. 145. Univ. Pennsylvania Press, Philadelphia, Pennsylvania.

Reynolds, M. (1970). *Physiologist* **13**, 292.

Reynolds, M., Linzell, J. L., and Rasmussen, F. (1968). *Amer. J. Physiol.* **214**, 1415.

Riis, P. M., Luick, J. R., and Kleiber, M. (1960). *Amer. J. Physiol.* **198**, 45.

Sapirstein, L. A. (1956). *Circ. Res.* **4**, 689.

Sapirstein, L. A. (1958). *Amer. J. Physiol.* **193**, 161.

Schoefl, G. I., and French, J. E. (1968). *Proc. Roy. Soc. London B* **169**, 153.

Seldinger, S. I. (1953). *Acta Radiol. Stockholm* **39**, 368.

Setchell, B. P., and Waites, G. M. H. (1962). *J. Physiol. London* **164**, 200.

Sham, G. B., White, F. C., and Bloor, C. M. (1970). *J. Appl. Physiol.* **28**, 510.

Shaw, J. C. (1942). *J. Biol. Chem.* **142**, 53.

Shaw, J. C. (1946). *J. Dairy Sci.* **29**, 183.

Shaw, J. C., and Petersen, W. E. (1939). *Proc. Soc. Exp. Biol. Med.* **42**, 520.

Shaw, J. C., Boyd, W. L., and Petersen, W. E. (1938). *Proc. Soc. Exp. Biol. Med.* **38**, 579.

Snedecor, G. W. (1950). "Statistical Methods," 4th ed., p. 214. Iowa State Press, Ames, Iowa.

Soemarwoto, I. N., and Bern, H. A. (1958). *Amer. J. Anat.* **103**, 403.

Spincer, J., Rook, J. A. F., and Towers, K. G. (1969). *Biochem. J.* **111**, 727.

Srukov, M. N. (1962). *Bull. Leningrad Univ.* **21**, 113.

Stegall, R. F., Rushmer, R. F., and Baker, D. W. (1966). *J. Appl. Physiol.* **21**, 707.

Tarten, M., and Schalm, O. W. (1964). *Amer. J. Vet. Res.* **25**, 501.

Tavenor, W. D. (1969). *Amer. J. Vet. Res.* **30**, 1881.

Tindal, J. S. (1957). *Amer. J. Physiol.* **151**, 287.

Tsakhaev, G. A. (1959). *Akad. Sci. Lithuanian S.S.R. Inst. Biol.* **57**.

Turkington, R. W., and Topper, Y. J. (1966). *Endocrinology* **79**, 175.

Twarog, J. M., and Larson, B. L. (1964). *Exp. Cell. Res.* **34**, 88.

Van Leersum, E. C. (1911). *Pflügers Arch.* **142**, 377.

Verbeke, R., and Peeters, G. (1964). *Biochem. J.* **94**, 183.

Verbeke, R., Peeters, G., Cocquyt, G., and Lauryssens, M. (1965). *Meded. Landb. Hoogesch. Opzolkstus. Gent.* **30**, 743.

Vladimirova, A. D. (1954). *Bull. Leningrad Univ.* **97**.

Vladimirova, A. D. (1955). *Bull. Leningrad Univ.* **83**.

Vladimirova, A. D. (1958). *Bull. Leningrad Univ.* **97**.

Vuorenkoski, V., Wasz-Hockert, O., Koivisto, E., and Lind, J. (1969). *Experientia* **25**, 1286.

Wahl, H. M. (1915). *Amer. J. Anat.* **18**, 515.

Watkins, W. M., and Hassid, W. Z. (1962). *J. Biol. Chem.* **237**, 1432.

Weirich, W. E., Will, J. A., and Crumpton, C. W. (1970). *J. Appl. Physiol.* **28**, 117.

West, C. E., Bickerstaffe, R., Annison, E. F., and Linzell, J. L. (1972). *Biochem. J.* **126**, 477.

Wood, H. G., Siu, P., and Schambye, P. (1957). *Arch. Biochem. Biophys.* **69**, 390.

Ziegler, H. (1959). *Schweiz. Akad. Med. Wissenshaft.* **15**, 105.

Zierler, K. L. (1961). *J. Clin. Invest.* **40**, 2111.

Zietzschmann, O. (1917). *Deut. tierärztl. Worschr.* **25**, 361.

Zweifach, B. W. (1939). *Anat. Rec.* **73**, 475.

CHAPTER FOUR

Neural and Hormonal Control of Milk Secretion and Milk Ejection

C. E. Grosvenor and F. Mena

I. Introduction 227
II. Innervation of the Mammary Gland 228
  A. Sensory Nerve Endings 228
  B. Efferent Innervation 231
  C. Neural Pathways from the Mammary Glands to the Brain 232
III. Removal of Milk from the Mammary Glands 236
  A. General 236
  B. Factors Affecting Rate of Milk Ejection 237
  C. Inhibition of the Milk Ejection Reflex 238
IV. Neuroendocrine Mechanisms in Milk Secretion 243
  A. General 243
  B. Neuroendocrine Mechanisms in Lactogenesis 243
  C. Neuroendocrine Mechanisms in Galatopoiesis 245
V. Decline and Cessation of Lactation 266
  References 268

I. INTRODUCTION

This account of the neuroendocrine control of milk secretion and milk ejection is in no way meant to be an exhaustive treatment of the subject. We have not discussed at length many areas of the subject, particularly those which have been subjected to recent review. The reader is referred to these throughout the text. Instead we have focused on the way the neuroendocrine mechanisms which influence the pituitary gland and mammary gland function to initiate and to maintain lactation. We have also briefly discussed the functioning of these mechanisms at the end of lactation and have considered how their level of function in combination with some other factors contribute to the decline and cessation of lactation.

If it appears that great emphasis is placed upon the physiology of prolactin it is because prolactin appears to be of paramount importance both in the initiation and in the maintenance of milk secretion in many species. Also the incorporation of pituitary culture and of radioimmunoassay techniques have provided great impetus to the study of prolactin. Certainly what is known concerning the neuroendocrine regulation of prolactin secretion during lactation will prove useful in investigations of other adenohypophyseal hormones.

Little new information is available in regard to milk ejection since last reviewed. We have emphasized that the efferent innervation of the mammary gland through alterations in ductal resistance may be an important controlling influence over the rate and extent of milk ejection.

II. INNERVATION OF THE MAMMARY GLAND

A. Sensory Nerve Endings

We possess very few details concerning the structure and arrangement of sensory receptors and even less in regard to their electrophysiological characteristics. Whereas there is good evidence for a profuse innervation of the teat, there is no unanimity of opinion regarding the type of receptor found there. The walls of the teats are thought by some to contain superficial and deep nerve plexuses with numerous encapsulated ends, including Merkels, Golgi-Mazzoni, and Pacini corpuscles (see Cross, 1961a; Denamur, 1965; Linzell, 1959, for references). Free nerve endings are abundant in the smooth muscles and in the walls of the blood vessels of the teat. In some species, e.g., the cow and the human, very few specifically differentiated receptors have been noted in the walls of the teat though numerous free nerve endings exist (Cathcart *et al.*, 1948; Giacometti and Montagna, 1962; Miller and Kasahara, 1959; Niggli-Stokar, 1961). The richly innervated areola apparently does not contain any corpuscular formations.

It is well established that the nerve endings in the teat respond to stimulation and that a variety of neural and hormonal events result from such stimulation. Among these, the secretion of oxytocin from the neurohypophysis and the secretion of prolactin from the adenohypophysis will be discussed at a later point in this paper. The properties of teat receptors have been examined in the rabbit by Findlay (1966) using electrophysiological afferent nerve recording techniques. He demonstrated that the teat contains mechanical receptors that are responsive to suction and to pressure, some of which were slowly adapting though most of which appeared to be of the rapidly adapting type.

A full coverage of the earlier histological work on the innervation of the mammary gland is available (Cross, 1961a). Reliable histochemical methods have recently been used to study the innervation of rabbit and cow mammary tissue (Ballantyne and Bunch, 1966; Hebb and Linzell, 1966; Lukášová and Lukáš, 1965). The rich nerve supply of the teat region has been confirmed in these species. In the cow, Lukášová and Lukáš (1965) described nerve fibers branching in the connective tissue of the cistern but found only small amounts of cholinesterase in the parenchyma and none at all in the alveoli. Hebb and Linzell (1966) demonstrated nerve fibers in intralobular connective tissue, often near ducts, in the rabbit gland, but they found no fibers within the lobules. Ballantyne and Bunch (1966), Edwardson (1968), and Hebb and Linzell (1970) have described cholinesterase-containing fibers in mammary tissue sections. Hebb and Linzell (1970) noted in the rabbit that the majority of nerve fibers followed the arteries and arterioles and formed a network in the walls of these vessels. Some fibers were found to lie near the mammary duct walls but none terminated at the mammary secretory cell, the myoepithelial cell or at the junctures of the ducts. Lassmann (1964) reported that many nerve fibers were found in the areolar and nipple areas of the human but that some fibers ended in the ducts. The epithelium of the large ducts were stated to occasionally contain organs of Ruffini. In an electron microscopic study of the innervation of the rabbit mammary gland, Findlay (1967) found many nerve fibers, both myelinated and unmyelinated, in the teat. He was able to demonstrate similar fibers in the parenchyma, but only in those areas of parenchyma immediately underlying the teat. He assumed that most of these fibers would be passing through the parenchyma to supply the teat. No nerve fibers were seen in areas of the parenchyma remote from the teat. Although sparse innervation could well go undetected in an ultrastructural study, there are certainly no clear indications that the innervation of the parenchyma is profuse.

The existence of receptors sensitive to changes in intramammary pressure has been established. Subjective sensations occurring in human lactation associated with the "draught reflex" were described by Isbister (1954). Forbes *et al.* (1955) found that similar sensations usually accompanied the injection of posterior pituitary extract. Grachev (1949) performed experiments on goats in which the entire udder, with the exception of the nerves, was separated from the animal and perfused through its blood vessels with oxygenated Tyrode solution at 38°C. Systemic blood pressure, heart rate, and respiration were recorded. Artificial distension of the udder with air, milk, or water brought about a rise in blood pressure and respiration rate which he believed to be due to the activation of the pressure receptors in the gland. The existence of chemoreceptors was also postulated on the basis of an increase in blood pressure and inhibition of respiration, which was elicited by the injection of 1% KOH into the cistern. Similar changes were elicited when KCl solutions were injected into the udder circulation. The nonphysiological nature of the injections of KOH and KCl makes the interpretation of these results difficult, but clearly afferent nerves from the udder were stimulated.

Grachev (1964) later investigated the effect of intramammary pressure changes on the production of conditioned reflexes in the goat. He introduced fluid or air into the udder at a pressure of 40 mm Hg. It was found that higher pressures elicited signs of acute discomfort. Grachev concluded that goats can discriminate between the stimulation of the left and the right mammary glands when stimulation of one is used as a positive, and the other as a negative, reinforcing stimulus. Cobo et al. (1967) found that in humans both suckling by the baby and duct dilation of the mammary gland produced a clear milk-ejection response. The characteristic waves of mammary contraction seen with suckling and duct dilation could be simulated by intermittent injections of oxytocin. There is also evidence that mammary distension can affect nursing behavior in the rabbit (Cross, 1952; Findlay, 1969). Mammary fullness appears to be a sufficient, but not a necessary condition for the display of nursing behavior in this species.

Cross and Findlay (1969) and Findlay (1966, 1967) recorded afferent discharges in mammary nerves of lactating rabbits which were produced by rises of intramammary pressure caused by the intravenous injection of oxytocin or by the introduction of fluid through a cannulated teat duct. After removal of the skin overlying the gland, receptors could still be detected which discharged in response to increases in intramammary pressure. Most of these were located in the teat region, but a small minority survived teat removal and were inactivated only by introduction of lignocaine into the mammary parenchyma itself. Receptors which were sensitive to intramammary pressure were found to be more responsive to increases in pressure than to either steady levels of or decreases in pressure.

B. Efferent Innervation

Peeters *et al.* (1949) stimulated the inguinal nerve of a perfused bovine mammary gland and recorded strong teat contractions, vasoconstriction, and slightly decreased intramammary pressures. Injection of the adrenergic blocking agent, Dibenamine, inhibited partly or completely the effect of nerve stimulation on the teat smooth muscle. In a later study Peeters *et al.* (1952) removed the right lumbar sympathetic trunk from lactating sheep. This was followed by a vasodilation which lasted about 3 days, although milk secretion and milk ejection were at no time affected. Teat contraction still followed stimulation of the inguinal nerves in normal glands but not in the sympathetically denervated glands. Milk expulsion never followed such stimulation. Tverskoi (personal communications) performed ipsilateral sympathectomy in the goat and noted that teat flaccidity resulted on the side that the sympathetic nerves were excised. Linzell (1950) noted that the vasoconstriction, which followed stimulation of the external spermatic nerve and the cutaneous nerves of cats and dogs, was not affected by atropine but was prevented by ergot preparations. The vasoconstriction was mimicked by epinephrine. Linzell (1959) observed also that teat contraction and vasoconstriction followed stimulation of both the perineal and external spermatic nerves in sheep and goats. These responses were abolished by Dibenamine. Linzell concluded as did Peeters that the efferent innervation of the mammary gland consisted of sympathetic fibers, which, when stimulated, caused vasoconstriction and teat contraction.

Recently, Hebb and Linzell (1970) studied the innervation of the mammary glands of the rabbit utilizing catecholamine and cholinesterase histochemical methods. They found that noradrenaline-containing fibers were abundant among the smooth muscles of the teat between the media and adventitia of the arteries. They obtained no evidence that cholinergic fibers supplied any part of the gland. These data thus agree with the physiological experiments, which demonstrated that the efferent nerves to both structures are of sympathetic origin.

Zaks (1951) working with sheep and goats and Baryshnikov *et al.* (1951) working with guinea pigs showed that stimulation of the peripheral end of the external spermatic nerve, which supplies the udder, suppresses the removal of milk through an udder catheter for a varying length of time. This was accompanied by a loss of color in the stimulated udder. Baryshnikov *et al.* (1953) stimulated the peripheral end of the spermatic nerve in goats and observed that if the stimulation was applied before milk ejection that milk ejection was promptly terminated. Cross

(1955) stimulated the external spermatic nerve of rabbits, which conveyed sympathetic fibers to the inguinal mammary glands, or the splanchnic nerve supply to the adrenal glands. He found that stimulation of either of these fibers inhibited the milk ejection response to injected oxytocin.

In summary, the available evidence indicates that the efferent innervation of the mammary gland is by way of the sympathetic division of the autonomic nervous system [see Findlay and Grosvenor (1969) for further discussion].

C. Neural Pathways from the Mammary Glands to the Brain

The analysis of the neural afferent connections between the mammary glands and the brain in different species with respect to the pathway of (1) the milk ejection reflex and (2) prolactin release by suckling has been the subject of several recent reviews (Averill, 1966; Beyer and Mena, 1969a,b; Bisset, 1968; Cross, 1966; Denamur, 1965; Tindal, 1967; Tindal and Knaggs, 1970). In the present section we shall be concerned mainly with recent developments in this field.

At present, it is considered that paraventricular (PV) and supraoptic (SO) neurons of the hypothalamus constitute the last relay, i.e., final common pathway, of the milk ejection reflex (see Cross, 1966, for discussion). Recently, in the guinea pig, destruction of an area including the PV, but not the SO nucleus, blocked the release of oxytocin induced by electrical stimulation of a discrete region in the midbrain (Tindal and Knaggs, 1971). Moreover, it has been shown that in the cat PV neurons increase their rate of discharge by peripheral stimulation of the nipple area. This indicates that PV neurons are activated by suckling during lactation (Brooks et al., 1966). On the other hand, much evidence indicates that these neurons are sensitive to a variety of stimuli, including tactile stimuli (see Beyer and Sawyer, 1969, for discussion). This knowledge is important when considering hypothalamic integration of the afferent influences, internal and external, that modify pituitary secretions during lactation. With respect to prolactin release, however, the existing information is not as clear as for oxytocin release. This, perhaps, is partly because the hypothalamic control of the adenohypophysis is more complicated than that of the neurohypophysis. The hypothalamic control of prolactin release is discussed in a subsequent section.

Afferent nerve fibers connect the mammary glands to the central nervous system through the dorsal roots. Destruction of these elements at appropriate levels has been found to suppress lactation in rats (Eayrs and Baddeley, 1956) and milk ejection in goats (Denamur and Martinet, 1959b). At the level of the spinal cord, transection of this structure has been shown to block the milk ejection reflex in all the species so far studied (Beyer *et al.*, 1962a; Denamur and Martinet, 1959b; Eayrs and Baddeley, 1956; Mena and Beyer, 1963; Tsakhaev, 1953). Within the spinal cord, however, variation among species has been found with respect to the location of the main component of fibers conducting impulses from the mammary glands. In ruminants, lesion experiments suggest that fibers of the milk ejection pathway ascend without crossing in the dorsal funiculus (Denamur and Martinet, 1959b; Popovici, 1963; Tsakhaev, 1953) either through the dorsal column-medial lemniscal, or through the spino-cervico-thalamic system (Richard *et al.*, 1970), whereas fibers related to cistern baroceptors have crossed representatives in the lateral funiculus (Popovici, 1963). In the rat (Eayrs and Baddeley, 1956) and the rabbit (Mena and Beyer, 1968a), on the other hand, the location of lesions effective for blocking milk ejection indicates that the spino-thalamic system of fibers is most likely related to the conduction of impulses for oxytocin release and that these fibers have a predominant ipsilateral distribution (see Beyer and Mena, 1969a,b; Denamur, 1965; Tindal and Knaggs, 1970, for further discussion).

The course of the afferent pathway for oxytocin and for prolactin release, at the level of the brainstem, has been studied by several workers. At the level of the medulla, electrical stimulation of the medial lemniscus but not of the reticular formation, resulted in milk ejection in the goat (Andersson, 1951). In the lactating rabbit, Cross (1961b) found that electrical stimulation of the central gray, midbrain reticular formation and medial lemniscus provoked milk ejection. On the basis of these results, it was suggested that the milk ejection pathway was diffusely distributed throughout the brainstem.

In lactating cats, localized lesions in the extreme rostral mesencephalic central gray interrupting the dorsal longitudinal fasciculus blocked oxytocin release by suckling. It was proposed that an important proportion of the fibers related to oxytocin release by suckling join the dorsal longitudinal fasciculus at the level of the rostral mesencephalon (Beyer and Mena, 1965a; Beyer *et al.*, 1962b). In the guinea pig and the rabbit, at the caudal mesencephalon, electrical stimulation of a discrete region in the dorsolateral mesencephalic tegmentum which corresponds to the location of the spinothalamic and spinotectal tracts, was associated with milk ejection. Further rostrally, positive points were detected also in the central gray. At the level of the rostral mesencephalon, the sensitive points were located in both a dorsal and a ventral position. The dorsally placed points extended medially to the extreme rostral central gray, the periventricular region at the mesodiencephalic zone and the parafascicular thalamic nucleus. The ventral component entered the subthalamus and lateral hypothalamus between the medial lemniscus and cerebral peduncle (Tindal *et al.*, 1967b, 1968, 1969). At the level of the lateral hypothalamus, both dorsal and ventral components were reunited and passed dorsomedially to relay with the lateral tip of the ipsilateral PV nucleus (Tindal and Knaggs, 1971).

From the results of other electrical stimulation experiments, the suggestion has been made that alternative routes to the neurohypophysis may exist in the brainstem. Thus, stimulation of some structures, e.g., mammillary peduncle (Mena *et al.*, 1961) and medial forebrain bundle (Cross, 1961b; Tindal *et al.*, 1967b) elicits oxytocin release. However, the destruction of some of these structures (Beyer and Mena, 1969b) does not impair normal milk ejection provoked by suckling. It is possible that these afferent tracts to the neurohypophysis are related to the release of oxytocin by other stimuli. However, such interpretations are necessarily speculative since the degree of information obtained through stimulation experiments is limited to a potential relation of a structure to a given function, and not to its functional significance.

In the hypothalamus, the periventricular diencephalic region has been implicated in different species as the site through which pass an important proportion of fibers related to milk ejection. Lesions in this area at the caudal hypothalamus in the cat (Beyer and Mena, 1965a) and the rat (Stutinsky and Terminn, 1964) or at the medial hypothalamus (dorsomedial and ventromedial nuclei) in the rat (Yokoyama and Ota, 1959) and the rabbit (Ban *et al.*, 1958) interfere with normal milk ejection. The principal system of fibers interrupted by these lesions was the periventricular diencephalic system of fibers, which is considered to be the hypothalamic extension of the dorsal longitudinal fasciculus or bundle of Schutz (Beyer and Mena, 1969b). It appears that both lesions and electrical stimulation experiments coincide in indicating that the dorsal longitudinal fasciculus and its hypothalamic extension, i.e., the periventricular diencephalic system of fibers, is the main pathway followed by the afferent impulses generated by suckling. Apparently, the dorsal component detected by Tindal *et al.* by electrical stimulation in the guinea pig and the rabbit, corresponds to the approximate sites of the effective lesions in the periventricular diencephalic system that were found to block milk ejection in the other species. Recently, Tindal and Knaggs (1971) reported that the response of a discrete region in the midbrain, i.e., the level at which the sensitive fibers are concentrated, was blocked to a higher degree when the ventral component was sectioned at the hypothalamic level than after sectioning of the dorsal component. From this, they inferred that the ventral is more important than the dorsal component in terms of oxytocin release. This, however, is contradictory to the results of lesion experiments in which a complete blockage of milk ejection was obtained after destruction of the periventricular region. It is possible that the different experimental conditions employed by each type of study may account for this discrepancy. On the other hand, it is perhaps premature to draw conclusions based on such a comparison of results. This is particularly true since the conclusion derived from the electrical stimulation experiments were based on the finding that only partial interference of the response was obtained after the selective destruction of the dorsal and ventral components. In the case of the lesion experiments complete blockage of the milk ejection reflex was obtained in spite of the fact that the neural elements corresponding to the location of the ventral component were not destroyed (Beyer and Mena, 1969a). It would be of interest to analyze the effect of small lesions of the pathway at the hypothalamus upon the release of oxytocin provoked by normal suckling stimulation.

Tindal and Knaggs (1969) found that in the pseudopregnant rabbit, electrical stimulation of the same discrete regions in the mesencephalon provoked oxytocin (Tindal *et al.,* 1969) and prolactin (Tindal and Knaggs, 1969) release. From this, they proposed that at the mesencephalic level, the same pathway was related to oxytocin and prolactin release. Further rostrally, however, only the dorsal portion of the milk ejection pathway was related with prolactin release.

In conclusion it would appear in the laboratory animals studied that two systems of fibers, the spinothalamic tracts and the dorsal longitudinal fasciculus, are involved in the afferent flow of impulses from the mammary glands to the hypothalamic–hypophyseal system.

Evidence has been obtained in several species with electrical stimulation and lesion techniques, which suggests that the functioning of the neurohypophysis is influenced by several extrahypothalamic regions. Thus, stimulation of the anterior cingulate gyrus, septum, hippocampus, and amygdala elicits oxytocin discharge (see Beyer and Mena, 1969a; Denamur, 1965, for review), while bilateral lesions in the amygdala have been reported to block lactation in the rat by interference with milk ejection (Stutinksy and Terminn, 1965). The importance of these structures for oxytocin release during lactation is, however, not clear and apparently they are not essential for normal milk ejection. Recently, it has been reported that removal of the entire telencephalon, including cerebral cortex, hippocampi, amygdala, and other parts, did not affect the release of oxytocin induced by electrical stimulation of the milk ejection pathway in the midbrain. These data raise the possibility that within the forebrain the pathway is entirely diencephalic (Tindal and Knaggs, 1971). Nevertheless, it is possible that the limbic forebrain participates in the conditioned release of oxytocin described by some workers (see Cross, 1966; Tindal and Knaggs, 1970; Zaks, 1962).

III. REMOVAL OF MILK FROM THE MAMMARY GLANDS

A. General

The milk in the alveoli and in the small ducts of the mammary gland must be ejected in contrast to that contained in the sinuses, cisterns, or other dilations of the large ducts which can be withdrawn passively, i.e., drained through a teat cannula. The amount of milk that can be withdrawn passively may comprise a large percentage of the total milk in cows and goats whose glands have large cisterns, but constitutes only a small percentage of that in such species as the rat, rabbit, and mouse whose glands lack a cistern or other dilation of the major ducts (see Cross, 1961a; Linzell, 1959).

The contractile tissues of the mammary gland have been shown by Richardson (1949) to be of two types: myoepithelium, which covers the stromal surface of the epithelium of the alveoli, ducts, and cisterns of the entire gland, and smooth muscle, which is found in the teat and forms scattered interlobular bundles closely associated with the blood vessels. On the alveoli the myoepithelial cells are arranged in a stellate form so that their contraction in response to oxytocin compresses the alveoli and raises the pressure within the gland. On the small ducts the cells are disposed longitudinally and the effect of their contraction in response to oxytocin is to widen and shorten the ducts (Linzell, 1955).

The ejection of milk is mediated via a neurohumoral reflex. Oxytocin is released from the neurohypophysis by suckling or milking stimuli and is carried by the circulation to the mammary gland, where a few seconds after it has been released, it causes the contraction of alveolar myoepithelium and expels the alveolar milk (Cross and Harris, 1952; Ely and Petersen, 1941)—under pressure—into the larger ducts or cisterns where it is available for withdrawal. The stimulation provided by the acts of suckling or milking is of a very complex nature and probably involves the simultaneous activation of various types of mammary receptors such as touch and heat. The frequency characteristics that mammary stimulation must fulfill in order to induce milk ejection have been studied in the goat (Grachev, 1953). He found that milk ejection is not produced at frequencies of milking below 12 per minute whereas rates of stimulation between 84 and 142 stimuli per minute were found to be maximally effective.

The release of oxytocin also may follow conditioned auditory and visual stimuli (Baryshnikov and Kokorina, 1959; Cleverley, 1968; Deis, 1968; Momongan and Schmidt, 1970) and stimulation of the vulva, vagina, and perianal regions of the female reproductive tract (Debackere *et al.,* 1961; Fitzpatrick, 1961; Knaggs, 1963; Roberts and Share, 1968). Some evidence exists in the rat (Mena and Grosvenor, 1968) and in the rabbit (Fuchs and Wagner, 1963) that the amount of oxytocin released by suckling is roughly directly proportional to the number of pups suckling. From the studies of Whittlestone (1951), Whittlestone *et al.* (1952), and Folley and Knaggs (1966) it would appear that oxytocin may be released at least in two packets, the first as a result of the premilking stimulus, e.g., the presence of the milker, and the other during the actual milking process.

B. Factors Affecting Rate of Milk Ejection

The rate of ejection of milk from the lactating mammary gland depends not only upon the pressure generated within the secretory alveoli as the myoepithelium that surrounds them contracts but also upon the resistance to flow within the ducts of the parenchyma and teats. There is some evidence that the duct system of the mammary gland can alter its resistance to the flow of milk from the alveoli to the exterior (see Findlay and Grosvenor, 1969; Zaks, 1962, for review). The alterations in resistance appear to be due in part to passive changes in diameter of the ducts. Thus, smaller ducts have been observed with the light microscope to shorten and widen in response to oxytocin (Linzell, 1955) presumably as the result of contraction of the myoepithelial cells and in the cow, goat, and rat, the resistance of parts of the duct system is overcome when the alveoli have accumulated a certain quantity of milk (DeNuccio and Grosvenor, 1971; Tverskoi and Dyusembin, 1955; Zaks and Pavlov, 1952). The mammary myoepithelial cells of a variety of species have been shown to contract in response to mechanical stimulation (see Findlay and Grosvenor, 1969, for references). It was first suggested by Cross (1954) and later analyzed by Grosvenor (1965c) that the mechanically induced contraction of the mammary gland may constitute a subsidiary system for the expulsion of milk. Findlay and Grosvenor (1967) demonstrated, however, that mechanical stimulation of the mammary gland of the rat and the rabbit results first in a transient decrease in intramammary pressure, which precedes the more easily observed mechanically induced rise in pressure. The reduction in pressure was thought to be the result of passive stretching of the ducts and/or contraction of the ductal myoepithelium since the effect persisted in lignocaine-filled glands and in glands that had been denervated. They suggested (Findlay and Grosvenor, 1967) that during active suckling, mechanical and oxytocic stimulation could act together to dilate ducts and to contract alveoli; both effects should assist in the attainment of a high rate of milk flow to the exterior. The resistance of the ducts also may be actively controlled to a certain extent by the efferent innervation, which, since there is the absence of both voluntary musculature and a parasympathetic innervation in the mammary gland, seems to be mainly by fibers of the sympathetic nervous system. The importance of this system in the maintenance of tone of the teat and larger ducts of the mammary gland has already been studied to some extent in the mouse, sheep, goat, and cow (see Findlay and Grosvenor, 1969, for references).

C. Inhibition of the Milk Ejection Reflex

The milk ejection reflex appears to be easily inhibited by various somatic and psychological stressors. Ely and Petersen (1941) reported that a reduction of milk yield occurred in cows when paper bags filled with air were exploded or when a cat was placed on the back of the cow during milking. Similar inhibition was obtained in cows by Whittlestone (1951) when faradic shocks were applied shortly before milking. Newton and Newton (1948) have reported that embarrassment, fear, or discomfort while nursing partially inhibited milk ejection in women. A reduction in milk ejection also has been shown to occur in rabbits (Cross, 1955) and guinea pigs (Chaudhury et al., 1961) when the mothers were forcibly restrained in a supine position during suckling. Severe stresses, e.g., a leg break or an open wound under ether anesthesia (Taleisnik and Deis, 1964) or milder stresses such as the odor of the oil of peppermint, intermittent low-intensity sounds, or intermittent bright light (Grosvenor and Mena, 1967) have been shown to drastically reduce milk ejection in rats.

1. Central and Peripheral Mechanisms

The mechanisms underlying emotional inhibition of milk ejection were first studied by Cross (1955) who concluded that one of the main factors in the emotional disturbance of the milk ejection reflex is a partial inhibition of oxytocin release from the neurohypophysis. Aulsebrook and Holland (1969) found that in the rabbit the release of oxytocin elicited by stimulation of the forebrain could be suppressed by simultaneous excitation of some regions of the brainstem, e.g., mesencephalic tegmentum, central gray, pretectal region, etc. The participation of the cerebral cortex in the emotional inhibition of oxytocin release also has been demonstrated by Taleisnik and Deis (1964) who found that cortical spreading depression prevented the inhibition of the milk ejection reflex produced by painful stimuli. Koizumi et al. (1964) found that electrical or chemical excitation of the anterior lobe of the cerebellum and the mesencephalic reticular formation inhibited the discharge rate of many of the neurosecretory neurons in the supraoptic and paraventricular nuclei.

There is little doubt, however, that activation of the sympathetic-adrenal system also can reduce the contractile response of the gland through one of several peripheral mechanisms including constriction of the mammary blood vessels, increased resistance of the mammary ducts (Findlay and Grosvenor, 1969; Grosvenor and Findlay, 1968; Hebb and Linzell, 1951), and direct inhibition of the effect of oxytocin on mammary myoepithelial cells (Bisset et al., 1967; Chan, 1965; Houvenaghel, 1969). The existence of adrenergic receptors in the mammary gland blood vessels and in the myoepithelial cells has been described in the smooth muscles of most organ systems Koelle (1965) and Vorherr (1971) recently concluded that α receptors are present in the mammary blood vessels and that β receptors are present in the myoepithelium. The epinephrine and norepinephrine inhibition of milk ejection thus may be due to stimulation to vascular α receptors and to myoepithelial β receptors.

Grosvenor et al. (1972) using an isometric recording system in the anesthetized lactating rat found that the ascending slope and amplitude of the intrammary pressure response to intravenously injected oxytocin increased following administration of either α- or β-adrenergic blocking agents or ganglionic blocking agents. The latency of the response, however, was not measurably affected. The high amplitude, steeply ascending pressures which occurred after adrenergic blockade often were accompanied by a slower than usual descent of the pressure to the preexisting basal pressure level and the responses frequently oscillated. These changes in the profile of the intramammary pressure response indicated that ductal resistance had been decreased following adrenergic blockade and suggested that the sympathetic system normally exerts a measure of control over the tone of the duct system. Grosvenor and Findlay (1968) earlier showed that ductal resistance was increased by catecholamines. However, the blockade of α receptors also leads to an increase in blood flow and to an increase in the concentration of oxytocin at the myoepithelium (see Bisset *et al.*, 1967; Vorherr, 1971).

Evidence is accumulating that oxytocin at certain high doses may actually inhibit milk secretion and/or milk ejection. Though the doses required admittedly are well above the physiological range, large doses of oxytocin frequently are injected routinely either to obtain the residual milk or to facilitate normal milk removal. Inhibitory effects of oxytocin upon milk yield have been observed in the cow (Carroll *et al.*, 1968; Donker *et al.*, 1954; Morag, 1967; Morag and Griffin, 1968), ewe (Morag and Fox, 1966), and in women (Beller *et al.*, 1958). Similar inhibitory effects have been observed in conscious rodents along with data indicating that the inhibitory effect of oxytocin upon milk ejection is dose-dependent and may be due to central and/or to peripheral inhibitory mechanisms (Deis, 1971; Kuhn and McCann, 1970; Mizuno and Shiiba, 1969; Mizuno and Satoh, 1970). Grosvenor and Mena (unpublished) found that the intramammary pressure responses to physiological doses of oxytocin in anesthetized rats were reduced to one-third of control values following the sustained contracture (12–55 minutes), which resulted from injection of 160–320 mU oxytocin intravenously. An average of 50 minutes was required before the responses returned to previous control values; the glands frequently ruptured following the 320 mU dose. Blockade of the sympathetic nervous system by prior administration of either phenoxybenzamine (Dibenzyline) or propranolol or pentolinium protected against rupture of the gland and completely prevented the fall in pressure, which normally occurred following the large dose of oxytocin. Similar protection followed section of the spinal cord at T-10, i.e., above the level of the recorded gland. Thus, supraphysiological doses of oxytocin impair the contractile functions of the gland of the rat in part through activation of the sympathetic nervous system. Kuhn and McCann (1970) noticed that some of their rats exhibited piloerection following intraventricular injection of 50 mU of oxytocin, and Mena and Beyer (1969) reported complete blockade of the inhibitory effect of oxytocin on milk secretion by spinal cord section and partial blockade following administration of either α- or β-adrenergic blocking agents (Mena *et al.*, unpublished).

These results further suggest that high doses of oxytocin may stimulate sympathetico-adrenal discharge.

Grosvenor *et al.* (1972) found that administration of KCl to the cerebral cortices of anesthetized lactating rats or section of the spinal cord greatly increased the slope and amplitude of the intramammary pressure response to intravenously injected oxytocin. In the case of spinal cord section, only the glands caudal to the section were affected. The effect of KCl persisted in rats which were pretreated either with Dibenzyline or with pentolinium. These data would seem to implicate a central mechanism in the regulation of ductal resistance within the mammary gland.

2. Activation of Inhibitory Mechanisms

There is evidence that the inhibitory systems operating in the mammary gland may be activated during the course of a normal suckling situation. A fall in neutrophils and lymphocytes has been observed subsequent either to intense suckling in rats (Emmel *et al.*, 1926) or machine milking in cows (Paape and Guidry, 1969), which suggests that suckling may have irritating effects that could activate the sympathetico-adrenal system. Cochrane (1949) milked a cow that had a teat fistula that allowed the escape of milk from the teat cistern. When the cow was milked at the other teats, milk streamed out through the fistula, but merely touching the injured teat caused abrupt cessation of the flow from the fistula, which lasted approximately 30 seconds while the other teats milked normally. Kokorina (1966) noticed that a slight change in milking routine in cows markedly reduced the amount of milk that would flow after introduction of the calf to the teat. Grachev (1949) separated the goat udder from the body, left it connected by way of the nerves, and perfused the isolated but innervated gland. He found that distension of the udder by air, water, or milk brought about an increase in blood pressure and respiration rate, effects that are clearly sympathetic effects. Dyusembin (1958) found that the inhibition of milk ejection by stress was weakened by udder denervation in cows and completely abolished when the adrenal glands were denervated.

Recently, Grosvenor and King (unpublished) found that the amplitude and slope of the intramammary pressure responses to intravenously injected oxytocin were reduced in an abdominal mammary gland of the anesthetized lactating rat following a few seconds of palpating or lightly squeezing of the upper thoracic glands. The compression of the glands was performed so as to simulate the butting and kneading action of rat pups during suckling. The intramammary pressure response was reduced—often to very great extent—within 1–3 minutes in the majority of rats tested after the squeezing took place. The length of the inhibitory period varied anywhere from 1 to 12 minutes, then returned to normal. Interestingly, the intramammary pressure responses then usually "overshot" in that the amplitude and slope of the responses each increased considerably above that of the level seen prior to squeezing of the gland. Injection of lignocaine into the squeezed glands or section of the segmental nerve supplying the abdominal gland abolished the effects of squeezing of the thoracic glands. Administration of ether by inhalation for a period of 1 minute induced a pattern of response similar to that following manual compression of the mammary glands, which suggested that the changes in pressure response following manual compression of other glands were not due to activation of a specific receptor and neural arc, but probably were due to activation of the sympathetic system.

Unilateral dorsal root section was shown by Grosvenor et al. (1972a) to increase the amplitude and slope of the oxytocin-induced intramammary pressure rise in each contralateral as well as ipsilateral gland that was caudal to the level of section. The responses of mammary glands above (i.e., cranial to) the segment of dorsal root section, however, were not affected. The increased slope and amplitude of the intramammary pressure responses following dorsal root section persisted in either dibenzyline or propranolol pretreated rats, which suggests that alterations in ductal resistance may occur also by mechanisms not under sympathetic domination.

Deis (1968) and Grosvenor and King (unpublished) found that the amount of milk obtained by the pups during the first 10–15 minutes of suckling, following several hours of nonsuckling, comprised only a small percentage of the total amount of milk extractable from the mammary gland with exogenous oxytocin. In the Grosvenor and King study 7% was obtained in the first 10 minutes of suckling and about 30% of the extractable milk was obtained during the subsequent 10 minutes of suckling. These data suggest that milk ejection partially was inhibited during the first 10 minutes of suckling, an interval of time that is in accord with that period of inhibition of intramammary pressure that followed manual compression of the mammary gland (see above). Grosvenor and King (unpublished) then found that, if they applied a mild stress (picking up the rat and injecting it subcutaneously with corn oil) 40 minutes prior to replacement of the pups, that the pups obtained 100% of the extractable milk within 15 minutes of suckling. This contrasted with 15–30% of the milk obtained by 15 minutes of suckling either if no stress was applied or if the stress was applied 10 minutes prior to suckling. These data suggested that 40 minutes after the onset of the stress the rats had passed through the period of inhibition and now were in the overshoot period.

IV. NEUROENDOCRINE MECHANISMS IN MILK SECRETION

A. General

At present, there is general agreement that the mammary epithelium is activated to synthesize milk by the action of prolactin and other pituitary hormones (ACTH, TSH, STH) discharged into the circulation at about the time of parturition. Emphasis has been given recently to the study of cellular and biochemical changes that occur during lactogenesis. As a result of this emphasis, progress has been made concerning the relationships between cell proliferation, biochemical development, and other factors, such as blood supply in the initiation of lactation. These aspects are treated separately elsewhere in this book. In the present section we will be concerned with the neuroendocrine mechanisms of lactogenesis and galactopoiesis with particular emphasis on recent developments in certain neurological and physiological aspects.

B. Neuroendocrine Mechanisms in Lactogenesis

Lactogenesis is yet not fully understood. This is because of insufficient knowledge of both the neuroendocrine mechanisms involved and of the secretion rates and mechanisms of action of those hormones, which control mammary growth and secretion during this period. The theories to explain lactogenesis can be divided into two general groups according to the importance given to neural or endocrine factors in the control of the secretion of the pituitary hormones. Among those theories that emphasize neural aspects is the one proposed by Selye *et al.* (1934). They suggested that suppression of milk secretion during pregnancy resulted from inhibitory afferent stimuli generated by distension of the uterus. Lactogenesis occurred when this restraining influence was withdrawn at the time of parturition. Subsequent workers (Bradbury, 1941; Greene, 1941), however, demonstrated that the experimental design did not warrant the conclusion of Selye *et al.* Recent work suggests that the uterus may influence the life span of the corpus luteum either through the secretion of a luteolysin or through possible neural influences on pituitary gonadotropin secretion (e.g., see Bland and Donovan, 1966). Thus, the possibility exists that the uterus may participate indirectly in lactogenesis by modifying ovarian and/or pituitary secretions.

Petersen (1944) suggested that the stimulus of suckling is the main factor in initiating lactation. He observed that lactation becomes established only after the first colostrum or milk is ejected from the alveoli by suckling or milking. In this respect, Cowie *et al.* (1968) reported that twice-daily milking for several weeks brought about mammary growth, lactogenesis, and galactopoiesis in ovariectomized virgin goats. Since these effects were absent in animals that had the pituitary stalk transected, one of the conclusions reached was that the autonomous capacity of the disconnected pituitary for prolactin secretion was not sufficient by itself to induce lactogenesis and, therefore, it was necessary for the milking stimulus to activate the secretion from the pituitary of the lactogenic and galactopoietic complex of hormones. These, as well as other similar studies (see Cowie *et al.*, 1968, for references), emphasize the importance of suckling in lactogenesis. On the other hand, several reports indicate that suckling or milking is only one of several possible factors that may participate in lactogenesis. Thus, in several species, suckling stimulation does not not seem to be necessary for the immediate postpartum rise in pituitary prolactin content (Meites, 1954; Meites and Turner, 1948). Moreover, Beyer and Mena (1970) reported that lactation is initiated and maintained in the rabbit after spinal cord transection. The importance of the suckling stimulus for the maintenance of milk secretion is discussed in a subsequent section.

Roth and Rosenblatt (1966, 1968) observed that the pregnant rat licks her own nipples and urogenital area and that such behavior intensifies during the last half of pregnancy. When licking was prevented by the use of specially fitted collars, mammary growth during pregnancy was retarded. These findings have been confirmed (McMurtry and Anderson, 1971). According to these investigators, self-stimulation of the ventral body surface including the nipples and genital region, plays a physiological role in normal mammary growth during pregnancy probably through the release of adenohypophysial hormones. Self-licking has not been studied in other species and, therefore, its role in mammary growth in species other than the rat is unknown (see Richards, 1967; Blaxter, 1971, for discussion).

Among the second group of theories are those of Meites and Turner (see Meites, 1959, 1966) and Folley *et al.* (see Folley, 1956; Folley and Malpress, 1948), which stress the importance of circulating levels of gonadal, placental, and corticoid steroids as the most important aspects for consideration. These theories consider that lactogenesis does not occur during pregnancy in part because (1) there is a strong inhibitory action exerted by a high progesterone to estrogen ratio upon the pituitary secretion of prolactin and (2), during gestation, the heightened secretion of estrogen and progesterone stimulates intense growth of the mammary gland thereby rendering the mammary parenchyma relatively refractory to the milk secretion-stimulating effects of prolactin. Toward the end of pregnancy the progesterone:estrogen ratio is altered and estrogen is able to increase prolactin secretion by the pituitary. During pregnancy also, adrenal steroids are bound more tightly to the serum protein, transcortin, thereby reducing the amount of steroid free to exert biological effects. The endocrine basis of lactogenesis has been the subject of recent reviews (Benson *et al.*, 1959; Cowie, 1969, 1971; Kuhn, 1971; Meites, 1966) and the reader is referred to them for further details.

In all likelihood each of the endocrine and neural factors stressed in the above theories participates partially in the mechanisms of the release of the lactogenic complex of hormones. Therefore, one should expect that the complete picture of lactogenesis will be obtained only when the role of each factor and their interactions are determined.

C. Neuroendocrine Mechanisms in Galactopoiesis

1. Hypothalamic and Extrahypothalamic Influences on the Secretion of the Pituitary Lactogenic and Galactopoietic Hormones

Many workers in the field of neuroendocrinology of lactation consider prolactin as perhaps the most important component of the lactogenic and galactopoietic pituitary complex of hormones. As a consequence, the analysis of the mechanism of prolactin secretion during lactation has received relatively greater attention than that for other hormones in the complex.

Prolactin secretion is maintained in several species following disconnection of the pituitary from the hypothalamus either by section of the pituitary stalk (Dugger *et al.*, 1962; Eckles *et al.*, 1958; Ehni and Eckles, 1959; Jacobsohn, 1949; Nikitovitch-Winer, 1957) or transplantation of the pituitary to a site remote from its normal location (Desclin, 1950; Everett, 1954). These observations led to the hypothesis that the pituitary acidophils possess the intrinsic or autonomous capacity to secrete prolactin in the absence of influences from the brain (see Everett, 1964, 1966; Everett and Nikitovitch-Winer, 1963). Strong experimental support for this concept came from experiments in which the secretion of prolactin was shown to occur without restraint when the pituitary was cultured *in vitro* (Meites *et al.*, 1961, 1962; Pasteels, 1961, 1962). The concept of the autonomous secretory capacity of the prolactin cell has been extended to include a large number of mammalian and nonmammalian species, though the absence of this capacity exists in some species (see Bern and Nicoll, 1968; Meites and Nicoll, 1966; Nicoll, 1971).

Evolving simultaneously to the hypothesis that the prolactin cell may have an autonomous secretory capability was the hypothesis that the control normally exerted by the CNS on prolactin secretion is of an inhibitory type (Everett, 1954, 1956).

This hypothesis gained strong support from *in vitro* work made initially by Pasteels (1961, 1962) and Meites *et al.* (1962) in which it was shown that the addition of hypothalamic tissue to pituitary cultures depressed both the synthesis and the release of prolactin. On the basis of these results it was suggested that there exists in the hypothalamus an inhibitory neurohumoral factor for prolactin secretion (PIF, or prolactin inhibiting factor), which passes by way of the hypophyseal stalk to the pituitary (see Meites *et al.*, 1963). This concept was subsequently confirmed *in vivo* (see Grosvenor *et al.*, 1968b, for earlier work). The use of sophisticated techniques that include collection of blood from the portal vessels and determinations of circulating levels of prolactin (see Porter *et al.*, 1971) also have supported this hypothesis.

The control exerted by the CNS on prolactin secretion, i.e., both synthesis and release, has been interpreted by some—in the rat, at least—almost exclusively in terms of the existence of PIF. However, Fiorindo and Nicoll (1969) described that after the initial well-known decrease in prolactin secretion had occurred, a stimulatory action of the hypothalamic tissue upon prolactin secretion *in vitro* became evident. The inhibitory action was not present in hypothalamic extract from estrogen-treated rats whereas the stimulatory action was unaffected (see Nicoll *et al.*, 1970). The stimulatory effect upon prolactin secretion *in vitro* had been interpreted previously by Ratner and Meites (1964) exclusively in terms of a suppression by estrogen of PIF concentration in the hypothalamus. The results obtained by Nicoll *et al.* have been supported by the *in vivo* and *in vitro* results of Arimura *et al.* (1969) and have been challenged by Meites (1970). At present the subject is still a matter of controversy. Nicoll *et al.* (1970) have critically analyzed the available *in vivo* and *in vitro* evidence obtained in regard to hypothalamic influences upon prolactin secretion in different species.

Grosvenor *et al.* (1970c) reported that injection of hypothalamic extracts immediately after suckling, at which time the pituitary prolactin content is low, increased the rate at which prolactin reaccumulated in the pituitary of the lactating rat. Since the prolactin that reaccumulated was considered as representing the hormone synthesized by the gland during the postsuckling period, their results were tentatively interpreted as suggestive of a stimulatory action of the hypothalamic extract upon prolactin synthesis. In their study, controls were taken to exclude the possibility that the effects may have been due to gonadal steroids, to oxytocin or to PIF.

Grosvenor *et al.* (1970c) found that the injection of prolactin immediately after suckling stimulated prolactin reaccumulation in the rat pituitary to a similar extent as after injection of hypothalamic extract, an effect that, unlike that of hypothalamic extract, was blocked by central anesthesia (Grosvenor and Mena, unpublished). These data suggested that prolactin may have an indirect influence via the hypothalamus upon its own synthesis.

Recently Convey and Reece (1969) reported that pituitaries removed from lactating rats after suckling behaved *in vitro* differently with regard to prolactin secretion, than has been observed thus far in most *in vitro* studies. In their study, the cultured glands not only did not release significant amounts of prolactin into the media but also failed to reaccumulate it, whereas the glands *in situ* reaccumulated approximately one-half of the prolactin discharged by suckling within 2 hours after suckling. The gland thus appeared to lack the autonomous capacity either for synthesis or for release. They inferred that after the discharge of prolactin by suckling, a hypothalamic influence was necessary to permit normal prolactin reaccumulation by the rat pituitary. In similar context, Yanai and Nagasawa (1969) noted that the rat pituitary released more prolactin *in vitro* if the rat was nonsuckled for 8 hours than if it was nonsuckled for either 0 or 16 hours prior to removal of its pituitary. This important finding suggests that the extent of the nonsuckling interval may directly influence the autonomous secretory activity of the prolactin cell.

The above studies (Convey and Reece, 1969; Yanai and Nagasawa, 1969) point up the importance of the physiological status of the donors of pituitaries in the interpretation of *in vitro* data. Most *in vitro* work on prolactin secretion, designed to test either the autonomous capacity of the gland or the effect of hypothalamic extracts, has employed male pituitaries. The resulting data have been extrapolated and generalized to particular physiological situations in the female. Female pituitaries have been considered unsuitable for such studies in part because of the variations they show in the secretion of the hormone, yet paradoxically such variations perhaps constitute the very reason for their usage.

The results of many investigations indicate that maintaining a high level of prolactin either in the circulation or in the hypothalamus leads to a reduction in prolactin secretion by the *in vitro* pituitary (see review by Nicoll, 1971). This is manifest in a reduction in serum prolactin levels (Niswender *et al.*, 1969; Voogt and Meites, 1970) and pituitary content (Chen *et al.*, 1967; Clemens and Meites, 1968; MacCleod *et al.*, 1966; MacCleod and Abad, 1968; Mena *et al.*, 1968; Sinha and Tucker, 1968; Welsch *et al.*, 1968) and in retarded mammary development (Clemens and Meites, 1968; Sinha and Tucker, 1968). The mechanism of the effect is unknown though the reduced responsiveness of the hypothalamo-adenohypophyseal system to stimuli that normally act to release prolactin, such as suckling (Clemens *et al.*, 1969; Mena *et al.*, 1968; Voogt and Meites, 1970), cervical stimulation, and deciduoma formation (Averill, 1968; Chen *et al.*, 1968; Clemens and Meites, 1968; Clemens *et al.*, 1969) suggest that prolactin at certain levels may depress the release mechanism possibly through modifications in the secretions of PIF. There is no evidence that prolactin synthesis is directly impaired by chronic high levels of prolactin. A chronic dysfunction of the mechanisms normally activated to release prolactin could by itself eventually lead to involutive changes in the pituitary comparable for example, to those that occur after removal of the suckling stimulus.

In spite of the unequivocal nature of the effect of chronic high levels of prolactin upon prolactin secretion, there has been no evidence to date that the hour by hour, day by day control of prolactin release by the pituitary is mediated by the circulating prolactin level. Although what would appear to be reasonable—that the uptake of prolactin from the circulation by the mammary gland would stimulate prolactin secretion, i.e., via a negative feedback control mechanism—a transient reduction in the circulating level of prolactin has not been shown to stimulate prolactin release (see Nicoll, 1971), nor has a transient increase in the circulation been shown to exert a depressant effect.

The finding (Chen *et al.*, 1967) that PIF is increased in rats with chronic high circulating levels of prolactin does not necessarily implicate PIF in the regulation of acute changes in prolactin secretion. We have observed (Grosvenor and Mena, unpublished) that in rats in which high levels of exogenous prolactin have been administered for 8 hours prior to suckling, that suckling is capable of provoking normal prolactin depletion, an effect which should not have occurred if an increased PIF concentration had been present.

The experiments referred to above (Grosvenor *et al.*, 1970c) in which acute exogenous administration of prolactin stimulated prolactin reaccumulation, indicate that a positive feedback effect of prolactin upon its own synthesis may occur. In these studies (Grosvenor *et al.*, 1970c) prolactin stimulated only the *rate* of prolactin reaccumulation following its discharge from the pituitary. The absolute level in prolactin in the pituitary was not altered when prolactin was injected repeatedly at high doses during an 8-hour period (Grosvenor and Mena, 1971a). Thus, it appears that in order for the prolactin-synthesis stimulatory effect of prolactin to be manifest, the pituitary first must release its prolactin.

The location of the cellular elements in the hypothalamus responsible for the production of factors controlling prolactin secretion has not been fully clarified. Both the mechanism of action of these factors at the pituitary level and that of neurotransmitters at the hypothalamic level are at present a matter of discussion (see reviews by Geschwind, 1969, 1970; McCann, 1971).

Evidence obtained in different species implicates the tuberal region of the hypothalamus in the control of prolactin secretion by the pituitary. The suggestion that this region is related to the production of an inhibitory factor for prolactin release was based on the results that destruction (Haun and Sawyer, 1960, 1961; Kanematsu *et al.*, 1963a) or implantation of reserpine (Kanematsu and Sawyer, 1963a) into this region provoked mammary growth and lactogenesis associated with a depletion of pituitary prolactin content. Moreover, systemic or intraventricular administration of reserpine failed to produce these effects in animals that had previously been lesioned in this region (Kanematsu *et al.*, 1963b). Implantation of estrogen into this region and into the anterior pituitary produced different results. Hypothalamic implants resulted in increased prolactin content and no mammary effects whereas pituitary implants were associated with low prolactin content and with lactogenesis (Kanematsu and Sawyer, 1963b). These results were interpreted as indicative of a stimulatory action of estrogen on prolactin synthesis at the hypothalamic level and on prolactin release at the pituitary level.

Evidence exists in the rat that both agrees and disagrees with data obtained in the rabbit. On the one hand, abundant evidence exists, both *in vivo* and *in vitro*, that estrogen directly stimulates the pituitary to secrete prolactin (Chen *et al.*, 1970; Desclin, 1949, 1950; Desclin and Grégoire, 1936; Desclin and Koulischer, 1960; Nicoll and Meites, 1962; Ramirez and McCann, 1964; Welsch *et al.*, 1968). At the level of the hypothalamus, apart from the possibility of diffusion or of transport of the steroid by the portal vessels (Bogdanove, 1964), the effects reported at the mammary gland level and at the pituitary level (Deis, 1967; Ramirez and McCann, 1964; Zambrano and Deis, 1970) suggest an action on both synthesis and release of the hormone mediated either through a suppression of PIF (Ratner and Meites, 1964) and/or through a stimulation of a prolactin-synthesis stimulating factor (Fiorindo and Nicoll, 1969). It is difficult, at present, to determine the reason for the discrepancy in the results obtained in the rat and rabbit. Perhaps species differences in the autonomous capacity of the prolactin cell are important.

Recently, Nicoll (1971) has reported that female rat pituitaries secrete much more prolactin *in vitro* than do female rabbit pituitaries. According to this, in spite of obvious limitations (see Nicoll *et al.*, 1970), it would be tempting to speculate that the sensitivity of the hypothalamic system controlling pituitary function to estrogen and perhaps to other substances varies according to the autonomous capacity of the prolactin cell. Species differences also become evident when analyzing the effect of reserpine. In the rabbit, it appears that this substance facilitates only the release of prolactin with no apparent effect upon the synthesis. In the rat, the evidence points to an action of reserpine similar to that of estrogen, i.e., an action on both synthesis and release of prolactin. Transplanted pituitaries respond to systemic reserpine administration by increasing their secretion rate of prolactin (Desclin, 1957, 1960), an effect that implicates a stimulatory action on prolactin synthesis. More recently, Desclin and Flament-Durand (1969) reported that prolactin cells in pituitaries grafted in the hypothalamus were highly stimulated in reserpine-treated rats. These authors interpreted their results as suggesting the presence of a stimulating factor in the hypothalamus rather than the depression of PIF by reserpine, as responsible for the stimulation of the grafts.

Hypothalamic lesions of different magnitudes in areas that included the median eminence and other hypothalamic areas (see Beyer and Mena, 1969a,b; Everett, 1964, 1966, 1969, for references) as well as electrical or electrochemical stimulation of localized regions have been made in rats in an attempt to define hypothalamic regions related to prolactin secretion. The end points employed have been peripheral effects indicative of prolactin release by the pituitary such as mammary growth and lactogenesis (DeVae *et al.*, 1966; McCann and Friedman, 1960), prolonged periods of diestrus (Anand *et al.*, 1957; Everett, 1966; Hillarp, 1949), "hyperluteinization" (Flerkó and Bárdos, 1959), and pseudopregnancy (Everett and Quinn, 1966; Flerkó, 1959; McCann and Friedman, 1960; Nikitovitch-Winer, 1960; Quinn and Everett, 1967), as well as changes in the circulating levels of the hormone (Chen *et al.*, 1970). Recently, localization of inhibitory and stimulatory activities of male hypothalamus have been reported (Krulich *et al.*, 1971) with use of a technique similar to that of Mess *et al.* (1967) of sectioning the hypothalamus and testing its effects on prolactin secretion *in vitro*. According to these workers the region of the lateral preoptic nucleus is related to PIF production whereas the median eminence and basal portion of the preoptic area contained prolactin-stimulating-type activity.

That hypothalamic cells controlling prolactin secretion are functionally related with other neural elements located in and out of the hypothalamus is suggested by lesion and estrogen implantation experiments in different neural structures. Averill and Purves (1963) reported that in the rat, lactogenesis was prevented by bilateral lesions in the lateral hypothalamus or lateral preoptic region. This effect apparently was due to interference with prolactin secretion since administration of this hormone permitted lactogenesis and subsequent galactopoiesis (Averill, 1965). These results suggest that extrahypothalamic structures, probably telencephalic, project on the hypothalamus to influence prolactin secretion at the time of parturition.

A possible telencephalic regulation of prolactin secretion was suggested by Beyer and Mena (1965c) who found that removal of this structure in spayed, estrogen-primed, or intact nonlactating rabbits was associated with mammary growth and milk secretion. Lesions in the neocortex and olfactory bulbs did not induce these effects. In a subsequent study more bilateral removal of the basal portion of the temporal lobes, including the enthorhinal cortex and amygdala, elicited milk secretion in a majority of spayed estrogen-primed rabbits (Mena and Beyer, 1968b). Similar results, i.e., lactogenesis induced by temporal lobe lesions, were independently obtained by Tindal *et al.* (1967a) in the same species. This same group reported also that estrogen implants in the amygdala and periamygdaloid cortex can induce milk secretion in pseudopregnant rabbits (Tindal *et al.*, 1967a), which suggests that estrogen sensitive neural elements within the basal temporal region may be functionally related to the hypothalamic cells controlling prolactin secretion.

The neural pathways through which the telencephalon may exert its action on prolactin secretion have not been determined. However, other lesions in the lateral part of the anterior hypothalamic preoptic area in cats (Grosz and Rothballer, 1961) and rats (Lantos and Tramezzani, 1962) or chronic electrical stimulation of the anterior hypothalamus can induce lactogenesis in rats and cats (Mishkinsky *et al.*, unpublished), which suggests that fibers related to prolactin secretion course through this diencephalic region. The main system of fibers traversing this region is the medial forebrain bundle, which contains a strong component of fibers from the amygdala (Knook, 1965).

2. Influence of Suckling

a. GENERAL. The most important stimuli that the mother receives during lactation are those that enter the CNS through receptors in the nipple region at the time of suckling and those that are perceived through special sense organs, i.e., exteroceptive stimulation. These stimuli are responsible for many of the endocrine, metabolic, and behavioral adaptations that develop in the lactating animal to provide the conditions to foster the development of the litter.

Following parturition, periodic suckling of the teats by the litter is necessary to maintain the progressive increase in growth and secretory function of the mammary glands as well as to build up the typical mother–infant interaction which occurs during the normal period of lactation. Separation of the mother and her young, particularly in early lactation, is known to be detrimental to milk secretion and to maternal behavior in different species (Collias, 1956; Findlay, 1971; Rosenblatt and Lehrman, 1963). Milk secretion (Ota and Yokoyama, 1965) and maternal behavior (Rosenblatt and Lehrman, 1963) in rats may be reinstated, however, providing the period of nonsuckling is only a few days in length. Conversely, prolongation of milk secretion and maternal behavior occurs past the normal time of weaning providing a succession of younger foster pups is given to the mother (Bruce, 1958; Kurz, 1967; Nicoll and Meites, 1959; Wiesner and Sheard, 1933).

Toward the end of the lactation period, not only do the mammary glands change their capacity for milk secretion but also less intimate relationships develop between mother and young. These changes lead to a gradual independence of the young for the milk of the mother for their caloric needs. In some species, these changes are reflected in the incidence of suckling during the lactation period. Thus, in mice, the time spent on the nest by the mother decreases during the period from parturition to about 15 days postpartum. This decrease is paralleled by a decrease in the average length of the nursing episode (Bateman, 1957). Similar observations have been made on dogs, which, as lactation declines, assume the nursing posture progressively less frequently (Martins, 1949). In rats a decline has been observed also in the frequency of suckling as lactation progresses. Substitution of young pups every 5 days, however, maintains the high incidence of suckling characteristic of the first part of lactation, whereas substitution of 12-day-old pups on postpartum day 5 mimics the rapid decline in suckling incidence normally seen during the last part of lactation (Grosvenor and Mena, 1971a).

b. INFLUENCE OF SUCKLING ON MILK SECRETION. The influence of suckling on adenohypophyseal function was first suggested by Selye (1934) and Selye *et al.*, (1934) who found that suckling retarded the atrophy of the alveolar epithelium and the glandular involution of mammary glands of rats, which follows ligation of the main mammary ducts. From these results it was postulated that the suckling stimulus provoked the adenohypophysis to release prolactin, which maintained the secretory activity of the gland (Selye, 1934; Selye *et al.*, 1934). The results of Selye *et al.* subsequently were confirmed by other workers. Thus, the retarding effect of suckling on mammary involution was mimicked by systemic injections of prolactin (Hooker and Williams, 1941; Williams, 1945). In mice a retardation of involution in all of the glands, indicating a central effect, occurred following sensory irritation of some of the nipples by turpentine (Hooker and Williams, 1940). Moreover, Ingelbrecht (1935) demonstrated in rats with midthoracic spinal cord transection that lactation was suppressed when the young were allowed to suckle only the glands located below the level of the spinal section, whereas lactation continued when the nipples anterior to the spinal section were suckled. These results indicated that nervous connections between the mammary glands and the brain were essential for the maintenance of lactation and that the effect of mechanical and tactile stimuli applied to the nipple was not a local one upon the mammary gland.

The theory of Selye *et al.* (1934) has been generally accepted although it was subsequently suggested that a complex of pituitary hormones rather than prolactin alone is released by suckling during galactopoiesis (Folley, 1947). At present, there is little doubt that suckling has a very pronounced effect on the functioning of the pituitary and that most, if not all, of the pituitary hormones are influenced by this stimulus in one way or the other. Thus, in addition to causing discharge of both neurohypophyseal hormones (Bisset, 1968; Meites, 1966), the suckling stimulus provokes the release of prolactin (Grosvenor and Turner, 1957, 1958a; Holst and Turner, 1939; Reece and Turner, 1937; Selye, 1934), STH (Grosvenor *et al.*, 1968a; Sar and Meites, 1969), TSH (Grosvenor, 1964a), ACTH (Denamur *et al.*, 1965; Gregoire, 1947; Tabaschnik and Trentin, 1951; Voogt *et al.*, 1969), and MSH (Taleisnik and Orias, 1966) in different species while it inhibits the secretion of gonadotropins in rats and other species (Everett, 1969; Rothchild, 1965). The methods employed in the analysis of suckling effects on hormone release have involved biological, chemical, and radioimmunological determinations of serum and pituitary hormone levels. These observations have also been correlated with microscopic and electron microscopic observations of the pituitary cells themselves (many of these studies are discussed in detail in the following recent reviews: Averill, 1966; Beyer and Mena, 1969b; Grosvenor and Mena, 1971a; Grosvenor et al., 1968b; Meites, 1966; Nicoll, 1971; Tindal, 1967; Tindal and Knaggs, 1970).

c. INFLUENCE OF NONSUCKLING STIMULI ON MILK SECRETION. The most important influence of suckling stimulation on galactopoiesis clearly is that of promoting the release of hypophyseal hormones which maintain milk secretion and milk ejection at an adequate level to meet the demands imposed by the litter. However, it appears clear that in the absence of suckling, the mammary glands of most species thus far studied are capable of continued milk secretion provided that oxytocin is given to evacuate the milk. The degree of maintenance of milk secretion following the removal of suckling, however, varies considerably among species. In rats, partial to complete blockade of galactopoiesis has been reported following interruption of afferent impulses to the hypothalamus from the mammary glands either by pharmocological (Beyer and Mena, 1965b; Eayrs and Baddeley, 1956; Edwardson and Eayrs, 1967; Ingelbrecht, 1935; Tindal et al., 1963; Yokoyama and Ota, 1965) or surgical means (Eayrs and Baddeley, 1956; Edwardson and Eayrs, 1967; Grosvenor, 1964b; Ingelbrecht, 1935; Tverskoi, 1968). In rabbits and cats the degree of interference with milk secretion following blockade of suckling varies according to the method employed. Partial or complete blockade of milk secretion followed spinal transection (Beyer et al., 1962a; Mena and Beyer, 1963), whereas normal milk yields were obtained in anesthetized suckled animals (Beyer and Mena, 1965b; Tindal et al., 1968). The reduced milk yields of the spinal animals have been ascribed in part to the different side effects of the surgical trauma upon the general condition of the experimental animals, particularly upon food intake (Mena and Beyer, 1963; see also Tindal, 1967).

In contrast to the effect of spinal lesions, transection of the pituitary stalk or lesions in the tuberal region which destroyed the hypothalamic pituitary portal vessels were compatible with normal milk yields in rabbits, provided that oxytocin was administered (Donovan and Van der Werff Ten Bosch, 1957; Jacobsohn, 1949). In the rat, the effect of transecting the pituitary stalk on milk secretion apparently has not been studied. However, it has been found that pituitary transplants maintain milk secretion in the rat, albeit at a reduced level, provided frequent injections of oxytocin are given (Cowie *et al.*, 1960; Rothchild, 1960).

In goats and sheep total disconnection between the mammary glands and the brain by means of mammary gland denervation or transplantation, spinal cord transection (Denamur and Martinet, 1959a,b,c; Linzell, 1963; Tsakhaev, 1953; Tverskoi, 1953), as well as milkings performed under anesthesia (Yokoyama and Ota, 1965) were compatible with normal milk yields. This suggests that stimuli other than suckling maintained the secretion of the galactopoietic hormones from the pituitary. However, interruption of suckling pathways at a higher level (in contrast to similar experiments in rabbits) did affect milk secretion. Thus, large lesions in the tuberal region or transection of the pituitary stalk in goats substantially reduced milk secretion (Cowie *et al.*, 1964; Denamur and Martinet, 1961; Gale, 1963; Tsakhaev, 1959; Tverskoi, 1960).

Partial or complete restoration of reduced milk yields was obtained by exogenous administration of a combination of somatotropin, triiodothyronine, insulin, and corticosteroids to goats either with pituitary stalk section (Cowie *et al.*, 1964) or with lesions in the tuberal region (Gale, 1963). These results suggest that the level of milk production attained after the operation was the result of prolactin secreted autonomously by the pituitary. The lack of secretion of the other hormones, in turn, was the cause of the reduced milk production.

In rats and rabbits with spinal cord transection or mammary gland denervation, exogenous prolactin (Eayrs and Edwardson, 1965; Grosvenor, 1966; Mena and Beyer, 1963; Tverskoi, 1968), cortisol (Eayrs and Edwardson, 1965), hydrocortisone (Tverskoi, 1968), or ACTH (Mena and Beyer, 1963), results in rapid and significant improvements of milk secretion. Interestingly, in the spinal rabbits, high milk yields were maintained after withdrawal of ACTH or prolactin, particularly after withdrawal of prolactin (Mena and Beyer, 1963). This result is similar to that recently reported by Gachev (1969) who found that a single injection of prolactin to rabbits with poor lactational performance significantly increased milk yields within a 24-hour period; the animals continued to secrete milk at levels comparable to those seen in normal lactating rabbits. Gachev suggested that exogenous prolactin exerted a positive feedback action upon prolactin secretion by the pituitary. The observation of Grosvenor *et al.* (1970c) that injection of prolactin into postsuckled rats stimulates a faster reaccumulation of the hormone within the adenohypophysis, is consistent with this interpretation.

It appears, therefore, that among the species there exists different integrative mechanisms that control adenohypophyseal galactopoietic hormones. Since only some of the adenohypophyseal hormones that are released by suckling (which one depends on the species) directly participate in milk secretion, as judged by substitutive therapy studies in hypophysectomized animals (Cowie, 1966, 1969; Cowie and Folley, 1961), it could be considered that the degree of maintenance of milk secretion after removal of suckling depends upon (a) the complexity of integration at the central level of the neuroendocrine mechanisms activated by suckling and (b) on the degree to which each adenohypophyseal galactopoietic hormone is dependent upon the neural stimulus of suckling for its own secretion.

If the supposition is made that suckling is capable of activating the secretion of all the pituitary hormones needed for galactopoiesis, then the influence of stimuli other than suckling on the maintenance of milk secretion in animals deprived of suckling will have to receive serious consideration. The role of these stimuli would be complementary to suckling for the secretion of the galactopoietic complex and to the autonomous capacity of the pituitary to secrete prolactin. There is evidence that external stimuli other than those of suckling or milking can provoke the release of prolactin and ACTH in rats and other species (see below).

A number of alternative neural and humoral mechanisms have been proposed to explain the maintenance of function of the mammary gland and the adenohypophysis in the absence of suckling stimulation. These mechanisms have been discussed in several recent reviews (Beyer and Mena, 1969b; Nicoll, 1971; Tindal, 1967) and will not be discussed here, particularly since experimental support is lacking for most of them (see Nicoll, 1971).

d. Influence of Suckling on Prolactin Secretion. Cogent, albeit indirect information concerning the physiological role of suckling during galactopoiesis through its actions on adenohypophyseal secretion came from direct measurements of prolactin content or concentration in the pituitary of lactating rats, rabbits, and guinea pigs under different experimental situations. Thus, a few years after Selye *et al.* (1934) proposed their hypothesis it was demonstrated (Meites and Turner, 1942a, 1948; Reece and Turner, 1937) that the pituitary content of prolactin was higher in rats and rabbits that had been suckled for several days than in animals that had their pups removed at birth. The prolactin content also declined to the prepartum level faster in nonsuckled than in suckled mothers (Meites and Turner, 1942b, 1948). Moreover, it was shown in rats, rabbits, and guinea pigs (Holst and Turner, 1939; Reece and Turner, 1937) that an acute suckling episode following a period of nonsuckling reduced the pituitary prolactin content to one-half of that of nonsuckled animals. Not only did these observations constitute a direct proof of the theory of Selye *et al.* (1934) that suckling was capable of influencing prolactin secretion, they also have provided, as subsequent research has demonstrated, an adequate experimental approach to determine the physiological importance of suckling stimulation on the function of the mammary gland and the adenohypophysis during lactation.

In 1957, both phases of the phenomenon of prolactin secretion, i.e., prolactin depletion and reaccumulation, were analyzed in rats. It was found that 30 minutes of suckling following 10 hours of nonsuckling in postpartum day 14 rats reduced prolactin concentration from one-half to one-third of that of rats nonsuckled for 10 hours, but that the reaccumulation of the hormone occurred slowly, having a similar duration as that of the previous nonsuckling interval (Grosvenor and Turner, 1957). These observations have been extended to both earlier and later phases of the lactation period (Grosvenor and Mena, 1971a; Grosvenor and Turner, 1958a).

The release of prolactin from the pituitary by short-term suckling has been confirmed many times both with bioassay and gel electrophoresis techniques and has been correlated, by light and electron microscopy, with the secretion of prolactin granules from prolactin cells of the pituitary, as well as with sudden increases in the circulating levels of the hormone as detected by radioimmunoassay methods (see Grosvenor and Mena, 1971a; Nicoll, 1971, for references).

The mechanisms by which the neural signal of suckling effects prolactin release from the pituitary during lactation is at present a matter of controversy. Clear *in vitro* and *in vivo* evidence has demonstrated the capacity of either crude or partially purified hypothalamic extracts of different species to depress the autonomous capacity of the pituitary to secrete prolactin *in vitro* and to block the suckling-induced depletion of prolactin *in vivo*. Ratner and Meites (1964) found that hypothalami from suckled rats were devoid of prolactin-inhibiting activity (PIF) *in vitro* and suggested that suckling depleted the hypothalamus of PIF. On the other hand, systemic injection of only one-third of a hypothalamus obtained from either pre- or postsuckled or stressed lactating rats was able to inhibit the suckling-induced or stress-induced discharge of prolactin in the lactating rat *in vivo* (Grosvenor, 1965a). This latter observation as well as the fact that 2 minutes of suckling were sufficient to induce prolactin release (Grosvenor *et al.*, 1967a) were the basis of the suggestion that the suckling stimulus elicits prolactin release in the rat, not by inhibiting the synthesis of PIF but by temporary inhibition of the tonic

release of PIF (Grosvenor, 1965a; Grosvenor and Mena, 1971a; Grosvenor et al., 1968b). To explain prolactin release through suckling by
suppression of an inhibitory factor would imply that following such
suppression the rapidity of the discharge of prolactin into the circulation
is dependent upon the autonomous capacity of the prolactin cell to
extrude the hormone from the cell into the circulation.

The possibility exists as proposed 10 years ago by Turner and Griffith
(1962) and supported recently by evidence (Arimura et al., 1969; Fiorindo and Nicoll, 1969; Krulich et al., 1971) that the suckling-induced
release of prolactin is through the mediation of a hypothalamic prolactin
releasing factor. The problem of the mechanism of prolactin release has
been discussed in a previous section on the problem of the hypothalamic
control of prolactin secretion. Also, several recent reviews discuss these
aspects at length (Grosvenor and Mena, 1971a; Meites, 1966, 1970;
Nicoll et al., 1970).

Following the release of the hormone into the circulation in response
to the stimulus of suckling, there is a gradual restoration of the hormone
within the pituitary (Grosvenor and Turner, 1957). Until recently, it was
considered that prolactin synthesis following release occurred passively
since the pituitary continued to synthesize prolactin either when separated from its normal location or cultured in vitro. However, as already
discussed in a previous section, in vivo and in vitro evidence have shown
that the autonomous capacity of the gland to synthesize prolactin may be
under the stimulatory influence of the hypothalamus (Convey and Reece,
1969; Grosvenor et al., 1970c). Moreover, it has recently been shown in
the rat that the amount of prolactin secreted autonomously by the transplanted pituitary does not reach the level in the circulation secreted by
the lactating pituitary gland in situ; in fact, the levels of the hormone in
the circulation were below those normally found at estrus (Chen et al.,
1970).

It is clear, however, that the secretory capacity of the prolactin cell
is able to adapt to the physiological situation of the lactating animal
suggesting the existence of control mechanisms superimposed upon the
autonomous capacity. Thus, in rats, the demands of the litter through the
intensity of suckling are reflected in the amount of the hormone present
in the gland. Tucker et al. (1967) reported in rats that raising the number
of pups from two to six increased the prolactin concentration 42% in the
pituitary of the mothers. Similarly, Mena and Grosvenor (1968) found in
rats that pituitary prolactin concentration increased threefold following
8 hours of nonsuckling as the litter size increased from two to ten pups.
In a recent study, it was demonstrated that maximum prolactin reac-

cumulation was achieved in the pituitary within 4 hours postsuckling in rats previously nonsuckled for 4 hours and with six pups per litter, whereas reaccumulation continued to increase over an 8-hour period in rats with eight pups per litter (Grosvenor and Mena, 1971a). The influence of suckling strength upon prolactin concentration, however, appears to be different in the rabbit since according to Meites *et al.* (1941) pituitary prolactin content was unaffected by the size of the litter.

The nonsuckling interval which precedes the application of an acute suckling period has been shown to influence prolactin release and prolactin reaccumulation as well as milk secretion. These studies have provided information not only on the physiological significance of the stimulus of suckling but also upon the importance of parallel functioning of the pituitary and the mammary gland during lactation. Thus, it has been found that the extent of prolactin release produced by 30 minutes of suckling on postpartum day 7 in the rat is smaller following 4 hours of nonsuckling than following 8 hours of nonsuckling, and this, in turn, is smaller than that following 10 hours of nonsuckling (Grosvenor and Mena, 1971a). These data suggest that the amount of prolactin released by suckling is related to the length of the previous nonsuckling period.

With respect to prolactin reaccumulation by the pituitary, rats nonsuckled for 8 hours prior to 30 minutes suckling did not fully reaccumulate prolactin in the pituitary within 8 hours postsuckling whereas those nonsuckled for 4 hours prior to suckling reaccumulated maximal amounts within 4 hours (Grosvenor and Mena, 1971a). The extent of the release to be sure was greater in the rats nonsuckled for 8 hours, and this apparently influenced the time required for full accumulation. Following 10 hours of nonsuckling, the pituitary failed also to reach presuckled levels (Grosvenor and Turner, 1957). These data suggest that there may be an impairment of postsuckling prolactin restoration if the previous nonsuckling period is sufficiently long. Short nonsuckling intervals would appear to be associated with small prolactin turnovers and, as a consequence, a more or less constant level of the hormone is maintained within the gland. The levels of prolactin in the lactating rat pituitary are similar after 4, 8, and 16 hours of nonsuckling on postpartum days 7 and 14 (Grosvenor and Mena, 1971a). From these results it can be deduced that prolactin is not secreted tonically in the lactating rat, but phasically, in response to stimulation. Very low circulating titers of the hormone are to be found in the absence of suckling stimulation (Amenomori *et al.*, 1970; Krulich *et al.*, 1970).

Nonsuckling periods of 4–12 hours appear to be compatible with the activation by suckling of the prolactin release mechanism in rats. However, shortening or lengthening the nonsuckling interval beyond these limits results in the inability of suckling to release detectable amounts of prolactin. Thus, when second suckling periods of 30 minutes duration were applied either immediately or 2 hours after an initial 30 minutes of suckling (which followed 8 hours of nonsuckling), no prolactin depletion was detected (Grosvenor and Mena, 1971a,b). At the time in which the second sucklings were applied, large poststimulation stores of prolactin remained in the pituitary, indicating that the lack of depletion was not due to insufficient hormone in the pituitary. Moreover, to further exclude this possibility, prolactin release was blocked at the first suckling by injection of purified ovine PIF. A second suckling 2 hours after the initial suckling still was unable to provoke the release of prolactin. The possibility was excluded that the injection of PIF carried over $2\frac{1}{2}$ hours to block the second stimulus of suckling (Grosvenor and Mena, 1971b). These results suggested that a neural refractoriness develops shortly after a stimulus, e.g., suckling, is applied, which protects the prolactin stores from further depletion and which lasts long enough to insure adequate resynthesis of the hormone.

A refractoriness also occurs when the nonsuckling interval is extended to more than 12 hours on postpartum days 7 or 14. Thus, suckling did not provoke prolactin release when the preceding interval was 16 hours in length (Grosvenor et al., 1967a), though prolactin release was restored if one or two short periods of suckling were provided to the mammary glands during the first 8 hours of an otherwise 16-hour nonsuckling period. This result suggested that during this period of lactation suckling stimulation must be applied periodically, at least at 8-hour intervals, to maintain the functioning of the prolactin discharge mechanism.

It appears clear that the functioning of the pituitary for prolactin secretion during lactation is extremely dependent upon the frequency of the afferent neural inflow from the periphery.

As might be expected, many of the changes in prolactin turnover in the pituitary are reflected in the functioning of the mammary glands for milk secretion. Thus, it has been demonstrated that deep anesthesia in rats blocks the suckling-induced release of prolactin (Grosvenor and Turner, 1958b) and that this in turn results in a drastic reduction in milk secretion (Grosvenor and Turner, 1959). Moreover, a selective blockade of prolactin release by suckling has been accomplished by the injection of crude and partially purified hypothalamic extracts from different species (Grosvenor, 1965a; Grosvenor et al., 1965). The injection of these extracts prior to suckling and following 8 hours of nonsuckling, coupled with the complete removal of milk by the pups with the aid of supplemental oxytocin, depressed milk synthesis to 44–51% of normal during the subsequent 16 hours. The reduction of milk secretion in these rats was overcome with a single injection of 3 mg prolactin (Grosvenor *et al.,* 1970c).

The milk secretory response of the mammary gland to prolactin is reduced gradually as the interval between suckling increases. Thus, full reaccumulation (100%), following emptying of the mammary glands, occurs within 8 hours if the preceding nonsuckling interval is not longer than 4 hours (Grosvenor and Mena, 1971c). When the preceding non-suckling interval is extended from 4 to 8 hours, only 50% reaccumulation results in the 8 hours following emptying, and it takes another 8 hours to reach full reaccumulation (Grosvenor and Mena, 1971c; Grosvenor *et al.,* 1970b). In animals nonsuckled for 12–24 hours full reaccumulation is never reached and the levels remain at about 30% of full capacity at the end of 16 hours (Grosvenor *et al.,* 1970b). Exogenous prolactin was only partially effective (70% of full reaccumulation) in stimulating milk secretion in the 12-hour nonsuckled group and completely ineffective in the 16- to 24-hour nonsuckled groups (Grosvenor and Mena 1971c; Grosvenor *et al.,* 1970b). In this last group, it was necessary either to administer other galactopoietic hormones (TSH, STH, hydrocortisone, and oxytocin) in addition to prolactin, or to provide a period of suckling midway during the 16-hour nonsuckling period in order to restore normal refilling of the glands (Grosvenor *et al.,* 1970b).

The injection of prolactin midway during an 8-hour nonsuckling period, i.e., 4 hours prior to suckling, resulted in the complete reaccumulation of milk within 8 rather than within 16 hours (Mena and Grosvenor, 1972). This led to further experiments from which it was concluded that once prolactin is discharged into the circulation, there is a time delay of several hours for the physiological expression of the effect of the hormone in terms of milk secretion. In other words the milk secreted following emptying of the glands at a given suckling is the result of prolactin released at earlier sucklings (Grosvenor, 1971; Grosvenor and Mena, 1971c).

It is inferred from the above data that in the rat the capacity of the mammary gland for milk secretion is adversely affected when the non-suckling interval increases beyond 4 hours, and, as in the case of the prolactin secretion mechanism of the pituitary, normal functioning is possible only when periodic suckling is maintained. Therefore, it appears that a clear functional parallelism exists between the pituitary, at least as far as prolactin secretion is concerned, and the mammary glands. Unfortunately, similar information is lacking for other species than the rat and for other hormones than prolactin. It is hoped that this void can be filled in the near future.

3. Influence of Exteroceptive Stimulation on Prolactin Secretion during Lactation

Evidence has been obtained that demonstrates that throughout the reproductive life of the animal the functioning of the prolactin releasing mechanism may be under the stimulatory or inhibitory influences of external, nontactile exteroceptive stimuli. Thus, stimulation or inhibition of prolactin release has been demonstrated in response to exteroceptive signals in cyclic (Van der Lee and Boot, 1955, 1956) or newly mated female mice (Bruce, 1959; Bruce and Parrot, 1960), in postparturient (Alloiteau, 1962) or lactating rats (Grosvenor, 1965b), goats (Bryant et al., 1970), and cows (Johke, 1970; Tucker, 1971), and in pigeons and doves (Witschi, 1935; Patel, 1936). These effects have been treated at length and their mechanisms of action amply discussed in recent reviews (Bronson, 1969; Whitten, 1966). Here, we wish to analyze only the physiological implications of some of these effects during lactation.

The first experimental evidence on the influence of exteroceptive stimulation (ECS) from the litter upon the secretion of prolactin by the maternal pituitary was obtained in 1965 (Grosvenor, 1965b). It was found that placement of rat pups beneath their mother, but separated from her by a wire screen, for 30 minutes following a 10-hour interval of isolation on postpartum day 14 resulted in a fall in pituitary prolactin concentration of the mother similar in extent to that following 30 minutes of actual suckling. Self-licking of mammary gland areas, though demonstrated indirectly to possibly cause prolactin release in the pregnant rat (McMurtry and Anderson, 1971; Roth and Rosenblatt, 1968), was shown to be ineffective in directly eliciting the acute fall in pituitary prolactin concentration of the lactating rat when exposed to her pups (Grosvenor and Mena, 1969). In another study (Grosvenor et al., 1967b), following suckling and emptying of the mammary glands, milk reaccumulation was significantly reduced over the next 16 hours in rats injected with PIF. Placement of the pups under their mother during the milk reaccumulation period restored milk secretion to normal. These studies demonstrated then, that ECS from the litter exerts a strong stimulatory influence upon prolactin release and thus indirectly upon milk secretion.

In subsequent studies (Mena and Grosvenor, 1971) the type of sensory information from the litter responsible for the release of prolactin from the maternal pituitary was determined to be mainly one of olfaction. It is noteworthy that these results agree with those found in mice (see Whitten, 1966, for references) upon the essential role of olfaction for the stimulation or inhibition of prolactin release by exteroceptive stimulation. In the studies in female mice, it was concluded that the effects of ECS on prolactin are mediated by a pheromone produced by the male of the same species. Pheromones from the pups may be instrumental in the ECS-induced release of prolactin in the lactating rat though crucial information still has to be obtained. In the experiments referred to above (Mena and Grosvenor, 1971), olfactory, visual, and auditory stimuli from the pups were blocked either singly or in combination during the period of exposure to the mother. In another series of experiments, the stimuli from the pups were not blocked, rather there was surgical elimination during pregnancy of two of the three sense organs of the mother. When the mothers were exposed on postpartum day 14 to their pups, a decrease in prolactin concentration occurred not only in those mothers that had only a functional olfactory sense remaining, but also in those in which only the optic sense was intact (Mena and Grosvenor, 1971). This latter result was interpreted as suggestive that in the absence of the specific mediator, i.e., olfaction, the optic sense was able to mediate the stimulus for prolactin release. This interpretation also suggested that visual cues from the pups may potentially influence prolactin release in normal rats under particular physiological situations. Auditory cues also may prove to be important, since in a recent study it was found that oxytocin release occurs in rats through mediation of the auditory sense (Deis, 1968).

Exteroceptive stimuli from the pups may influence the secretion of other galactopoietic hormones from the pituitary. Zarrow *et al.* (1972) recently found that plasma corticosterone levels in lactating rats increased after exposure, without suckling, to their pups. Olfactory cues from the pups apparently were involved since olfactory bulbectomy abolished the response as did placing the pups in a sealed transparent container. Vision was not indispensable since blinding the mothers by enucleation did not block the effect.

The significance of ECS from the litter as a stimulus for prolactin release from the mother apparently varies throughout the normal 21-day period of lactation in the rat. Thus, in the primiparous rat the exteroceptive mechanism for prolactin release is not functioning in early lactation, i.e., day 7, though it is in mid- (day 14) and late (day 21) lactation

(Grosvenor et al., 1970a). Apparently, this function develops somewhere between early and midlactation, although the precise mechanism involved as yet is not known.

Whatever the mechanism of this development, it is clear that by postpartum day 14 the configuration of the exteroceptive cues from the pups is well established as a stimulus, since the mother rats on day 14 can discriminate between those cues emanating from much older or younger pups that are placed under them (Grosvenor et al., 1970a). Moreover, these rats do not respond to exteroceptive cues either from her own or from variously aged pups of other lactating rats that are housed in adjacent or nearby cages in the same room (Grosvenor et al., 1970a). This observation suggests that the spatial relationship of mothers and pups during suckling may be important for the exteroceptive release of prolactin.

On the other hand, the changing characteristics of the pups and/or the changing behavioral interrelationships between pups and mother as the pups grow, possibly contribute to the onset of function of the exteroceptive mechanism in the primiparous rat. This is suggested by the finding that prolactin release occurred in primiparous rats by ECS on day 7 providing the mother was given 7- to 8-day-old foster pups on day 2 (Grosvenor et al., 1970a). The fact that primiparous rats on day 7 did not show a reduction in prolactin when exposed for the first time to 14-day-old pups further indicates that the development of the exteroceptive mechanism is a gradual one.

Once the stimuli configuration is established, it is apparently retained through a second pregnancy following a normal first lactation, since exposure of the mother to the pups on day 7 of a second lactation elicited prolactin release to the same extent as that following suckling (Grosvenor et al., 1970a).

The observation that lactating rats do not release prolactin by ECS from the litter in early lactation has been contradicted by the report of Moltz et al. (1969). These workers found that in the postpartum rat whose nipples have been removed before pregnancy the mere physical presence of the pups provoked prolactin release as determined by the deciduoma response and the arrest of the estrus cycle. However, apart from important differences in experimental procedures, it is possible that either postsurgical irritation of the proximal ends of the severed mammary nerves or the tactile stimuli of nuzzling, etc, from the pups could have excited the release of prolactin via receptors in the mammary gland area, which in addition to those in the nipple, send afferent information to the brain via the segmental nerve (Findlay, 1966; Relkin, 1967).

Between mid- and late lactation, the exteroceptive mechanism for prolactin release undergoes two further modifications. The first change involved is in the direction of an increased sensitivity of the mother to exteroceptive signals. Results recently obtained indicate that in contrast to the 14-day postpartum rat in which the exteroceptive mechanism is activated only when the pups are underneath the mother, the 21-day postpartum rat releases her prolactin in response to exteroceptive signals emanating from the general environment of the animal room. The causative exteroceptive stimuli in the animal room environment apparently emanates from other lactating rats and/or their litters (Mena and Grosvenor, 1972). Thus, in order to demonstrate the effect of a stimulus such as suckling on prolactin release on day 21, it was necessary first to isolate the mothers from the general animal room environment (Mena and Grosvenor, 1972).

The changing characteristics of the pups from 14 to 21 days of age in some manner is involved in the increasing responsiveness of the exteroceptive mechanism for prolactin release, which occurs from day 14 to 21 postpartum. A release of prolactin occurs in response to animal room environmental stimuli in the day 14 primiparous rat provided 13- and 14-day-old foster pups were inserted in place of mother's own pups on day 7 (Mena and Grosvenor, 1972).

The second modification is the generation by the pups of a peripheral inhibitory influence upon the action of prolactin in stimulating milk secretion. In contrast to day 14 in which exposure of the mothers to their litters leads to depletion of pituitary prolactin which then stimulates milk secretion, the same procedure on isolated 21 day postpartum rats resulted in a normal depletion of prolactin but was accompanied by an inhibition rather than a stimulation to milk secretion (Grosvenor and Mena, 1972). These observations suggest that simultaneous to the stimulatory influence of ECS from the pups on prolactin release, as evidenced by the depletion of the hormone by the pituitary, a blocking influence is exerted by stimuli emanating from the pups on the hormone, perhaps at the level of the mammary gland, which prevents it from stimulating milk secretion.

The normal spatial relationship of the mother and her pups at the time of suckling, i.e., the pups under the mother, in late lactation (day 21) is required before the stimuli from the pups are inhibitory for milk secretion. No inhibition of milk secretion occurred, for example, if the pups were placed alongside the mother in another cage. These observations may provide a mechanism whereby galactopoiesis is reduced at the time the litter is less dependent on the milk of the mother for survival though the pituitary and mammary glands are still quite functional. The mechanism of the inhibitory effect is unknown at present, but may be related to sympathetic adrenal activation.

It is apparent, therefore, as with the stimulus of suckling, ECS from the litter plays a decisive role in prolactin secretion during lactation in the rat. The importance of each type of stimuli, however, varies throughout the lactation period. Thus, the fact that the exteroceptive mechanism has not yet developed in the primiparous rat in early lactation suggests that suckling constitutes the major mechanism for release of prolactin, which is necessary for the maintenance of milk secretion during this period. During the later stages of lactation, although suckling stimuli maintain their effectivenesss as in the previous stages, the increasing responsiveness of the exteroceptive mechanism may shift the major role from suckling to the exteroceptive mechanism as the principal regulator of prolactin release.

V. DECLINE AND CESSATION OF LACTATION

It is commonly appreciated that milk secretion slows or ceases altogether if the frequency and/or extent of milk removal is reduced. However, the secretory activity of the mammary gland declines and eventually ceases, though the milk is removed regularly, and also in spite of an adequate level of nutrition. The natural decline in milk secretion often coincides with a reduction in the dependency of the young for the mother's milk, i.e., with the weaning of the young.

The mechanisms underlying the gradual cessation of milk secretion at weaning are largely unknown. However, speculations regarding this process can be made based upon two separate lines of evidence obtained mainly in the rat and described in detail in Section IV. Whether or not the information obtained from the lactating rat has any bearing on the mechanisms of decline and cessation of lactation in other species remains to be investigated.

Firstly, altering either the frequency of stimulation of the pituitary or the frequency of hormonal stimulation of the mammary gland can result in changes in the level of milk secretory function of the mammary gland. Decreasing the frequency of stimulation of the pituitary by increasing the length of the nonsuckling interval has been shown (1) to retard the time it takes for prolactin to reaccumulate in the pituitary after suckling; (2) to first increase the extent of prolactin release, but as the nonsuckling interval lengthens (beyond about 12 hours) to block the release of prolactin in response to suckling; (3) to reduce the autonomous capacity of the pituitary to secrete prolactin; (4) to retard the rate and extent of milk reaccumulation by the mammary gland following suckling, and (5) to reduce the milk secretory response of the mammary gland to exogenous prolactin.

It is important also to relate the timing, alignment, or phasing of the stimuli arriving at either the pituitary or mammary gland to their stage of functional receptivity. An analysis of this, however, is confounded by the fact that the timing of the signals to the response appears normally to be out of phase. Thus, a release of prolactin does not occur each time a stimulus (suckling or exteroceptive) is applied. Instead, the release of prolactin appears to occur at some frequency which is set by the length of the refractoriness, which develops in the prolactin release mechanism following suckling or exteroceptive stimulation. Also, once prolactin release occurs, the function of the hormone is not expressed in terms of milk secretion until several hours afterwards. In other words, that milk secreted after the gland has been emptied of milk by suckling is the result of prolactin that has been released at some previous suckling.

These points taken together imply that the functional capacity of the mammary gland is dependent upon a rather specific relationship between stimulus input, hormone release, and responsivity of the target organ. When this relationship is disrupted by changes in either the timing or the nature of the stimuli, the functional capacity of the system breaks down at all levels. As examples, a change either in the length of the refractory period, which follows suckling or exteroceptive stimulation, or in the length of time between prolactin release and its expression in terms of milk secretion in each instance would eventually result in a decline in milk secretion.

Secondly, specific inhibitory systems may commence to function in late lactation though the frequency of stimulation of the pituitary and mammary gland may be unaltered or, perhaps, even increased. Recently, we have found that placement of pups under their mother but without physical contact on postpartum day 21, i.e., during the normal time of weaning, stimulates the mother in a manner that results in an inhibition of the normal stimulatory effects of prolactin upon milk secretion. Such inhibition does not occur if the pups are placed alongside the mother. This inhibition occurs in spite of the fact that not only do the mother's own pups but also those of other lactators easily provoke the discharge of prolactin from the maternal pituitary. Thus, an inhibition of the normal galactopoietic effects of prolactin that has been discharged into the circulation apparently has occurred. This finding may help to explain the paradox in the lactating rate of the occurrence of weaning though up to that time milk secretion is still quite intense.

ACKNOWLEDGMENTS

Supported by USPHS HD 04358 to CEG and by Grant 710–0099 to FM from the Ford Foundation.

REFERENCES

Alloiteau, J. J. (1962). *Biol. Méd.* **51**, 250.
Amenomori, Y., Chen, C. L., and Meites, J. (1970). *Endocrinology* **86**, 506.
Anand, B. K., Malkani, P. K., and Kand, S. S. (1957). *Indian J. Med. Res.* **45**, 503.
Andersson, B. (1951). *Acta Physiol. Scand.* **23**, 8.
Arimura, A., Saito, M., and Wakabayashi, I. (1969). *Program Endocrine Soc.* (Abstr.), p. 46.
Aulsebrook, L. H., and Holland, R. C. (1969). *Amer. J. Physiol.* **216**, 830.
Averill, R. L. W. (1965). *J. Endocrinol.* **31**, 191.
Averill, R. L. W. (1966). *Brit. Med. Bull.* **22**, 261.
Averill, R. L. W. (1968). *Neuroendocrinology* **5**, 121.
Averill, R. L. W., and Purves, H. D. (1963). *J. Endocrinol.* **26**, 463.
Ballantyne, B., and Bunch, G. A. (1966). *J Comp. Neurol.* **127**, 471.
Ban, T., Shimizu, S., and Kurotsu, T. (1958). *Med. J. Osaka Univ.* **8**, 345.
Baryshnikov, I. A., and Kokorina, E. P. (1959). *Proc. Int. Dairy Congr., 15th* **1**, 46.
Baryshnikov, I. A., Zaks, M. G., Zotikova, I. N., Levitskaya, E. S., Pavlov, G. N., Pavlov, E. F., Tverskoi, G. B., Tolbukhin, V. I., and Tsakhaev, G. A. (1951). *Zh. Obshch. Biol.* **12**, 423.
Baryshnikov, I. A., Borsuk, V. N., Zaks, M. G., Zotikova, I. N., Pavlov, G. N., and Tolbukhin, V. I. (1953). *Zh. Obshch. Biol.* **14**, 257.
Bateman, V. (1957). *J. Argr. Sci.* **49**, 60.
Beller, T. K., Krumholz, K. H., and Zuminiger, K. (1958). *Acta Endocrinol.* **29**, 1.
Benson, G. K., Cowie, A. T., Folley, S. J., and Tindal, J. S. (1959). *In* "Recent Progress in the Endocrinology of Reproduction" (C. W. Lloyd, ed.), pp. 457–490. Academic Press, New York.
Bern, H. A., and Nicoll, C. S. (1968). *In* "Recent Progress in Hormone Research," Vol. 24, pp. 681–720. Academic Press, New York.
Beyer, C., and Mena, F. (1965a). *Amer. J. Physiol.* **208**, 585.
Beyer, C., and Mena, F. (1965b). *Bol. Inst. Estud. Méd. Biol.* (*México*) **23**, 89.
Beyer, C., and Mena, F. (1965c). *Amer. J. Physiol.* **208**, 289.
Beyer, C., and Mena, F. (1969a). *In* "Progress in Endocrinology" (C. Gual, ed.), pp. 952–958. Excerpta Medica Int. Congr. Ser. No. 184.
Beyer, C., and Mena, F. (1969b). *In* "Physiology and Pathology of Adaptation Mechanisms" (E. Bajusz, ed.), pp. 310–344. Pergamon, Oxford.
Beyer, C., and Mena, F. (1970). *Endocrinology* **87**, 195.
Beyer, C., and Sawyer, C. H. (1969). *In* "Frontiers in Neuroendocrinology" (W. F. Ganong and L. Martini, eds.), pp. 255–287. Oxford Univ. Press, London and New York.

Beyer, C., Mena, F., Pacheco, P., and Alcaraz, M. (1962a). *Fed. Proc. Fed. Amer. Soc. Exp. Biol.* **21**, 353.

Beyer, C., Mena, F., Pacheco, P., and Alcaraz, M. (1962b). *Amer. J. Physiol.* **202**, 465.

Bisset, G. W. (1968). *In* "Handbook of Experimental Pharmacology" (B. Berde, ed.), Vol. XXIII, pp. 475–544. Springer-Verlag, Berlin.

Bisset, G. W., Clark, B. J., and Lewis, G. P. (1967). *Brit. J. Pharmacol. Chemotherap.* **31**, 550.

Bland, K. P., and Donovan, B. T. (1966). *Advan. Reproductive Physiol.* **1**, 179–214.

Blaxter, K. L. (1971). *In* "Lactation" (I. R. Falconer, ed.), pp. 51–69. Butterworths, London and Washington, D.C.

Bogdanove, E. M. (1964). *Vitam. Horm.* **22**, 205.

Bradbury, J. T. (1941). *Endocrinology* **29**, 393.

Bronson, F. H. (1969). *In* "Pheromonal Influences on Mammalian Reproduction" (M. Diamond, ed.), pp. 341–361. Indiana Univ. Press.

Brooks, C. Mc.C., Ishikawa, T., Koizumi, K., and Lu, H. H. (1966). *J. Physiol.* **182**, 217.

Bruce, H. M. (1958). *Proc. Roy. Soc. Biol.* **149**, 421.

Bruce, H. M. (1959). *Nature (London)* **184**, 105.

Bruce, H. M., and Parrot, D. M. V. (1960). *Science* **131**, 1526.

Bryant, G. D., Linzell, J. L., and Greenwood, F. C. (1970). *Hormones* **1**, 26.

Carroll, E. J., Jacobsen, M. S., Kassouny, M., Smith, N. E., and Armstrong, D. T. (1968). *Endocrinology* **82**, 179.

Cathcart, E. P., Gairns, F. W., and Garven, H. S. D. (1948). *Trans. Roy. Soc. Edinburgh* **61**, 699.

Chan, W. Y. (1965). *J. Pharmacol. Exp. Therap.* **147**, 48.

Chaudhury, R. R., Chaudhury, M. R., and Lu, F. C. (1961). *Brit. J. Pharmcol.* **17**, 305.

Chen, C. L., Minaguchi, H., and Meites, J. (1967). *Proc. Soc. Exp. Biol. Med.* **126**, 317.

Chen, C. L., Voogt, J. L., Meites, J. (1968). *Endocrinology* **83**, 1273.

Chen, C. L., Amenomori, Y., Lu, K. H., Voogt, J. L., and Meites, J. (1970). *Neuroendocrinology* **6**, 220.

Clemens, J. A., and Meites, J. (1968). *Endocrinology* **82**, 876.

Clemens, J. A., Sar, M., and Meites, J. (1969). *Endocrinology* **84**, 868.

Cleverley, J. D. (1968). *J. Endocrinol.* **40**, ii.

Cobo, E., Bernal, M., Gaitan, E., and Quintero, C. A. (1967). *Amer. J. Obstet. Gynecol.* **97**, 519.

Cochrane, E. R. (1949). *Brit. Vet. J.* **105**, 320.

Collias, N. E. (1956). *Ecology* **37**, 228.

Convey, E. M., and Reece, R. P. (1969). *Proc. Soc. Exp. Biol. Med.* **131**, 543.

Cowie, A. T. (1966). *In* "The Pituitary Gland" (G. W. Harris and B. T. Donovan, eds.), Vol. 2, pp. 412–443. Butterworths, London and Washington, D.C.

Cowie, A. T. (1969). *In* "Lactogenesis, the Initiation of Milk Secretion" (M. Reynolds and S. J. Folley, eds.), pp. 157–169. Univ. of Pennsylvania Press, Philadelphia, Pennsylvania.

Cowie, A. T. (1971). *In* "Lactation" (I. R. Falconer, ed.), pp. 123–140, Butterworths, London and Washington, D.C.

Cowie, A. T., and Folley, S. J. (1961). *In* "Sex and Internal Secretions" (W. C. Young, ed.), Vol. 1, pp. 590–642. Williams and Wilkins, Baltimore, Maryland.

Cowie, A. T., Tindal, J. S., and Benson, G. K. (1960). *J. Endocrinol.* **21**, 115.
Cowie, A. T., Daniel, P. M. Knaggs, G. S., Pritchard, M. L., and Tindal, J. S. (1964). *J. Endocrinol.* **28**, 253.
Cowie, A. T., Knaggs, G. S., Tindal, J. S., and Turvey, A. (1968). *J. Endocrinol.* **40**, 243.
Cowie, A. T., Hartmann, P. E., and Turvey, A. (1969). *J. Endocrinol.* **43**, 651.
Cross, B. A. (1952). *J. Endocrinol.* **8**, xiii.
Cross, B. A. (1954). *Nature (London)* **173**, 450.
Cross, B. A. (1955). *J. Endocrinol.* **12**, 15.
Cross, B. A. (1961a). *In* "Milk: the Mammary Gland and Its Secretion" (S. K. Kon and A. T. Cowie, eds.), Vol. 1, pp. 229–277. Academic Press, New York.
Cross, B. A. (1961b). *In* "Oxytocin" (R. Caldeyro-Barcia and H. Heller, eds.), pp. 24–46. Pergamon, Oxford.
Cross, B. A. (1966). *In* "Neuroendocrinology" (L. Martini and F. Ganong, eds.), Vol. 1, pp. 217–259. Academic Press, New York.
Cross, B. A., and Findlay, A. L. R. (1969). *In* "Lactogenesis" (M. Reynolds, and S. J. Folley, eds.), pp. 245–252. Univ. of Pennsylvania Press, Philadelphia, Pennsylvania.
Cross, B. A., and Harris, G. W. (1952). *J. Endocrinol.* **8**, 148.
Debackere, M., Peeters, G., and Tuyttens, N. (1961). *J. Endocrinol.* **22**, 321.
Deis, R. P. (1967). "A Study of Certain of the Central Effects of Sexual Hormones," pp. 1–111, Ph.D. thesis. Univ. of Edinburgh, Edinburgh, Scotland.
Deis, R. P. (1968). *J. Physiol.* **197**, 37.
Deis, R. P. (1971). *Proc. Soc. Exp. Biol. Med.* **137**, 1006.
Denamur, R. (1965). *Dairy Sci. Abstr.* **27**, 193.
Denamur, R., and Martinet, J. (1959a). *C. R. Acad. Sci.* **248**, 743.
Denamur, R., and Martinet, J. (1959b). *Arch. Sci. Physiol.* **13**, 271.
Denamur, R., and Martinet, J. (1959c). *C. R. Acad. Sci.* **248**, 860.
Denamur, R., and Martinet, J. (1961). *Ann. Endocrinol.* **22**, 760.
Denamur, R., Stoliaroff, M., and Desclin, J. (1965). *C. R. Hebd. Séances Acad. Sci.* **260**, 3175.
DeNuccio, D. J., and Grosvenor, C. E. (1971). *J. Endocrinol.* **51**, 437.
Desclin, L. (1949). *C. R. Soc. Biol.* **143**, 1154.
Desclin, L. (1950). *Ann. Endocrinol.* **11**, 656.
Desclin, L. (1957). *C. R. Soc. Biol.* **151**, 1774.
Desclin, L. (1960). *Anat. Rec.* **136**, 182.
Desclin, L., and Flament-Durand, J. (1969). *J. Endocrinol.* **43**, lix.
Desclin, L., and Grégoire, C. (1936). *C. R. Soc. Biol.* **121**, 1366.
Desclin, L., and Koulischer, L. (1960). *C. R. Séances Soc. Biol.* **154**, 1515.
De Vae, W. F., Ramírez, V. D., and McCann, S. M. (1966). *Endocrinology* **78**, 158.
Donker, J. D., Koshi, J. H., and Petersen, W. E. (1954). *Science* **119**, 67.
Donovan, B. T., and Van der Werff Ten Bosch, J. J. (1957). *J. Physiol.* **137**, 410.
Dugger, G. S., Van Wyk, J. J., Newsome, J. F. (1962). *J. Neurosurg.* **19**, 589.
Dyusembin, Kh. (1958). *Izv. Akad. Nauk Kazakh. SSR (Ser. Med. Fiziol.)* **1**, 25.
Eayrs, J. T., and Baddeley, R. M. (1956). *J. Anat.* **90**, 161.
Eayrs, J. T., and Edwardson, J. A. (1965). *Acta Endocrinol. Suppl.* **100**, **50**, 154.
Eckles, N. E., Ehni, G., and Kirschbaum, A. (1958). *Anat. Rec.* **130**, 295.
Edwardson, J. A. (1968). *J. Anat.* **103**, 188.
Edwardson, J. A., and Eayrs, J. T. (1967). *J. Endocrinol.* **38**, 51.

Ehni, G., and Eckles, N. E. (1959). *J. Neurosurg.* **16**, 628.

Ely, F., and Petersen, W. E. (1941). *J. Dairy Sci.* **24**, 211.

Emmel, V. E., Weatherford, H. L., and Streicher, M. H. (1926). *Amer. J. Anat.* **38**, 1.

Everett, J. W. (1954). *Endocrinology* **54**, 685.

Everett, J. W. (1956). *Endocrinology* **58**, 786.

Everett, J. W. (1964). *Physiol. Rev.* **44**, 373.

Everett, J. W. (1966). *In* "The Pituitary Gland" (G. W. Harris and B. T. Donovan, eds.), Vol. II, pp. 166–194. Butterworths, London and Washington, D.C.

Everett, J. W. (1969). *Ann. Rev. Physiol.* **31**, 383.

Everett, J. W., and Nikitovitch-Winer, M. (1963). *In* "Advances in Neuroendocrinology" (A. V. Nalbandov, ed.), pp. 289–304. Univ. of Illinois Press, Urbana, Illinois.

Everett, J. W., and Quinn, D. L. (1966). *Endocrinology* **78**, 141.

Findlay, A. L. R. (1966). *Nature (London)* **211**, 1183.

Findlay, A. L. R. (1967). "Studies on the Sensory Innervation of the Mammary Gland and the Neural Control of Mammary Motor Function." Ph.D. thesis, Univ. of Cambridge, Cambridge, England.

Findlay, A. L. R. (1969). *J. Comp. Physiol. Psychol.* **69**, 115.

Findlay, A. L. R. (1971). *In* "Lactation" (I. R. Falconer, ed.), pp. 75–91. Butterworths, London and Washington, D.C.

Findlay, A. L. R., and Grosvenor, C. E. (1967). *Proc. Soc. Exp. Biol. Med.* **127**, 637.

Findlay, A. L. R., and Grosvenor, C. E. (1969). *Dairy Sci. Abstr.* **3**, 109.

Fiorindo, R. P., and Nicoll, C. S. (1969). *Fed. Proc. Fed. Amer. Soc. Exp. Biol.* **28**, 437.

Fitzpatrick, R. J. (1961). *J. Endocrinol.* **22**, xix.

Flerkó, B. (1959). *Acta Physiol. Acad. Sci. Hung.* **16**, 108.

Flerkó, B., and Bárdos, V. (1959). *Acta Neuroveg.* **20**, 248.

Folley, S. J. (1947). *Brit. Med. Bull.* **5**, 142.

Folley, S. J. (1956). "The Physiology and Biochemistry of Lactation." Oliver and Boyd, Edinburgh.

Folley, S. J., and Knaggs, G. S. (1966). *J. Endocrinol.* **34**, 197.

Folley, S. J., and Malpress, F. H. (1948). *In* "The Hormones" (G. Pincus and K. V. Thimann, eds.), Vol. 1, Chapter 16. Academic Press, New York.

Forbes, A., Forbes, A. P., and Neyland, M. (1955). *J. Appl. Physiol.* **7**, 675.

Fuchs, A. R., and Wagner, G. (1963). *Acta Endocrinol.* **44**, 581.

Gachev, E. P. (1969). *C. R. Acad. Bulg. Sci.* **22**, 217.

Gale, C. C. (1963). *Acta Physiol. Scand.* **59**, 269.

Geschwind, I. I. (1969). *In* "Frontiers in Neuroendocrinology" (L. Martini and W. F. Ganong, eds.), pp. 389–432. Oxford Univ. Press, London and New York.

Geschwind, I. I. (1970). *In* "Hypophysiotrophic Hormones of the Hypothalamus: Assay and Chemistry" (J. Meites, ed.), pp. 289–319. Williams and Wilkins, Baltimore, Maryland.

Giacometti, L., and Montagna, W. (1962). *Anat. Rec.* **144**, 191.

Grachev, I. I. (1949). *Zh. Obshch. Biol.* **10**, 401.

Grachev, I. I. (1953). *Endocrinology* **29**, 1026.

Grachev, I. I. (1964). "Reflex Regulation of Lactation." Izdatel stvo Leningradskogo Univ., Leningrad.

Greene, R. R. (1941). *Endocrinology* **29**, 1026.

Grégoire, C. (1947). J. Endocrinol. 5, 68.
Grosvenor, C. E. (1964a). Endocrinology 75, 15.
Grosvenor, C. E. (1964b). Endocrinology 74, 548.
Grosvenor, C. E. (1965a). Endocrinology 77, 1037.
Grosvenor, C. E. (1965b). Endocrinology 76, 340.
Grosvenor, C. E. (1965c). Amer. J. Physiol. 208, 214.
Grosvenor, C. E. (1966). Proc. Soc. Exp. Biol. Med. 121, 366.
Grosvenor, C. E. (1971). J. Dairy Sci. 54, 769.
Grosvenor, C. E., and Findlay, A. L. R. (1968). Amer. J. Physiol. 214, 820.
Grosvenor, C. E., and Mena, F. (1967). Endocrinology 80, 840.
Grosvenor, C. E., and Mena, F. (1969). Horm. Behav. 1, 85.
Grosvenor, C. E., and Mena, F. (1971a). LX Bi. Symp. Anim. Reprod. 32, 115.
Grosvenor, C. E., and Mena, F. (1971b). Endocrinology 88, 355.
Grosvenor, C. E., and Mena, F. (1971c). Fed. Proc. Fed. Amer. Soc. Exp. Biol. 30, 474.
Grosvenor, C. E., and Mena, F. (1972). Fed. Proc. Fed. Amer. Soc. Exp. Biol. 31, 275.
Grosvenor, C. E., and Turner, C. W. (1957). Proc. Soc. Exp. Biol. Med. 96, 723.
Grosvenor, C. E., and Turner, C. W. (1958a). Endocrinology 63, 535.
Grosvenor, C. E., and Turner, C. W. (1958b). Proc. Soc. Exp. Biol. Med. 97, 463.
Grosvenor, C. E., and Turner, C. W. (1959). Proc. Soc. Exp. Biol. Med. 101, 699.
Grosvenor, C. E., McCann, S. M., and Nallar, R. (1965). Endocrinology 76, 883.
Grosvenor, C. E., Mena, F., Schaefgen, D. A. (1967a). Endocrinology 81, 449.
Grosvenor, C. E., Mena, F., Dhariwal, A. P. S., and McCann, S. M. (1967b). Endocrinology 81, 1021.
Grosvenor, C. E., Krulich, L., and McCann, S.M. (1968a). Endocrinology 82, 617.
Grosvenor, C. E., Mena, F., Schaefgen, D. A., Dhariwal, A. P. S., Antunes-Rodriguez, J., and McCann, S. M. (1968b). In "Pharmacology of Hormonal Polypeptides and Proteins" (N. Back, L. Martini, and R. Paoletti, eds.), pp. 242–253. Plenum Press, New York.
Grosvenor, C. E., Maiweg, H., and Mena, F. (1970a). Horm. Behav. 1, 111.
Grosvenor, C. E., Maiweg, H., and Mena, F. (1970b). Amer. J. Physiol. 219, 403.
Grosvenor, C. E., Mena, F., Maiweg, H., Dhariwal, A. P. S., and McCann, S. M. (1970c). J. Endocrinol. 47, 339.
Grosvenor, C. E., DeNuccio, D. J., King, S. F., Maiweg, H., and Mena, F. (1972). J. Endocrinol. 55, 299.
Grosz, H. J., and Rothballer, A. B. (1961). Nature (London) 190, 349.
Haun, C. K., and Sawyer, C. H. (1960). Endocrinology 67, 270.
Haun, C. K., and Sawyer, C. H. (1961). Acta Endocrinol. 38, 99.
Hebb, C., and Linzell, J. L. (1951). Quart. J. Exp. Physiol. 36, 159.
Hebb, C., and Linzell, J. L. (1966). J. Physiol. 186, 82P.
Hebb, C., and Linzell, J. L. (1970). Histochem. J. 2, 491.
Hillarp, N. A. (1949). Acta Endocrinol. 2, 11.
Holst, V., and Turner, C. W. (1939). Proc. Soc. Exp. Biol. Med. 42, 479.
Hooker, C. W., and Williams, W. L. (1940). Yale J. Biol. Med. 12, 559.
Hooker, C. W., and Williams, W. L. (1941). Endocrinology 28, 42.
Houvenaghel, A. (1969). Mëm Acad. Mëd. Belg. 7, 47.
Ingelbrecht, P. (1935). C. R. Soc. Biol. 120, 1369.
Isbister, C. (1954). Arch. Dis. Childh. 29, 66.
Jacobsohn, D. (1949). Acta Physiol. Scand. 19, 10.

Johke, T. (1970). *Endocrinol. Jap.* **16**, 179.

Kanematsu, S., and Sawyer, C. H. (1963a). *Acta Endocrinol.* **44**, 467.

Kanematsu, S., and Sawyer, C. H. (1963b). *Endocrinology* **72**, 243.

Kanematsu, S., Hilliard, J., and Sawyer, C. H. (1963a). *Endocrinology* **73**, 345.

Kanematsu, S., Hilliard, J., and Sawyer, C. H. (1963b). *Acta Endocrinol.* **44**, 467.

Knaggs, G. S. (1963). *J. Endocrinol.* **26**, xxiv.

Knook, H. L. (1965). "The Fibre Connections of the Forebrain." Van Gorcum, Assen.

Koelle, G. B. (1965). *In* "The Pharmacological Basis of Therapeutics" (L. S. Goodman and A. Gilman, eds.), p. 399. Macmillan, New York.

Koizumi, K., Ishikawa, T., and Brooks, Mc C. (1964). *J. Neurophysiol.* **27**, 878.

Kokorina, E. P. (1966). *In* "Neiro-gormonal'naya regulyatsiya laktatsii" (I. A. Barȳshnikov and G. B. Tverskoi, eds.), p. 152. Izdatel'stov 'Nauka,' Moscow.

Krulich, L., Kühn, E. Illner, P., and McCann, S. M. (1970). *Fed. Proc. Fed. Amer. Soc. Exp. Biol.* **29**, 579.

Krulich, L., Quijada, M., and Illner, P. (1971). *Program Endocrine Soc.* (Abstr.) p. 82.

Kühn, E. R., and McCann, S. M. (1970). *Endocrinology* **87**, 1266.

Kuhn, N. J. (1971). *In* "Lactation" (I. R. Falconer, ed.), pp. 161–177. Butterworths, London and Washington, D.C.

Kurz, M. (1967). *In* "Symposium on Reproduction" (K. Lissak, ed.), p. 175–211. Akademiai Kiado, Budapest.

Lantos, C. P., and Tramezzani, H. J. (1962). *Acta Physiol. Lat. Amer.* **12**, 101.

Lassmann, G. (1964). *Acta Anat.* **58**, 131.

Linzell, J. L. (1950). *Quart. J. Exp. Physiol.* **35**, 295.

Linzell, J. L. (1955). *J. Physiol.* **130**, 257.

Linzell, J. L. (1959). *Physiol. Rev.* **39**, 534.

Linzell, J. L. (1963). *Quart. J. Exp. Physiol.* **48**, 34.

Lukášová, J., and Lukáš, Z. (1965). *Vet. Med. Praha.* **10**, 293.

MacCleod, R. M., and Abad, A. (1968). *Endocrinology* **83**, 799.

MacCleod, R. M., Smitt, M. C., and De Witt, G. W. (1966). *Endocrinology* **79**, 1149.

Martins, T. (1949). *Physiol. Zool.* **22**, 169.

McCann, S. M. (1971). *In* "Frontiers in Neuroendocrinology" (L. Martini and W. F. Ganong, eds.), pp. 209–235. Williams and Wilkins, Baltimore, Maryland.

McCann, S. M., and Friedman, H. M. (1960). *Endocrinology* **67**, 597.

McMurtry, J. P., and Anderson, R. R. (1971). *Proc. Soc. Exp. Biol. Med.* **137**, 354.

Meites, J. (1954). *Rev. Can. Biol.* ·**13**, 359.

Meites, J. (1959). *In* "Reproduction in Domestic Animals" (H. H. Cole and P. T. Cupps, eds.), Vol. 1, pp. 539–593. Academic Press, New York.

Meites, J. (1966). *In* "Neuroendocrinology" (L. Martini and W. F. Ganong, eds.), Vol. 1, pp. 664–708. Academic Press, New York.

Meites, J. (1970). *In* "Hypophysiotrophic Hormones of the Hypothalamus. Assay and Chemistry" (J. Meites, ed.), Chapter 9. Williams and Wilkins, Baltimore, Maryland.

Meites, J., and Nicoll, C. S. (1966). *Ann. Rev. Physiol.* **28**, 57.

Meites, J., and Turner, C. W. (1942a). *Endocrinology* **30**, 726.

Meites, J., and Turner, C. W. (1942b). *Endocrinology* **31**, 1340.

Meites, J., and Turner, C. W. (1948). *Res. Bull. Mo. Agr. Exp. Sta.* No. 416.

274   C. E. Grosvenor and F. Mena

Meites, J., Bergman, A. J., and Turner, C. W. (1941). Proc. Soc. Exp. Biol. Med. 46, 670.
Meites, J., Kahn, R. H., and Nicoll, C. W. (1961). Program Endocrine Soc. (Abstr.) p. 6.
Meites, J., Nicoll, C. S., and Talwalker, P. K. (1962). Program Endocrine Soc. (Abstr.) p. 39.
Meites, J., Nicoll, C. S., and Talwalker, P. K. (1963). Advan. Neuroendocrinol. 238–277.
Mena, F., and Beyer, C. (1963). Amer. J. Physiol. 205, 313.
Mena, F., and Beyer, C. (1968a). Endocrinology 83, 615.
Mena, F., and Beyer, C. (1968b). Endocrinology 83, 618.
Mena, F., and Beyer, C. (1969). Physiologist 12, 300.
Mena, F., and Grosvenor, C. E. (1968). Endocrinology 82, 623.
Mena, F., and Grosvenor, C. E. (1971). Horm. Behav. 2, 107.
Mena, F., and Grosvenor, C. E. (1972). J. Endocrinol. 52, 11.
Mena, F., Anguiano, G., and Beyer, C. (1961). Bol. Inst. Estud. Méd. Biol. Méx. 19, 119.
Mena, F., Maiweg, H., and Grosvenor, C. E. (1968). Endocrinology 83, 1359.
Mess, B., Fraschini, F., Motta, M., and Martini, L. (1967). Proc. Int. Congr. Horm. Steroids, 2nd, Milan, 1966 Excerpta Medica Int. Congr. Ser. 132, 1009.
Miller, M. R., and Kasahara, M. (1959). Anat. Rec. 135, 153.
Mizuno, H., and Satoh, K. (1970). Endocrinol. Japan 17, 15.
Mizuno, H., and Shiiba, N. (1969). Endocrinol. Japan 16, 547.
Moltz, H., Levin, R., and Leon, M. (1969). Science 163, 1083.
Momongan, V. G., and Schmidt, G. H. (1970). J. Dairy Sci. 53, 747.
Morag, M. (1967). Life Sci. 6, 1513.
Morag, M., and Fox, S. (1966). Ann. Biol. Anim. Biochem. Biophys. 6, 467.
Morag, M., and Griffin, T. K. (1968). Ann. Biol. Anim. Biochem. Biophys. 8, 235.
Newton, M., and Newton, N. R. (1948). J. Pediat. 33, 698.
Nicoll, C. S. (1971). In "Frontiers in Neuroendocrinology" (L. Martini and W. F. Ganong, eds.), pp. 291–330. Oxford Univ. Press, London and New York.
Nicoll, C. S., and Meites, J. (1959). Proc. Soc. Exp. Biol. Med. 101, 81.
Nicoll, C. S., and Meites, J. (1962). Endocrinology 70, 272.
Nicoll, C. S., Fiorindo, R. P., McKennee, C. T., and Parsons, J. T. (1970). In "Hypophysiotrophic Hormones of the Hypothalamus: Assay and Chemistry" (J. Meites, ed.), Chapter 9. Williams and Wilkins, Baltimore, Maryland.
Niggli-Stokar, U. Von. (1961). Acta Anat. 46, 104.
Nikitovitch-Winer, M. (1957). "Humoral Influence of the Hypothalamus on Gonadotrophin Secretions." Ph.D. dissertation. Duke Univ., Durham, North Carolina.
Nikitovitch-Winer, M. (1960). Mem. Soc. Endocrinol. 9, 70.
Niswender, G. P., Chen, C. L., Midgley, A. R., Jr., Meites, J., and Ellis, S. (1969). Proc. Soc. Exp. Biol. Med. 130, 793.
Ota, K., and Yokoyama, A. (1965). J. Endocrinol. 33, 185.
Paape, M. J., and Guidry, A. J. (1969). Dairy Sci. 52, 998.
Pasteels, J. L. (1961). C. R. Acad. Sci. 253, 2140.
Pasteels, J. L. (1962). C. R. Acad. Sci. 254, 4083.
Patel, M. D. (1936). Physiol. Zool. 9, 129.
Peeters, G. Bouckaert, J. H., and Oyaert, W. (1952). Arch. Int. Pharmacodyn. Thérap. 88, 197.

Peeters, G., Coussens, R., and Oyaert, W. (1949). *Arch. Int. Pharmacodyn. Thérap.* **79**, 113.

Petersen, W. E. (1944). *Physiol. Rev.* **24**, 340.

Popovici, D. G. (1963). *Rev. Biol.* **8**, 75.

Porter, J. C., Kamberi, I. A., and Grazia, Y. R. (1971). *In* "Frontiers in Neuroendocrinology" (L. Martini and W. F. Ganong, eds.), pp. 145–175. Oxford Univ. Press, London and New York.

Quinn, D. L., and Everett, J. W. (1967). *Endocrinology* **80**, 155.

Ramírez, V. D., and McCann, S. M. (1964). *Endocrinology* **75**, 206.

Ratner, A., and Meites, J. (1964). *Endocrinology* **75**, 377.

Reece, R. P., and Turner, C. W. (1937). *Proc. Soc. Exp. Biol. Med.* **35**, 621.

Relkin, R. (1967). *Dis. Nerv. Syst.* **28**, 94.

Richard, P. H., Urban, I., and Denamur, R. (1970). *J. Endocrinol.* **47**, 45.

Richards, M. P. M. (1967). *Advan. Reproduct. Physiol.* **2**, 53–110.

Richardson, R. C. (1949). *Proc. Roy. Soc. London B* **136**, 30.

Roberts, J. S., and Share, L. (1968). *Endocrinology* **83**, 272.

Rosenblatt, J. S., and Lehrman, D. S. (1963). *In* "Maternal Behavior in Mammals" (H. L. Reingold, ed.), pp. 8–57. Wiley, New York.

Roth, L. L., and Rosenblatt, J. S. (1966). *Science* **151**, 1403.

Roth, L. L., and Rosenblatt, J. S. (1968). *J. Endocrinol.* **42**, 363.

Rothchild, I. (1960). *Endocrinology* **67**, 9.

Rothchild, I. (1965). *Vitam. Horm.* **23**, 209.

Sar, M., and Meites, J. (1969). *Neuroendocrinology* **4**, 25.

Selye, H. (1934). *Amer. J. Physiol.* **107**, 535.

Selye, H., Collip, J. B., and Thomson, D. L. (1934). *Endocrinology* **18**, 237.

Sinha, Y. N., and Tucker, H. A. (1968). *Proc. Soc. Exp. Biol. Med.* **128**, 84.

Stutinsky, F., and Terminn, Y. (1964). *C. R. Séances Soc. Biol.* **158**, 833.

Stutinsky, F., and Terminn, Y. (1965). *J. Physiol.* **57**, 279.

Tabaschnik, I. I. A., and Trentin, J. J. (1951). *Fed. Proc. Fed. Amer. Soc. Exp. Biol.* **10**, 339.

Taleisnik, S., and Deis, R. P. (1964). *Amer. J. Physiol.* **207**, 1394.

Taleisnik, S., and Orias, R. (1966). *Endocrinology* **78**, 522.

Tindal, J. S. (1967). *In* "Reproduction in the Female Mammal" (G. E. Lamming and E. C. Amoroso, eds.), pp. 79–107. Butterworths, London and Washington, D.C.

Tindal, J. S., and Knaggs, G. S. (1969). *J. Endocrinol.* **45**, 111.

Tindal, J. S., and Knaggs, G. S. (1970). *In* "Hormones and the Environment" (G. K. Benson and J. G. Phillips, eds.), pp. 239–256. Cambridge Univ. Press, London and New York.

Tindal, J. S., and Knaggs, G. S. (1971). *J. Endocrinol.* **50**, 135.

Tindal, J. S., Beyer, C., and Sawyer, C. H. (1963). *Endocrinology* **72**, 720.

Tindal, J. S., Knaggs, G. S., and Turvey, A. (1967a). *J. Endocrinol.* **37**, 279.

Tindal, J. S., Knaggs, G. S., and Turvey, A. (1967b). *J. Endocrinol.* **38**, 337.

Tindal, J. S., Knaggs, G. S., and Turvey, A. (1968). *J. Endocrinol.* **40**, 205.

Tindal, J. S., Knaggs, G. S., and Turvey, A. (1969). *J. Endocrinol.* **43**, 663.

Tucker, H. A. (1971). *LX Bi. Symp. Amer. Rep.* **32**, 137.

Tucker, H. A., Paape, M. J., and Sinha, Y. N. (1967). *Amer. J. Physiol.* **213**, 262.

Turner, C. W., and Griffith, D. R. (1962). *Proc. Int. Union Physiol. Sci.* **1**, 97.

Tsakhaev, G. A. (1953). *Dokl. Akad. Nauk. SSSR* **93**, 1131.

Tsakhaev, G. A. (1959). *In* "Problems of the Physiology of Farm Animals," pp. 39–46. Akad. Nauk. Lit. SSR., Moscow.

Tverskoi, G. B. (1953). *Zh. Obshch. Biol. Mosk.* **14**, 349.

Tverskoi, G. B. (1960). *Nature (London)* **186**, 782.

Tverskoi, G. B. (1968). *Proc. Int. Un. Physiol. Sci.* **6**, 211.

Tverskoi, G. B., and Dyusembin, Kh. (1955). *Tr. Inst. Fiz. I.P. Pavlova.* **4**, 95.

Van der Lee, S., and Boot, L. M. (1955). *Acta Physiol. Pharmacol. Neerl.* **4**, 442.

Van der Lee, S., and Boot, L. M. (1956). *Acta Physiol. Pharmacol. Neerl.* **5**, 213.

Voogt, J. L., and Meites, J. (1970). *Program Endocrine Soc.* (Abstr.) p. 125.

Voogt, J. L., Sar, M., and Meites, J. (1969). *Amer. J. Physiol.* **216**, 655.

Vorherr, H. (1971). *Acta Endocrinol. Suppl.* **154**. 57.

Welsch, C. W., Negro-Vilar, A., and Meites, J. (1968). *Neuroendocrinology* **3**, 238.

Whitten, W. K. (1966). *Advan. Reproduct. Physiol.* **I**, 154–177.

Whittlestone, W. G. (1951). *New Zealand J. Sci. Technol.* **32**, 1.

Whittlestone, W. G., Perrin, D. R., Parkinson, R. D., and Turner, C. W. (1952). *J. Dairy Sci.* **35**, 11.

Wiesner, B. P., and Sheard, N. M. (1933). "Maternal Behavior in the Rat," p. 55. Oliver and Boyd, Edinburgh.

Williams, W. L. (1945). *Anat. Rec.* **93**, 171.

Witschi, E. (1935). *Wilson Bull.* **47**, 177.

Yanai, R., and Nagasawa, H. (1969). *Proc. Soc. Exp. Biol. Med.* **131**, 167.

Yokoyama, A., and Ota, K. (1959). *Endocrinol. Jap.* **6**, 14.

Yokoyama, A., and Ota, K. (1965). *J. Endocrinol.* **33**, 341.

Zaks, M. G. (1951). Cited by Zaks (1962).

Zaks, M. G. (1962). "The Motor Apparatus of the Mammary Gland." Oliver and Boyd, Edinburgh.

Zaks, M. G., and Pavlov, E. F. (1952). *Tr. Sovesheh. Biol. Osnovam Povȳsh. Prod. Zhivot.* **18**, (cited by Zaks, 1962).

Zambrano, D., and Deis, R. P. (1970). *J. Endocrinol.* **47**, 101.

Zarrow, M. X., Schlein, P. A., and Denenberg, V. H. and Cohen, H. A. (1972) *Endocrinology* **21**, 191.

CHAPTER FIVE

General Endocrinological Control of Lactation

H. Allen Tucker

I.	Introduction	277
II.	Hormonal Control of Mammary Secretory Activity before Pregnancy	278
III.	Mammary Secretory Activity during Pregnancy...........	279
IV.	Hormonal Control of Lactogenesis	280
	A. Anterior Pituitary	281
	B. Adrenal Cortex	285
	C. Ovary	289
	D. Other Factors Associated with Lactogenesis	292
	E. Experimental Lactogenesis in Farm Animals	293
V.	The Lactation Curve	294
VI.	Hormonal Maintenance of Lactation	296
	A. Anterior Pituitary	297
	B. Posterior Pituitary	304
	C. Adrenal Cortex	305
	D. Thyroid	308
	E. Parathyroid	311
	F. Endocrine Pancreas	312
	G. Ovary	313
	H. Pineal	315
VII.	Effect of Nursing Intensity and Pregnancy on Lactation ...	315
VIII.	Conclusions	317
	References	318

I. INTRODUCTION

The function of the mammary gland is to secrete milk for the nourishment of the young. This secretory process, lactation, includes intracellular synthesis of milk, the subsequent expulsion of milk from the mammary secretory cell, and the ejection of milk from the mammary gland. Initiation

277

and maintenance of lactation are dependent on hormones from several endocrine glands. Furthermore, mammary secretory activity normally is associated with changes in the reproductive status of the animal. While small quantities of lacteal fluids may accumulate earlier, secretion of large quantities of milk occurs only after formation of the mammary lobule-alveolar system, a process that also requires hormones (see Anderson, Chapter 2). For earlier comprehensive reviews of the endocrinological control of lactation the reader is referred to Folley (1956), Reece (1958), Cowie (1961), Cowie and Folley (1961), Meites (1966), Reynolds and Folley (1969), and Falconer (1971).

II. HORMONAL CONTROL OF MAMMARY SECRETORY ACTIVITY BEFORE PREGNANCY

Visible evidence of secretion in mammary tissue sometimes occurs in the newborn human and is called "witches milk" (Mayer and Klein, 1961). This type of secretion may occur also in the neonatal rabbit, cat, goat, and horse. The specific hormones involved are not known nor is it known with certainty if they originate from the maternal or fetal endocrine system or from the placenta. Support for fetal hormone participation comes from the finding that adrenal glucocorticoids, hormones known to play a major role in inducing normal lactation at parturition in the dam, increase markedly in the fetus shortly before birth and remain elevated for a short time after birth (Bassett and Thorburn, 1969). Further indirect evidence that these secretions are related to hormonal changes associated with parturition is provided by the observation that they subside shortly after birth, a time when the adrenal secretions in the neonate decline and the reproductive system is relatively inactive.

Accumulation of secretion within the mammary gland does not occur again in the growing animal until the estrous cycles commence. At this time, a small quantity of a colostral-like secretion often appears around the time of estrus, but it disappears during the luteal phase of the estrous cycle (Hammond, 1927; Grynfeltt, 1937). Metabolic activity of mammary tissue of heifers and rats, as measured by ribonucleic acid (RNA) content, was significantly increased during estrus relative to values obtained during the luteal phase of the cycle. These changes in mammary RNA content were associated with changes in pituitary prolactin concentrations (Sinha and Tucker, 1969a,b). Furthermore, serum concentrations of prolactin are greatest during the estrogenic phase and lowest during the luteal phase of the estrous cycle in heifers (Swanson and Hafs, 1971) and rats (Fig. 1; Amenomori *et al.*, 1970; Neil, 1972).

Growth hormone synthesis and release do not change during the estrous cycle of the rat (Ieiri *et al.*, 1971), but in mice Sinha *et al.* (1972) observed elevated serum growth hormone concentrations during proestrus. Koprowski and Tucker (1973b) observed maximum serum growth hormone during estrus in cows. More direct evidence that other hormones interact with prolactin to induce the lacteal secretions during estrus is lacking at the present time.

III. MAMMARY SECRETORY ACTIVITY DURING PREGNANCY

Histological studies during pregnancy showed that mammary secretory activity gradually increases (Jeffers, 1935), but the most rapid shift from the nonlactational to the lactational state occurs around the time of parturition. Quantification of the secretory activity pattern during pregnancy using total RNA content of the mammary glands of rats (Tucker and Reece, 1963a) is shown in Fig. 2. The gradual increase in total secretory activity is probably related to the total amount of secretory tissue present as well as the ability of these cells to secrete milk. As a result, milk production that may follow abortion in cows is greater if the abortion occurs late in gestation.

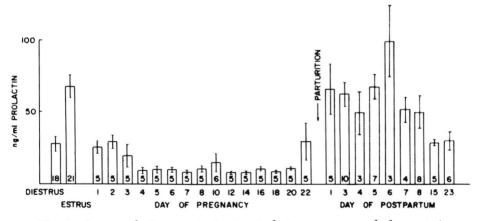

Fig. 1.   Serum prolactin concentration in rats during pregnancy and after parturition. Mean and standard error of mean are indicated at top of each bar. Number of rats in each group is indicated at bottom of each bar. (From Amenomori *et al.*, 1970.)

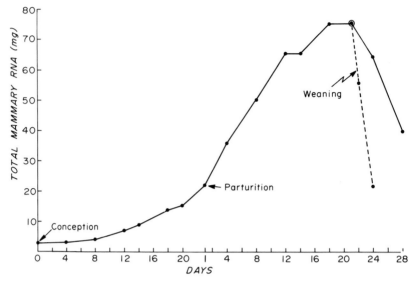

Fig. 2.   Mammary RNA content in rats from pregnancy through lactation. (Data from Tucker and Reece, 1963a,b,d.)

IV.   HORMONAL CONTROL OF LACTOGENESIS

The sudden surge in the secretion of milk at parturition, lactogenesis, is caused by an interaction among several hormones. Lactogenesis is usually measured in terms of gross or histological appearance of mammary tissue or in terms of the induction of a specific component of milk or mammary tissue such as RNA, α-lactalbumin, lactose, or casein. With the exception of a few studies in ruminants, evidence for lactogenesis has not included measurement of milk removed from the mammary gland.

Specific hormonal requirements vary among species, but, in general, minimal needs include prolactin and adrenal glucocorticoids and the relative absence of progesterone. The lactogenic properties of a hormone are usually tested in animals having well-developed mammary glands as a result of pregnancy, pseudopregnancy, or pretreatment with hormones that stimulate mammary growth. In recent years, *in vitro* systems have provided additional insights into hormonal control of lactogenesis (see Topper and Oka, Chapter 6). Reynolds and Folley (1969) and Denamur (1971) have presented recent reviews of the hormonal requirements for lactogenesis.

A. Anterior Pituitary

Grueter (1928) and Stricker and Grueter (1929) were first to show that aqueous extracts of the anterior pituitary would induce lactation in pseudopregnant rabbits. Lyons (1942) extended these observations when he demonstrated that a purified anterior pituitary preparation, which caused local proliferation of the pigeon crop-sac mucosa, also induced a local lactation at the site of injection in the rabbit mammary gland. This hormone is commonly called "prolactin" although the terms "luteotropin (LTH)," "mammotropin," and "lactogen" are also used.

Although systemic injections of anterior pituitary extracts induced milk secretion in pregnant rats, guinea pigs, rabbits, and goats, the exact role of these hormones in lactogenesis could not be determined because death of the fetuses always preceded lactogenesis (Nelson, 1934; Defremery, 1936; Meites and Turner, 1947). In experiments utilizing injections of more highly purified prolactin preparations, lactation was not initiated in rats (Talwalker *et al.*, 1961), mice (Nandi and Bern, 1961), or ewes (Delouis and Denamur, 1967), although pregnancy was not affected. Reece (1939) induced lactation in pseudopregnant rats by using an adrenal cortical extract in conjunction with prolactin. This strongly suggests that the difference in response between crude pituitary extracts and purified prolactin is caused by a lack of adrenocorticotropic hormone (ACTH) in the purified prolactin preparations. ACTH and glucocorticoids will also induce lactation in intact pseudopregnant rabbits (Chadwick and Folley, 1962; Chadwick, 1971). The next section contains a further discussion of the role of the adrenal in lactogenesis.

Studies in hypophysectomized animals, with and without hormonal replacement therapy, have contributed additional knowledge of pituitary factors regulating lactogenesis. Hypophysectomy during pregnancy restricts lactogenesis at parturition to a transient secretion (Selye *et al.*, 1933a,b; Nelson and Gaunt, 1936), which is probably caused by fetal or placental hormones. Analogous to the initial results obtained in intact animals, studies in hypophysectomized animals showed that, although crude extracts of the anterior pituitary were lactogenic, highly purified prolactin was inactive unless combined with ACTH (Gomez and Turner, 1937) or cortisone (Nelson *et al.*, 1943). Using hypophysectomized, adrenalectomized, and ovariectomized (triply operated) rats, Lyons (1958) determined that the minimal requirements for initiating lactation were prolactin and adrenal glucocorticoids.

Results similar to those in rats were observed in triply operated mice except that growth hormone could completely replace prolactin in certain strains of mice (Nandi and Bern, 1961). There is little conclusive evidence to suggest that growth hormone from infraprimate sources is lactogenic by itself; it must be combined with a corticoid or a corticoid plus prolactin. Some strains of mice are completely refractory to the lactogenic properties of growth hormone, and this fact appears to be related to genetic differences in the mammary tissue and not to differences in the hormone secretion patterns (Nandi, 1958).

In goats hypophysectomized during lactation, prolactin and adrenal corticoids are lactogenic, but complete restoration of milk yields requires the addition of growth hormone and triiodothyronine (Cowie, 1969a).

In contrast to other species, secretion of copious quantities of milk can be induced in hypophysectomized rabbits with prolactin alone (Fredrikson, 1939; Kilpatrick et al., 1964). Cowie and Watson (1966) induced lactation with prolactin in adrenalectomized or adrenalectomized-ovariectomized rabbits during pseudopregnancy, suggesting that although adrenal cortical hormones may normally play a role, they are not absolutely essential to lactogenesis in the rabbit.

Special mention should be made of the lactogenic hormones isolated from the pituitaries of humans. Because growth hormone derived from infraprimates will not promote growth in primates, there has been a considerable research effort to isolate, purify, and eventually to synthesize human growth hormone for clinical use. Li et al. (1966, 1969a) have now determined the primary structure of human growth hormone (Fig. 3). However, all preparations of human growth hormone contain intrinsic prolactinlike activities (Forsyth, 1969). That is, they stimulate growth of pigeon crop-sac mucosa, promote mammary growth, and induce a local lactogenesis after intraductal injection into pseudopregnant rabbits (Lyons et al., 1960). This overlapping biological function may now have been explained by the finding that there are three homologous segments of amino acids in ovine prolactin and human growth hormone molecules and that this homology represents about 45% of the two peptide chains (Li et al., 1969b; Brewley and Li, 1970).

To date prolactin has not been isolated chemically from primate pituitaries as a hormone completely free of growth hormone activity, but there is considerable immunologic and electrophoretic evidence (Frantz and Kleinberg, 1970; Friesen and Guyda, 1971; Guyda et al., 1971; Lewis et al., 1971) to suggest that primate prolactin is a separate entity. Furthermore, when human pituitaries are cultured in vitro, the growth hormone activity disappears with time whereas the prolactinlike function remains (Pasteels, 1969; Forsyth, 1969). Also, addition of hypothalamic extracts

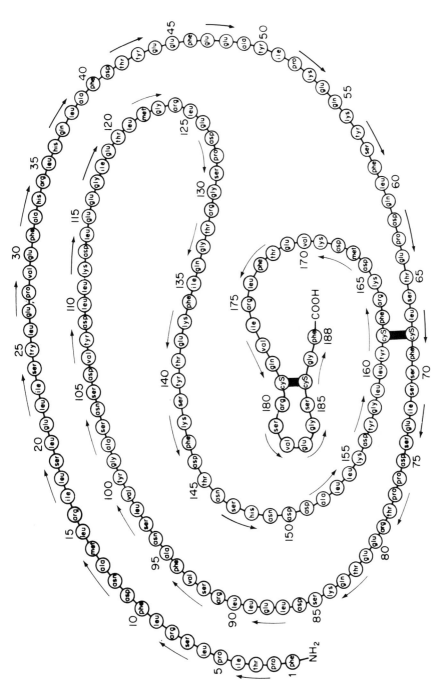

Fig. 3. The amino acid sequence of human growth hormone. (From Li *et al.*, 1969a.)

to monkey pituitaries stimulated growth hormone release but either inhibited or was without effect on prolactin release (Nicoll et al., 1970).
Furthermore, Forsyth (1970) found that the prolactin activity of serum
from lactating women exceeds the serum growth hormone concentrations.

Another aspect of this problem is the fact that the human placenta
produces a hormone that partially cross reacts with primate growth
hormone (Josimovich and MacLaren, 1962). This hormone is called
"human placental lactogen" or "human chorionic somatomammotropin." It
is luteotropic in the rat, has slight pigeon crop-sac-stimulating activity, is
lactogenic when injected intraductally into pseudopregnant or pregnant
rabbits (Josimovich and MacLaren, 1962; Friesen, 1966), and can sub-
stitue for ovine prolactin in stimulating cultured mammary cells to secrete
casein (Turkington and Topper, 1966). Human placental lactogen and
human growth hormone possess similar amino acid sequences (Catt et al.,
1967) with about 85% of the positions being identical in the two molecules (Sherwood et al., 1971). The precise role that human growth
hormone or human placental lactogen plays in lactogenesis in the normal
woman is not clear, although it is known that the hormone passes to the
maternal and not to the fetal vascular system (Kaplan and Grumbach,
1965). Varma et al. (1971) devised a method to correct for cross reactivity
between human growth hormone and human placental lactogen. They
discovered that growth hormone remains constant at about 4.3 ng/ml
throughout pregnancy whereas human placental lactogen increases
steadily from 0.4 µg/ml at 8 weeks to 6.2 µg/ml at 38 weeks of pregnancy. Possibly, the transitory lactation that occurs at parturition in
primates previously hypophysectomized during pregnancy may be related
to the secretion of human placental lactogen (Forsyth, 1969). However,
the action of human placental lactogen on lactogenesis normally must be
inhibited, otherwise one would expect lactogenesis to occur much earlier
in gestation because the hormone is present for the greater part of
pregnancy.

Pregnant rats also secrete a hormone from the placenta into the maternal blood (Matthies, 1967) which has mammotropic, lactogenic, luteotropic, and pigeon crop-sac activity when injected into the appropriate
test animals (Ray et al., 1955). It is not certain if this material is
identical with prolactin, but it probably has little influence in normal
lactogenesis because it disappears from the serum after the twelfth day
of pregnancy (Cohen and Gala, 1969). Placentas from mice also secrete
a mammotropic hormone (Newton and Beck, 1939) until at least day 19
of pregnancy (Yanai and Nagasawa, 1971). But it is not clear whether or
not mouse placental mammotropins play a part in lactogenesis.

Analyses of pituitary and serum concentrations of hormones at parturition have provided additional information concerning the endocrinological control of lactogenesis. Reece and Turner (1937) showed that prolactin content of the pituitary of rats was low during pregnancy but increased markedly after parturition. Grosvenor and Turner (1960) showed that pituitary prolactin increased during the first two-thirds of pregnancy but decreased during the last trimester to only 8% of that present at mid-pregnancy. These data were interpreted to reflect an increased rate of release of prolactin during the interval of lactogenesis.

In confirmation of the pituitary content data, prolactin concentration in the serum of rats (Amenomori *et al.*, 1970) was reduced for the greater portion of pregnancy until shortly before parturition (Fig. 1). Measurements of prolactin in the serum of several species amply confirm that concentrations of prolactin are markedly elevated around the time of parturition (Amenomori *et al.*, 1970; Arai and Lee, 1967; Davis *et al.*, 1971; Bryant *et al.*, 1968; Schams and Karg, 1970; Ingalls *et al.*, 1973). Data for cows are shown in Fig. 4.

Little change in the circulating level of growth hormone has been observed during pregnancy and through lactation in rats (Schalch and Reichlin, 1966) or ewes (Bassett *et al.*, 1970). Similarly, Oxender *et al.* (1972) found relatively constant amounts of growth hormone for the greater part of gestation, but Ingalls *et al.* (1973) observed that growth hormone increased markedly but briefly at parturition, about 24 hours after prolactin was released (Fig. 4). Thus, these data fit the theory that growth hormone may synergize with prolactin and/or the adrenal corticoids to initiate lactation in the bovine.

However, measurements of circulating concentrations of hormones do not necessarily reflect tissue utilization of the hormone. In this writer's opinion our understanding will be markedly enhanced from studies of mammary tissue uptake of the hormones and their relationship to the induction of specific events at lactogenesis.

B. Adrenal Cortex

The importance of the adrenal cortical hormone in lactogenesis has already been suggested in the previous section. Injections of glucocorticoids into pregnant rats (Talwalker *et al.*, 1961), mice (Nandi and Bern, 1961), rabbits (Meites *et al.*, 1963; Friesen, 1966), ewes (Delouis and Denamur, 1967), or cows (Fig. 5; Tucker and Meites, 1965) initiate lactation. However, in all instances the combination of prolactin and

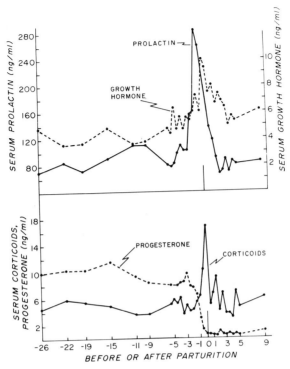

Fig. 4. Serum prolactin, growth hormone, corticoid, and progesterone concentrations in cows before and after parturition. (Data from Ingalls *et al.*, 1973; Smith *et al.* 1973.)

glucocorticoid has produced a more marked milk secretion than if either hormone was given alone (Reece, 1939; Meites *et al.*, 1963; Friesen, 1966).

Except for the work in ewes and cows where the milk was weighed (Fig. 5), gross or histological appearance of the mammary tissue was used as the criteria for lactogenesis. But more specific criteria such as appearance of caseinlike proteins, enhanced RNA synthesis, or lactose in the mammary glands failed to support the idea that glucocorticoids initiate lactation in rats (Davis and Liu, 1969; Kuhn, 1969a). Ferreri and Griffith (1969) observed a small increase in mammary RNA of rats during late pregnancy in response to hydrocortisone acetate, but the increase was much less than that observed after normal parturition. Whether these negative findings reflect species or strain differences with respect to glucocorticoid sensitivity is yet to be resolved.

Nonetheless, the adrenal secretions must play some role in lactogenesis

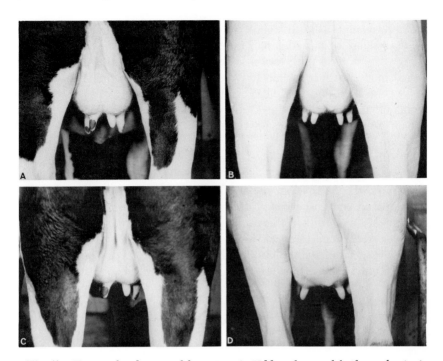

Fig. 5. Hormonal induction of lactation. A, Udder of control heifer at beginning of treatment. B, Udder of control heifer after 6 days of no treatment. C, Udder of experimental heifer at beginning of experiment. D, Udder of experimental heifer after 6 days injection with synthetic glucocorticoid (9α-fluoroprednisolone acetate). At the first milking on day 7 controls produced no milk whereas corticoid-treated heifers averaged 10 pounds of milk. (From Tucker and Meites, 1965.)

because adrenalectomy prevents induction of synthesis of caseinlike proteins and RNA, which occurs after ovariectomy of normal pregnant rats (Davis and Liu, 1969). Similarly, Ben-David *et al.* (1965a) induced lactation with the tranquilizing drug, perphenazine, but this response will not occur in adrenalectomized animals (Ben-David and Sulman, 1970). Since perphenazine elevates prolactin concentration in the blood, the failure of lactogenesis in adrenalectomized, perphenazine-treated animals must reflect a lack of corticosteroids at the mammary gland (Ben-David *et al.*, 1971).

Further support for the idea that adrenal cortical steroids play an important role in lactogenesis has been forthcoming from studies designed to measure adrenal cortical activity. Various indirect measurements suggest that adrenal cortical activity increases in many species as pregnancy advances (Poulton and Reece, 1957; Anderson and Turner,

1962a; Kamoun, 1970). In recent years the development of highly sensitive assays has permitted direct assessment of circulating concentrations of adrenal steroids. With the onset of gestation, corticosteroids decrease in the blood and they remain low until the onset of lactation in rats and mice (Gala and Westphal, 1965a, 1967; Voogt et al., 1969). Studies in ruminants also suggest reduced adrenal cortical activity for the greater part of gestation (Lindner, 1964; Paterson and Hills, 1967; Bassett and Thorburn, 1969).

With the onset of lactation circulating corticosteroids rise during the last few days of pregnancy in the rat (Milkovic and Milkovic, 1963; Kamoun et al., 1965; Voogt et al., 1969). Kamoun (1970) observed that the increased corticosteroids were caused by an increased secretion rate from the adrenal rather than a decrease in metabolic clearance rate. However, the prepartum rise in corticosteroids is not greater than the changes associated with circadian rhythms in the rat during late pregnancy (Kuhn, 1969a). Increased serum corticosteroid concentrations have also been observed during late pregnancy in the mouse (Gala and Westphal, 1967), guinea pig (Gala and Westphal, 1967; Rosenthal et al., 1969), dog (Seal and Doe, 1963), cow (Heitzman et al., 1970; Adams and Wagner, 1970; Ingalls et al., 1973; Fig. 4), and woman (Stewart et al., 1961; Friedman and Beard, 1966; Scholz and Huther, 1971). In contrast, there may be no elevated secretion of corticosteroids before parturition in ewes (Paterson and Harrison, 1967, 1968; Bassett and Thorburn, 1969) or monkeys (Wolf and Bowman, 1966). Whether this represents species specificity or failure to sample the animals at sufficiently frequent intervals is not known. Sampling frequency is especially pertinent in view of the marked variation as to whether the burst of adrenal activity is of relatively short or long duration. For example, in women adrenal activity increases during the last trimester of pregnancy, whereas in cattle the increase commences only 1–5 days before parturition (Adams and Wagner, 1970; Ingalls et al., 1973).

The fetus may be the source of some of the corticosteroids found in the serum of pregnant females. Hypophysectomy (Liggins et al., 1967) or adrenalectomy (Drost and Holm, 1968) of fetal lambs prolongs gestation, and injection of exogenous ACTH or corticoids into the fetus (van Rensburg, 1967; Liggins, 1969) or into the mother (Adams and Wagner, 1970) induces premature parturition. The concentration of corticosteroids in the near-term fetal lamb exceeds that of the ewe (Bassett and Thorburn, 1969), and in the rat corticosterone secretion rates are equivalent in the fetus and adult animal (Milkovic and Milkovic, 1962). But evidence presented by Bassett and Thorburn (1969) suggests that high concentrations of corticoids in fetal lambs at term may not affect the maternal concentrations. However, in rats (a species known to have an increased concentration of corticosteroids in the maternal blood near parturition) corticosterone can pass from the fetus to the mother (Kamoun and Stutinsky, 1968), and adrenalectomy of the mother at this time reduces corticosterone about 50% (Milkovic and Milkovic, 1963). This information in rats supports the idea that the fetal adrenal may be an important source of corticosteroids in the dam near parturition. The concept of the fetal endocrine contribution to lactogenesis in the mother should be investigated further in species with elevated maternal gluco-corticoid secretion around the time of lactogenesis.

Another factor influencing lactogenesis is binding of corticosteroids (and progesterone, Section IV, C) to corticosteroid-binding globulin (CBG) and to a lesser extent serum albumin. When the steroid hormones are bound to these proteins they are biologically inactive. Increased binding to these proteins may explain why hyperadrenalism does not occur in species with increased corticosteroid blood levels during late pregnancy. The association between the blood proteins and steroids may represent a storage mechanism (Hoffmann *et al.*, 1969) from which the supply of free, biologically active steroids can be increased. A marked fall in CBG values and a coincidental increase in free corticosteroids between late pregnancy and the first few days of lactation in the rat (Gala and Westphal, 1965a), mouse, and rabbit (Gala and Westphal, 1967) suggests that such a mechanism participates in lactogenesis. In contrast, changes do not appear in corticosteroid-binding capacity during pregnancy in ewes (Lindner, 1964; Paterson and Hills, 1967) or cows (Krulik and Svobodova, 1969).

C. Ovary

Injections of estrogens into animals with well-developed mammary glands will induce milk secretion (Meites, 1961). These effects probably are mediated through the ability of estrogens to stimulate secretion of prolactin (Tindal and Knaggs, 1966; Minaguchi *et al.*, 1968; Nagasawa *et al.*, 1969) and ACTH (Gemzell, 1952). Although estrogens may counteract lactogenesis in humans by stimulating CBG synthesis (Yates and Urguhart, 1962), estrogen does not affect CBG in female rats (Gala and Westphal, 1965b), dogs (Plager *et al.*, 1963), or sheep (Lindner, 1964).

In rats the ovarian venous plasma concentrations of estrogen remain low during pregnancy until just before parturition, when a sharp increase occurs (Yoshinaga *et al.*, 1969). On the other hand, in cattle there is a gradual increase throughout pregnancy in the excretion of estrogens into urine (Erb *et al.*, 1971). Similar to the rapid increase in estrogen in rats, there is a marked elevation in estrone concentration within 5 days of parturition in cattle, followed by a rapid decline postpartum (Robinson *et al.*, 1970). The rapidly changing patterns of estrogen excretion and progesterone concentration in the plasma around the time of parturition were monitored by Hunter *et al.* (1970) and are summarized in Fig. 6. At the present time it is not clear why the greater blood levels of estrone within 5 days of parturition are not reflected in greater concentrations of this steroid in the urine. But the sharp increase in 17β-estradiol and total

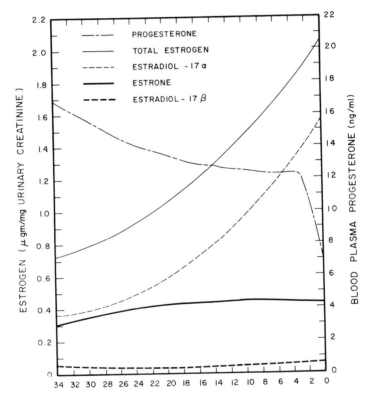

DAYS BEFORE CALVING

Fig. 6. Changes in excretion of estrogen in urine and progesterone concentration in blood plasma of cows during the last 34 days of pregnancy. (From Hunter *et al.*, 1970.)

estrogens in urine (Fig. 6) is consistent with the theory that estrogens stimulate pituitary hormone secretions which in turn initiate lactation at parturition.

All of the hormones discussed to this point can be stimulatory to lactogenesis, yet lactation is not induced by the normal secretion of these hormones during the greater part of pregnancy. Although some of the lactogenic hormones may be inactive or secreted in insufficient quantities during pregnancy to initiate lactation, there is also evidence that inhibitory substances have a direct role in lactogenesis.

Most of the interest in inhibitory hormones has centered on progesterone. The most direct evidence of the inhibitory nature of progesterone was generated from studies utilizing progesterone injections which block the induction of α-lactalbumin (Turkington and Hill, 1969), lactose (Kuhn, 1969a), as well as affecting the histological appearance of milk (Herrenkohl, 1971) during late pregnancy. Also progesterone partially inhibits the stimulatory effects of estrogen on prolactin concentration in the serum of rats (Chen and Meites, 1970).

Ovariectomy or other means of removing progesterone from the circulation will induce lactation in mid- or late-pregnant rats (Astwood and Greep, 1938; Yokoyama *et al.*, 1969; Kuhn, 1969a; Davis and Liu, 1969). However, ovariectomy of pregnant rats also induces abortion, but this occurs about 1 day after some of the chemical criteria for lactogenesis have commenced to rise in the mammary tissue. Deis (1971) showed that exogenous administration of prostaglandin, PGF_{2a}, induces lactogenesis followed by abortion in pregnant rats. Although the mode of action was not studied, these effects are probably mediated through the luteolytic action of PGF_{2a} on the corpus luteum to reduce circulating progesterone (Pharris and Wyngarden, 1969).

Other evidence of the inhibitory role of progesterone in lactogenesis has come from measurements of the circulating quantities of the steroid. For example, progesterone increases during early pregnancy and is maintained at relatively high concentrations for the greater part of gestation in the ewe, sow, cow (Erb *et al.*, 1971), rat (Fajer and Barraclough, 1967; Hashimoto *et al.*, 1968), hamster (Leavitt and Blaha, 1970), and guinea pig (Heap and Deanesley, 1966). In guinea pigs the increased progesterone during pregnancy is caused by increased secretion from the ovaries (and/or adrenals, placenta) as well as by a decreased metabolic clearance rate of the hormone (Illingworth *et al.*, 1970). Since CBG has an even greater affinity for progesterone than for glucocorticoids, the exact role this blood protein plays with respect to progesterone physiology during pregnancy is not known with certainty because biological activity of progesterone is reduced by complex formation with CBG (Hoffmann et al., 1969).

Shortly before parturition, however, there is a marked decrease in circulating progesterone in cows (Figs. 4, 6). The timing of this event has been closely followed in rats where appearance of lactose in mammary tissue commences 30 hours prepartum. This coincides with the rapid decline in progesterone secretion and an increased secretion of 20α-hydroxypregn-4-ene-3-one (Kuhn, 1969a; Kuhn and Briley, 1970). This metabolite of progesterone will not prevent lactogenesis (Kuhn, 1969b).

Simply removing the progesterone block to lactogenesis is not sufficient to induce lactation, however, because ovariectomy during pregnancy in the rat does not induce synthesis of caseinlike proteins or RNA in mammary tissue in the absence of the adrenal (Davis and Liu, 1969). Also copious amounts of milk are not secreted at parturition in hypophysectomized animals. Again this reinforces the concept that positive as well as negative factors are involved in lactogenesis.

D. Other Factors Associated with Lactogenesis

Milk secretion, based on histological evidence, can be induced with nonspecific stresses, drugs, and neural stimuli (Meites, 1966). Generally, most of these effects probably are mediated through the hypothalamus and pituitary, resulting in increased secretion of prolactin and ACTH (see Grosvenor and Mena, Chapter 4). Direct neural connections to the mammary gland are not essential for lactogenesis, because transplanted mammary glands can secrete milk (Linzell, 1963). Nor is the suckling stimulus required for lactogenesis since Reece and Turner (1937) observed that mammary glands of rats were distended with milk within 6 hours after parturition in the complete absence of suckling. On the other hand lactation can be induced by prepartum milking cows (Tucker and Meites, 1965). Presumably this is the result of stimulating prolactin and ACTH secretion.

There is rapid mammary cell division throughout gestation and early lactation (Tucker, 1969). This cell division may be essential for lactogenesis because results from in vitro cultures of mammary cells have shown that the cells must divide before they can synthesize casein (Topper, 1970; Topper and Oka, Chapter 6). Furthermore, a specific sequence of hormones is required to induce lactation in vitro. In this system mammary cell division is caused by insulin and hydrocortisone, and casein synthesis is induced with insulin, hydrocortisone, and prolactin. However, hydrocortisone exposure must precede prolactin to initiate casein synthesis. Addition of progesterone to the normal lactogenic complex of hormones *in vitro* blocks induction of α-lactalbumin synthesis (Turkington and Hill, 1969) which appears similar to the progesterone blockage of lactogenesis *in vivo*.

Evidence to support the sequential nature of the hormonal induction of lactation *in vivo* has come from hormone assays of blood from the bovine immediately preceding parturition (Ingalls *et al.*, 1973; Smith *et al.*, 1973; Fig. 4). Serum estradiol and estrone were the first hormones observed to increase during lactogenesis, rising tenfold during the month before parturition and achieving maximal values 2 days before parturition (Smith *et al.*, 1973). Both estrogens decreased precipitously from the serum during the last 2 days of pregnancy. Progesterone decreases concurrently with a sharp increase in prolactin beginning about 2 days before parturition. Prolactin is maximal 1 day before parturition and then declines to basal levels by parturition. Next, adrenal corticosteroids were released about 12 hours before parturition, reached a peak at parturition, but quickly decreased to baseline by 12 hours after parturition. Last, growth hormone was released starting at parturition and remained elevated for 36 hours. Luteinizing hormone concentrations did not vary significantly during this interval. It remains to be tested whether these hormone spurts are essential for lactogenesis, or for that matter whether they are of any more importance than the basal concentrations of the same hormones that continuously bathe the mammary cells.

E.   Experimental Lactogenesis in Farm Animals

The comprehensive review of Meites summarized the status of attempts through 1961 to stimulate mammary development and to initiate lactation with exogenous hormones in farm animals. In most studies estrogen or a combination of estrogen and progesterone was given. However, resulting milk yields were always variable among cows and were usually low. It is uncertain whether the poor lactation reflected inadequate mammary growth or inadequate lactogenic stimuli. More recently, development of the udder almost equal to that during normal pregnancy in cows was achieved with more effective doses of estrogen and progesterone (Sud *et al.*, 1968). Lactation can be initiated with glucocorticoids in these animals, but again milk yields are low and variable (Sud, Tucker, and Meites, unpublished data). Similarly, Hindery and Turner (1968) initiated lactation in nulliparous and multiparous dairy cows with high doses of estradiol benzoate, but the quantity of milk produced was not equivalent to normal lactation. Injections of 17 β-estradiol (0.1 mg/kg body weight) and progesterone (0.25 mg/kg body weight) for 7 days will initiate lactation in about 60% of infertile cows (Smith and Schanbacher, 1973). Milk production in the cows that responded to treatment produced an average of 5069 kg in 305 days of lactation. To this author the most remarkable finding is that such a large proportion of cows acquired the capacity to produce milk within 7 days, a process that normally requires a 9-month gestation. This approach of using short-term injection sequences is certainly an area worthy of continued research in an effort to salvage additional quantities of milk from infertile cows that would otherwise be slaughtered.

V. THE LACTATION CURVE

Precise measurements of milk yields in various species is dependent primarily upon whether or not milk removed from the mammary gland can be weighed directly and repetitively throughout lactation. Thus, better estimates of lactational performance are obtained in larger species of domestic animals from which milk is easily removed and weighed.

Removal of milk from cattle in the Western hemisphere is most often accomplished with milking machines. Although experimental milking machines have been devised for litter-bearing mammals, their use has not been extensive, and milk yields are most frequently measured as some function of litter weight gain. Daggs (1935) suggested the use of a lactation index for rats based upon logarithmic transformation of daily litter weight gains between the fourth to tenth and tenth to seventeenth day of lactation. Cowie and Folley (1946) proposed the use of a litter-growth index for rats which was calculated from the daily litter weight gain between days 6 and 11 of lactation, the period when daily gain is greatest. More recently, litter weight gains between the first and second week of lactation have been used as indices of lactational performance (Tucker, 1966; Reddy and Donker, 1965). However, daily milk yields cannot be calculated precisely from litter growth data because of variable losses in excreta and perspiration. Nor does each offspring or litter have identical abilities to convert milk to body weight at the same rate.

In an effort to circumvent some of these problems in rats, Grosvenor and Turner (1959a) proposed to measure lactational performance as the amount of milk removed after a single 10-hour separation of litter and mother on day 14 of lactation. At the time of reunion, mothers were anesthesized and injected with oxytocin to facilitate complete evacuation of milk, and the stomach contents were weighed after nursing. Later, this method was expanded to include several individual milk yield measurements based on litter weights before and after nursing between days 14 and 20 of lactation (Djojosoebagio and Turner, 1964a,b). Results from the use of individual measurements have not always agreed with analyses based on litter weight gains in experiments identical in most other respects (e.g., Meites, 1957; Grosvenor and Turner, 1959a). Sometimes within the same experiment the two methods do not agree (Kumaresan and Turner, 1965a). In general, more hormones appear to stimulate lactation (galactopoiesis) and the magnitude of the response is greater with the individual milk yield method than with the litter gain measurements. This dichotomy may be explained in part by our finding (Tucker *et al.*, 1967a) that different conclusions can be drawn from the same experiment depending upon whether the *total* litter weight or the litter weight gain, a measure of *rate,* is used to express lactational performance.

Tucker and Reece (1963b) observed that RNA content of mammary tissue changed markedly throughout lactation (Fig. 2) and that RNA might parallel changes in functional activity of the mammary gland. Later, Tucker (1966) found that RNA content was highly correlated ($r = > 0.93$) with litter weight gain and that mammary RNA was a good estimator of lactational potential, especially where milk removal was not possible.

Lactation in cows commences at a relatively high rate immediately after parturition, increases at a decreasing rate to a peak 3–6 weeks later, and then decreases exponentially until the animal ceases to lactate, which may be anywhere from several months to several years later (Fig. 7). Concurrent pregnancy accounts for the faster decline in milk yield after the eighth month of lactation. Usually modern dairy cows lactate for 10–12 months at which time dairymen terminate lactation in preparation for a subsequent parturition and lactation. In goats lactation usually increases for 4–6 weeks and lasts for 40–60 weeks. Various physiological, nutritional, environmental, and genetic factors affecting the lactational performance of ruminants are described in Volume III, Chapters 8, by Flatt and Moe, and 9, by Touchberry.

In rats, milk secretion rate increases steadily during early lactation and reaches a peak sometime during the second half of the lactation period which is normally about 21 days. Forced weaning or reduced nursing intensity (by using litters older than 21 days) cause rapid declines in mammary secretory activity (Fig. 2). However, by repeated fostering of

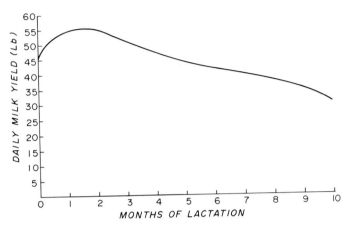

Fig. 7. Lactation curve of the dairy cow.

young litters, rats will lactate well beyond 21 days, but the secretion rate gradually declines (Nicoll and Meites, 1959; Tucker and Reece, 1963c; Thatcher and Tucker, 1968). Thus the shape of the lactation curve of the rat can be experimentally manipulated to mimic that of the cow. Lactation reaches a maximum in mice about 11 days postpartum and then gradually decreases until approximately day 21 of lactation when the litters are weaned by the mother.

Lactation in women is initiated shortly after parturition, but the quantities of milk produced are extremely variable. In fact, Newton (1961) suggested that lactation in women should not be deemed successful until 4–6 weeks postpartum. Thereafter, milk production usually is maintained at a fairly constant rate until weaning several months later, but there are many reports of women who have nursed continuously for several years. Newton (1961) summarized the factors affecting lactation in woman.

VI. HORMONAL MAINTENANCE OF LACTATION

Removal of milk complicates our interpretation of the hormonal requirements for milk synthesis, because without frequent emptying of the mammary gland, milk synthesis will not persist in spite of an adequate hormonal status (Tucker and Reece, 1963e). Conversely, maintenance of intense suckling to provide adequate milk removal will not maintain lactation indefinitely (Thatcher and Tucker, 1968). Thus, milk removal and milk synthesis are closely associated processes. Oxytocin is required for milk removal whereas several other hormones are essential for maintenance of intense milk synthesis. Although there are species variation, in general prolactin, growth hormone, ACTH (or glucocorticoids), TSH (or thyroid hormones), and parathyroid hormone are included in this latter category.

A. Anterior Pituitary

1. Studies in Hypophysectomized Mammals

Selye *et al.* (1933a,b) showed that hypophysectomy of rats or mice caused cessation of milk synthesis. This was confirmed in several laboratory species (Folley, 1952) and recently observed in hypophysectomized goats (Cowie *et al.*, 1964; Cowie, 1969a). The harmful effects of hypophysectomy on milk synthesis are evident shortly after hypophysectomy (Fig. 8). Hypophysectomy of lactating rats reduces mammary cell num-

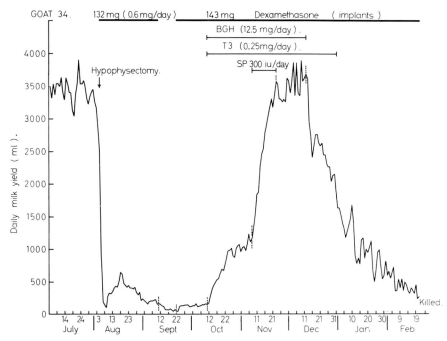

Fig. 8.   Daily milk yields of a goat before and after complete hypophysectomy and during replacement therapy. BGH, Bovine growth hormone; T_3, triiodothyronine; SP, sheep prolactin. (From Cowie, 1969a.)

bers, deoxyribonucleic acid (DNA), RNA, and several enzymes essential for milk synthesis (Baldwin and Martin, 1968).

Hormonal replacement studies using hypophysectomized rats revealed that the minimal requirements to maintain lactation at a level sufficient to rear litters were an adrenal corticoid or ACTH and prolactin (Bintarningsih *et al.*, 1957, 1958; Cowie, 1957). Supplementation of the above combination with growth hormone may improve lactational performance of the hypophysectomized rat (Lyons, 1958). In no instance, however, has lactational performance in rats been restored to normal prehypophysectomy levels. In goats, on the other hand, Cowie (1969a) obtained a complete return of lactation to prehypophysectomy levels with the administration of prolactin, growth hormone, adrenal corticoids, and triiodothyronine (Fig. 8). Also, in the hypophysectomized rabbit, prolactin alone is sufficient to completely reestablish milk synthesis (Cowie *et al.*, 1969).

2. Studies in Intact Mammals

Administration of a hormone that stimulates lactation of intact animals has been interpreted to indicate that the hormone is secreted in suboptimal quantities (Grosvenor and Turner, 1959a,b). However, in itself, such a response may be pharmacological and unrelated to the normal properties of the hormone. Furthermore, this approach does not permit assessment as to whether a hormone directly or indirectly affects the mammary gland. Despite these restrictions, however, experiments with intact animals have provided useful information concerning the hormonal control of lactation.

During early lactation, daily injections of 1 mg of prolactin does not stimulate litter weight gains of rats (Talwalker *et al.*, 1960; Kumaresan *et al.*, 1966) but increasing the dose to 3 mg prolactin daily stimulates milk secretion primarily by increasing metabolism rather than size of the mammary gland (Kumaresan *et al.*, 1966). More recently, Grosvenor *et al.* (1970) reported that prolactin may reduce the time required to fill the mammary gland of the rat. Collectively, the data suggest that prolactin may limit milk synthesis during early lactation.

Fostering litters of rats extends lactation well beyond its normal length (Nicoll and Meites, 1959; Tucker and Reece, 1963c), but maximal milk secretion rates are not maintained (Thatcher and Tucker, 1968). Nor were Thatcher and Tucker (1970a) able to prevent the declines in litter weight gains during prolonged lactation with twice daily injections of sheep prolactin (total daily dose = 2 mg) although mammary DNA was

TABLE I

AVERAGE LITTER WEIGHT GAIN (LWG) AND NUCLEIC ACID CONTENT OF MAMMARY
GLANDS OF INTENSELY SUCKLED RATS[a] INJECTED DURING LACTATION[b]

Treat-ment[c]	LWG[d]			DNA (mg)[e] per 100 gm body wt	RNA (mg)[e] per 100 gm body wt
	8–16 days	16–24 days	24–32 days		
Saline	80	71	32	9.2	51.6
P	80	90	44	12.1	57.7
G	79	78	38	11.4	50.2
G, P	82	80	41	9.4	57.2
C	85	88	64	15.0	71.9
C, P	79	91	62	12.2	78.0
C, G	84	102	74	15.1	78.4
C, P, G	83	99	76	11.5	89.2

[a] Litters 16 days old replaced with 8-day-old foster litters.
[b] From Thatcher and Tucker (1970a). Injected from day 16 to day 32 of lactation.
[c] Cortisol-21-acetate (C), prolactin (P), and growth hormone (G).
[d] Cumulative litter weight gain, in grams, recorded between days 8 and 16 of age for all litters.
[e] Measured on day 32 of lactation.

stimulated (Table I). Since the prolactin was from sheep and injected only twice daily, we attempted to determine if the chronic secretion of rat prolactin from pituitaries isotransplanted under the kidney capsule (Meites and Nicoll, 1966) would prevent declines in milk synthesis during prolonged lactation. But similar to the results observed with prolactin injections, isotransplanted pituitaries did not prevent the decline in litter weight gains during extended lactation (Thatcher and Tucker, 1970b). Furthermore, the pituitary content of prolactin at the peak of lactation (day 16) was not different from that at the thirty-sixth day (Thatcher and Tucker, 1968). We concluded that although prolactin is essential for lactation, it is probably not rate limiting to milk synthesis during prolonged lactation in the rat.

Although definitive studies have not been performed in ruminants because of a lack of sufficient quantities of prolactin, the available evidence suggests that prolactin has little effect on milk yields of lactating cows (Folley and Young, 1940; Cotes *et al.*, 1949) or ewes (Denamur and Martinet, 1970; Morag *et al.*, 1971). Similarly prolactin had little effect in milk yields of guinea pigs during the declining phase of lactation (Nagasawa and Naito, 1963). In contrast, the rabbit's lactational performance is markedly enhanced by exogenous prolactin during late lactation (Cowie, 1969b). Perhaps this high dependency of the rabbit on prolactin during lactation is not surprising in view of the ease in initiating lactation in this species with this hormone alone.

Meites (1957) and Macdonald and Reece (1961) reported that growth hormone injections were not galactopoietic during early lactation in rats although the mothers' body weights increased. In direct contrast to these results, Grosvenor and Turner (1959a), von Berswordt-Wallrabe et al. (1960), and Moon (1965) observed that administration of growth hormone resulted in a marked increase in the milk obtained by the litter within 30 minutes after a 10-hour separation from the mother. They suggested that one reason why others have failed to find galactopoietic properties for growth hormone was that litter weight gain method for measuring milk yields did not sufficiently challenge the lactational potential of the mother. However, Cowie et al. (1957) failed to observe any galactopoietic responses to growth hormone with 16 pups per lactating mother. Similarly, Thatcher and Tucker (1970a) increased nursing intensity to one pup per functional mammary gland and exchanged foster litters frequently, yet exogenous administration of growth hormone alone or in combination with prolactin failed to prevent the normal declines in milk synthesis during advanced lactation (Table I). Nagasawa and Naito (1963) also observed a lack of response to growth hormone or prolactin in guinea pigs.

In contrast to the results in rats, growth hormone is clearly galactopoietic in ruminants (Cowie, 1961; Meites, 1961). Since growth hormone preparations used in earlier experiments were possibly contaminated with prolactin and thyroid stimulating hormone (TSH), Bullis et al. (1965) compared commercial and highly purified growth hormone. The increase in milk yields averaged 7.6, 3.4, and −4.4% for cows injected with commercial growth hormone, highly purified growth hormone, and saline, respectively; thus confirming the earlier galactopoietic properties for growth hormone in cows. Recently, Machlin (1973) observed that injections of highly purified growth hormone for 10 weeks stimulate lactation for the total period and that the elevated milk yields persist for a time following cessation of the growth hormone injections. Growth hormone is also galactopoietic in goats (Tomov, 1963) and ewes (Denamur and Martinet, 1970).

Lyons et al. (1968) injected human growth hormone into lactating women who had complained of lactational insufficiency, and lactation was stimulated approximately threefold over that in mothers given placebo. In light of the difficulties involved in chemically separating prolactin and growth hormone activities in humans (see Section IV,A), it cannot be determined with certainty which hormonal activity (or both) is responsible for the galactopoietic response.

ACTH injections into intact cows depress milk secretion (Cowie, 1961), whereas in rats ACTH is stimulatory to lactation (Johnson and Meites, 1958). TSH is also galactopoietic in cows (Wrenn and Sykes, 1953; Brumby and Hancock, 1955) and goats (Owen and Darroch, 1957). However, there is no evidence to suggest that either ACTH or TSH are acting in a fashion other than through their respective target endocrine glands. Thus, further discussion of this topic will be covered in the adrenal and thyroid sections of this chapter.

3. Endogenous Concentrations of Pituitary Hormones

Suckling causes a rapid release of prolactin from the anterior pituitary of rats (Reece and Turner, 1937; Grosvenor and Turner, 1957). Convey and Reece (1969) observed that pituitary prolactin is restored in 8–9 hours, and Grosvenor and Mena (1971) found that the amount of prolactin released and its subsequent rate of reaccumulation was dependent upon intensity of the suckling stimulus and duration of the previous nonsuckling interval. Although acute suckling temporarily reduces pituitary prolactin, increasing the frequency of nursing over a prolonged period of time increases the concentration of pituitary prolactin (Tucker *et al.*, 1967a,b). Since mammary nucleic acid content and litter weight gains also were increased, the increased pituitary hormone content was interpreted to indicate increased synthesis and release of prolactin.

Yanai and Nagasawa (1971) found greater pituitary concentration of prolactin and growth hormone during the estrous cycle and during pregnancy in mice with superior milk-producing capabilities. Except that the superior strain released more prolactin during suckling, there were negligible differences between the superior and inferior strains in either prolactin or growth hormone during lactation. This may suggest that the primary difference in milk production between these two strains of mice was associated with the number of mammary cells produced during pregnancy rather than associated with the metabolic activity of the cells during lactation.

With the advent of sensitive radioimmunoassays it is now possible to test directly whether these interpretations of pituitary hormone content changes were correct. It has been shown in rats (Amenomori *et al.*, 1970), goats (Bryant and Greenwood, 1968), and cows (Johke, 1970; Tucker, 1971; Koprowski and Tucker, 1971) that milking causes a sharp release of prolactin. In cattle this increase occurred within 5 minutes after the stimulus was applied, remained elevated for at least 5 minutes after it was withdrawn, and returned to baseline about 35 minutes after the milking machine was removed (Table II). Prolactin release can be elicited by washing the udder without removing milk, by simulated venipuncture (Tucker, 1971), by washing the brisket (Koprowski et al., 1971), by feeding (Johke, 1970), or by injecting thyrotropin releasing hormone (Convey et al., 1973a). Prolactin concentration varies according to circadian rhythms (Koprowski et al., 1972), being higher at night and lower during the day in lactating cows and is higher in the summer than in the winter months in both cows and bulls (Koprowski and Tucker, 1973a; unpublished data). A number of these stimuli also release prolactin in women (Frantz et al., 1972; Tyson et al., 1972). The most potent releaser of prolactin used in cows and women has been thyrotropin-releasing hormone, and administration of this releasing hormone to cows (Convey et al., 1973b) or women (Tyson et al., 1972) stimulates milk production. Whether the enhanced lactation is due to increased availability of prolactin, growth hormone, or thyroxine (Convey et al., 1973a), acting independently or in concert is not known.

The changes throughout lactation in prolactin taken 1 hour before, 5 minutes after, and 1 hour after milking and the corresponding milk yields are plotted in Fig. 9 (Koprowski and Tucker, 1973a). Although the prolactin in postmilking blood samples remained rather stable throughout lactation the prolactin in premilking samples increased steadily

TABLE II

SERUM LEVELS OF PROLACTIN AND GROWTH HORMONE AFTER NORMAL MILKING[a]

Sample taken	Prolactin (ng/ml)	Growth hormone (ng/ml)
10 min. before wash	45	2.1
5 min. before wash	38	1.8
5 min. after wash[b]	52	1.6
10 min. after wash[c]	119	2.1
15 min. after wash	82	1.9
20 min. after wash	71	1.7
25 min. after wash	55	1.7
30 min. after wash	48	1.7
35 min. after wash	51	1.7

[a] From Tucker, 1971.
[b] Milking machine placed on udder.
[c] Milking machine removed from udder.

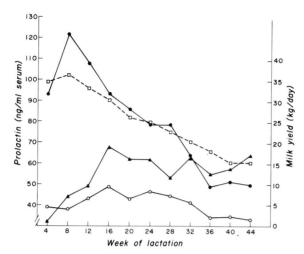

Fig. 9. Serum prolactin concentration in cows during lactation. Blood samples collected 1 hour before milking (○), 5 minutes after milking (●), and 1 hour after milking (▲). (□), Average daily milk yields. (From Koprowski and Tucker, 1973a.)

from the fourth to sixteenth week of lactation until it stabilized at 50–60 ng/ml serum. In contrast, the prolactin in samples collected immediately after milking paralleled the changes in milk yield. Thus, as lactation advances the prolactin response to the milking stimulus decreases. Correlation analyses between milk yield and prolactin concentration within each month of lactation revealed that there is practically no relationship between the two variables until after the twelfth week where the correlations ranged between 0.08 and 0.48 (Table III). We conclude that serum concentrations of prolactin are associated with changes in milk yield in the bovine, but cause–effect relationships remain to be established. It should be emphasized that many known stimuli will elicit prolactin release, but perhaps more intriguingly we and others have observed markedly fluctuating serum concentrations of prolactin when no known stimuli were being applied to the animals. What relationship these spontaneous fluctuations in prolactin have to milk secretion is unknown at the present time.

Acute nursing also releases growth hormone in rats (Grosvenor *et al.*, 1968), but application of chronic nursing decreases the concentration of growth hormone in the pituitary (Tucker and Thatcher, 1968). In cows, on the other hand, we have been unable to alter significantly the circulating level of growth hormone with milking (Table II; Tucker, 1971). Furthermore, serum growth hormone is negatively associated with milk

TABLE III

CORRELATION COEFFICIENTS BETWEEN SERUM PROLACTIN AND MILK YIELDS DURING LACTATION[a]

Week of lactation	Correlation coefficients
4	0.02
8	0.09
12	0.31
16	0.19
20	0.17
24	0.28
28	0.13
32	0.26
36	0.48
40	0.39
44	0.08

[a] From Koprowski, Ph.D. thesis, Michigan State University, 1972. Blood samples taken 1 hour after milking.

yield, especially after 24 weeks of lactation (Koprowski and Tucker, 1973b). This response is puzzling especially since growth hormone stimulates lactation in cattle. However, stage of concurrent pregnancy also advanced as lactation progressed in these cows, and there was a coincident increase in serum growth hormone associated with advancing pregnancy. Perhaps the negative correlations reflect a change in serum growth hormone which is associated with pregnancy rather than lactation. Spellacy et al. (1970) also failed to detect differences in human growth hormone concentrations of blood from lactating or nonlactating women subjected to resting or insulin-induced hypoglycemia. But whether these data mean that growth hormone is not rate limiting to lactation must await further investigation.

B. Posterior Pituitary

The importance of the posterior pituitary lobe in regulating lactational performance was recognized much later than the importance of the anterior lobe. But, as previously discussed, without the active participation of the milk ejection reflex, milk secretion will soon decline.

Injections of oxytocin to rats during early lactation stimulated milk yields 13% (Kumaresan and Turner, 1966), but, when injected during later phases of lactation, oxytocin failed to retard the normal decline in litter weight gains although declines in mammary cell numbers and metabolic activity were retarded (Thatcher and Tucker, 1970a). Considering the short half-life of oxytocin and the probable lack of synchronism between nursing and the oxytocin injections perhaps it is not surprising that oxytocin's effect on milk yield is not more dramatic in rats. In fact when oxytocin is given and cows are milked immediately afterwards, there is little question that oxytocin is galactopoietic (Knodt and Petersen, 1944).

Oxytocic activity in the blood increases markedly in response to nursing (Bisset *et al.*, 1970) or milking (Momongan and Schmidt, 1970). The amount of oxytocin released appears to be related to the nursing intensity, but it is not affected by the amount of milk present in the mammary gland (Fitzpatrick, 1961). There is a tendency for the amount of oxytocin released at milking to decrease as lactation advances (Momongan and Schmidt, 1970). Cleverley and Folley (1970) reported that only 68% of the cows tested released oxytocin, and about one-half of these cows released oxytocin to auditory or visual stimuli associated with milking. Since milk production was not affected in those cows which failed to release detectable oxytocin, it seems pertinent to question whether the assays of oxytocin are sufficiently sensitive, or whether some cows can expel milk from the udder without the participation of the neuroendocrine milk-ejection reflex.

C. Adrenal Cortex

1. Studies in Adrenalectomized Mammals

Many studies have shown that adrenalectomy impairs milk secretion (Cowie and Tindal, 1958; Anderson and Turner, 1962b, 1963a,b), and the cessation in lactation occurs much sooner if the ovaries are simultaneously removed (Flux, 1955; Anderson and Turner, 1963b). Use of individual gluco- or mineralocorticoids will partially restore milk secretion, but a combination of the two steroids is more effective (Cowie and Tindal, 1958; Anderson and Turner, 1963b). This suggests that the reduced lactation following adrenalectomy is due to impaired electrolyte, protein, and carbohydrate metabolism.

2. Studies in Intact Mammals

Several reports (Cotes *et al.*, 1949; Flux *et al.*, 1954; Shaw *et al.*, 1955; Brush, 1960; Campbell *et al.*, 1964; Braun *et al.*, 1970) strongly suggest that ACTH or glucocorticoids cause temporary decreases in milk production in cows. In contrast, injections into rats of optimal doses of either corticosterone (Hahn and Turner, 1966), cortisone acetate (Johnson and Meites, 1958), or cortisol acetate (Talwalker *et al.*, 1960) stimulated lactational performance 12–27% during early lactation. However, even in the rat, inhibitory responses can be obtained readily if the dosage is too high (Hahn and Turner, 1966; Kowalewski, 1969). During the late phases of lactation in rats, Thatcher and Tucker (1970a,b) reduced markedly the decline in lactational performance with either cortisol acetate (Table I) or 9α-fluoroprednisolone acetate. In fact by manipulating the dose of glucocorticoids (Thatcher and Tucker, 1970b) or, if they are administered in combination with high fat diets (Emery *et al.*, 1971), lactational performance and mammary nucleic acid content can be maintained at maximum values for at least 32 days.

3. Endogenous Concentrations of ACTH and Adrenal Steroids

Suckling or milking will cause release of ACTH from the pituitary of rats (Voogt *et al.*, 1969), sheep, or goats (Denamur *et al.*, 1965). In turn, this results in increased circulating adrenal corticoids (Voogt *et al.*, 1969; Smith and Convey, 1971; Paape and Desjardins, 1971). In contrast to our finding that the milking induced release of prolactin gradually disappears as lactation advances (Fig. 9), cows do not lose their ability to discharge corticoids (Koprowski and Tucker, 1973b) as lactation proceeds. Increasing the suckling stimulus in rats from two to six pups reduced the ACTH content of the pituitary (Tucker *et al.*, 1967a), but this probably represents an increased release from the pituitary because several workers recorded increased concentrations of corticosterone in response to increased litter sizes (Gala and Westphal, 1965a; Kamoun, 1970; Smith and Convey, 1971). Additionally, Voogt *et al.* (1969) and Paape and Desjardins (1971) have shown that exteroceptive stimuli associated with nursing will evoke corticosterone release in lactating rats.

That the adrenal secretions are rate limiting to milk synthesis during advanced lactation is supported by our finding that ACTH in the pituitary decreases about 68% during extended lactation (Thatcher and Tucker, 1968). Similarly adrenal corticosterone content, which has been used as an index of secretory activity (Holzbauer, 1957), decreased linearly between day 16 and 32 of lactation (Table IV; Thatcher and Tucker, 1970c). In fact, the adrenal corticosterone content is highly correlated with the mammary nucleic acid content during lactation; in contrast, the concentration of corticosterone in the blood remained unaltered during lactation although there is a marked increase between the virginal and the lactating state (Table IV). During early lactation there is a marked

TABLE IV

CORTICOSTERONE CHANGES IN INTENSELY SUCKLED RATS[a] DURING EXTENDED
LACTATION AND IN VIRGIN RATS[b]

Corticosterone	Virgin rats	16[c]	24[c]	32[c]
μg/2 adrenals	1.2	2.0	1.7	1.4
μg/100 ml plasma	10.6	18.8	18.3	16.0
μg bound/100 ml plasma	—	63	58	75

[a] Litters 16 days old replaced with 8-day-old foster litters.
[b] From Thatcher and Tucker (1970c).
[c] Days of lactation.

decrease in CBG (Gala and Westphal, 1965a; Koch, 1969), but as lactation advances it rises gradually (Table IV; Thatcher and Tucker, 1970c).
ACTH and adrenal functions decrease simultaneously with decreases in
milk synthesis and glucocorticoid supplementation will prevent the
reduced milk synthesis, strongly suggesting that adrenal secretions are
rate limiting to milk synthesis during prolonged lactation in the rat.

Heitzman *et al.* (1970) showed that, except for high values around
parturition, corticosteroid values during lactation do not differ from those
of nonlactating cows. Furthermore, there does not appear to be any
reduction in CBG activity during lactation in cattle (Krulik and Svobodova, 1969). These observations, coupled with the previously described
inhibitory actions of corticoids on milk yields in cattle, suggest that the
corticoids are not rate limiting to milk secretion in this species.

Although the adrenal corticoids may not be rate limiting to lactation in
cattle, this does not mean that they are unessential for lactation. Paterson
and Linzell (1971) observed that the mammary glands of pregnant goats
took up about 0.2 μg cortisol per minute whereas mammary glands of
preparturient and early lactating goats removed an average of 1.3 μg
cortisol per minute. Metabolic clearance rates of corticoids did not change
appreciably, but adrenal secretion rates were almost fourfold greater in
lactating goats compared with pregnant goats. They calculated that the
mammary gland removes about 2.8% of the secreted cortisol and about
two-thirds of the unbound cortisol entering the gland. Furthermore, we
have recently observed a specific binding mechanism in bovine mammary
cells which has a very high affinity ($K_d \simeq 5 \times 10^{-8}$ M to 2×10^{-9} M)
for cortisol (Tucker *et al.*, 1971). Each mammary cell contains about 7500
specific binding sites for cortisol. The uptake of cortisol by the mammary
cells could be inhibited by many (but not all) corticoids, by progesterone, by 17α-hydroxypregn-4-ene-3-one, and by heating to 100° C for 10
minutes. Uptake was not affected by 17β-estradiol, testosterone, or 20α-

hydoxypregn-4-ene-3-one. However, there are no data to relate binding capacity with a specific physiological response in the mammary secretory cell.

D. Thyroid

1. Studies in Thyroidectomized Mammals

Graham (1934) observed a marked decrease in milk yields in cows following thyroidectomy, but cows given sham operations also fell in milk production. More definitive results were obtained by Ekman (1965) who showed that by specifically eliminating the thyroid cells with ^{131}I milk yields were reduced markedly.

In the rat, the parathyroid glands are located on the surface of the thyroid glands, thus surgical removal of the thyroid also eliminates the parathyroid gland. Folley (1942) stimulated litter growth in thyroidectomized rats with parathyroid extracts alone suggesting much of the inhibitory response of thyroidectomy was in fact due to the simultaneous removal of the parathyroid glands. Furthermore, Cowie and Folley (1945) observed that surgical removal of only the parathyroid glands inhibited lactation almost as much as removal of both thyroid and parathyroid glands. Although destroying the thyroid with ^{131}I did not affect lactational performance of rats (Bruce and Sloviter, 1957), feeding of the goitrogen, propylthiouracil, which suppresses endogenous secretion of thyroxine, markedly reduced milk yields (Ben-David et al., 1965b). The general conclusion to be reached is that the thyroid strongly influences milk synthesis, but its secretions are not absolutely essential for the process.

2. Studies in Intact Mammals

There is little question that exogenous administration of thyroxine (T_4) or triiodothyronine (T_3) will markedly stimulate lactational performance in both ruminants and nonruminants (Blaxter et al., 1949; Desclin, 1949; Grosvenor and Turner, 1959b; von Berswordt-Wallrabe et al., 1960). For example, the experiments of Hindery and Turner (1965) indicate that daily injection of T_4 into lactating dairy cows for 7 weeks at 25% above their thyroid secretion rate stimulated milk yields an average of 27%. However, it seems doubtful if this procedure will produce a permanent elevation in milk yields, because increasing T_4 to 150% of the thyroid secretion rate for an additional 7 weeks resulted in minimal responses and several of the cows did not respond at all.

Although T_3 and T_4 are biologically active when fed to cattle, their effectiveness relative to injections is markedly reduced (Bauman and Turner, 1965). The usual approach is to feed the synthetic product, iodinated casein (thyroprotein). This topic has been investigated and extensive reviews have been published (Meites, 1961; Moore, 1958).

Feeding thyroprotein to cows during early lactation boosts milk production about 10% (Tucker and Reece, 1961), but if it is fed during the declining phases milk yields are often increased 15–20% (Blaxter *et al.*, 1949; Moore, 1958). Although there is wide variation in response among cows, usually older cows and higher-yielding cows respond best. The beneficial effects, however, usually only last 2–4 months, and subsequent yields are often below that normally expected (Schmidt *et al.*, 1971). The net result is often that there is no benefit over the entire lactation in terms of increased milk production.

Milk yield usually declines any time thyroprotein is taken away abruptly from the cow. Feed intake must be increased during thyroprotein feeding, and current recommendations are that it should be fed only to cows gaining in weight and its use should be discontinued if milk yields are not increased within 2 weeks after the feeding is started. Possibly, the failure to maintain high milk production with thyroprotein represents a situation whereby other hormones become limiting. Also Gala and Westphal (1966) observed that TSH acting through thyroxine stimulates CBG production in rats. If cattle respond similarly, it would seem reasonable to speculate that this factor may play a role in subsequent reduced milk yield response of cows to thyroprotein.

The site of action of the thyroid hormones in stimulating milk secretion is not known completely, but Nicoll and Meites (1963) have shown in *in vitro* studies that T_3 and T_4 can stimulate the anterior pituitary to release prolactin. More recently, Chen and Meites (1969) reported that T_4 stimulates and thiouracil reduces prolactin content of the pituitary without altering the prolactin-inhibiting factor content of the hypothalamus of rats. This suggests that at least part of the site of action of the thyroid hormone is directly on the anterior pituitary to release prolactin in rats. In contrast, Shaw *et al.* (1972) observed that in cows fed thyroprotein, although serum thyroxine doubled, serum concentrations of prolactin, growth hormone, and total corticoids were unaltered. Thus, the cause of the failure of long-term thyroprotein feeding to stimulate lactation remains unknown.

Thyrocalcitonin is another hormone released from the thyroid in response to high levels of blood calcium. Thyrocalcitonin inhibits resorption of calcium from bone thereby lowering blood calcium (and phosphorus). Overproduction of thyrocalcitonin may be involved in the parturient paresis (milk fever) syndrome of dairy cows (Capen and Young, 1967). However, Baksi and Anderson (1969, 1971) showed that thyrocalcitonin was not a critical hormone needed by the mammary gland to maintain serum calcium levels or lactation in rats.

3. Secretion Rates of Thyroid Hormones

Several methods have been developed to measure thyroxine secretion rates starting with the goitrogen technique of Dempsey and Astwood (1943). With the availability of ^{131}I, a thyroxine degradation procedure was developed (Sterling *et al.*, 1954; Ingbar and Freinkel, 1955). Henneman *et al.* (1952) and Reineke and Singh (1955) were first to apply a thyroxine substitution method to estimate daily thyroid secretion rates in individual animals. These methods have been used widely (e.g., see Turner, 1969), and the general conclusion based on the substitution method is that thyroid hormone secretion rates increase during lactation relative to the thyroid secretion rate of nonlactating animals (Grosvenor, 1961; Turner, 1969) and that the thyroxine secretion rate is positively related to milk production (Anderson, 1971). In response to the nursing stimulus in rats, Grosvenor (1964) observed elevated thyroid activity, but Sar and Meites (1969) failed to detect TSH release from the anterior pituitary.

Research by Reineke (1964) cast doubt on the reliability of thyroxine substitution methods as a precise measure of thyroid hormone secretion rates in situations where iodine may be in limited supply, such as during lactation where large quantities of iodine are trapped by the mammary gland and excreted into the milk (Flamboe and Reineke, 1959; Grosvenor, 1960). The implication of these findings is that a functional thyroid hormone deficiency state may exist during lactation. In 1967, Reineke and Lorscheider described a "direct output" method for determining thyroid secretion rate, applicable to cases where iodine is limited. Using this method, Lorscheider and Reineke (1972) observed that thyroid secretion rate is reduced during lactation, and this reduction is reflected in lowered concentrations of serum thyroxine. Furthermore, there was an inverse correlation between serum thyroxine and nursing intensity (Fig. 10) that could not be reversed by increasing the dietary iodine content in rats (Lorscheider and Reineke, 1971). Injections of prolactin do not alter serum thyroxine, suggesting that elevated concentrations of serum prolactin associated with nursing are not directly involved in lowering serum thyroxine during lactation (Lorscheider and Reineke, 1971).

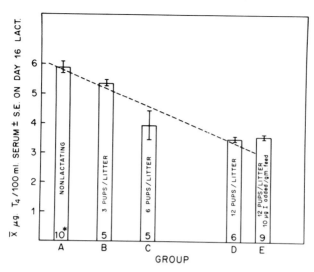

Fig. 10. Rat serum thyroxine versus lactational intensity and elevated iodine intake. Mean and standard error of mean are indicated at top of each bar, number of rats per group is indicated at the bottom of each bar. Groups A–D: r = −.83 (p < 0.001). (From Lorscheider and Reineke, 1971.)

There is no change in the thyroxine binding globulin, the major thyroxine carrying blood protein, during lactation in cows, but again serum thyroid was significantly reduced (Etta and Reineke, 1971). This suggests that the lactating animal is in a functional hypothyroid state because of reduced availability of thyroxine, rather than altered thyroxine-binding globulin activity. If lactating animals are functionally hypothyroid, one would expect an increase in thyroid function and possibly milk production if iodine was supplemented to their diet. Swanson (1972) increased plasma total iodine, PBI, and T_4 with supplemental iodine, but unfortunately this did not result in greater milk yield in cows.

E. Parathyroid

1. Studies in Parathyroidectomized Mammals

As reviewed by Cowie (1961), there is evidence that parathyroidectomy reduces the intensity of milk secretion in several species. von Berswordt-Wallrabe and Turner (1960) removed both thyroid and parathyroid glands of lactating rats, and when only thyroxine was replaced the milk yield was 1.6 gm on day 14. When both thyroxine and parathyroid hormone were given, milk yield increased to within a normal range (10.6 gm). Administration of substitutes for the parathyroid hormone (dihydrovitamin D_2 II, dihydrotachysterol, vitamin D_2, or vitamin D_3) in conjunction with injections of thyroxine will also maintain normal lactation in thyro-parathyroidectomized animals (von Berswordt-Wallrabe and Turner, 1960; Djojosoebagio and Turner, 1964a; Srivastava and Turner, 1966). Apparently these substitutes mobilize blood calcium sufficiently to maintain calcium concentrations in milk and permit contraction of the myoepithelial cells of the mammary gland in response to oxytocin thereby facilitating milk removal (Djojosoebagio and Turner, 1964c).

2. Studies in Intact Mammals

Administration of parathyroid hormone, dihydrovitamin D_2 II, or vitamin D_2 stimulated milk yields of normal rats 10 and 56% when measured between days 14 and 20 of lactation (Djojosoebagio and Turner, 1964b). These studies have not been extended to other species.

F. Endocrine Pancreas

Surgical removal of the pancreas (Cuthbert et al., 1936) or administration of the diabetogenic agent, alloxan (Kumaresan and Turner, 1965b), reduce the growth rate of the litters of rats. Alloxan depresses synthesis of lactose, casein, and lipid by mammary tissue slices, and these deleterious effects are associated with impairment of glucose utilization (Martin and Baldwin, 1971a). Acute experiments using antiinsulin serum suggest that the impaired glucose utilization may be attributed to reduced activity of the electron transport system (Martin and Baldwin, 1971b). The reduced synthetic capacity of mammary tissue of diabetic rats can be reversed with insulin.

Administration of insulin to intact lactating rats increased milk yields on day 14 of lactation following a 10-hour separation from the litter, but the significance of this is doubtful because litter weight gains were unaffected (Kumaresan and Turner, 1965a). There is almost universal agreement that administration of insulin to lactating dairy cows decreases milk production (Cowie, 1961; Kronfeld et al., 1963; Rook et al., 1965; Schmidt, 1966). However, if blood glucose is maintained, insulin will not inhibit lactation (Kronfeld et al., 1963) suggesting that it is hypoglycemia rather than a direct effect of insulin that is the cause of the reduced milk yields. During normal conditions we have observed a consistent negative correlation between serum insulin concentration and milk yield (Koprowski and Tucker, 1973b). We also found that milking causes release of insulin, but what triggers this release is not known although changes in serum glucose, volatile fatty acids, or other metabolites would be likely candidates in view of their known roles in affecting serum insulin.

G. Ovary

1. Studies in Ovariectomized Mammals

Ovariectomy of a variety of species has failed to alter significantly lactational performance (Kuramitsu and Loeb, 1921; Richter, 1936; Folley and Kon, 1938; Barsantini and Masson, 1947; Flux, 1955; Griffith and Turner, 1962). We confirmed these results with respect to litter weight gains in rats between day 7 and 16 of lactation; however, total litter weights were reduced (Tucker *et al.*, 1967a). The depressed litter weights may have reflected a partial failure of the mammary gland to undergo maximal mitotic activity during early lactation. This was supported by the finding that ovariectomy significantly reduced the DNA and RNA contents of the mammary gland on day 8 of lactation, but by day 16 the difference in nucleic acid content had largely disappeared, especially in rats nursing larger litters. Thus any inhibitory effects of ovariectomy on lactation was overcome with greater nursing intensities applied for longer times. That any effects of ovariectomy on lactation are of a secondary nature was reinforced by Knox and Griffith (1970) who observed that weights of litters of ovariectomized rats were reduced only 5% on the sixteenth day of lactation in comparison with normal rats.

2. Studies in Intact Mammals

The inhibitory effects of estrogens on lactation in several species have been summarized by Cowie (1961) and Meites (1961), and there are several reports of the inhibitory effects of synthetic estrogens on lactation in women (Morris, 1967; McGlone, 1969; Watson, 1969). On the other hand, even massive doses of progesterone do not affect lactation (Folley, 1942). But if combined with estrogen, the reduction of lactation is more marked than if only estrogen is used (Barsantini *et al.*, 1936). Griffith and Turner (1962) confirmed these results in intact rats, but when the steroids were given to lactating, ovariectomized animals there was little or no effect on lactation. They suggested that the steroids interfered in some manner with the milk ejection reflex because the glands remained engorged with milk in spite of administering exogenous oxytocin. Bruce and

Ramirez (1970) observed that the inhibitory site of estrogen action in rats was at the mammary tissue because local implants of estrogen into the mammary gland reduced lactation whereas similar implants in the anterior pituitary stimulated lactation.

There is considerable evidence in cows (Meites, 1961) and rats (Ben-David *et al.*, 1966) that low doses of estrogens can stimulate milk production. More recently the effects of progestins, which have been used for estrous cycle synchronization, have been tested in lactating cows. Most of these studies involve the oral administration of the steroid for a period of less than 3 weeks, and it should be noted that the only compound tested in lactating cows, 17α-acetoxy-6-methyl-16-methylene-pregna-4,6-diene-3,20-dione (melengestrol acetate), results in both progestogenic and estrogenic responses in the cow (Zimbelman and Smith, 1966). This compound did not affect milk production (Roussel and Beatty, 1969; Boyd, 1970). Two other progestins, 6α-methyl-17α-acetoxyprogesterone (MAP) and 17α-acetoxy-9α-fluoro-11β-hydroxyprogesterone (flurogestone acetate), also had no effect on lactation in ewes (Smith and Inskeep, 1970).

With the widespread use of oral contraceptive agents, which are usually composed of synthetic progestins and estrogens, an examination of their effects on lactation is warranted. Joshi and Rao (1968) reported that Enovid reduced litter growth rates of rats 10–20% whereas it stimulated litter growth of rabbits but was without effect in mice. Others (Saunders, 1967; Clancy and Edgren, 1968) failed to confirm the inhibitory effects in rats even when enormous doses were used, although various abnormalities of the reproductive system of the female offspring were noted. When these agents are administered to lactating women, especially in higher dosages, there is a strong tendency for milk yields to be diminished (Pincus, 1965; Kora, 1969; Miller and Hughes, 1970; Borglin and Sandholm, 1971). In fact the use of combination as well as sequential oral contraceptives have been used successfully to reduce postpartum breast engorgement in women (Booker *et al.*, 1970). On the other hand there are a few reports that administration of low doses of certain steroid contraceptives has no effect on lactation (Garcia and Pincus, 1964; Semm, 1966) or may even stimulate milk yields (Kamal *et al.*, 1970; Karim *et al.*, 1971). Perhaps, as new compounds are developed, a combination of consistent ovulation prevention and unaltered lactation will be discovered.

Oral administration of radioactively labeled norethynodrel (Pincus *et al.*, 1966; Laumas *et al.*, 1967) or lynestrenol (van der Molen *et al.*, 1969) to lactating mothers results in the excretion of a small quantity of steroid in the milk. Although most reports are negative with respect to altered physiology in nursing infants whose mothers were taking oral contraceptives, a few isolated cases of abnormal breast (Curtis, 1964) or vaginal development (Lauritzen, 1967) have been observed in the infants. However, there is no proof that these abnormalities were caused by the steroids.

H. Pineal

The pineal gland contains several biogenic amines of which melatonin, serotonin, and catecholamines are perhaps the most notable. Melatonin is uniquely found in the pineal and has been implicated in the pigmentation response. The concentration of serotonin is greater in the pineal than in any other tissue of the rat (Snyder *et al.*, 1965) and serotonin has been shown to inhibit the suckling-induced release of oxytocin (Mizuno *et al.*, 1967). Recently catecholamines have been implicated as neurotransmitters which stimulate the prolactin-inhibiting factor thereby reducing prolactin secretion (Kamberi *et al.*, 1970; Koch *et al.*, 1970; Donoso *et al.*, 1971). Thus, one might suspect that the pineal could affect lactation, but pinealectomy (Nir *et al.*, 1968; Mizuno and Sensui, 1970) or injections of melatonin had no effect on the milk ejection reflex of rats (Mizuno and Sensui, 1970). On the other hand, injections of four biogenic amines (noradrenaline, dopamine, serotonin, and melatonin) reduced the milk yields of rabbits as measured by litter weight gains (Shani *et al.*, 1971). Thus, we may anticipate that elucidation of the relationships between biogenic amines, pituitary hormones, and the mammary response will be pursued vigorously in the near future.

VII. EFFECT OF NURSING INTENSITY AND PREGNANCY ON LACTATION

By increasing litter size during early lactation, mitotic activity in the mammary gland during lactation is prolonged to the point where the total amount of mammary development produced during lactation exceeds that produced during pregnancy (Fig. 11; Tucker, 1966). Although there is a corresponding increase in the total metabolism of the gland, eventually lactational intensity declines. Edwardson and Eayrs (1967) showed that increasing the litter size of rats up to 10 pups resulted in greater quantities of milk, but more than 10 pups had no further effect. Tucker

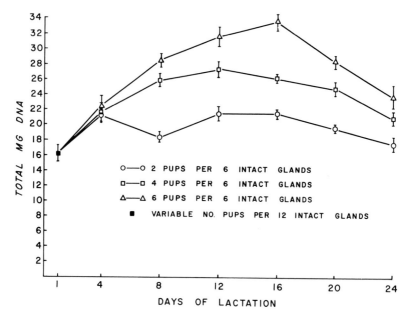

Fig. 11. Total DNA content of 6 abdominal–inguinal mammary glands of rats suckling 2, 4, or 6 pups per 6 glands. Points are means ± standard error of mean. There were 12 lactating rats per point. On day 3 of lactation, litter size was adjusted and thoracic teats were ligated. (From Tucker, 1966.)

et al. (1967b) found that nursing frequency had to be greater than 4 times per day to maintain mammary DNA and RNA content.

Removal of the litter results in a rapid loss in mammary cells and in the metabolic activity of the remaining cells (Tucker and Reece, 1963d), but Ota and Yokoyama (1965, 1967) claimed that lactation could be reestablished with foster litters if the period of nonsuckling did not exceed 5 days. In contrast, Walsh and Tucker (1972) observed that interruption of the nursing stimulus for intervals as short as 24 hours resulted in a permanent reduction in litter weight gains and mammary RNA content, although mammary DNA was not affected. These results agree with those of Walsh and Downey (1967) and those of Wheelock *et al.* (1967) in cattle who showed that omission of several milkings results in a permanent reduction of milk synthesis. Since the milking stimulus exerts such a pronounced effect on milk synthesis (also see Grosvenor and Mena, Chapter 4), these experiments on milking frequency emphasize that frequent removal of milk is essential for the hormones to express themselves in terms of maximal milk synthesis.

In addition to the milking stimulus, pregnancy concurrent with lactation also can influence milk yields and mammary gland metabolism. Early stages of concurrent pregnancy during lactation do not alter milk yield or mammary cell numbers, but litter weight gains are reduced during later stages of pregnancy as a result of both reduced mammary cell numbers and milk synthesis capacity of the remaining cells (Tucker and Reece, 1964; Paape and Tucker, 1969). This pregnancy-caused reduction in milk yield also occurs in cattle (Fig. 7; Ragsdale *et al.*, 1924), but it is not known if the inhibition is associated with hormones such as estrogen and progesterone or with the nutrient demands of the fetus.

VIII.   CONCLUSIONS

The hormonal control of mammary development (Chapter 2), lactogenesis, and maintenance of milk secretion are closely related processes, yet some hormones that stimulate one process may inhibit another. There are species differences with respect to endocrinological involvement in initiation and maintenance of lactation, and these differences need further clarification. The following might be adopted as a working hypothesis. Initiation of lactation occurs when progesterone secretion is low, and prolactin and adrenal corticoid secretions are elevated. Maintenance of milk secretion at a high level requires oxytocin, prolactin, growth hormone, thyroxine, adrenal corticoids, and parathyroid hormone.

With the development of sensitive and specific methods for determining most lactogenic and galactopoietic hormones in blood, many questions associated with bioassays of hormone content of the various endocrine glands have been resolved. From future studies of the hormonal changes in the blood during various physiological states we should expect further clarification of the endocrine control mechanisms associated with initiation and maintenance of lactation. For example, it may be possible to resolve the hormonal causes of reduced milk production in domestic animals and to provide methods whereby the intensity of milk synthesis can be readily controlled.

ACKNOWLEDGMENTS

I wish to thank Drs. E. M. Convey and H. D. Hafs of Michigan State University and Dr. R. P. Reece of Rutgers—The State University for valuable criticisms of this manuscript. The studies in our laboratory were supported by grants-in-aid from the Michigan Agricultural Experiment Station, National Institutes of Health, and The Upjohn Company.

REFERENCES

Adams, W. M., and Wagner, W. C. (1970). *Biol. Reprod.* 3, 223.
Amenomori, Y., Chen, C. L., and Meites, J. (1970). *Endocrinology* 86, 506.
Anderson, R. R. (1971). *J. Dairy Sci.* 54, 1195.
Anderson, R. R., and Turner, C. W. (1962a). *Endocrinology* 70, 796.
Anderson, R. R., and Turner, C. W. (1962b). *Proc. Soc. Exp. Biol. Med.* 110, 349.
Anderson, R. R., and Turner, C. W. (1963a). *Amer. J. Physiol.* 205, 1077.
Anderson, R. R., and Turner, C. W. (1963b). *Proc. Soc. Exp. Biol. Med.* 112, 997.
Arai, Y., and Lee, T. H. (1967). *Endocrinology* 81, 1041.
Astwood, E. B., and Greep, R. O. (1938). *Proc. Soc. Exp. Biol. Med.* 38, 713.
Baksi, S. N., and Anderson, R. R. (1969). *J. Anim. Sci.* 29, 184.
Baksi, S. N., and Anderson, R. R. (1971). *Proc. Soc. Exp. Biol. Med.* 137, 215.
Baldwin, R. L., and Martin, R. J. (1968). *J. Dairy Sci.* 51, 748.
Barsantini, J. C., and Masson, G. M. C. (1947). *Endocrinology* 41, 299.
Barsantini, J. C., Masson, G., and Selye, H. (1936). *Rev. Can. Biol.* 5, 407.
Bassett, J. M., and Thorburn, G. D. (1969). *J. Endocrinol.* 44, 285.
Bassett, J. M., Thorburn, G. D., and Wallace, A. L. C. (1970). *J. Endocrinol.* 48, 251.
Bauman, T. R., and Turner, C. W. (1965). *J. Dairy Sci.* 48, 1353.
Ben-David, M., and Sulman, F. G. (1970). *Acta Endocrinol.* 65, 361.
Ben-David, M., Dikstein, S., and Sulman, F. G. (1965a). *Proc. Soc. Exp. Biol. Med.* 118, 265.
Ben-David, M., Roderig, H., Khazen, K., and Sulman, F. G. (1965b). *Proc. Soc. Exp. Biol. Med.* 120, 620.
Ben-David, M., Dikstein, S., and Sulman, F. G. (1966). *Proc. Soc. Exp. Biol. Med.* 121, 873.
Ben-David, M., Danon, A., Benveniste, R., Weller, C. P., and Sulman, F. G. (1971). *J. Endocrinol.* 50, 599.
von Berswordt-Wallrabe, R., and Turner, C. W. (1960). *Proc. Soc. Exp. Biol. Med.* 104, 113.
von Berswordt-Wallrabe, R., Moon, R. C., and Turner, C. W. (1960). *Proc. Soc. Exp. Biol. Med.* 104, 530.
Bintarningsih, Lyons, W. R., Johnson, R. E., and Li, C. H. (1957). *Anat. Rec.* 127, 266.
Bintarningsih, Lyons, W. R., Johnson, R. E., and Li, C. H. (1958). *Endocrinology* 63, 540.
Bisset, G. W., Clark, B. J., and Haldar, J. (1970). *J. Physiol.* 206, 711.
Blaxter, K. L., Reineke, E. P., Crampton, E. W., and Petersen, W. E. (1949). *J. Anim. Sci.* 8, 307.
Booker, D. E., Pahl, I. R., and Forbes, D. A. (1970). *Amer. J. Obstet. Gynecol.* 108, 240.
Borglin, N. E., and Sandholm, L. E. (1971). *Fert. Ster.* 22, 39.
Boyd, L. J. (1970). *J. Anim. Sci.* 31, 751.
Braun, R. K., Bergman, E. N., and Albert, T. F. (1970). *J. Amer. Vet. Med. Ass.* 157, 941.
Brewley, T. A., and Li, C. H. (1970). *Science* 168, 1361.
Bruce, H. M., and Sloviter, H. A. (1957). *J. Endocrinol.* 15, 72.

Bruce, J. O., and Ramirez, V. D. (1970). *Neuroendocrinology* **6**, 19.

Brumby, P. J., and Hancock, J. (1955). *New Zealand J. Sci. Tech. A* **36**, 417.

Brush, M. G. (1960). *J. Endocrinol.* **21**, 155.

Bryant, G. D., and Greenwood, F. C. (1968). *Biochem. J.* **109**, 831.

Bryant, G. D., Greenwood, F. C., and Linzell, J. L. (1968). *J. Endocrinol.* **40**, IV.

Bullis, D. D., Bush, L. J., and Barto, P. B. (1965). *J. Dairy Sci.* **48**, 338.

Campbell, I. L., Davey, A. W. F., McDowall, F. H., Wilson, G. F., and Munford, R. E. (1964). *J. Dairy Res.* **31**, 71.

Capen, C. C., and Young, D. M. (1967). *Science* **157**, 205.

Catt, K. J., Moffat, B., and Niall, H. D. (1967). *Science* **157**, 321.

Chadwick, A. (1971). *J. Endocrinol.* **49**, 1.

Chadwick, A., and Folley, S. J. (1962). *J. Endocrinol.* **24**, XI.

Chen, C. L., and Meites, J. (1969). *Proc. Soc. Exp. Biol. Med.* **131**, 576.

Chen, C. L., and Meites, J. (1970). *Endocrinology* **86**, 503.

Clancy, D. P., and Edgren, R. A. (1968). *Int. J. Fert.* **13**, 133.

Cleverley, J. D., and Folley, S. J. (1970). *J. Endocrinol.* **46**, 347.

Cohen, R. M., and Gala, R. R. (1969). *Proc. Soc. Exp. Biol. Med.* **132**, 683.

Convey, E. M., and Reece, R. P. (1969). *Proc. Soc. Exp. Biol. Med.* **131**, 543.

Convey, E. M., Tucker, H. A., Smith, V. G., and Zolman, J. (1973a). *Endocrinology,* **92**, 471.

Convey, E. M., Thomas, J. W., Tucker, H. A., and Gill, J. L. (1973b). *J. Dairy Sci.* **56**, 484.

Cotes, P. H., Crichton, J. A., Folley, S. J., and Young, F. G. (1949). *Nature (London)* **164**, 992.

Cowie, A. T. (1957). *J. Endocrinol.* **16**, 135.

Cowie, A. T. (1961). *In* "Milk: The Mammary Gland and its Secretion" (S. K. Kon and A. T. Cowie, eds.), Vol. I, pp. 163–203. Academic Press, New York.

Cowie, A. T. (1969a). *In* "Lactogenesis: The Initiation of Milk Secretion at Parturition" (M. Reynolds and S. J. Folley, eds.), pp. 157–169. Univ. Penn. Press, Philadelphia, Pennsylvania.

Cowie, A. T. (1969b). *J. Endocrinol.* **44**, 437.

Cowie, A. T., and Folley, S. J. (1945). *Nature (London)* **156**, 719.

Cowie, A. T., and Folley, S. J. (1946). *J. Endocrinol.* **5**, 9.

Cowie, A. T., and Folley, S. J. (1961). *In* "Sex and Internal Secretions" (W. C. Young, ed.), 3rd ed., Vol. I, pp. 590–642. Williams and Wilkins, Baltimore, Maryland.

Cowie, A. T., and Tindal, J. S. (1958). *J. Endocrinol.* **16**, 403.

Cowie, A. T., and Watson, S. C. (1966) *J. Endocrinol.* **35**, 213.

Cowie, A. T., Cox, C. P., and Naito, M. (1957). *Rep. Nat. Int. Dairy, Reading* p. 55.

Cowie, A. T., Knaggs, G. S., and Tindal, J. S. (1964). *J. Endocrinol.* **28**, 267.

Cowie, A. T., Hartmann, P. E., and Turvey, A. (1969). *J. Endocrinol.* **43**, 651.

Curtis, E. M. (1964). *Obstet. Gynecol.* **23**, 295.

Cuthbert, F. P., Ivy, A. C., Isaacs, B. L., and Gray, J. (1936). *Amer. J. Physiol.* **115**, 480.

Daggs, R. G. (1935). *J. Nutr.* **9**, 575.

Davis, J. W., and Liu, T. M. Y. (1969). *Endocrinology* **85**, 155.

Davis, S. L., Reichert, L. E., and Niswender, G. D. (1971). *Biol. Reprod.* **4**, 145.

De Fremery, P. (1936). *Proc. Physiol. Soc.* **87**, 10.

Deis, R. P. (1971). *Nature (London)* **229**, 568.

Delouis, C., and Denamur, R. (1967). *C. R. Acad. Sci.* **264D**, 2493.
Dempsey, E. W., and Astwood, E. B. (1943). *Endocrinology* **32**, 509.
Denamur, R. (1971). *J. Dairy Res.* **38**, 237.
Denamur, R., and Martinet, J. (1970). *Arch. Int. Pharmacodyn. Therap.* **186**, 185.
Denamur, R., Stoliaroff, M., and Desclin, J. (1965). *C. R. Acad. Sci. Paris* **260**, 3175.
Desclin, L. (1949). *C. R. Soc. Biol. Paris* **143**, 1156.
Djojosoebagio, S., and Turner, C. W. (1964a). *Endocrinology* **74**, 554.
Djojosoebagio, S., and Turner, C.W. (1964b). *Proc. Soc. Exp. Biol. Med.* **116**, 213.
Djojosoebagio, S., and Turner, C. W. (1964c). *Proc. Soc. Exp. Biol. Med.* **117**, 667.
Donoso, A. O., Bishop, W., Fawcett, C. P., Krulich, L., and McCann, S. M. (1971). *Endocrinology* **89**, 774.
Drost, M., and Holm, L. W. (1968). *J. Endocrinol.* **40**, 293.
Edwardson, J. A., and Eayrs, J. T. (1967). *J. Endocrinol.* **38**, 51.
Ekman, L. (1965). *Acta Physiol. Scand.* **64**, 331.
Emery, R. S., Benson, J. D., and Tucker, H. A. (1971). *J. Nutr.* **101**, 831.
Erb, R. E., Randel, R. D., and Callahan, C. J. (1971). *J. Anim. Sci. Suppl. I* **32**, 80
Etta, K. M., and Reineke, E. P. (1971). *J. Dairy Sci.* **54**, 767.
Fajer, A. B., and Barraclough, C. A. (1967). *Endocrinology* **81**, 617.
Falconer, I. R. (ed.) (1971). "Lactation." Pennsylvania State Univ. Press, University Park, Pennsylvania.
Ferreri, L. F., and Griffith, D. R. (1969). *Proc. Soc. Exp. Biol. Med.* **130**, 1216.
Fitzpatrick, R. S. (1961). *In* "Oxytocin" (R. Caldeyro-Barcia and H. Heller, eds.), pp. 358–379. Pergamon, Oxford.
Flamboe, E. E., and Reineke, E. P. (1959). *J. Anim. Sci.* **18**, 1135.
Flux, D. S. (1955). *J. Endocrinol.* **12**, 57.
Flux, D. S., Folley, S. J., and Rowland, S. J. (1954). *J. Endocrinol.* **10**, 333.
Folley, S. J. (1942). *Nature (London)* **150**, 266.
Folley, S. J. (1952). *In* "Marshall's Physiology of Reproduction" (A. S. Parkes, ed.), Vol. II, pp. 525–647. Longmans, Green, London.
Folley, S. J. (1956). "The Physiology and Biochemistry of Lactation." Oliver and Boyd, Edinburgh.
Folley, S. J., and Kon, S. K. (1938). *Proc. Roy. Soc. London, Ser. B* **124**, 476.
Folley, S. J., and Young, F. G. (1940). *J. Endocrinol.* **2**, 226.
Forsyth, I. A. (1969). *In* "Lactogenesis: The Initiation of Milk Secretion at Parturition" (M. Reynolds and S. J. Folley, eds.), pp. 195–205. Univ. Pennsylvania Press, Philadelphia, Pennsylvania.
Forsyth, I. A. (1970). *J. Endocrinol.* **46**, IV.
Frantz, A. G., and Kleinberg, D. L. (1970). *Science* **170**, 745.
Frantz, A. G., Klienberg, D. L., and Noel, G. L. (1972). *Recent Prog. Hormone Res.* **28**, 527.
Fredrikson, H. (1939). *Acta Obstet. Gynecol. Scand. Suppl. I* **19**, 1.
Friedman, M., and Beard, R. W. (1966). *J. Obstet. Gynaecol. Brit. Commonw.* **73**, 123.
Friesen, H. G. (1966). *Endocrinology* **79**, 212.
Friesen, H. G., and Guyda, H. (1971). *Endocrinology* **88**, 1353.
Gala, R. R., and Westphal, U. (1965a). *Endocrinology* **76**, 1079.
Gala, R. R., and Westphal, U. (1965b). *Endocrinology* **77**, 841.
Gala, R. R., and Westphal, U. (1966). *Endocrinology* **79**, 55.
Gala, R. R., and Westphal, U. (1967). *Acta Endocrinol.* **55**, 47.

Garcia, C., and Pincus, G. (1964). *Intern. J. Fert.* **9**, 95.

Gemzell, C. A. (1952). *Acta Endocrinol.* **11**, 221.

Gomez, E. T., and Turner, C. W. (1937). *Proc. Soc. Exp. Biol. Med.* **36**, 78.

Graham, W. R. (1934). *J. Nutr.* **7**, 407.

Griffith, D. R., and Turner, C. W. (1962). *Proc. Soc. Exp. Biol. Med.* **110**, 862.

Grosvenor, C. E. (1960). *Amer. J. Physiol.* **199**, 419.

Grosvenor, C. E. (1961). *Amer. J. Physiol.* **200**, 483.

Grosvenor, C. E. (1964). *Endocrinology* **75**, 15.

Grosvenor, C. E., and Mena, F. (1971). *J. Anim. Sci. Suppl. I* **32**, 115.

Grosvenor, C. E., and Turner, C. W. (1957). *Proc. Soc. Exp. Biol. Med.* **96**, 723.

Grosvenor, C. E., and Turner, C. W. (1959a). *Proc. Soc. Exp. Biol. Med.* **100**, 158.

Grosvenor, C. E., and Turner, C. W. (1959b). *Proc. Soc. Exp. Biol. Med.* **100**, 162.

Grosvenor, C. E., and Turner, C. W. (1960). *Endocrinology* **66**, 96.

Grosvenor, C. E., Krulich, L., and McCann, S. M. (1968). *Endocrinology* **82**, 617.

Grosvenor, C. E., Maiweg, H., and Mena, F. (1970). *Amer. J. Physiol.* **219**, 403.

Grueter, F. (1928). *C. R. Soc. Biol.* **98**, 1215.

Grynfeltt, J. (1937). *Arch. Anat. Microsc.* **33**, 177.

Guyda, H., Hwang, P., and Friesen, H. (1971). *J. Clin. Endocrinol. Metab.* **32**, 120.

Hahn, D. W., and Turner, C. W. (1966). *Proc. Soc. Exp. Biol. Med.* **121**, 1056.

Hammond, J. (1927). "The Physiology of Reproduction in the Cow." Cambridge Univ. Press, London and New York.

Hashimoto, I., Henricks, D. M., Anderson, L. L., and Melampy, R. M. (1968). *Endocrinology* **82**, 333.

Heap, R. B., and Deanesley, R. (1966). *J. Endocrinol.* **34**, 417.

Heitzman, R. J., Adams, T. C., and Hunter, G. D. (1970). *J. Endocrinol.* **47**, 133.

Henneman, H. A., Griffin, S. A., and Reineke, E. P. (1952). *J. Anim. Sci.* **11**, 794.

Herrenkohl, L. R. (1971). *Proc. Soc. Exp. Biol. Med.* **138**, 39.

Hindery, G. A., and Turner, C. W. (1965). *J. Dairy Sci.* **48**, 596.

Hindery, G. A., and Turner, C. W. (1968). *Mo. Univ. Exp. Sta. Res. Bull.* No. 932.

Hoffman, W., Forbes, T. R., and Westphal, U. (1969). *Endocrinology* **85**, 778.

Holzbauer, M. (1957). *J. Physiol.* **139**, 294.

Hunter, D. L., Erb, R. E., Randel, R. D., Garverick, H. A., Callahan, C. J., and Harrington, R. B. (1970). *J. Anim. Sci.* **30**, 47.

Ieiri, T., Akikusa, Y., and Yamamoto, L. (1971). *Endocrinology* **89**, 1553.

Illingworth, D. V., Heap, R. B., Perry, J. S. (1970). *J. Endocrinol.* **48**, 409.

Ingalls, W. G., Convey, E. M., and Hafs, H. D. (1973). *Proc. Soc. Exp. Biol. Med.* **143**, 161.

Ingbar, S. H., and Freinkel, N. (1955). *J. Clin. Invest.* **34**, 808.

Jeffers, K. R. (1935). *Amer. J. Anat.* **56**, 257.

Johke, T. (1970). *Endocrinol. Japon.* **17**, 393.

Johnson, R. M., and Meites, J. (1958). *Endocrinology* **63**, 290.

Joshi, U. M., and Rao, S. S. (1968). *J. Reprod. Fert.* **16**, 15.

Josimovich, J. B., and MacLaren, J. A. (1962). *Endocrinology* **71**, 209.

Kamal, I., Hefnawi, F., Ghoneim, M., Abdallah, M., and Abdel Razek, S. (1970). *Amer. J. Obstet. Gynecol.* **108**, 655.

Kamberi, I. A., Mical, R. S., and Porter, J. C. (1970). *Fed. Proc. Fed. Amer. Soc. Exp. Biol.* **29**, 378.

Kamoun, A. (1970). *J. Physiol. Paris* **62**, 5.

Kamoun, A., and Stutinsky, F. (1968). *J. Physiol. Paris Suppl. 2* **60**, 475.

Kamoun, A., Mialhe-Voloss, C., Stutinsky, F. (1965). *C. R. Soc. Biol.* **159**, 469.

Kaplan, S. L., and Grumbach, M. M. (1965). *J. Clin. Endocrinol. Metab.* **25**, 1370.

Karim, M., Ammar, R., El Mahgoub, S., El Ganzoury, B., Fikri, F., and Abdou, I. (1971). *Brit. Med. J.* **1**, 200.

Kilpatrick, R., Armstrong, D. T., and Greep, R. O. (1964). *Endocrinology* **74**, 453.

Knodt, C. B., and Petersen, W. E. (1944). *J. Dairy Sci.* **27**, 449.

Knox, F. S., and Griffith, D. R. (1970). *Proc. Soc. Exp. Biol. Med.* **133**, 135.

Koch, B. (1969). *Horm. Metab. Res.* **1**, 129.

Koch, Y., Lu, K. H., and Meites, J. (1970). *Endocrinology* **87**, 673.

Koprowski, J. A., and Tucker, H. A. (1971). *J. Dairy Sci.* **54**, 1675.

Koprowski, J. A., and Tucker, H. A. (1973a). *Endocrinology* **92**, 1480.

Koprowski, J. A., and Tucker, H. A. (1973b). *Endocrinology* **93**, 645.

Koprowski, J. A., Convey, E. M., and Tucker, H. A. (1971). *J. Dairy Sci.* **54**, 769.

Koprowski, J. A., Tucker, H. A., and Convey, E. M. (1972). *Proc. Soc. Exp. Biol. Med.* **140**, 1012.

Kora, S. J. (1969). *Fert. Ster.* **20**, 419.

Kowalewski, K. (1969). *Endocrinology* **84**, 432.

Kronfeld, D. S., Mayer, G. P., Robertson, J. M., and Raggi, F. (1963). *J. Dairy Sci.* **46**, 559.

Krulik, R., and Svobodova, J. (1969). *Physiol. Bohemoslov.* **18**, 141.

Kuhn, N. J. (1969a). *J. Endocrinol.* **44**, 39.

Kuhn, N. J. (1969b). *J. Endocrinol.* **45**, 615.

Kuhn, N. J., and Briley, M. S. (1970). *Biochem. J.* **117**, 193.

Kumaresan, P., and Turner, C. W. (1965a). *Proc. Exp. Biol. Med.* **119**, 415.

Kumaresan, P., and Turner, C. W. (1965b). *Proc. Soc. Exp. Biol. Med.* **119**, 1133.

Kumaresan, P., and Turner, C. W. (1966). *Proc. Soc. Exp. Biol. Med.* **123**, 70.

Kumaresan, P., Anderson, R. R., and Turner, C. W. (1966). *Proc. Soc. Exp. Biol. Med.* **123**, 581.

Kuramitsu, C., and Loeb, L. (1921). *Amer. J. Physiol.* **56**, 40.

Laumas, K. R., Malkani, P. K., Bhatnagar, S., and Laumas, V. (1967). *Amer. J. Obstet. Gynecol.* **98**, 411.

Lauritzen, C. (1967). *Acta Endocrinol. Suppl.* **124**, 87.

Leavitt, W. W., and Blaha, G. C. (1970). *Biol. Reprod.* **3**, 353.

Lewis, U. J., Singh, R. N. P., Sinha, Y. N., and Vander Laan, W. P. (1971). *J. Clin. Endocrinol. Metab.* **33**, 153.

Li, C. H., Liu, W. K., and Dixon, J. S. (1966). *J. Amer. Chem. Soc.* **88**, 2050.

Li, C. H., Dixon, J. S., and Liu, W. K. (1969a). *Arch. Biochem. Biophys.* **133**, 70.

Li, C. H., Dixon, J. S., Lo, T. B., Pankov, Y. A., and Schmidt, K. D. (1969b). *Nature (London)* **224**, 695.

Liggins, G. C. (1969). *J. Endocrinol.* **45**, 515.

Liggins, G. C., Kennedy, P. C., and Holm, L. W. (1967). *Amer. J. Obstet. Gynecol.* **98**, 1080.

Lindner, H. R. (1964). *J. Endocrinol.* **28**, 301.

Linzell, J. L. (1963). *Quart. J. Exp. Physiol.* **48**, 34.

Lorscheider, F. L., and Reineke, E. P. (1971). *Proc. Soc. Exp. Biol. Med.* **138**, 1116.

Lorscheider, F. L., and Reineke, E. P. (1972). *J. Reprod. Fertil.* **30**, 269.

Lyons, W. R. (1942). *Proc. Soc. Exp. Biol. Med.* **51**, 308.

Lyons, W. R. (1958). *Proc. Roy. Soc. London B* **149**, 303.

Lyons, W. R., Li, C. H., and Johnson, R. E. (1960). *Acta Endocrinol. Suppl.* **51**, 1145.

Lyons, W. R., Li, C. H., Ahmad, N., and Rice-Wray, E. (1968). *Excerpta Med. Int. Congr. Series No. 158*, p. 349.

Macdonald, G. J., and Reece, R. P. (1961). *J. Anim. Sci.* **20**, 196.

Machlin, L. J. (1973). *J. Dairy Sci.* **56**, 575.

Martin, R. J., and Baldwin, R. L. (1971a). *Endocrinology* **88**, 863.

Martin, R. J., and Baldwin, R. L. (1971b). *Endocrinology* **88**, 868.

Matthies, D. L. (1967). *Anat. Rec.* **159**, 55.

Mayer, G., and Klein, M. (1961). *In* "Milk: The Mammary Gland and its Secretion" (S. K. Kon and A. T. Cowie, eds.), Vol. I, pp. 47–126. Academic Press, New York.

McGlone, J. (1969). *Practitioner* **203**, 187.

Meites, J. (1957). *Proc. Soc. Exp. Biol. Med.* **96**, 730.

Meites, J. (1961). *In* "Milk: The Mammary Gland and its Secretion" (S. K. Kon and A. T. Cowie, eds.), Vol. I, pp. 321–367. Academic Press, New York.

Meites, J. (1966). *In* "Neuroendocrinology" (L. Martini and W.F. Ganong, eds.), Vol. I, pp. 669–707. Academic Press, New York.

Meites, J., and Nicoll, C. S. (1966). *Ann. Rev. Physiol.* **28**, 57.

Meites, J., and Turner, C. W. (1947). *Amer. J. Physiol.* **150**, 394.

Meites, J., Hopkins, T. F., and Talwalker, P. K. (1963). *Endocrinology* **73**, 261.

Milkovic, K., and Milkovic, S. (1962). *Endocrinology* **71**, 799.

Milkovic, K., and Milkovic, S. (1963). *Endocrinology* **73**, 535.

Miller, G. H., and Hughes, L. R. (1970). *Obstet. Gynecol.* **35**, 44.

Minaguchi, H., Clemens, J. A., and Meites, J. (1968). *Endocrinology* **82**, 555.

Mizuno, H., and Sensui, N. (1970). *Endocrinol. Japon.* **17**, 417.

Mizuno, H., Talwalker, P. K., and Meites, J. (1967). *Neuroendocrinology* **2**, 222.

van der Molen, H. J., Hart, P. G., and Wymenga, H. G. (1969). *Acta Endocrinol.* **61**, 255.

Momongan, V. G., and Schmidt, G. H. (1970). *J. Dairy Sci.* **53**, 747.

Moon, R. C. (1965). *Proc. Soc. Exp. Biol. Med.* **118**, 181.

Moore, L. A. (1958). *J. Dairy Sci.* **41**, 452.

Morag, M., Shani, J., Sulman, F. G., and Yagil, R. (1971). *J. Endocrinol.* **49**, 351.

Morris, J. A. (1967). *Int. J. Fert.* **12**, 261.

Nagasawa, H., and Naito, M. (1963). *Jap. J. Zootech. Sci.* **34**, 174.

Nagasawa, H., Chen, C. L., and Meites, J. (1969). *Proc. Soc. Exp. Biol. Med.* **132**, 859.

Nandi, S. (1958). *Science* **128**, 772.

Nandi, S., and Bern, H. A. (1961). *Gen. Comp. Endocrinol.* **1**, 195.

Neil, J. D. (1972). *Endocrinology* **90**, 568.

Nelson, W. O. (1934). *Endocrinology* **18**, 33.

Nelson, W. O., and Gaunt, R. (1936). *Proc. Soc. Exp. Biol. Med.* **34**, 671.

Nelson, W. O., Gaunt, R., and Schweizer, M. (1943). *Endocrinology* **33**, 325.

Newton, M. (1961). *In* "Milk: The Mammary Gland and its Secretion" (S. K. Kon and A. T. Cowie, eds.), Vol. I, pp. 281–320. Academic Press, New York.

Newton, W. H., and Beck, N. (1939). *J. Endocrinol.* **1**, 65.

Nicoll, C. S., and Meites, J. (1959). *Proc. Soc. Exp. Biol. Med.* **101**, 81.

Nicoll, C. S., and Meites, J. (1963). *Endocrinology* **72**, 544.

Nicoll, C. S., Parsons, J. A., Fiorindo, R. P., Nichols, C. W., and Sakuma, M. (1970). *J. Clin. Endocrinol. Metab.* **30**, 512.

Nir, I., Mishkinsky, J., Eshchar, N., and Sulman, F. G. (1968). *J. Endocrinol.* **42**, 161.

Ota, K., and Yokoyama, A. (1965). *J. Endocrinol.* **33**, 185.

Ota, K., and Yokoyama, A. (1967). *J. Endocrinol.* **38**, 251.

Owen, E. C., and Darroch, R. A. (1957). *J. Dairy Res.* **24**, 157.

Oxender, W. D., Hafs, H. D., and Edgerton, L. A. (1972). *J. Anim. Sci.* **35**, 51.

Paape, M. J., and Desjardins, C. (1971). *Proc. Soc. Exp. Biol. Med.* **138**, 12.

Paape, M. J., and Tucker, H. A. (1969). *J. Dairy Sci.* **52**, 380.

Pasteels, J. L. (1969). *In* "Lactogenesis: The Initiation of Milk Secretion at Parturition" (M. Reynolds and S. J. Folley, eds.), pp. 207–216. Univ. Pennsylvania Press, Philadelphia, Pennsylvania.

Paterson, J. Y. F., and Harrison, F. A. (1967). *J. Endocrinol.* **37**, 269.

Paterson, J. Y. F., and Harrison, F. A. (1968). *J. Endocrinol.* **40**, 37.

Paterson, J. Y. F., and Hills, F. (1967). *J. Endocrinol.* **37**, 261.

Paterson, J. Y. F., and Linzell, J. L. (1971). *J. Endocrinol.* **50**, 493.

Pharris, B. B., and Wyngarden, L. J. (1969). *Proc. Soc. Exp. Biol. Med.* **130**, 92.

Pincus, G. (1965). "The Control of Fertility," p. 261. Academic Press, New York.

Pincus, G., Bialy, G., Layne, D. S., Paniagua, M., and Williams, K. I. H. (1966). *Nature (London)* **212**, 924.

Plager, J. E., Knopp, R., Slaunwhite, W. R., and Sandberg, A. A. (1963). *Endocrinology* **73**, 353.

Poulton, B. R., and Reece, R. P. (1957). *Endocrinology* **61**, 217.

Ragsdale, A. C., Turner, C. W., and Brody, S. (1924). *J. Dairy Sci.* **7**, 24.

Ray, E. W., Averill, S. C., Lyons, W. R., and Johnson, R. E. (1955). *Endocrinology* **56**, 359.

Reddy, R. R., and Donker, J. D. (1965). *J. Dairy Sci.* **48**, 978.

Reece, R. P. (1939). *Proc. Soc. Exp. Biol. Med.* **40**, 25.

Reece, R. P. (1958). *In* "The Endocrinology of Reproduction" (J. T. Velardo, ed.), pp. 213–240. Oxford Univ. Press, London and New York.

Reece, R. P., and Turner, C. W. (1937). *Mo. Univ. Agr. Exp. Sta. Res. Bull.*, No. 266.

Reineke, E. P. (1964). *Fed. Proc. Fed. Amer. Soc. Exp. Biol.* **23**, 203.

Reineke, E. P., and Lorscheider, F. L. (1967). *Gen. Comp. Endocrinol.* **9**, 362.

Reineke, E. P., and Singh, O. N. (1955). *Proc. Soc. Exp. Biol. Med.* **88**, 203.

van Rensburg, S. J. (1967). *J. Endocrinol.* **38**, 83.

Reynolds, M., and Folley, S. J. (eds.) (1969). "Lactogenesis: The Initiation of Milk Secretion at Parturition." Univ. Pennsylvania Press, Philadelphia, Pennsylvania.

Richter, J. (1936). *Berl. Tierarztl. Worschr.* **277**, 293.

Robinson, R., Baker, R. D., Anastassiadis, P. A., and Common, R. H. (1970). *J. Dairy Sci.* **53**, 1592.

Rook, J. A. F., Storry, J. E., and Wheelock, J. V. (1965). *J. Dairy Sci.* **48**, 745.

Rosenthal, H. E., Slaunwhite, W. R., and Sandberg, A. A. (1969). *Endocrinology* **85**, 825.

Roussel, J. D., and Beatty, J. F. (1969). *J. Dairy Sci.* **52**, 2020.

Sar, M., and Meites, J. (1969). *Neuroendocrinology* **4**, 25.

Saunders, F. J. (1967). *Endocrinology* **80**, 447.

Schalch, D. S., and Reichlin, S. (1966). *Endocrinology* **79**, 275.

Schams, D., and Karg, H. (1970). *Zentbl. Vet. Med.* **A17**, 193.

Schmidt, G. H. (1966). *J. Dairy Sci.* **49**, 381.

Schmidt, G. H., Warner, R. G., Tyrrell, H. F., and Hansel, W. (1971). *J. Dairy Sci.* 54, 481.

Scholz, H. R., and Huther, K. J. (1971). *Horm. Metab. Res.* 3, 215.

Seal, U. S., and Doe, R. P. (1963). *Endocrinology* 73, 371.

Selye, H., Collip, J. B., and Thomson, D. L. (1933a), *Proc. Soc. Exp. Biol. Med.* 30, 589.

Selye, H., Collip, J. B., and Thomson, D. L. (1933b). *Proc. Soc. Exp. Biol. Med.* 31, 82.

Semm, K. (1966). *In* "Social and Medical Aspects of Oral Contraception" (M. N. G. Dukes, ed.), Int. Congr. Series 130, pp. 98–101. Excerpta Med. Found., Amsterdam.

Shani, J., Knaggs, G. S., and Tindal, J. S. (1971). *J. Endocrinol.* 50, 543.

Shaw, J. C., Chung, A. C., and Bunding, I. (1955). *Endocrinology* 56, 327.

Shaw, G. H., Reineke, E. P., Convey, E. M., Tucker, H. A., and Thomas, J. W. (1972). *J. Dairy Sci.* 55, 664.

Sherwood, L. M., Handwerger, S., McLaurin, W. D., and Lanner, M. (1971). *Nature New Biol.* 233, 59.

Sinha, Y. N., and Tucker, H. A. (1969a). *J. Dairy Sci.* 52, 507.

Sinha, Y. N., and Tucker, H. A. (1969b). *Proc. Soc. Exp. Biol. Med.* 131, 908.

Sinha, Y. N., Selby, F. W., Lewis, U. J., and Vanderlaan, W. P. (1972). *Endocrinology* 91, 784.

Smith, L. W., and Inskeep, E. K. (1970). *J. Anim. Sci.* 30, 957.

Smith, K. L., and Schanbacher, F. L. (1973). *J. Dairy Sci.* 56, 738.

Smith, V. G., and Convey, E. M. (1971). *Proc. Soc. Exp. Biol. Med.* 136, 588.

Smith, V. G., Edgerton, L. A., Hafs, H. D., and Convey, E. M. (1973). *J. Anim. Sci.* 36, 301.

Snyder, S. H., Zweig, M., Axelrod, J., and Fischer, J. E. (1965). *Proc. Nat. Acad. Sci.* 53, 301.

Spellacy, W. N., Buhi, W. C., and Birk, S. A. (1970). *Amer. J. Obstet. Gynecol.* 107, 244

Srivastava, L. S., and Turner, C. W. (1966). *J. Dairy Sci.* 49, 1459.

Sterling, K., Laslof, J. C., and Man, E. B. (1954). *J. Clin. Invest.* 33, 1031.

Stewart, C. P., Albert-Recht, F., and Osman, L. M. (1961). *Clin. Chim. Acta* 6, 696.

Stricker, P., and Grueter, F. (1929). *Presse Med.* 37, 1268.

Sud, S. C., Tucker, H. A., and Meites, J. (1968). *J. Dairy Sci.* 51, 210.

Swanson, E. W. (1972). *J. Dairy Sci.* 55, 1763.

Swanson, L. V., and Hafs, H. D. (1971). *J. Anim. Sci.* 33, 1038.

Talwalker, P. K., Meites, J., and Nicoll, C. S. (1960). *Amer. J. Physiol.* 199, 1070.

Talwalker, P. K., Nicoll, C. S., and Meites, J. (1961). *Endocrinology* 69, 802.

Thatcher, W. W., and Tucker, H. A. (1968). *Proc. Soc. Exp. Biol. Med.* 128, 46.

Thatcher, W. W., and Tucker, H. A. (1970a). *Endocrinology* 86, 237.

Thatcher, W. W., and Tucker, H. A. (1970b). *Proc. Soc. Exp. Biol. Med.* 134, 705.

Thatcher, W. W., and Tucker, H. A. (1970c). *Proc. Soc. Exp. Biol. Med.* 134, 915.

Tindal, J. S., and Knaggs, G. S. (1966). *J. Endocrinol.* 34, ii.

Tomoy, T. (1963). *Nauch. Trud. Vissh. Vet. Med. Inst. G. Pavlov* 11, 71. In *J. Dairy Sci.* (abstr.) 26, 272 (1964).

Topper, Y. J. (1970). *Recent Progr. Hormone Res.* 26, 287.

Tucker, H. A. (1966). *Amer. J. Physiol.* 210, 1209.

Tucker, H. A. (1969). *J. Dairy Sci.* 52, 721.

Tucker, H. A. (1971). *J. Anim. Sci. Suppl. I* 32, 137.
Tucker, H. A., and Meites, J. (1965). *J. Dairy Sci.* 48, 403.
Tucker, H. A., and Reece, R. P. (1961). *J. Dairy Sci.* 44, 1751.
Tucker, H. A., and Reece, R. P. (1963a). *Proc. Soc. Exp. Biol. Med.* 112, 370.
Tucker, H. A., and Reece, R. P. (1963b). *Proc. Soc. Exp. Biol. Med.* 112, 409.
Tucker, H. A., and Reece, R. P. (1963c). *Proc. Soc. Exp. Biol. Med.* 112, 688.
Tucker, H. A., and Reece, R. P. (1963d). *Proc. Soc. Exp. Biol. Med.* 112, 1002.
Tucker, H. A., and Reece, R. P. (1963e). *Proc. Soc. Exp. Biol. Med.* 113, 717.
Tucker, H. A., and Reece, R. P. (1964), *Proc. Soc. Exp. Biol. Med.* 115, 885.
Tucker, H. A., and Thatcher, W. W. (1968). *Proc. Soc. Exp. Biol. Med.* 129, 578.
Tucker, H. A., Paape, M. J., and Sinha, Y. N. (1967a). *Amer. J. Physiol.* 213, 262.
Tucker, H. A., Paape, M. J., Sinha, Y. N., Pritchard, D. E, and Thatcher, W. W. (1967b). *Proc. Soc. Exp. Biol. Med.* 126, 100.
Tucker, H. A., Larson, B. L., and Gorski, J. (1971). *Endocrinology* 89, 152.
Turkington, R. W., and Hill, R. L. (1969). *Science* 163, 1458.
Turkington, R. W., and Topper, Y. J. (1966). *Endocrinology* 79, 175.
Turner, C .W. (1969). *Mo. Univ. Exp. Sta. Res. Bull.* No. 969.
Tyson, J. E., Frieson, H. G., and Anderson, M. S. (1972). *Science* 177, 897.
Varma, S. K., Sonksen, P. H., Varma, K., Soeldner, J. S., Selenkow, H. A., and Emerson, K. (1971). *J. Clin. Endocrinol. Metab.* 32, 328.
Voogt, J. L., Sar, M., and Meites, J. (1969). *Amer. J. Physiol.* 216, 655.
Walsh, J. P., and Downey, W. K. (1967). *Biochem. J.* 103, 41 P.
Walsh, J. P., and Tucker, H. A. (1972). *Proc. Soc. Exp. Biol. Med.* 140, 13.
Watson, P. S. (1969). *Practitioner* 203, 184.
Wheelock, J. V., Smith, A., and Dodd, F. H. (1967). *J. Dairy Res.* 34, 151.
Wolf, R. C., and Bowman, R. E. (1966). *Proc. Soc. Exp. Biol. Med.* 121, 986.
Wrenn, T. R., and Sykes, J. F. (1953). *J. Dairy Sci.* 36, 1313.
Yanai, R., and Nagasawa, H. (1971). *Horm. Behav.* 2, 73.
Yates, F. E., and Urquhart, J. (1962). *Physiol. Rev.* 42, 359.
Yokoyama, A., Shinde, Y., and Ota, K. (1969). *In* "Lactogenesis: The Initiation of Milk Secretion at Parturition" (M. Reynolds and S. J. Folley, eds.), pp. 65–71. Univ. Pennsylvania Press, Philadelphia, Pennsylvania.
Yoshinaga, K., Hawkins, R. A., and Stocker, J. F. (1969). *Endocrinology* 85, 103.
Zimbelman, R. G., and Smith, L. W. (1966). *J. Reprod. Fert.* 11, 193.

CHAPTER SIX

Some Aspects of Mammary Gland Development in the Mature Mouse

Yale J. Topper and Takami Oka

I.	Introduction	327
II.	Insulin and Serum Factor(s) Insensitivity	328
III.	Dynamics of Insulin Action	329
IV.	Cryptic Insulin Apparatus	330
V.	Insulin and Serum Factor(s) Sensitivity in Different States of Development	331
VI.	Sensitization by Prolactin	332
VII.	Protein Markers of Highly Developed Mammary Cells	334
VIII.	Requirement for Mitosis	335
IX.	Selection of a System for Further Study	336
X.	Developmental Status of Mammary Epithelial Cells in the Midpregnant Mouse	337
XI.	Synchronization of Midpregnancy Alveolar Cells	339
	A. Incubation in the Presence of Insulin	339
	B. Incubation in the Presence of Insulin and Hydrocortisone	341
	C. Incubation in the Presence of Prolactin	342
XII.	Additional Considerations	344
	References	346

I. INTRODUCTION

The epithelial component of the mammary gland in the adult, virgin mouse consists of an arboreal ductal system with alveoli at the termini of the branches. This system, formed largely between the third and sixteenth postnatal weeks (period of puberty), is embedded in the mammary fat pads. At this time the fat cells are the major component of the tissue in terms of volume. Several hormones, including estrogen and progesterone, seem to be involved as mitogenic and morphogenetic agents during puberty (Prop, 1961; Ichinose and Nandi, 1964), but the interrelationships among them have not been clearly defined.

With maturity at the age of 3–4 months, epithelial cell proliferation virtually stops, except for a low level of activity during estrus. The reason is not known. Functional development of the gland is also arrested as long as the animal remains nonpregnant. Very little α-lactalbumin occurs in this state (Turkington et al., 1968; Palmiter, 1969a; McKenzie et al., 1971). The minute amount of casein formation that has been observed (Lockwood et al., 1966; Stockdale and Topper, 1966) is probably a reflection of hormonal changes during estrus.

The majority of mammary epithelial cells in the adult, virgin mouse have a nonsecretory appearance (Sekhri et al., 1967). They have a rudimentary Golgi apparatus situated laterally to the nucleus and are almost devoid of rough endoplasmic reticulum (RER). The small percentage of epithelial cells that has a supply of RER probably represents the site of the low-level casein synthesis (Mills and Topper, unpublished).

This chapter is concerned with efforts to understand the reasons for the dormancy of the mature virgin mammary gland. We try to unravel the network of events that leads to further growth and development during pregnancy. In order to simplify the problem, isolated tissue from C3H/ Hen mice has been studied. Under these circumstances, of course, care must be taken to insure that observed changes reflect relevant phenomena occurring in vivo.

II. INSULIN AND SERUM FACTOR(S) INSENSITIVITY*

In the mature, nonpregnant state, mammary growth and development are essentially halted. However, when explants from the abdominal mammary glands of adult, virgin mice are cultured in the presence of insulin or insulin-free serum using the technique of Elias (1957, 1959), epithelial proliferation occurs after 1 or 2 days (Stockdale and Topper, 1966; Friedberg et al., 1970). When such explants are exposed to insulin, glucocorticoid, and prolactin, casein synthesis increases markedly (Stockdale and Topper, 1966), and α-lactalbumin emerges (Vonderhaar et al., 1973). The formation of these secretory proteins is dependent upon the fabrication and accumulation of RER, which, in turn, reflects a synergistic action of insulin and glucocorticoid (Mills and Topper, 1969; Oka and Topper, 1971a). If these effects of insulin, insulin-free serum, and glucocorticoid have a physiological counterpart, why do these humoral

---

* Abbreviations: I, insulin; F, the glucocorticoid, hydrocortisone; P, prolactin.

agents not exert similar influences on the gland in the intact, non-pregnant mouse (Topper, 1968)?

The evidence adduced indicates that these factors probably *do* elicit the described responses in the intact *pregnant* mouse because the mammary epithelial cells in such an animal are sensitive to insulin (Friedberg *et al.*, 1970; Oka and Topper, 1972a; Oka unpublished) and insulin-free serum (Majumder and Turkington, 1971). In contrast, the cells in the adult, nonpregnant mouse are not sensitive to these agents in the circulation (Friedberg *et al.*, 1970; Oka unpublished). This probably accounts largely for the failure of the epithelial cells in adult, virgin gland to proliferate. These cells are, in fact, sensitive to glucocorticoid (Topper and Oka, 1971). Thus, insensitivity to insulin alone can account for their lack of RER (Friedberg *et al.*, 1970). Actually, the virgin cells, unlike pregnant cells, are unresponsive to insulin in other respects also. Thus, insulin-sensitive, pregnant mammary cells are stimulated promply by the hormone in terms of the synthesis of the intracellular enzyme glucose-6-phosphate dehydrogenase (Leader and Barry, 1969) and the rate of accumulation of the nonmetabolizable amino acid, α-aminoisobutyric acid (AIB); insulin-insensitive virgin cells are not (Friedberg *et al.*, 1970).

It is fortunate from the standpoint of the investigator that the virgin cells can acquire insulin sensitivity after about 24 hours in culture (Friedberg *et al.*, 1970). Otherwise the dormant virgin gland would not develop *in vitro* in response to insulin, glucocorticoid, and prolactin, as described above. The mechanism by which sensitivity develops in the isolated tissue is not known. But it is clear that no exogenous hormones are required and that no contribution from the fat cells is necessary (Friedberg *et al.*, 1970). Similar considerations relating to sensitivity and insensitivity of mammary cells to serum factor(s) will be discussed later.

The results indicate that the presence of a stimulus is no guarantee that an effective tissue-stimulus interaction will ensue. Furthermore, it appears that development of the ability to respond to a signal, such as a hormone, is not necessarily dependent on the presence of the signal.

III. DYNAMICS OF INSULIN ACTION

At this point a brief consideration of the dynamics of insulin action will lead us into another interesting aspect of the development of the mammary cell. In contrast to steroid hormones, such as 17β-estradiol, which enter cells and form complexes with receptor proteins (Jensen *et al.*,

1968) before eliciting their characteristic biological responses, protein hormones can effect changes in their target cells without entering the cells, by impinging on the cell membrane. This concept was most recently established by studies in which the protein hormones used are covalently bound to large, biologically inert particles, such as sepharose beads (Cuatrecasas, 1969; Selinger and Civen, 1971; Johnson *et al.*, 1972). The particles are so large that they could not possibly enter the cell. Furthermore, several lines of evidence indicate that the biological responses are not a consequence of release of the free hormone from the particulate (Cuatrecasas, 1969; Oka and Topper, 1971b). Clearly, protein hormones can affect cellular events through contact with the outer cell membrane. In this context, it has been demonstrated that insulin-sepharose complexes can simulate the stimulatory effects of insulin on RNA synthesis (Turkington, 1970b), and AIB accumulation (Oka and Topper, 1971b) by insulin-sensitive mammary epithelial cells from pregnant mice. In the course of these studies it was discovered (Oka and Topper, 1972b) that tight binding between the hormone and mammary cell is not necessary for elicitation of a biological response. Transient contact in the form of collisions that result from shaking the suspended cells and insulin-sepharose beads will suffice. Similar considerations seem to apply to the interaction between ACTH-sepharose and adrenal cells (Selinger and Civen, 1971).

IV. CRYPTIC INSULIN APPARATUS

Mammary cells from pregnant mice, therefore, respond to insulin sepharose as they do to free insulin. Even though we knew that the cells in virgin mice do not respond to circulating insulin, and that the cells in explants from virgin mice are initially insensitive to insulin, it was conceivable that these cells might respond promptly to insulin sepharose *in vitro*. Accordingly, a suspension of epithelial cells, contaminated with a small percentage of connective tissue cells, but free from fat cells, was prepared by treating mammary tissue from virgin mice with crude collagenase (Friedberg *et al.*, 1970; Oka and Topper, 1971b). Again, it was observed that the cells do not respond to insulin during the first day of culture in terms of the rate of AIB accumulation but acquire insulin sensitivity subsequently. Surprisingly, the cells *do* respond almost immediately to insulin sepharose (Oka and Topper, 1971b). They act toward insulin sepharose in this respect as cells from pregnant mice act toward both free insulin and insulin sepharose. Prior exposure of the virgin cells to free insulin eradicates the response to insulin sepharose. This effect is quite specific, since a number of other proteins tested, such as bovine serum albumin, and the A- and B-chains of insulin, do not block this stimulatory activity of insulin sepharose.

We do not understand why the virgin cells can interact effectively with insulin sepharose, but not with free insulin. Two interpretations have been presented recently (Oka and Topper, 1971b). It is apparent that the mammary cells in adult, virgin mice do possess at least part of the insulin apparatus, but it is associated with the cell membrane in a cryptic form.

V. INSULIN AND SERUM FACTOR(S) SENSITIVITY IN DIFFERENT STATES OF DEVELOPMENT

Insulin sensitivity has been discussed with respect to mammary cells in mature virgin and pregnant mice. What is the status of this cellular property as a function of other developmental states? Does a dissociation between the stimulatory effect on DNA synthesis and AIB accumulation ever occur? Do serum factors other than insulin elicit similar stimulatory responses?

Insulin-free serum from several sources has been shown to stimulate epithelial DNA synthesis by mammary explants from pregnant mice (Majumder and Turkington, 1971). A more recent report (Oka unpublished) has confirmed this finding and has also shown that cells in tissue from mature virgin mice are unresponsive to the serum factor(s). As with insulin, the virgin cells acquire serum sensitivity, in terms of DNA synthesis, after about 24 hours in culture. There will be more discussion of insulin and insulin-free serum as mitogenic agents in a later section.

Insulin sensitivity has been studied more extensively than serum sensitivity. Epithelial cells in the gland of the 3-week-old mouse proliferate rapidly *in vivo*. In organ culture the cells are initially insensitive to insulin, but they acquire sensitivity by the second day of culture in terms of both DNA synthesis and AIB accumulation (Oka *et al.*, unpublished). It should be noted, however, that considerable cell proliferation does occur *in vitro* in the absence of exogenous insulin (Voytovich and Topper, 1967).

Insulin insensitivity of the cells in the mature, virgin mouse was discussed in an earlier section. In this state, sensitivity to insulin in terms of the several responses cited appear to develop almost synchronously *in vitro*.

Insulin sensitivity in respect to both DNA synthesis and AIB accumulation first becomes detectable by the second day of pregnancy in the mouse (Oka *et al.*, unpublished). All the mammary epithelial cells that are potentially capable of responding to insulin appear to be sensitive by the tenth to twelfth day (midpregnancy). Sensitivity in both respects is maintained during the remainder of pregnancy.

Lactating mouse cells require insulin for maintenance of the initial high rate of AIB accumulation (unpublished). But they are not sensitive to the hormone in terms of DNA synthesis, and so the two responses seem to be dissociated from each other in this state. They can acquire sensitivity in regard to DNA formation after 1–2 days in culture (Oka *et al.*, unpublished).

The cells in the involuted gland are insensitive to insulin in regard to DNA synthesis and AIB accumulation. Therefore, the multiparous nonpregnant gland is as developmentally dormant as the virgin gland (Oka *et al.*, unpublished). Sensitivity can be acquired *in vitro*. The cycle is repeated with the start of another pregnancy.

VI. SENSITIZATION BY PROLACTIN

It was pointed out that sensitization to insulin is probably necessary in order for mammary cells in the gland of mature virgin mice to develop further. Such sensitization can occur *in vitro* in the absence of added hormones. This makes it possible to study the development of tissue from mature, nonpregnant mice *in vitro*. However, the sensitizing factor that operates during pregnancy was yet to be discovered.

Recent evidence (Oka and Topper, 1972a) strongly implicates prolactin as the agent which converts insulin- and serum factor(s)-insensitive mammary cells into sensitive ones. There is good correlation between elevation of serum prolactin levels and the advent of sensitivity in the mouse and rat. The cells in the 3-week-old and mature, nonpregnant mouse are insensitive, while the circulating prolactin level is relatively low. The small degree of cell proliferation and casein synthesis which occurs in the adult mouse probably reflects transient elevations of prolactin during estrus. The prolactin level is thought to increase shortly after coitus in the mouse (Browning *et al.*, 1962; Bronson *et al.*, 1966) and sensitivity emerges during the second day of pregnancy in this species (Oka *et al.*, unpublished). In contrast, except for an early spike, the level does not rise in the rat until late pregnancy (Amenomori *et al.*, 1970;

Linkie and Niswender, 1972) and sensitivity does not appear until late pregnancy (Oka and Topper, 1972a). These observations are consistent with others that indicate a wave of mammary epithelial proliferation during the second day of pregnancy in the mouse (Oka *et al.*, unpublished) but no increase in epithelial-DNA concentration until late pregnancy in the rat (Oka and Topper, 1972a). Incidentally, insulin-insensitive rat mammary cells, like those from mice, can acquire sensitivity *in vitro* regarding both DNA synthesis and AIB accumulation (Oko and Topper, 1972a).

Prolactin administration to mature virgin mice and rats increases the epithelial DNA concentration of the mammary gland (Lyons *et al.*, 1958; Oka and Topper, 1972a). This does not necessarily mean that prolactin itself is the mitogenic agent. In fact, prolactin has no proliferative effect *in vitro*, either by itself or in combination with insulin or with serum (Stockdale and Topper, 1966; Oka and Topper, 1972a). But prolactin administration to virgin mice and rats renders their mammary epithelium sensitive to the mitogenic actions of insulin and serum *in vitro*. It is proposed, on this basis, that prolactin leads to proliferation of mammary cells *in vivo* by sensitizing the cells to serum and/or to insulin. This effect appears to be direct, not systemic. Injection of a small amount of the hormone directly into one abdominal gland of virgin mice rendered that gland sensitive to insulin as measured by [³H]thymidine incorporation into DNA, whereas the placebo-injected contralateral gland remained insensitive to insulin. This finding is consistent with an earlier report by Lyons *et al.* (1967), who found that local injection of prolactin resulted in proliferation only in the injected mammary gland. Also, the effect is reversible, since within 10 days after withdrawal of the hormone the cells reverted to an insulin-insensitive condition (Oka and Topper, unpublished).

Addition of prolactin to the culture medium does not accelerate the development of sensitivity. How can one rationalize this in terms of the direct sensitization by prolactin of the epithelium *in vivo*? Since the hormone-independent sensitization *in vitro* requires about the same time as the prolactin-dependent sensitization *in vivo* (Oka and Topper, 1972a), it may be that the time factor precludes manifestation of a prolactin effect *in vitro*. Alternatively, the experimental conditions *in vitro* may not be suitable for expression of this effect of prolactin.

The control of proliferation of mammary epithelium may thus be visualized as follows: the cells in the mature virgin female undergo virtually no proliferation, despite the fact that potentially mitogenic agents, such

as insulin and serum factors, are in the circulation. This may be ascribed
to the fact that such cells are insensitive to these agents (Friedberg *et al.*,
1970; Oka and Topper, 1972a). Insulin and serum sensitivity and proliferation are observable as a consequence of elevation of circulating prolactin.
Prolactin, then, is not itself a mitogenic agent, but it enables the cells
to respond to mitogens such as insulin and/or serum. Placental lactogen
may play a similar role in some species, such as the rat.

VII. PROTEIN MARKERS OF HIGHLY DEVELOPED MAMMARY CELLS

The mammary gland is at its developmental peak during lactation. In
this state it manufactures and secretes a variety of unique products, including proteins. Two of the most abundant milk proteins are casein and
α-lactalbumin, and the synthesis of these substances has served as a
convenient criterion of functional maturation in the studies to be described.

Mouse casein is a family of three to four phosphoproteins that can be
identified by their electrophoretic mobility (Turkington *et al.*, 1965) after
precipitation in the presence of rennin and calcium ions. Their synthesis
in vitro requires the presence of insulin, glucocorticoid, and prolactin. In
some instances, to be described later, other humoral factors can substitute
for insulin and prolactin. The synthesis of these phosphorproteins in the
organ culture system used appears to be coordinate (Turkington *et al.*,
1967b). Most, if not all, of the phosphate groups are introduced into the
molecules after the polypeptides have been formed (Turkington and
Topper, 1966a).

Lactose synthetase is the enzyme complex that synthesizes lactose from
uridine diphosphogalactose and glucose (Watkins and Hassid, 1962;
Bartley *et al.*, 1966). The complex consists of two proteins, A and B. The
A-protein is a galactosyltransferase that is not unique to the mammary
gland (Fleischer *et al.*, 1969). The B-protein was found to be identical to
α-lactalbumin (Brodbeck *et al.*, 1967). Unlike the A-protein, B-protein
has no known enzymic activity by itself, but it lowers the apparent K_m for
glucose so that glucose becomes a physiologically significant acceptor of
the galactosyl portion of uridine diphosphogalactose (Brodbeck *et al.*,
1967; Brew *et al.*, 1968). In essence, B-protein directs A-protein to catalyze
lactose formation. Maximal synthesis of B-protein has the same triple-
hormone requirement as that of casein (Turkington *et al.*, 1968; Palmiter,
1969a).

VIII. REQUIREMENT FOR MITOSIS

One of the early effects of prolactin on the development of mammary cells during pregnancy, as we have seen, is to make it possible for them to respond to insulin and/or serum factor(s). Once this occurs, the floodgates to further development are open. Epithelial proliferation ensues, and this, in turn, makes it possible for glucocorticoid and prolactin to ultimately elicit milk protein formation.

It was pointed out that many generations of mammary epithelial cells arise during puberty. At this time, the cells are insensitive to insulin and serum factor(s), and the identity of the mitogenic agents(s) has not been clearly delineated. In any case, the cells so formed (those present in the adult, virgin mouse) are not *themselves* competent to fabricate milk proteins under the influence of insulin, glucocorticoid, and prolactin. A progression thru mitosis to generate competent daughter cells is necessary for further development. This requirement has been suspected for some years. However, the pertinent experiments were performed with tissue from midpregnant mice, using colchicine and androgens as inhibitors of cell proliferation. It will be shown that the conclusion drawn is unjustified because the wrong model system was used, and because the inhibitors used have serious side effects. Nevertheless, results of a recent study, using a different model system and other inhibitors, do indicate that a mitosis is necessary in virgin tissue.

In earlier studies (Stockdale and Topper, 1966) it was shown that colchicine blocks an increase in milk protein formation by explants from midpregnant mice in the presence of insulin, hydrocortisone, and prolactin. However, since colchicine arrests dividing cells in metaphase, and, since metaphase cells usually have a limited capacity to make proteins (Pfeiffer, 1968; Martin *et al.*, 1969) one cannot conclude that a colchicine block of milk protein production indicates a necessary coupling between cell proliferation and synthesis of milk proteins.

Androgens have been shown to inhibit mammary epithelial DNA synthesis and casein production by midpregnancy explants (Turkington and Topper, 1967). It cannot be concluded from this observation, either, that DNA and casein synthesis are necessarily coupled, because it has been subsequently demonstrated (Owens *et al.*, 1973) that androgen inhibits casein synthesis even by postmitotic cells.

In fact, using inhibitors which do not have these side effects, it can be shown (Owens *et al.*, 1973) that by midpregnancy in the mouse, most of the mammary cells have, indeed, already achieved competence.

Cytosine arabinoside inhibits epithelial DNA synthesis and mitosis in midpregnancy explants almost completely. This agent does reduce the stimulatory effect of insulin, hydrocortisone, and prolactin on the synthesis of casein and α-lactalbumin. But, when the results are normalized to a per-cell basis, it is clear that each cell makes these secretory proteins, in response to the hormones, almost independently of the presence of the inhibitor (Owens *et al.*, 1973).

However, a mitosis is necessary for the mammary epithelial cells in the mature, virgin gland to manufacture milk proteins. Both cytosine arabinoside and fluorodeoxyuridine completely inhibit epithelial DNA synthesis in explants from virgin mice (Owens *et al.*, 1973). The three hormones markedly stimulate the synthesis of casein and cause the emergence of α-lactalbumin synthesis by this tissue. Both inhibitors completely prevent the hormonal stimulation of the formation of the milk proteins (Owens *et al.*, 1973). Neither inhibitor has any postmitotic effect on the synthesis of these proteins.

It is clear that the parent, virgin cells are not competent to make milk proteins in response to the hormones. It is not known whether DNA synthesis alone (leading to G-2 cells) is sufficient, or whether mitosis, which generates daughter cells, is necessary for development of competency. In the normal course of events, of course, daughter cells are indeed formed after DNA duplication and become the source of milk proteins. It is relevant to note that stimulation, by insulin, of the synthesis of glucose-6-phosphate dehydrogenase, a protein which is not unique to the mammary gland appears not to be dependent on mitosis (Owens *et al.*, 1973).

IX. SELECTION OF A SYSTEM FOR FURTHER STUDY

It has been established that after the mammary cells from virgin mice acquire insulin sensitivity *in vitro*, they can generate competent daughter cells. These cells can themselves manufacture casein and α-lactalbumin in response to actions of insulin, glucocorticoid, and prolactin. All the studies to be discussed represent attempts to understand the hormone-mediated events embodied in the basic experiment just described, which result in the transformation of nonsecretory into secretory mammary epithelial cells. Effective analysis of the system would obviously include determination of the changes wrought by each hormone, and delineation of permissible sequences of development. Dissection of this type requires that incomplete complements of the hormones be capable of evoking partial responses, which, in sum, are climaxed by fabrication of the milk proteins. Although explants from the mammary gland of virgin mice can make these proteins when all three hormones are added simultaneously, they had not been responding when the hormones were added sequentially in the various combinations tested. Quite recently, however, it has been possible to effect this response after sequential addition of the hormones (Vonderhaar and Topper, unpublished). Explants from mice in midpregnancy do make increased amounts of casein and α-lactalbumin after sequential addition of the hormones. The biological system used for further analysis, therefore, was mammary tissue derived from mice in the tenth to twelfth day of pregnancy.

X. DEVELOPMENTAL STATUS OF MAMMARY EPITHELIAL CELLS IN THE MIDPREGNANT MOUSE*

Comparison of whole mounts prepared from mammary glands of mature virgin mice and mice in midpregnancy reveals that considerable alveolar epithelial proliferation occurs during the first half of pregnancy. This is consistent with the fact that the mouse mammary cells become sensitive to mitogens such as insulin and serum factor(s) early in pregnancy. One round of cell replication represents the critical mitosis, discussed above. Additional rounds obviously serve to increase the number of potential milk-producing units which will be available during lactation.

---

* *Abbreviations: I-alveoli* contain I-cells. (These comprise the major alveolar component in midpregnancy mouse mammary gland. The cells have undergone a critical mitosis *in vivo* in the presence of insulin. They have the least specialized ultrastructure, described in the text.) *I°-alveoli* contains I°-cells. (These are present *in vitro* after exposure to insulin alone, and have essentially the same ultrastructure as I-alveoli.) *IF-alveoli* contain IF-cells. [These comprise a minor alveolar component in midpregnancy mouse mammary gland. They have the intermediate ultrastructure (uniformly distributed RER, etc.) described in the text.] *IF°-alveoli* contain IF°-cells. (These are present *in vitro* after exposure to insulin and hydrocortisone and have essentially the same ultrastructure as IF-alveoli.) *IFP-alveoli* contain IFP-cells. (These comprise a minor alveolar component in midpregnancy mouse mammary gland. They have the secretory ultrastructure described in the text.) *IFP°-alveoli* contain IFP°-cells. (These are present *in vitro* after exposure to insulin, hydrocortisone, and prolactin and have essentially the same ultrastructure as IFP-alveoli.)

The initial rate of casein synthesis (per unit weight of wet tissue) by explants from midpregnancy tissue is 8–10 times that observed with explants from mature virgin mice, and 10–20% that from lactating mice (Lockwood et al., 1966). Furthermore, while the virgin gland exhibits barely detectable B-protein activity (Turkington et al., 1968; Palmiter, 1969a; McKenzie et al., 1971; Vonderhaar et al., 1973), the pregnant gland has about 1% of the amount present in lactating tissue (Vonderhaar and Topper, unpublished). It is apparent that some functional development occurs during the first half of pregnancy in the mouse and that the capacity to make casein evolves earlier than the capacity to make B-protein (Turkington et al., 1968; McKenzie et al., 1971).

It was pointed out earlier that rat mammary cells do not develop insulin sensitivity until late pregnancy. Consistent with this fact are the observations that rat mammary epithelial DNA concentration does not increase during the first half of pregnancy (Oka and Topper, 1972a), and that midpregnancy rat gland has no detectable B-protein activity (McKenzie et al., 1971).

Ultrastructural development of the alveoli is asynchronous in the first 12 days of pregnancy in the mouse, although within a given alveolus the epithelial cells have similar morphology (Mills and Topper, 1970). At midpregnancy a small percentage of alveoli (IFP-alveoli) have a characteristic secretory appearance (Hollmann, 1959; Wellings et al., 1966). They display a fairly discrete polarity of organelles. The well-developed rough endoplasmic reticulum (RER) and enlarged nuclei, containing enlarged nucleoli, are located at the base of the cell, while the engorged Golgi apparatus is in the apical cytoplasm. Numerous vacuoles containing protein granules are in the Golgi, and protein granules outside the Golgi are also seen in the apical cytoplasm. Many free ribosomes and lipid droplets are found throughout the cytoplasm. It is reasonable to suppose that most, if not all, of the milk proteins made by the gland during this stage are actually produced by these IFP-alveoli.

Another small percentage of alveoli (IF-alveoli) have a less advanced, nonsecretory ultrastructure. Their organelles are not geographically polarized. They have a rich supply of RER, but it is randomly distributed, and the nucleus occupies a position in the center of the cell. The Golgi apparatus usually is lateral to the nucleus, and its vesicles, vacuoles, and cisternae appear empty. Small lipid droplets are occasionally encountered, but protein granules are rarely seen.

Most of the alveoli (I-alveoli) in the midpregnancy gland are obviously nonsecretory. They have numerous free ribosomes throughout their cytoplasm, but the most dramatic difference between them and the nonsecretory IF-alveoli is that I-alveoli have virtually no RER. In fact, I-alveolar cells look very similar to those in the mature virgin. There are, however, two important differences, relevant to this discussion but not discernible in electron micrographs, between I-cells and alveolar cells in the virgin. I-cells are insulin sensitive, and are progeny of cells that have undergone critical mitosis. Cells in the gland of the virgin are insulin insensitive and have not experienced critical mitosis.

XI. SYNCHRONIZATION OF MIDPREGNANCY ALVEOLAR CELLS

A. Incubation in the Presence of Insulin

The minimal concentration of insulin necessary to elicit the changes to be described is 10^{-7} M when the previously reported organ culture technique is used (Rivera, 1964; Juergens *et al.*, 1965). However, when 2.5% bovine serum albumin is added to the chemically defined medium to minimize loss of hormone due to adsorption on glassware, the minimal effective concentration of insulin is 10^{-9} M (Friedberg *et al.*, 1970).

Insulin exerts a mitogenic effect on the epithelial component of midpregnancy explants similar to that described for sensitized explants from the virgin. In the presence of the hormone, epithelial DNA synthesis reaches a peak after about 24 hours of culture (Stockdale and Topper, 1966) and virtually ceases after 3–4 days. Microscopic examination reveals that the average number of cells per alveolar cross section has increased from an initial value of 8 to a value of 16 at this time (Mills and Topper, 1970). In the absence of the hormone the relatively high initial DNA synthetic activity declines precipitously (Friedberg *et al.*, 1970). Nothing is known about the mechanism by which insulin directs the mammary cells to enter the DNA synthetic phase (S-phase) of the cell cycle. In fact, almost nothing is known about the control of entry of any eucaryotic cell into S-phase.

Ultrastructural changes also occur during exposure to insulin. After 48 hours many additional alveolar cells develop a copious supply of randomly distributed RER (Mills and Topper, unpublished; Oka and Topper, 1971a). However, after 96 hours virtually all the alveolar cells exhibit the morphological features of I-alveoli described above (Mills and Topper, 1970). Thus, both the IFP-alveoli and the IF-alveoli initially present regress to a less specialized state, and the daughter cells are morphologically indistinguishable from the major fraction of alveolar cells present in the freshly excised tissue. It is clear that insulin alone is not capable of maintaining certain organelles and organellar configurations. The only structural difference, discernible by microscopy, between I-alveoli and I*-alveoli is that the latter contain more cells. However, chemical analysis reveals that I*-cells have more free ribosomes (Turkington and Riddle, 1970; Oka and Topper, 1971a).

Functional regression accompanies the structural regression. As the IFP-alveoli lose their secretory appearance, casein synthesis declines. After 4 days, formation of these phosphoproteins is no longer detectable (Turkington et al., 1967b). This synchronization, at a low level of specialization, provides operational advantages. It affords an opportunity to study the developmental ascent of a more homogeneous population of cells, and to demonstrate, as we shall see, that many of the developmental changes that these cells experience are reversible.

Insulin elicits other responses by the epithelial cells. It can, even in the absence of glucocorticoid and prolactin, stimulate the synthesis of glucose-6-phosphate dehydrogenase and gluconate-6-phosphate dehydrogenase (Leader and Barry, 1969; Friedberg et al., 1970). These enzymes of the oxidative pathway for glucose metabolism generate NADPH, a co-factor required for the synthesis of fatty acids. Augmentation of this pathway may, then, anticipate the eventual formation of milk lipids.

The formation of certain other nonsecretory proteins is also stimulated maximally by insulin in the absence of other added hormones (Lockwood et al., 1966). This is true in spite of the fact that in the presence of all three hormones the number of ribosomes is increased. It is clear that the hormonal requirements for the formation of many nonsecretory proteins by mammary cells are different from those for the secretory proteins.

Stimulation of epithelial RNA polymerase activity represents an early action of insulin (Turkington and Ward, 1969). It is not known whether this effect is relevant to the proliferative response evoked by the hormone, or to the ultimate synthesis of casein and α-lactalbumin. It is at least partly related to an insulin-induced increase in RNA synthesis including ribosome formation (Mayne et al., 1966; Stockdale et al., 1966; Palmiter, 1969b; Turkington, 1970a,b; Oka and Topper, 1971a) and augmented synthesis of certain nonsecretory proteins (Lockwood et al., 1966; Mayne et al., 1966).

As in many other cells, histone synthesis accompanies DNA synthesis in mammary epithelial cells (Irvin et al., 1963; Chalkley and Maurer, 1965). Insulin stimulates phosphorylation of certain mammary cell histones (Marzluff et al., 1969; Marzluff and McCarty, 1970). It remains to be determined if this effect is relevant to the ultimate formation of milk proteins.

B. Incubation in the Presence of Insulin and Hydrocortisone

1. After 96 Hours

Culture of midpregnancy explants for 4 days in the presence of insulin and hydrocortisone (F, minimal effective concentration, $10^{-8} M$) results in the same degree of alveolar cell proliferation as occurs in the presence of insulin alone (Mills and Topper, 1970). Thus, hydrocortisone has no proliferative effect on these cells (Stockdale and Topper, 1966). Again, casein synthesis becomes undetectable (Turkington *et al.*, 1967b), suggesting that the IFP-alveoli present initially have regressed after 4 days. In regard to cell number and lack of casein synthesis, then, I*-alveoli and IF*-alveoli are alike. Electron microscopy, however, reveals a dramatic difference (Mills and Topper, 1969). Essentially all of the IF*-cells have the rich supply of randomly distributed RER characteristic of the IF-alveolar cells described earlier. In this case, synchronization at an intermediate stage of development is a result of regression of the IFP-alveoli, and progression of the I-alveoli. I*- and IF*-cells have about the same increased total number of ribosomes (Oka and Topper, 1971a). However, most of the ribosomes are free in the cytoplasm in the I*-cells, while many are membrane-bound in the IF*-cells. RER, of course, is an important component of the translational machinery for the production of secretory proteins. Lack of casein synthesis indicates that this machinery is virtually nonfunctional in the stage of development represented by IF*-cells, for reasons to be discussed later.

2. Time Course of RER Development

The transient formation of RER after 48 hours with insulin was alluded to earlier. This has been observed in electron micrographs (Mills and Topper, unpublished) and by isolation of the microsomes on sucrose gradients (Oka and Topper, 1971a). Such membranes are not only labile, they are also deficient in a characteristic enzyme activity, NADH-cytochrome c reductase. It is not known whether deficiency of the enzyme is responsible for the ephemeral nature of the membranes.

Hydrocortisone alone causes almost no increase in isolatable RER, and only a small increase in the activity of NADH-cytochrome c reductase during the course of 96 hours of culture (Oka and Topper, 1971a).

Insulin and hydrocortisone together promote maximal formation of isolatable RER and NADH-cytochrome c reductase activity by 48 hours (Oka and Topper, 1971a). Both remain elevated after 96 hours in the presence of the two hormones. It is clear that these effects represent key functions of glucocorticoid on this system. [Similar effects of glucocorticoid have been confirmed *in vivo* (Banerjee and Banerjee, 1971).] But it is equally apparent that insulin is also required for these biological responses. Recall that insulin-insensitive virgin cells are almost devoid of RER in spite of the presence of circulating glucocorticoids.

3. Sequential Addition of Insulin and Hydrocortisone

Postmitotic I*-cells can be converted into the equivalent of IF*-cells by the addition of hydrocortisone (Oka and Topper, 1971a). There is some analytic advantage in creating IF*-cells by sequential addition, rather than by the simultaneous addition of the hormones. Events that are related to RER formation can be more easily distinguished from those related to DNA synthesis, for instance.

Within about 36 hours after addition of hydrocortisone to I*-cells (in the continued presence of insulin) an augmented epithelial content of RER can be observed, and this reaches a maximum after 60–72 hours (Oka and Topper, 1971a). During this time the total number of ribosomes remains approximately constant, but they become redistributed in the cell. As the ribosomal component of the RER increases there is a reciprocal fall in the free ribosomes within the cytoplasm. It is not known whether the hormones play a direct role in the translocation of the ribosomes. Hydrocortisone does not detectably increase the rate of total epithelial RNA synthesis (Green and Topper, 1970; Oka and Topper, 1971a). This observation is consistent with the fact that the steroid does not increase the total number of ribosomes but does not rule out the possibility that increased synthesis of a particular RNA species related to fabrication of RER occurs.

The RER formed under the conditions described is viable. It is potentially capable of synthesizing the milk proteins. This system appears to be a good model for study of the biogenesis of RER in greater detail.

C. Incubation in the Presence of Prolactin

1. Addition of Prolactin to IF*-cells (in the Continuing Presence of I and F)

Casein synthesis emerges and B-protein activity begins to increase 8–12 hours after the addition of prolactin to IF*-explants (Turkington *et al.*, 1967b, 1968; Turkington and Ward, 1969). Both syntheses reach a maximum after about 48 hours (Vonderhaar *et al.*, unpublished).

In concert with this functional maturation the ultrastructure of the cells changes from that of the IF*-type to the IFP*-type. Within about 48 hours virtually all of the alveolar cells are synchronized at the IFP* level (Mills and Topper, 1970). It is not known whether the translocation of organelles, largely under the influence of prolactin, is a prelude to, or a consequence of, secretory activity.

It is known that RNA synthesis is required in order that milk protein formation occur after the addition of prolactin (Turkington, 1968). Moreover, it has been shown that prolactin increases RNA synthesis (Turkington, 1969; Turkington and Ward, 1969; Green and Topper, 1970; Green *et al.*, 1971; Oka and Topper, 1971a) and the RNA content (Green and Topper, 1970; Oka and Topper, 1971a) of IF*-cells. The ribosomal component of the RER is augmented (Oka and Topper, 1971a), and formation of all detectable molecular species of RNA is increased. However, no selective effect on particular types of RNA has been observed, and no new species of RNA have yet been seen to emerge under the influence of prolactin (Green *et al.*, 1971).

It is not certain whether or not hydrocortisone need be present during the conversion of IF*- into IFP*-cells (Lockwood *et al.*, 1967), but it is clear that both insulin and prolactin are required for this conversion (Voytovich *et al.*, 1969). Do both hormones have to be present simultaneously, and if not, what is the sequence in which they operate? It has been shown (Voytovich *et al.*, 1969) that prolactin can execute at least part of its functions in the absence of insulin, but that insulin must be present terminally in order that casein synthesis can emerge.

2. Addition of Hydrocortisone and Prolactin to I*-cells

While it takes about 48 hours for most IF*-cells to be converted into IFP*-cells after the addition of prolactin, it takes about 96 hours for I*-cells to be converted into IFP*-cells after the simultaneous addition of hydrocortisone and prolactin. What additional information can be gained from the latter experiment? From observation of ultrastructural changes as a function of time (Mills and Topper, 1970) it is known that prolactin does not promote translocation of the Golgi apparatus or nucleus until hydrocortisone, in conjunction with insulin, has caused the accumulation of randomly distributed RER. Each process takes about 48 hours. This has been confirmed with biochemical techniques (Oka and Topper, 1971a). RER, isolatable on sucrose gradients, begins to increase after about 36 hours and reaches a maximum after 60–72 hours, while casein synthesis does not emerge until about 60 hours, reaching a maximum after about 120 hours. These studies demonstrate that the formation of secretory protein by mammary cells requires RER. This, of course, is also true for other secretory cells. In contrast, it will be recalled that maximal synthesis of certain nonsecretory proteins by mammary cells does not require RER. These studies show, in addition, that some of the modulations elicited by prolactin are dependent upon prior exposure of the cells to glucocorticoid.

3. Addition of Prolactin to I*-cells

It has been pointed out that some of the major ultrastructural and functional effects of prolactin must await the accumulation of RER in the mammary cell. This does not appear to represent a case of prolactin insensitivity analogous to the insulin insensitivity discussed earlier. I*-cells, which lack RER, do, in fact, seem to be capable of responding to prolactin initially, although casein synthesis is undetectable under these circumstances (Oka and Topper, 1971a), even after 5 days of culture. RNA synthesis is transiently increased. For about 24 hours after its addition, prolactin stimulates total RNA synthesis by both I*-cell and IF*-cells to almost the same extent. Subsequently, this effect falls precipitously in the I*-cells but is sustained for another 24 hours in the IF*-cells. When hydrocortisone is added to I*-cells concomitantly with prolactin, a second burst of RNA synthesis occurs after 48 hours, i.e., after RER has accumulated. It appears, then, that RNA formation which is promoted by prolactin is initially independent of RER, but that sustained formation of RNA under the influence of prolactin is dependent on the RER. The precise nature of the control that RER seems to exert on these transcriptional events is not known. In any case the I*-cells are initially competent to respond to prolactin in terms of total RNA synthesis, but the lack of the membranes somehow switches off such synthesis at a later time.

In two instances the mammary epithelial cell seems incipiently capable of undergoing development in the absence of glucocorticoid, only to have these changes aborted for lack of the steroid. The transient nature of the RER formed in the presence of insulin is one case in point. The short-lived burst of RNA synthesis after addition of prolactin to I*-cells is the second. The mechanisms by which glucocorticoids sustain these effects remain to be elucidated.

XII. ADDITIONAL CONSIDERATIONS

Discussion of some aspects of the development of the mammary gland has been deferred until this final section, not because they are more or less interesting than those considered earlier, but because inclusion in previous sections would have interrupted the continuity. Consideration of these aspects here will not only introduce additional information, but will also serve to summarize certain concepts discussed previously.

The development of a number of different types of embryonic epithelial cells is dependent upon the presence of diffusible factors derived from mesenchymal cells. Embryonic mammary cells also exhibit such dependency in terms of morphogenesis (Kratochwil, 1969). In this chapter, of course, we have considered development of mammary cells of the adult animal. It has been shown that acquisition of insulin and serum sensitivity is not dependent upon any contribution from the mammary fat cells. It has also been demonstrated that insulin can promote epithelial proliferation (Oka and Topper, unpublished) and stimulate epithelial RNA synthesis in the absence of the fat cells (Turkington, 1970b). However, it is not known whether or not the other developmental phenomena discussed are influenced by mesenchyme. In other words, it is not known whether milk protein synthesis can be induced by the hormones without the intervention of mesenchyme.

Nothing has been said about estrogen and progesterone in the context of development of the gland in the adult animal. This is because the cells from such a gland can, in fact, be induced to produce milk proteins in the presence of insulin, glucocorticoid, and prolactin, but in the absence of exogenous estrogen and progesterone. It may be, however, that the sex steroids play a morphogenetic role in the adult, similar to that which they appear to play in the development of mammary gland in the immature animal (Cowie and Folley, 1961; Jacobsohn, 1961; Ichinose and Nandi, 1964).

In the presence of insulin, glucocorticoid, and prolactin, mammary explants from mature virgin mice synthesize casein maximally after 3 days of culture (Stockdale and Topper, 1966; Vonderhaar et al., 1973), while the emergence of B-protein activity is retarded by 1–2 days (Vonderhaar et al., 1973). In contrast, explants from pregnant mice respond synchronously in terms of these proteins (Vonderhaar et al., 1973). Administration of a relatively small amount of prolactin to virgin mice, an amount insufficient to induce insulin and serum sensitivity, results in synchronous synthesis of these proteins by virgin explants (Vonderhaar et al., 1973). This synchronization effect of prolactin appears to be distinct from the sensitization effect, and from the terminal action of prolactin which leads, in the presence of insulin, to the prompt appearance of casein and B-protein activity.

Although mammary explants from pregnant mice produce casein and

B-protein synchronously, partly as a consequence of exposure to elevated levels of prolactin early during pregnancy in the mouse, the gland in the intact mouse does not form appreciable B-protein until about the time of parturition. Presumably, this is due to a repressive effect of progesterone (Turkington and Hill, 1969) superimposed upon the synchronization effect of prolactin (Vonderhaar *et al.*, 1973).

With the advent of insulin- and serum-sensitivity, the mammary cells can undergo a critical mitosis, and then proceed to develop further under the influence of the hormones. In the experiments described earlier, using Medium 199, insulin promoted only one round of alveolar cell division. When an organic buffer, N-2-hydroxyethylpiperazine-N-2-ethanesulfonic acid, is added to the medium, insulin promotes several rounds of DNA synthesis (Oka and Topper, upublished). Insulin-free serum also promotes several rounds of DNA synthesis (Majumder and Turkington, 1971). It is not known whether insulin [or serum factor(s), or both] is the mitogenic agent that operates during pregnancy. It appears, however, that only insulin can synergize with prolactin in regard to the terminal action of the pituitary hormone (Majumder and Turkington, 1971).

Hydrocortisone is not the only glucocorticoid which is effective on the mammary gland system *in vitro*. A number of other steroids with glucocorticoid activity, including aldosterone and corticosterone, the natural murine glucocorticoid, are also active (Turkington *et al.*, 1967a).

Human placental lactogen (Turkington and Topper, 1966b) and, to some extent, ovine growth hormone, can simulate the action of prolactin in regard to its terminal synergism with insulin. It is not yet known whether they can also synchronize mammary tissue in terms of casein and α-lactalbumin, or sensitize virgin cells to insulin and serum factor(s).

The analysis of the intricate interdependencies of hormone effects on the mammary gland system has been largely descriptive. Elucidation of these effects at a molecular level should be a major goal for the future.

REFERENCES

Amenomori, Y., Chen, C. L., and Meites, J. (1970). *Endocrinology* **86**, 506.
Banerjee, M. R., and Banerjee, D. N. (1971). *Exp. Cell Res.* **64**, 307.
Bartley, J. C., Abraham, S., and Chaikoff, I. L. (1966). *J. Biol. Chem.* **241**, 1132.
Brew, K., Vanaman, T. C., and Hill, R. L. (1968). *Proc. Nat. Acad. Sci. US* **59**, 491.
Brodbeck, U., Denton, W. L., Tanahashi, N., and Ebner, K. E. (1967). *J. Biol. Chem.* **242**, 1391.
Browning, H. C., Larke, G. A., and White, W. D. (1962). *Proc. Soc. Exp. Biol. Med.* **111**, 686.

Bronson, F. H., Dagg, C. D., and Snell, G. D. (1966). In "Biology of the Laboratory Mouse" (E. L. Green, ed.), pp. 187–204. McGraw-Hill, New York.

Chalkley, G. R., and Maurer, H. R. (1965). *Proc. Nat. Acad. Sci. US* **54**, 498.

Cowie, A. T., and Folley, S. J. (1961). In "Sex and Internal Secretions" (W. C. Young, ed.), 3rd ed., pp. 590–642. Williams and Wilkins, Baltimore, Maryland.

Cuatrecasas, P. (1969). *Proc. Nat. Acad. Sci. US* **63**, 450.

Elias, J. J. (1957). *Science* **126**, 842.

Elias, J. J. (1959). *Proc. Soc. Exp. Biol. Med.* **101**, 500.

Fleischer, B., Fleischer, S., and Ozawa, H. (1969). *J. Cell Biol.* **43**, 59.

Friedberg, S. H., Oka, T., and Topper, Y. J. (1970). *Proc. Nat. Acad. Sci. US* **67**, 1493.

Green, M. R., and Topper, Y. J. (1970). *Biochim. Biophys. Acta* **204**, 441.

Green, M. R., Bunting, S. L., and Peacock, A. C. (1971). *Biochemistry* **10**, 2366.

Hollmann, K. H. (1959). *J. Ultrastruct. Res.* **2**, 423.

Ichinose, R. R., and Nandi, S. (1964). *Science* **145**, 496.

Irvin, J. L., Holbrook, D. J., Jr., Evans, J. H., McAllister, H. C., and Stiles, E. P. (1963). *Exp. Cell Res. Suppl.* **9**, 359.

Jacobsohn, D. (1961). In "Milk: the Mammary Gland and its Secretion" (C. S. K. Kon and A. T. Cowie, eds.), Vol. 1, pp. 127–160. Academic Press, New York.

Jensen, E. V., Suzuki, T., Kawashima, T., Stumpf, W. E., Jungblut, P. W., and De-Sombre, E. R. (1968). *Proc. Nat. Acad. Sci. US* **57**, 632.

Johnson, C. B., Blecher, M., and Giorgio, N. A., Jr. (1972). *Biochem. Biophys. Res. Commun.* **46**, 1035.

Juergens, W. G., Stockdale, F. E., Topper, Y. J., and Elias, J. J. (1965). *Proc. Nat. Acad. Sci. US* **54**, 629.

Kratochwil, K. (1969). *Develop. Biol.* **20**, 46.

Leader, D. P., and Barry, J. M. (1969). *Biochem. J.* **113**, 175.

Linkie, D. M., and Niswender, G. D. (1972). *Endocrinology* **90**, 632.

Lockwood, D. H., Turkington, R. W., and Topper, Y. J. (1966). *Biochim. Biophys. Acta* **130**, 493.

Lockwood, D. H., Stockdale, F. E., and Topper, Y. J. (1967). *Science* **156**, 945.

Lyons, W. R., Li, C. H., and Johnson, R. E. (1958). *Recent Progr. Hormone Res.* **14**, 219.

Lyons, W. R., Li, C. H., Ahmad, N., and Rice-Wray, E. (1967). *Proc. Int. Symp. Growth Hormone, Milan, Italy* p. 349.

Majumder, G. C., and Turkington, R. W. (1971). *Endocrinology* **88**, 1506.

Martin, D., Jr., Tomkins, G. M., and Granner, D. (1969). *Proc. Nat. Acad. Sci. US* **62**, 248.

Marzluff, W. F., Jr., McCarty, K. S., and Turkington, R. W. (1969). *Biochim. Biophys. Acta* **190**, 517.

Marzluff, W. F., Jr., and McCarty, K. S. (1970). *J. Biol. Chem.* **245**, 5637.

Mayne, R., Barry, J. M., and Rivera, E. M. (1966). *Biochem. J.* **99**, 688.

Mayne, R., Forsyth, I. A., and Barry, J. M. (1968). *J. Endocrinol.* **41**, 247.

McKenzie, L., Fitzgerald, D. K., and Ebner, K. E. (1971). *Biochim. Biophys. Acta* **230**, 526.

Mills, E. S., and Topper, Y. J. (1969). *Science* **165**, 1127.

Mills, E. S., and Topper, Y. J. (1970). *J. Cell Biol.* **44**, 310.

Oka, T., and Topper, Y. J. (1971a). *J. Biol. Chem.* **246**, 7701.

Oka, T., and Topper, Y. J. (1971b). *Proc. Nat. Acad. Sci. US* **68**, 2066.

Oka, T., and Topper, Y. J. (1972a). *Proc. Nat. Acad. Sci. US* **69**, 693.

Oka, T., and Topper, Y. J. (1972b). *Nature New Biol.* **239**, 216.

Owens, I. S., Vonderhaar, B. K., and Topper, Y. J. (1973) *J. Biol. Chem.* **248**, 472.

Palmiter, R. D. (1969a). *Biochem. J.* **113**, 409.

Palmiter, R. D. (1969b). *Endocrinology* **85**, 747.

Pfeiffer, S. E. (1968). *J. Cell Physiol.* **71**, 95.

Prop, F. J. A. (1961). *Pathol. Biol.* **9**, 640.

Rivera, E. M. (1964). *Endocrinology* **74**, 853.

Sekhri, K. K., Pitelka, D. R., and DeOme, K. B. (1967). *J. Nat. Cancer Inst.* **39**, 459.

Selinger, R. C. L., and Civen, M. (1971). *Biochem. Biophys. Res. Commun.* **43**, 793.

Stockdale, F. E., and Topper, Y. J. (1966). *Proc. Nat. Acad. Sci. US* **56**, 1283.

Stockdale, F. E., Juergens, W. G., and Topper, Y. J. (1966). *Develop. Biol.* **13**, 266.

Topper, Y. J. (1968). *Trans. N. Y. Acad. Sci.* **30**, 869.

Topper, Y. J., and Oka, T. (1971). *In* "Effects of Drugs on Cellular Control Mechanisms" (B. R. Rabin and R. B. Freedman, eds.), pp. 131–150. Macmillan, New York.

Turkington, R. W. (1968). *Endocrinology* **82**, 575.

Turkington, R. W. (1969). *J. Biol. Chem.* **244**, 5140.

Turkington, R. W. (1970a). *J. Biol. Chem.* **245**, 6690.

Turkington, R. W. (1970b). *Biochem. Biophys. Res. Commun.* **41**, 1362.

Turkington, R. W., and Hill, R. L. (1969). *Science* **163**, 1458.

Turkington, R. W., and Riddle, M. (1970). *J. Biol. Chem.* **245**, 5145.

Turkington, R. W., and Topper, Y. J. (1966a). *Biochim. Biophys. Acta* **127**, 366.

Turkington, R. W., and Topper, Y. J. (1966b). *Endocrinology* **79**, 175.

Turkington, R. W., and Topper, Y. J. (1967). *Endocrinology* **80**, 329.

Turkington, R. W., and Ward, O. T. (1969). *Biochim. Biophys. Acta* **174**, 291.

Turkington, R. W., Juergens, W. G., and Topper, Y. J. (1965). *Biochim. Biophys. Acta* **111**, 573.

Turkington, R. W., Juergens, W. G., and Topper, Y. J. (1967a). *Endocrinology* **80**, 1139.

Turkington, R. W., Lockwood, D. H., and Topper, Y. J. (1967b). *Biochim. Biophys. Acta* **148**, 475.

Turkington, R .W., Brew, K., Vanaman, T. C. and Hill, R. L. (1968). *J. Biol. Chem.* **243**, 3382.

Vonderhaar, B. K., Owens, I. S., and Topper, Y. J. (1973) *J. Biol. Chem.* **248**, 467.

Voytovich, A. E., and Topper, Y. J. (1967). *Science* **158**, 1326.

Voytovich, A. E., Owens, I. S., and Topper, Y. J. (1969). *Proc. Nat. Acad. Sci. US* **63**, 213.

Watkins, W. M., and Hassid, W. Z. (1962). *J. Biol. Chem.* **237**, 1432.

Wellings, S. R., Cooper, R. A., and Rivera, E. M. (1966). *J. Nat. Cancer Inst.* **36**, 657.

CHAPTER SEVEN

Enzymatic and Metabolic Changes in the Development of Lactation

R. L. Baldwin and Y. T. Yang

I. Introduction 349
II. Mammary Enzyme Levels, Characteristics, and Relationships
    to Milk Synthesis 351
    A. Glucose Activation 364
    B. Lactose Synthesis 367
    C. Pentose Cycle 369
    D. Embden–Meyerhof Glycolysis 373
    E. Citric Acid Cycle and Related Functions 378
    F. Fatty Acid Synthesis: Metabolism and Esterification ... 383
    G. Other Enzymes 386
III. Regulation of Mammary Enzyme Activities 389
    A. Changes in Enzyme Activities during Secretory Cell De-
       velopment, Lactogenesis, Lactation, and Involution . 389
    B. Hormones and the Regulation of Mammary Enzyme
       Activities 399
IV. Summary 406
    References 407

I. INTRODUCTION

Mammary enzymes have been investigated with the objectives of proving the presence of specific metabolic pathways in mammary tissue, of studying mammary development and lactogenesis, of evaluating hormone actions upon the mammary gland, and of evaluating relationships between changes in enzyme activities and changes in metabolic activities and patterns. Different considerations and constraints are applied in interpreting enzyme data with regard to each of these objectives. Demonstration of the presence in mammary secretory cells of each enzyme in a pathway is an essential element of proof required to establish the participation of that pathway in mammary metabolism and milk synthesis. Other types (radioisotope tracer) of data are required to determine the extent to which a pathway contributes, but presence of the enzymes must be demonstrated to establish that the pathway can participate or is present. In the cases of mammary development and determinations of hormone actions on the mammary gland, interpretations of enzyme data are, on the surface, straightforward. If an enzyme is uniquely found in mammary secretory cells or its activity is much higher in mature mammary secretory cells than in other cell types, as is the case with many enzymes, then increases in the activities of these enzymes can be interpreted as reflecting either increases in mammary secretory cell numbers or the development of secretory cells. If mammary DNA levels are increasing at the same time enzyme levels are increasing, it seems reasonable to conclude that the enzyme changes reflect the formation and development of secretory cells. Similarly, if it is suspected that a given hormone acts upon the mammary gland to cause general or specific changes in enzyme levels in secretory cells, demonstrations of appropriate enzyme changes attributable to administration of a hormone or to hormone insufficiency can be applied as partial proof of the hypothesis as long as care is taken to assure that the hormone actions are direct and upon the mammary gland and to distinguish general from specific enzyme responses. Interpretations of enzyme data in relation to mammary metabolism and metabolic regulation are less straightforward. Although good relationships or correlations are often observed between changes in enzyme activities and changes in metabolism, numerous exceptions have been reported wherein metabolic changes occurred in the absence of enzyme changes or vice versa and where enzyme changes were not essential to or for a correlated metabolic change. Also, demonstration that an enzyme has metabolic regulatory properties does not establish the fact that these properties are expressed *in vivo*. For these reasons, it is not possible to relate enzyme and metabolic changes in a cause and effect fashion based on simple enzyme data. In recent years some progress has been made in developing additional or auxiliary techniques and approaches which, in part, enable further evaluation of relationships between enzyme levels and metabolism. In this chapter, specific attention has been directed at evaluations of mammary enzyme data with regard to the pathways of milk synthesis, mammary gland development and function, actions of several hormones *in vivo* and possible and/or probable relationships between changes in enzyme activities and mammary metabolism. In developing the first section of the chapter, "normal" activities of a number of mammary enzymes for several species in full lactation are tabulated. In addition, these enzymes are considered in terms of their metabolic role, their assay, their properties, and their roles in the regulation of mammary metabolism. In subsequent sections, enzyme changes related to mammary development and function, involution, and to hormone actions are considered.

II. MAMMARY ENZYME LEVELS, CHARACTERISTICS, AND RELATIONSHIPS TO MILK SYNTHESIS

In this section, an attempt is made to summarize a wide range of data relevant to the activities, metabolic roles, and regulatory characteristics of several mammary enzymes. In order to assure brevity and ready reference, a number of these data are presented in tabular form. A description of the reasoning behind and methods of summarization and computation of the tabular data are presented in subsequent paragraphs. These descriptions are followed by discussions of several enzymes in which nomenclature, assay methods, enzyme characteristics, and probable roles of the enzymes in the regulation of mammary metabolism are considered. Several enzymes are also discussed in the chapters on lactose synthesis (Chapter 3, Vol. II, by Ebner and Schanbacher) lipid metabolism and milk fat synthesis (Chapters 1 and 2, Vol. II) and amino acid metabolism and protein synthesis (Chapter 4, Vol. II, by Larson and Jorgensen). Discussion of these enzymes was kept at a minimum in this chapter to avoid repetition. However, it was felt that these should be considered briefly to maintain continuity in discussion relative to the role of enzymes and enzyme activity changes in the regulation of mammary metabolism.

The summarization of mammary enzyme levels at peak lactation in rats, cows, rabbits, sows, guinea pigs, and mice presented in Table I is based upon a survey of a number of publications in which mammary enzyme data were reported. Data relating to changes in enzyme activities occurring during pregnancy, lactation, and involution are summarized in Section III. The intent in summarizing mammary enzyme levels in this section was to enable interspecific comparisons, to provide for comparison of reported enzyme activities with *in vivo* flux at peak lactation (Table II), and to provide a convenient, tabular reference for comparison of new enzyme activity data with estimates obtained in previous studies. For these purposes and in view of time dependent differences between species and/or strains in patterns of change in enzyme activities during pregnancy and early and late lactation, it was considered that enzyme activ-

TABLE I

SUMMARIZATION OF RAT, COW, RABBIT, SOW, GUINEA PIG, AND MOUSE MAMMARY ENZYME ACTIVITIES AT PEAK LACTATION

Enzyme and pathway	Species and enzyme activity[a]						References[b]
	Rats	Cows	Rabbits	Sows	Guinea pig	Mice	
Glucose activation							
Hexokinase	1–3	0.1–0.5	0.3	0.44	2.1	1.0–1.5	2, 6, 7, 23, 24, 31, 35, 41, 44, 46, 49
Lactose synthesis							
P-Glucose mutase	2–4	0.5–2.5	1.3	7.8	7.0	1.9	2, 6, 13 15, 23, 24, 27, 33, 34, 35
UDPG-pyrophosphorylase	15–70	16.5	5.5–6.4	40.8	70	7.5	2, 6, 9, 13, 14, 15, 23, 24, 27, 33, 41
UDPglucose-4-epimerase	2–8	1.7	2.5–4.5	3.9	6.6	—	2, 6, 14, 15, 23, 24, 33, 41
Lactose synthetase (galactosyltransferase)	0.01–0.15	0.01–0.24	—	—	—	0.01–0.5	16, 20, 23, 24, 25, 30, 33
Pentose cycle							
Glucose-6-P dehydrogenase	20–50	1.0–7.0	26–54	25–35	20	15–20	2, 4, 5, 6, 7, 8, 15, 23, 24, 31, 32, 33, 35, 38, 42, 44, 50, 51
6-P-Gluconate dehydrogenase	3.5–8.5	1.1–1.7	3–5	1.6–2.8	5.0	3.1	2, 4, 6, 8, 13, 15, 19, 20, 23, 24, 31, 32, 33, 35, 38, 42, 43, 50, 51
Pentose-P-metabolizing activity	3–9	0.70	0.70	1.8	4.5	0.70	2, 6, 23, 24

							References
Embden–Meyerhof glycolysis							
P-Glucose isomerase	50–75	7	24	14.1	35	5.6	2, 6, 23, 24, 31, 34
Phosphofructokinase	2–14	2.7	0.7	—	—	—	3, 5, 13, 15, 19, 23, 24
Fructose-1,6-diphosphate adolase	3–9	0.9	4.5	1.5	4.5	3.2	2, 6, 23, 24
Triose phosphate isomerase	—	100	—	—	—	—	3
Glyceraldehyde-3-P dehydrogenase	30	2.3	1.6	3.0	7.0	1.6	2, 6
Pyruvate kinase	24–35	—	—	—	—	—	22, 23, 24
Lactate dehydrogenase	60–95	19–25	—	—	—	—	4, 21, 23, 24, 38
Citric acid cycle and related functions							
Acetyl-CoA synthetase	1.0–2.1	0.24	1.1	—	—	—	6, 13, 28, 36, 43, 47, 48
Citrate synthetase	—	3.3	—	—	—	—	3
Isocitrate dehydrogenase (NADP)	1–9	20–60	9.6	6.5–8.2	15.0	5.0	2, 6, 8, 23, 24, 33, 37, 38, 42, 47, 48
Glutamate dehydrogenase	2.52	0.3	—	—	—	—	3, 10
Aspartate aminotransferase	15–52	5–20	18.2	19.4	14.1	14.0	2, 3, 6, 10, 17, 23, 24
Succinate dehydrogenase	0.1–2.5	0.06	0.2	1.9	0.05	—	2, 6, 11
Malate dehydrogenase ($NADH_2$;OAA)	200–300	180	180	200–250	300	260	2, 4, 6, 8, 23, 24, 35, 37, 38, 40

TABLE I (*Continued*)

Enzyme and pathway	Species and enzyme activity^a				Guinea pig		References^b
	Rats	Cows	Rabbits	Sows		Mice	
Fatty acid synthesis, metabolism and esterification							
Malic enzyme	5.4–10	0.1–0.2	—	0.13	—	10–15	3, 7, 8, 23, 24, 31, 38, 44
Citrate cleavage enzyme	8–15	0.1–0.2	0.3–0.6	2.2–4.1	1.1	2.5–5.0	2, 7, 8, 13, 18, 19, 23, 24, 26, 35, 37, 44, 45, 47, 48
Acetyl-CoA carboxylase	0.5–1.2	0.20	0.02–0.12	—	—	0.9	13, 18, 19, 20, 26, 33, 43, 44
Fatty acid synthetase (NADPH$_2$ consumed)	2–10	0.12–1.3	2.9	3.6	0.9	1.6–10	2, 3, 6, 22, 33, 35, 44
α-Glycerol-P dehydrogenase	3.5–6.0	0.5–0.7	0.6	0.3	0.5	2.1–2.3	2, 4, 6, 23, 24, 26, 44
Lipoprotein lipase (μm fatty acid released)	1.5–3	10	—	—	25–40	—	1 2, 12, 29, 39, 42

^{a} Enzyme activity expressed as units per gram fresh tissue.

^{b} References coded as follows: (1) Askew et al., 1970; (2) Baldwin, 1966; (3) Baldwin (unpublished); (4) Baldwin et al., 1969b; (5) Baldwin and Martin, 1968; (6) Baldwin and Milligan, 1966; (7) Bartley et al., 1966; (8) Bauman et al., 1970; (9) Emery and Baldwin, 1967; (10) Greenbaum and Greenwood, 1954; (11) Greenbaum and Slater, 1957; (12) Hamosh et al., 1970; (13) Hartmann and Jones, 1970; (14) Heitzman, 1967; (15) Heitzman, 1969; (16) Helminen and Ericsson, 1971; (17) Herzfeld and Greengard, 1971; (18) Howanitz and Levy, 1965; (19) Jones, 1967; (20) Jones, 1972; (21) Karlsson and Carlsson, 1968; (22) Korsrud and Baldwin, 1969; (23) Korsrud and Baldwin, 1972a; (24) Korsrud and Baldwin, 1972b; (25) Kuhn, 1968; (26) Kuhn and Lowenstein, 1967; (27) Malpress, 1961; (28) Marinez and Cook, 1971; (29) McBride and Korn, 1963; (30) McKenzie et al., 1971; (31) McLean, 1958; (32) McLean, 1964; (33) Mellenberger et al., 1972; (34) Narayanan and Ganguli, 1965; (35) Opstvedt et al., 1967; (36) Ponto et al., 1969; (37) Raineri and Levy, 1970; (38) Rees and Huggins, 1960; (39) Robinson, 1963; (40) Saacke and Heald, 1969; (41) Shatton et al., 1965; (42) Shirley et al., 1971; (43) Smith et al., 1966; (44) Smith et al., 1969; (45) Spencer and Lowenstein, 1966; (46) Walters and McLean, 1967a; (47) Walters and McLean, 1967b; (48) Walters and McLean, 1968a; (49) Walters and McLean, 1968b; (50) Willmer, 1960; and (51) Willmer and Foster, 1965.

ities reported at peak lactation would be the most consistent or reliable base for comparison, reference, and tabulation. The common base for expression of enzyme data used in Table I is units per gram tissue. This base was selected because most of the available data are either expressed as units per gram tissue or could be converted to this form of comparison, evaluation, and summarization. Other bases of expression including, for example, total units per gland, units per milligram DNA, and units per milligram protein are preferred when indices of total gland capacity, enzyme activity per cell and specific enzyme inductions, respectively, are desired. The data in Table I can be easily converted to these bases in evaluating most studies. The major problem encountered in using units per gram tissue as a base for expression of mammary enzyme data is the unknown contribution of milk in the tissue to tissue weight. This problem is prominent in comparing data within a specific experiment or when amounts of residual milk are expected to vary significantly between experimental groups. The objective in preparing Table I was to provide an estimate of the normal range of enzyme levels. Effects of residual milk are likely accommodated within the ranges in enzyme levels tabulated. In comparing literature data and selecting a range of normal values for tabulation which included 80–100% of available data as was done in constructing Table I, a remarkable consistency in data was observed as evidenced by the fact that many of the values cited cover only a two- to threefold range. Differences within these narrow ranges are likely attributable to differences in level of lactation, sources of animals, diet and small methodological differences. In a few cases, very large differences between the values in Table I and data in an individual paper were noted. It was supposed that many of these discrepancies are attributable to computational errors and the data were ignored.

The summary data presented in Tables II and III and Figs. 1 and 2 were prepared for and are presented in support of the discussions of mammary enzymes presented in subsequent paragraphs. It should be noted and recognized at the outset that many of the data and calculations presented in Table II are tentative and speculative. The calculations are presented with the objectives of attempting to summarize and correlate a great many diverse data in a coherent quantitative or semiquantitative context and, by doing so, to assess the state of current knowledge of the roles of mammary enzymes in milk synthesis, the *in vivo* states of the reactions they catalyze, and the potential regulatory or metabolic significances of the enzymes and changes in their *in vivo* activities. Within our knowledge this is the first comprehensive effort undertaken directed at these objectives and, hence, this must be considered a tentative beginning

TABLE II

COMPARISON OF EQUILIBRIUM CONSTANTS AND MASS ACTION COEFFICIENTS AND V_{max}, FORWARD VELOCITY AND *in Vivo* NET MEASUREMENT FOR SELECTED RAT AND COW MAMMARY ENZYMES[a]

Enzyme and pathway	Species	Equilibrium	Constant[b]	Mass action coefficient[c]	V_{max}[a]	Forward velocity[a] in vivo	Net flux[a] in vivo
Glucose activation							
Hexokinase	Rat	$\dfrac{(ADP)(G6P)}{(ATP)(Glucose)}$	$= 1\text{–}5 \times 10^{3}$	$0.6 \sim 2.7 \times 10^{-1}$	172	86	68.7
	Cow			1.2×10^{-2}	60	30	7.0
Lactose synthesis							
P-Glucose mutase	Rat	$\dfrac{(G1P)}{(G6P)}$	$= 0.55\text{–}1.8 \times 10^{-1}$	0.13	58	51	3.8
	Cow			0.49	69	63	4.2
UDPG pyrophosphorylase	Rat	$\dfrac{(PPi)(UDGP)}{(UTP)(G1P)}$	$= 0.28\text{–}0.34$	0.39	1000	130	3.8
	Cow			5.4×10^{-2}	496	150	4.2
UDP glucose-4-epimerase	Rat	$\dfrac{(UDPGal)}{(UDPG)}$	$= 0.284$	—	115	88	3.8
	Cow			—	51	32	4.2
Lactose synthetase	Rat	Irreversible		Irrev.	2.2	1.5	3.8
	Cow				0.3–7.2	0.1	4.2
Pentose cycle							
Glucose-6-P dehydrogenase	Rat	$\dfrac{(6PG)(NADPH)(H^{+})}{(G6P)(NADP)}$	$= 6.0 \times 10^{-7} M$	—	720	590	37
	Cow			—	210	170	4.8

Enzyme	Species	Mass-action ratio	Equilibrium				
6-P-Gluconate dehydrogenase	Rat	$\frac{(RU5P)(NADPH)}{(6PG)(NADP)}$	$= 0.17\ M$	—	115	—	37
	Cow			—	51	—	4.8
Pentose-P metabolizing activity	Rat	—		—	129	—	37
	Cow	—		—	21	—	4.8
Embden-Meyerhof glycolysis							
P-Glucose isomerase	Rat	$\frac{(F6P)}{(G6P)}$	$= 0.28\text{–}0.47$	Assumed equil.	1080	337	27.9
	Cow				210	65	2.0
Phosphofructokinase	Rat	$\frac{(ADP)(F\text{-}1,6\text{-}DiP)}{(ATP)(F6P)}$	$= 0.91\text{–}1.2 \times 10^3$	2.9×10^{-2}	29–202	Complex kinetics	52.5
	Cow			1.5×10^{-1}	80		1.2
Fructose-1,6-diphosphate aldolase	Rat	$\frac{(DHAP)(GAP)}{(F\text{-}1,6\text{-}DiP)}$	$= 6.8\text{–}13 \times 10^{-5}\ M$	$7.3 \times 10^{-5}\ M$	130	0.25	52.5
	Cow			$1.05 \times 10^{-3}\ M$	27	0.60	1.2
Triose-P isomerase	Rat	$\frac{(GAP)}{(DHAP)}$	$= 4.52 \times 10^{-2}$	6.5×10^{-1}	—	—	44.4
	Cow			1.31×10^{-1}	3000	244	0.66
Glyceraldehyde-3-P dehydrogenase	Rat	$\frac{(1,3\ DiPGA)(NADH)}{(GAP)(Pi)(NAD)}$	$= 0.5\ M^{-1}$	—	430	16.4	109.2
	Cow			—	68	35.5	3.5

TABLE II (*Continued*)

Enzyme and pathway	Species	Equilibrium	Constant[b]	Mass action coefficient[c]	V_{max}[d]	Forward velocity[d] in vivo	Net flux[d] in vivo
Pyruvate kinase	Rat	$\dfrac{\text{(Pyruvate)(ATP)}}{\text{(PEP)(ADP)}}$	$= 0.2\text{--}2.0 \times 10^4$	$1.0 \sim 5.4$	335	75	109.2
	Cow			15.5	—	—	3.0
Lactate dehydrogenase	Rat	$\dfrac{\text{(Pyruvate)(NADH)}}{\text{(Lactate)(NAD)}}$	$= 1.11 \times 10^{-4}$	Assume equil.	1370	120	0.0
	Cow					750	24	0.0
Citric acid cycle and related functions							
Citrate synthetase	Rat	$\dfrac{\text{(Citrate)(CoA)}}{\text{(Acetyl CoA)(OAA)(H}_2\text{O)}}$	$= 8.38 \times 10^3\ M^{-1}$	—	—	—	109.2
	Cow			$1.1 \times 10^4\ M^{-1}$	100	29	12.8
Isocitrate dehydrogenase (NADP)	Rat	$\dfrac{\text{(}\alpha\text{KG)(CO}_2\text{)(NADPH)}}{\text{(Isocitrate)(NADP)}}$	$= 0.77\text{--}0.91\ M$	Assume equil.	58	58	0.0
	Cow				1500	1500	3.4
Glutamate dehydrogenase	Rat	$\dfrac{\text{(}\alpha\text{KG)(NAD)(NH}_4^+\text{)}}{\text{(Glutamate)(NADH)}}$	$= 3.87 \times 10^{-6}\ M$	—	37	—	0.0
	Cow				9	—	0.0
Aspartate amino transferase	Rat	$\dfrac{\text{(OAA)(Glutamate)}}{\text{(Aspartate)(}\alpha\text{KG)}}$	$= 0.15\text{--}0.17$	—	750	37	0.0
	Cow				600	37	0.3
Malate dehydrogenase	Rat	$\dfrac{\text{(OAA)(NAD)}}{\text{(Malate)(NADP)}}$	$= 2.8 \times 10^{-5}$	2.7×10^{-5}	2800–4300	86–130	78.3
	Cow				1.7×10^{-5}	5400	151	11.5

Fatty acid synthesis, metabolism and esterification

Enzyme	Species	Reaction			
Malic enzyme (NADP)	Rat	$\dfrac{(\text{Pyruvate})(CO_2)(\text{NADPH})}{(\text{Malate})(\text{NADP})} = 3.44\text{-}5.1 \times 10^{-2}\,M$ See text	144	100	98.8
	Cow		6.0	3.24	0.54
Citrate cleavage enzyme	Rat	—	44–215	38–187	98.8
	Cow	—	1.8–4.2	—	—
Acetyl-CoA synthetase	Rat	—	30	—	0.0
	Cow	—	7.2	—	15.7
Acetyl-CoA carboxylase	Rat	Irreversible	17.3	Complex	86.4
	Cow		6.0	kinetics	6.02
Fatty acid synthetase (FA formed)	Rat	Irreversible	10.7	—	12.4
	Cow		2.6	—	0.93
α-Glycerol-P dehydrogenase	Rat	$\dfrac{(\alpha\text{-glycerol-P})(\text{NAD})}{(\text{DHAP})(\text{NADH})} = 1.78 \times 10^4$ 9.6×10^4	87	55	8.2
	Cow	4.1×10^3	20	7.1	0.54

[a] Abbreviations include: glucose-6-P (G6P); glucose-1-P (G1P); pyrophosphate (PPi); UDPglucose (UDPG); UDPgalactose (UDPGAL); 6-P-gluconate (6PG); ribulose-5-P (RU5P); fructose-6-P (F6P); fructose-1,6-diP (F1,6DiP); dihydroxyacetone-3-P (DHAP); glyceraldehyde-3-P (GAP); 1,3-diP glycerate (1,3DiPGA); phosphoenolpyruvate (PEP); oxalacetate (OAA); and α-ketoglutarate (αKG).

[b] Tabulated from Barman (1969), Greenbaum et al. (1971), Veech et al. (1969a), and Williamson (1965).

[c] Levels of metabolites used for calculating mass action coefficient were taken from within specific experiments. In cases where large differences between experiments were noted two values were presented.

[d] Methods of calculation for individual values were given in the text.

TABLE III

SUMMARY OF INTERMEDIARY METABOLITE LEVELS IN RAT AND COW MAMMARY GLANDS

Metabolite[a]	Rat	Cow	Metabolite	Rat	Cow
ATP	440–550	529.0	α-Glycerolphosphate	443	143
ADP	460–610	227	Phosphoenolpyruvate	0.5–20	4.8
AMP	340–500	270	Pyruvate	28–60	32
PPi	16.0[b]	—	Lactate	1,300–1,800	1,300
Glucose	200–1,000	1911	α-Ketoglutarate	5–20	25.2
Glucose-6-phosphate	53	52	Isocitrate	40–280	800
Glucose-1-phosphate	6.6	25.2	Glutamate	1,200–1,500	2,800
UDPglucose	291	154	Aspartate	1,200–2,400	686
UTP	1,800.0[b]	—	Oxalacetate	1–5	1.5
UDPgalactose	82.5[c]	54.5[c]	Malate	126.2	406
Fructose-6-phosphate	21.2[d]	20.8[d]	Citrate	3,300	14,000
Fructose-1,6-diphosphate	0.6	7.2	CoASH	—	90
Dihydroxyacetone phosphate	8.0	76.8	Acetyl-CoA	—	14
Glyceraldehyde-3-phosphate	5.5	99	$NAD/NADH_2$[e]	174–402	220
			$NADP/NADPH_2$[e]	0.9–1.1×10^{-4}	4×10^{-5}

[a] Values expressed as μmoles per kilogram fresh tissue. When two values are cited they represent the range of values reported in different papers or for different stages of lactation. Data taken from Korsrud and Baldwin (1972b), Baldwin and Cheng (1968), Baldwin et al. (1969), and Martin and Baldwin (1971a).

[b] From Kuhn (1968).

[c] Calculated from K_{equil} assuming UDPglucose-4-epimerase was in equilibrium.

[d] Calculated from K_{equil} assuming P-glucose isomerase was in equilibrium.

[e] Calculated assuming lactate dehydrogenase and isocitrate dehydrogenase (NADP) are in equilibrium as indicated in Table II and text.

and not a dogmatic or final analysis of the role(s) of enzymes in the regulation of mammary metabolism or of the mechanisms of action of hormones that alter mammary metabolism by acting through enzymes. Equilibrium constants and *in vivo* mass action coefficients for a number of reactions are presented in Table II. The equilibrium constants (K_{equil}) were obtained from the references cited in Table II, footnote *b* and are

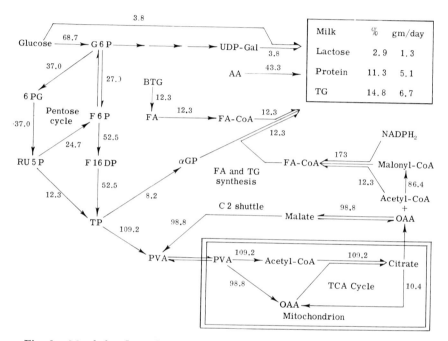

Fig. 1. Metabolite fluxes during milk synthesis in the rat. Metabolite fluxes through the several pathways were computed on the basis of carbon, $NADH_2$, $NADPH_2$, and ATP requirements for synthesis of 45 gm milk/day, with the composition indicated. Fluxes for each reaction and/or pathway are expressed in mmoles per day. Rounding errors in notating fluxes on arrows leads to slight imbalances but basically the system is in balance. Energy requirements for uptake, synthesis and/or secretion of minor milk components and for gland maintenance were not considered. The primary precursors of milk were considered to be blood glucose, triglycerides (BTG), and amino acids (AA). The computed flux rates through the several pathways are essentially in agreement with results of isotope tracer studies excepting that pentose cycle activity and $NADPH_2$ generation via this route may be low (Katz and Wals, 1972). Abbreviations include glucose-6-P (G6P), UDPgalactose (UDPGAL), 6-phosphogluconate (6PG), ribulose-5-P (RU5P), fructose-6-P (F6P), fructose-1,6-diphosphate (F1,6DP), triose phosphates (TP), α-glycerol-P (αGP), pyruvate (PVA), oxalacetic acid (OAA), fatty acid (FA), triglycerides (TG), tricarboxylic acid pathway (TCA), and Fatty acyl-CoA (FACoA).

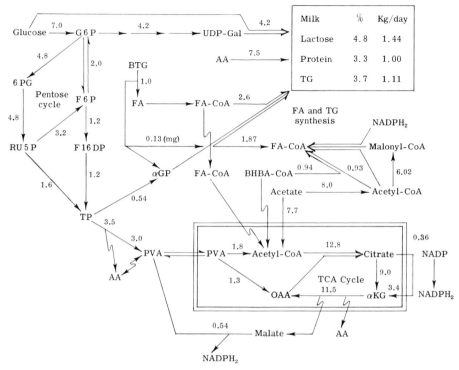

Fig. 2. Metabolite fluxes during milk synthesis in the cow. Fluxes were computed as described for rat in Fig. 1 excepting that the primary precursors considered were glucose, acetate, amino acids, ketone bodies (BHBA), and blood triglycerides. Milk yield was considered to be 30 kg/day. Some metabolism of amino acids was considered and the secretion of 0.36 moles/day of citrate in milk was accommodated. (From Baldwin and Smith, 1971.)

the result of efforts by these workers to determine or calculate K_{equil} for the reactions under physiological conditions. The mass action coefficients (K_{ma}) were calculated as the ratios of products to substrates as indicated for K_{equil} (Table II) using the estimates of mammary metabolite levels tabulated in Table III. If, upon comparison, it is found that tabulated values for K_{equil} and K_{ma} are identical or very close to one another, it can be concluded that the reaction being considered is at or very close to equilibrium *in vivo* (Williamson, 1965; Krebs and Veech, 1969; Krebs, 1969; Greenbaum *et al.*, 1971). Such a result strongly implies that the *in vivo* ΔF of the reaction is close to zero, that tissue levels of the enzyme which catalyzes the reaction are in excess, that the forward and reverse rates of the reaction *in vivo* are high relative to net flux through the reaction, and that the reaction is not a good candidate to consider in attempting to identify rate-limiting, regulatory sites. Also tabulated in Table II are estimates of maximum potential forward velocity (V_{max}), the result of a simplistic computation of forward velocity *in vivo* (v_f) and an estimate of net flux through the reaction *in vivo*. The estimates of V_{max} were obtained by converting the highest estimates of units (μmoles/minute)/gm tissue in Table I to mmoles/day/10 gm tissue for rats and moles/day/20.84 kg tissue for cows. *In vivo* forward velocities (v_f) were computed using the simple Michaelis-Menten equation $v_f = (V_{max} S)/ (S + K_m)$. For bisubstrate enzymes, the same equation was used thus considering the effect upon velocity of only one substrate. This is valid only in cases where the second substrate is in large excess (Mahler and Cordes, 1966). The primary reason for this simplification was that most of the bisubstrate enzymes considered are dehydrogenases, and the concentrations of free or unbound NAD, $NADH_2$, NADP, and $NADPH_2$ in the cell are not known. For the remaining enzymes considered, it was observed that one substrate was clearly limiting while the other was present in concentrations considerably above the K_m and, hence, in excess. In electing to present the v_f estimates, it was felt that a general indication of the influences of physiological concentrations of substrates on reaction rates would be of benefit in discussion and in considering probable relationships between substrate and enzyme levels, equilibria, net flux *in vivo* and metabolic regulation. In considering computation of v_f, we initially attempted to apply more sophisticated formulas that better accounted for concentrations of multiple substrates, orders of binding of substrates and release of products, concentrations of enzymes, compartmentation, etc. (Reiner, 1969). However, in view of lack of information regarding enzyme concentration *in vivo*, the difficulty and assumptions required in computing concentrations of enzyme-substrate complexes, and lack of data on concentrations of free pyridine nucleotides *in vivo*, it was decided not to imply sophistication but to select the simplest available index of the effect of *in vivo* substrate concentration on forward velocity.

The estimates of net flux *in vivo* presented in Table II were obtained from Figs. 1 and 2. The bases for formulation of these were, basically, input:output requirements for a cow producing 30 kg of milk per day and a rat producing 45 gm of milk per day (Baldwin and Smith, 1971). These should be considered minimal estimates since only carbon, hydrogen, and energy requirements for milk synthesis are accommodated. The use of carbon and energy for gland maintenance and basal functions was not considered (rat) or was considered only in part (cow) due to lack of relevant data.

In subsequent paragraphs, many of the enzymes involved in milk synthesis will be discussed briefly within the context of the data presented in Tables I and II with a view to pointing out some of their interesting and pertinent characteristics, their roles in milk synthesis, and their possible roles in the regulation of mammary gland metabolism. As were many of the computations summarized in Tables I and II and Figs. 1 and 2, many of the suggestions made in these paragraphs must be considered speculative. It is hoped, however, that in the overall, a coherent and realistic view of mammary enzymes and their functions is obtained through evaluation of the broad range of data tabulated and discussed.

A. Glucose Activation

1. Hexokinase (ATP:D-hexose-6-phosphotransferase; EC 2.7.1.1)

a. REACTION. $ATP + D\text{-hexose} \rightarrow ADP + D\text{-hexose-6-P}$

b. ASSAY. $D\text{-Glucose} + ATP \rightarrow glucose\text{-6-P} + ADP$

$glucose\text{-6-P}^* + NADP \rightarrow 6\text{-P gluconate} + NADPH_2$

c. COMMENTS AND DISCUSSION.   Several hexokinase isoenzymes designated I, II, III, and IV on the basis of their mobilities on vertical starch gel electrophoresis have been identified in several mammalian tissues (Grossbard and Schimke, 1966; Katzen, 1967; Katzen et al., 1970). The isoenzymes have similar molecular weights and pH optima and different Michaelis constants (K_m) for glucose. In rat mammary gland, types I and II hexokinase have been reported. The type I isoenzyme has a K_m for glucose of 4.5×10^{-5} and the type II, a K_m of 2.3×10^{-4} (Walters and McLean, 1967a). The ratio of type I to type II in mammary glands from pregnant and lactating rats, respectively, are 0.7 and 3.0 indicating a major increase in the amount of type II at lactogenesis. Because glucose concentrations in many tissues are greater than the K_m of type I hexokinase and often similar to or less than the K_m of type II hexokinase, it is often

---

* Rate of glucose-6-P formation determined in presence of excess glucose-6-P dehydrogenase by measuring rate of $NADPH_2$ formation at 340 nm. In crude extracts, levels of 6-P-gluconate dehydrogenase are high and the products of glucose-6-P oxidation are ribulose-5-P, CO_2 and 2 $NADPH_2$. In this case, rate of $NADPH_2$ formation divided by 2 equals rate of glucose-6-P formation (Korsrud and Baldwin, 1972a).

held that type I hexokinase is close to saturation with respect to glucose under normal conditions. It is also believed that increases in rates of glucose phosphorylation due to insulin reflect increases in cellular glucose concentrations or in glucose availability for binding to hexokinase type II (Hansen *et al.*, 1967a,b). Consistent with this view, it has been found that the activity of type II relative to type I is high in insulin-sensitive tissues such as diaphragm, skeletal muscle, fat pad, and heart and low in insulin insensitive tissues such as brain, liver, kidney, and lung (Katzen, 1967). On the basis of the large relative increase in mammary type II hexokinase during lactation and the above reasoning, Walters and McLean (1967a) suggested that the insulin responsiveness of mammary tissue should increase during lactation. On the other hand, studies of effects of insulin *in vitro* in mammary tissue slices and dispersed secretory cells indicate only marginal (20–50%) increases in glucose oxidation in the presence of insulin (Abraham *et al.*, 1957; Martin and Baldwin, 1971c) and, further, that the rate-limiting site of insulin action in mammary secretory cells is not at the level of glucose uptake and phosphorylation. This apparent lack of insulin responsiveness in mammary tissue may be explainable on the basis of observations that normal mammary glucose levels are in the range of $0.5–1.0 \times 10^{-3} M$ (Table III) and, hence, sufficient to almost saturate hexokinase type II with glucose. If this is the case, increases in tissue glucose concentration induced by insulin would not result in large increases in the rate of glucose phosphorylation.

A further complicating factor that must be considered in discussing hexokinase is the observation that hexokinase is found in both the soluble, nonparticulate or cytosolic fraction of tissue homogenates and in association with particulate—mostly mitochondrial—fractions prepared from tissue homogenates (Katzen, 1967; Walters and McLean, 1968b; Katzen *et al.*, 1970). An interesting difference between the particulate and nonparticulate hexokinase fractions is that the soluble form is more susceptible to glucose-6-P inhibition than the particulate form (Tuttle and Wilson, 1970). In general, there is a tendency for a greater proportion of hexokinase to be bound to mitochondria in active tissues with high glycolytic rates (Pilkis, 1970; Saito and Sato, 1971). This generalization appears to hold for rat mammary wherein the proportion of bound hexokinase increases from 10–20% during pregnancy to 60% during lactation (Walters and McLean, 1967a, 1968b). In addition, release of bound hexokinase from the mitochrondria to the cytosol was reported in rat mammary glands during insulin insufficiency.

Based upon extensive studies with many tissues and cells in mammalian and nonmammalian species it is clear that hexokinase fulfills a critical role in limiting and/or regulating the rate of glucose phosphorylation (Katzen, 1967; Pilkis, 1970). More limited data obtained with mammary tissue including the hexokinase isoenzyme and particle binding data mentioned above and the summary data in Tables I–III are consistent with the view that the hexokinase reaction is rate-limiting in the mammary gland, that the rate of the reaction can be regulated and, hence, that this reaction is a regulatory site in mammary tissue. Mammary hexokinase activity is low in all the species considered in Table I. There are no clear relationships between species attributable to differences in body weight, milk composition, or milk precursors. Comparisons of the equilibrium constant and mass action coefficients in Table II indicate that the hexokinase reaction is 10,000- or more fold out of equilibrium *in vivo*—a requirement that must be satisfied to conclude that a reaction is rate limiting *in vivo* but is, of course, easily satisfied in the case of essentially irreversible reactions such as the hexokinase reaction. Comparisons of the V_{max}, forward velocity, and net *in vivo* flux estimates in Table III indicate that hexokinase is acting at one-half maximum velocity *in vivo* in the rat. Despite the fact that these estimates must be considered with appropriate reservations as will be emphasized in subsequent sections, the comparison is consistent with the suggestion that the hexokinase reaction is potentially rate limiting. Some of the corrections applied in calculating the V_{max} and forward velocity estimates presented in Table II must be noted. Because most estimates of mammary hexokinase summarized in Table I were obtained in assays at $25°C$ using postmitochondrial supernatants and observations that hexokinase activity at $37°C$ is twice that at $25°C$ (England and Randle, 1967) and that in lactating rats 50% or more of the hexokinase is bound to mitochondria (Walters and McLean, 1968b), a correction factor of 4.0 was used in calculating V_{max}. Mammary glucose concentrations in rats and cows are 50–100 times greater than the composite hexokinase K_m for glucose while tissue ATP concentrations are approximately equal to the hexokinase K_m for ATP of 1.2×10^{-5} M. Therefore glucose was considered nonrate limiting and ATP values were used in calculating v_f. These simplistic assumptions or reasonings generally yield overestimates of forward velocity but were employed in calculating most of the forward velocity estimates presented in Table II. Our view in doing this, as stated in the introduction, was to present a simple estimate of the effect of physiological substrate concentrations on reaction velocity and not to present an oversophisticated estimate based on insufficient data.

B. Lactose Synthesis

1. Phosphoglucomutase (α-D-glucose-1,6-diphosphate:α-D-glucose-1-phosphate phosphotransferase; EC 2.7.5.1)

a. REACTION. Glucose-1-P $\rightleftharpoons$ glucose-6-P

b. ASSAY. Glucose-1-P $\rightarrow$ glucose-6-P

  glucose-6-P* + NADP $\rightarrow$ 6-P-gluconate + NADPH$_2$

c. COMMENTS AND DISCUSSION. Phosphoglucomutase is a cytoplasmic enzyme and catalyzes the first reaction in the pathway of lactose synthesis. The enzyme in cow mammary gland has K_m values for glucose-6-P and glucose-1-P of 5.0×10^{-6} and 8.5×10^{-6} M, respectively (Ray and Roselli, 1964). Based on metabolite data (Table III), the enzyme activity data in Table I, and these K_m data it can be calculated that the ratio of K_{equil} to mass action coefficient is close to 1 and that the forward velocity of the enzyme *in vivo* is in the order of 10 times the net flux required for lactose synthesis. Both of these observations are consistent with the view that phosphoglucomutase activity *in vivo* is nonlimiting.

2. UDPG pyrophosphorylase (UTP:α-D-glucose-1-phosphate uridylyltransferase; EC 2.7.7.9)

a. REACTION. UTP + α-D-glucose-1-phosphate $\rightleftharpoons$ PPi + UDPglucose

b. ASSAY. Determine rate of UDPglucose formation in reaction above by coupling to NAD-linked UDPglucose dehydrogenase and measuring rate of NADH$_2$ formation (Baldwin and Milligan, 1966). An alternate assay is to determine rate of glucose-1-P formation from UDPglucose by linking through phosphoglucomutase to glucose-6-P dehydrogenase and NADPH$_2$ formation (Korsrud and Baldwin, 1972a).

c. COMMENTS AND DISCUSSION. Mammary UDPglucose pyrophosphorylase levels are extremely high in all species that have been studied (Table I). In rats and cows the K_{equil}/K_{ma} ratio is close to 1 indicating that *in vivo*, the reaction is essentially in equilibrium (Table II). The estimate of forward velocity in Table II is 30–40 times greater than the net flux required for lactose synthesis. The estimate of forward flux (Table

---

* Assayed in presence of excess glucose-6-P dehydrogenase and by determination of NADPH$_2$ formation at 340 nm. The same precautions discussed for assay of hexokinase in crude homogenates apply (Korsrud and Baldwin, 1972a).

II) was calculated on the assumption that glucose-1-P concentration was rate limiting. This decision for computational purposes was made after comparison of the K_m values for UTP and glucose-1-P of 2.0×10^{-4} and 4×10^{-4} to 5×10^{-5} M, respectively (Emery and Baldwin, 1967; Aksamit and Ebner, 1972) with the concentrations of these substrates (Table III) indicating that glucose-1-P was the limiting substrate *in vivo*. According to these criteria, it appears clear that mammary enzymatic capacity for UDPglucose synthesis is in great excess of requirements. In this regard, it is interesting to note that mammary UDPglucose pyrophosphorylase activity is subject to significant hormonal regulation as will be documented in a later section of this chapter. This appears to be a clear example of a case where hormones regulate the activity of an enzyme with no metabolic consequences. Changes in the activity of an enzyme which is present in 100-fold excess according to V_{max} estimates and which catalyzes a reaction which is in equilibrium *in vivo* would not be expected to alter net flux through a pathway or have metabolic regulatory significance.

3. UDPglucose-4-epimerase (EC 5.1.3.2)

a. REACTION.   UDPglucose $\leftrightarrows$ UDPgalactose

b. ASSAY.   Using UDPgalactose as substrate determine rate of UDPglucose formation by linking to UDPglucose dehydrogenase and NAD as in the UDPglucose pyrophosphorylase assay (Baldwin and Milligan, 1966).

c. COMMENTS AND DISCUSSION.   UDPglucose-4-epimerase is a cytoplasmic enzyme and is present in mammary tissues at levels comparable to P-glucose mutase in all the species listed in Table I. K_m values for UDPglucose-4-epimerase isolated from calf liver and rat mammary are 9×10^{-5} and 5×10^{-5} M, respectively, for UDPglucose and UDPgalactose (Barman, 1969; Shatton *et al.*, 1965). Since tissue levels of UDPglucose are 3–4 times greater (Table III) than the K_m for this substrate it would appear that the enzyme is close to saturated with respect to substrate *in vivo* and that forward velocities are 10 times greater than net flux (Table II). Even though tissue UDPgalactose levels have not been determined enabling comparison of K_{equil} to the mass action coefficient, it seems safe, on the basis of amounts of enzyme and substrate available, to suggest that the activity of UDPglucose-4-epimerase is nonlimiting *in vivo*.

4. Lactose synthetase (UDPgalactose:D-glucose-1-galactosyltransferase; EC 2.4.1.22)

a. REACTION.   UDPgalactose + D-glucose $\rightarrow$ UDP + lactose

b. Assay. Usually assayed by determining rate of UDP-[^{14}C]galactose incorporation into lactose in presence of excess concentrations of α-lactalbumin (Korsrud and Baldwin, 1972b). In crude extracts care must be taken to correct for or avoid error due to UDP-[^{14}C]galactose hydrolysis (Kuhn, 1968).

c. Comments and Discussion. The lactose synthetase system is complex and is the likely rate limiting and regulatory site in the pathway of lactose synthesis. Ebner discusses this system in detail in his chapter (Chapter 3, Vol. II) and only minimum comment on the data tabulated in Tables I and II is appropriate here. It is noteworthy that all estimates of tissue lactose synthetase activity in mammary tissue are low (Table I) and, in fact, much lower than estimates that would be required to accommodate *in vivo* rates of lactose synthesis (Table III). This presumably reflects the difficulty of assessing, in a meaningful fashion, the activities of complex, particulate, multiprotein enzymes in homogenates.

Since in the above consideration of the other enzymes involved in lactose synthesis it was established that these reactions are at close to equilibrium *in vivo* and that enzymatic capacities are in excess, it follows that lactose synthetase which catalyzes the only irreversible reaction in the pathway and is subject to regulation (Chapter 3, Vol. II, by Ebner) is the rate-limiting enzyme in the pathway and the most likely site of regulation of lactose synthesis.

C. Pentose Cycle

1. Glucose-6-P dehydrogenase (D-glucose-6-phosphate:NADP oxidoreductase; EC 1.1.1.49)

a. Reaction. D-Glucose-6-P + NADP $\leftrightarrows$ D-glucono-δ-lactone-6-P + NADPH$_2$

D-glucono-δ-lactone-6-P → 6-P-gluconate (lactonase)

b. Assay. Glucose-6-P + NADP → 6-P-gluconate + NADPH$_2$

6-P-gluconate* + NADP → ribulose-5-P + CO$_2$ + NADPH$_2$

c. Comments and Discussion. Glucose-6-P dehydrogenase is the first enzyme of the hexose monophosphate pathway or pentose cycle. This pathway is one of the mechanisms of generation of NADPH$_2$ required for

---

* Determine rate of NADPH$_2$ formation at 340 nm. 6-P-gluconate dehydrogenase levels in crude homogenates are high, so that the yield of NADPH$_2$ from glucose-6-P

reductive synthesis in the mammary secretory cell. Because the glucono-lactone formed as a product by glucose-6-P dehydrogenase is rapidly and irreversibly converted to 6-P gluconate either spontaneously or by lacto-nase, the glucose-6-P dehydrogenase reaction can be considered essen-tially irreversible and, hence, the reaction which irreversibly commits glucose-6-P to the hexose monophosphate pathway. For this reason, the glucose-6-P dehydrogenase reaction is of considerable interest. Mammary glucose-6-P dehydrogenase has been studied in some detail (Emery and Baldwin, 1967; Levy, 1963; Levy *et al.* 1966; Raineri and Levy, 1970). Comparisons of the V_{max}, v_f, and net *in vivo* flux estimates in Table II imply that the amounts of glucose-6-P dehydrogenase and glucose-6-P present *in vivo* do not limit rate of glucose-6-P oxidation *via* the hexose monophosphate route. In calculating v_f, the high estimates for V_{max} (Table I) were used. The values for v_f for each species reflect estimates obtained from use of a K_m value for glucose-6-P of 1.2×10^{-5} (Raineri and Levy, 1970). It can be seen that mammary glucose-6-P levels (Table III) are sufficient to support *in vivo* rates of from 60–80% of V_{max} and that v_f estimates obtained considering glucose-6-P to be the limiting sub-strate are 10–30 times greater than actual *in vivo* fluxes. These estimates suggest that factors other than glucose-6-P dehydrogenase and glucose-6-P levels limit the rate of the reaction. Several observations indicate that free NADP concentrations limit the rate of this reaction. Walters and McLean (1968a), reported that addition of phenazine methosulfate, an artificial electron acceptor, to mammary slices *in vitro* increased [1-^{14}C]-glucose-oxidation twofold. This observation correlates well with the general observation that hexose monophosphate pathway flux is responsive to changes in rates of $NADPH_2$ utilization for fatty acid synthesis. Another evidence supporting the view that NADP availability limits glucose-6-P dehydrogenase flux is that mammary free $NADP/NADPH_2$ ratios are in the $10^{-3}–10^{-5}$ range (Table III). If one assumes that all the NADP and

---

is often greater than 1.0. Two approaches are utilized to avoid overestimates of glu-cose-6-P dehydrogenase activity in homogenates due to this fact. The most common approach is to add 6-P-gluconate to one cuvette and glucose-6-P plus 6-P-gluconate to a second cuvette. The rate of $NADPH_2$ formation in cuvette 1 provides an estimate of 6-P-gluconate dehydrogenase activity while the rate in cuvette 2 provides an esti-mate of the activities of 6-P gluconate dehydrogenase plus glucose-6-P dehydrogenase. Subtraction of the rate in cuvette 1 from the rate observed in cuvette 2 provides an estimate of glucose-6-P dehydrogenase activity (Korsrud and Baldwin, 1972a). An alternate approach is to add nonlimiting amounts of purified 6-P-gluconate dehydro-genase to the assay. In this case, rate of $NADPH_2$ formation divided by 2.0 provides an estimate of glucose-6-P dehydrogenase activity.

NADPH$_2$ in mammary tissue is free in the cytoplasm—a maximal and incorrect assumption due to extensive binding to proteins—and multiplies the total concentration of NADP + NADPH$_2$ in mammary tissue (10^{-4} M; Baldwin and Milligan, 1966) by 10^{-3} and 10^{-5} ($10^{-4} \times 10^{-3}$ or 10^{-5}), an estimate of free mammary NADP concentrations in the 10^{-7}–10^{-9} M range is obtained. Since the glucose-6-P dehydrogenase K_m for NADP is 10^{-6} M (Raineri and Levy, 1970), mammary NADP concentrations are 0.1–10% of K_m and, hence, NADP concentrations are rate limiting.

The isoenzymes of glucose-6-P dehydrogenase have been studied extensively in many tissues and species. The isoenzymes have been of particular interest in genetic studies because a gene for glucose-6-P dehydrogenase is located on the X chromosome (Trujillo *et al.*, 1965; Young *et al.*, 1964). Varying patterns of glucose-6-P dehydrogenase heterogeneity have been reported. One common difficulty encountered in interpreting multiple glucose-6-P dehydrogenase patterns is effects of sample treatments prior to and during electrophoresis. Active glucose-6-P dehydrogenase exists as a dimer, tetramer, and hexamer (Holten, 1972; Levy *et al.*, 1966; Taketa and Watanabe, 1971). Differences in pH and ionic strength, in availability of NADP and reducing agents, and due to aging of extracts lead to considerable variability in enzyme dissociation and association and in electrophoretic heterogeneity (Kirkman, 1962; Taketa and Watanabe, 1971). Richards and Russell (1971) reported two glucose-6-P isoenzymes present in virgin mammary glands. Increases in glucose-6-P dehydrogenase activity during early pregnancy were accounted for by an increase in one of these isoenzymes. In late pregnancy, a third electrophoretic component appeared which accounted for the bulk of the increase in glucose-6-P dehydrogenase activity that occurred during late pregnancy and lactation. This third component was rapidly lost at involution. It is not known whether these changes in mammary isoenzyme patterns reflect changes in prominent cell types (secretory versus adipose cells), secretory cell differentiation, hormone inductions, or other effects. Glucose-6-P dehydrogenase isoenzyme patterns in rat liver and pregnant mammary are affected by estrogen (Hori and Matsui, 1967; Richards and Russell 1971).

2. 6-P-Gluconate dehydrogenase (6-phospho-D-gluconate:NADP oxidoreductase [decarboxylating]; EC 1.1.1.44)

a. REACTION. 6-P-gluconate + NADP $\leftrightarrows$ D-ribulose-5-P + CO$_2$ + NADPH$_2$

b. ASSAY. Determine rate of NADPH$_2$ formation at 340 nm in the presence of 6-P-gluconate; usually assayed in connection with glucose-6-P dehydrogenase assays as stated above (Korsrud and Baldwin, 1972a).

c. Comments and Discussion. Mammary activities of 6-P-gluconate dehydrogenase are lower than but in the same order as glucose-6-P dehydrogenase. There are no data available regarding mammary 6-P gluconate levels and no v_f computation was done. It seems reasonable, however, to suggest that this enzyme is present in excess since V_{max} estimates are 4–10 times greater than net *in vivo* flux (Table II) and further, without data support, that intracellular concentrations of free NADP and the rate of 6-P-gluconate formation by the glucose-6-P dehydrogenase reaction, also determined by NADP concentration, are determinant of 6-P-gluconate dehydrogenase flux *in vivo*.

3. Other Pentose Cycle Enzymes

There are very few data available regarding mammary activities of the other enzymes of the hexose monophosphate pathway or the pentose cycle. When the hexose-monophosphate pathway is operating as a (pentose) cycle, 3 moles of ribulose-5-P formed from glucose-6-P are converted to 2 fructose-6-P and 1 glyceraldehyde-3-P by this group of enzymes which includes transaldolase and transketolase. The cycle is completed by the conversion of the fructose-6-P to glucose-6-P by hexose-P-isomerase. An important characteristic of these conversions to keep in mind in considering radioisotope tracer data is that labeled glyceraldehyde-3-P can be incorporated into or can exchange into fructose-6-P via this cycle leading to interesting labeling patterns in glucose-6-P and lactose formed therefrom (Wood *et al.*, 1958; Katz and Wood, 1963).

A few data obtained using a composite assay of "pentose phosphate metabolizing activity" are presented in Tables II and III. In this assay, the rate of conversion of ribose-5-P to ribulose-5-P (isomerase) to xylulose-5-P (epimerase) to glyceraldehyde-3-P (transketolase) is determined by measuring the rate of glyceraldehyde-3-P formation from ribose-5-P in the presence of excess glyceraldehyde-3-P dehydrogenase and NAD. Transketolase is probably the rate-limiting enzyme in the conversions (Benevenga *et al.*, 1964). V_{max} estimates obtained using this assay system are in significant excess of *in vivo* flux but not to an extent which allows an unequivocated conclusion that the enzymes of pentose-P metabolism are nonlimiting under all conditions. There are no data or analyses that suggest limitations or regulation in this portion of the cycle.

D. Embden–Meyerhof Glycolysis

1. Hexose-P isomerase (D-glucose-6-P ketal-isomerase; EC 5.3.1.9)

a. REACTION.   Glucose-6-P $\leftrightarrows$ fructose-6-P

b. ASSAY.   Determine rate of fructose-6-P conversion to glucose-6-P by measuring rate of $NADPH_2$ formation in the presence of excess NADP and glucose-6-P dehydrogenase.

c. COMMENTS AND DISCUSSION.   Enzyme capacities *in vivo* in rats and cows are in significant excess as indicated by comparison of the V_{max} and v_f (calculated using a K_m for glucose-6-P of 1.2×10^{-4} M; Hines and Wolfe, 1963) estimate with net flux. As indicated in Figs. 1 and 2 the net flux of the reaction *in vivo* can be in either direction depending upon the relative rate of glycolysis and pentose cycle activity. The primary concern with regard to this reaction *in vivo* is whether or not the reaction is in rapid equilibrium. The rate of equilibration of radioisotope label between glucose-6-P and fructose-6-P is very important in interpretations of tracer experiments (Katz and Wood, 1963).

2. Phosphofructokinase (ATP:D-fructose-6-phosphate-1-phospho-transferase; EC 2.7.1.11)

a. REACTION.   ATP + D-fructose $\leftrightarrows$ ADP + D-fructose-1,6-diP

b. ASSAY.   ATP + fructose-6-P → fructose-1,6-diP + ADP (NH_4^+ or AMP present as activator)

     fructose-1,6-diP → triose-P (x.s. aldolase and triose-P isomerase)

     triose-P + $NADH_2$ → α-glycerol-P + NAD (x.s. α-glycerol-P dehydrogenase)

or[*]   triose-P + NAD → 3-P glycerate + $NADH_2$ (x.s. glyceraldehyde-3-P dehydrogenase + ASO_4)

[*] Two systems are commonly used in assaying this enzyme. In the first, the rate of fructose-1,6-diP formation is determined by conversion to α-glycerol-P in the presence of aldolase, triose-P isomerase, α-glycerol-P dehydrogenase and $NADH_2$. In the other, fructose-1,6-diP formation is determined by linking to aldolase, triose-P isomerase, glyceraldehyde-3-P dehydrogenase, NAD and arsenate. The latter reaction is rendered irreversible when the initial product ($1-ASO_4-3-P$-glycerate) hydrolyzes spontaneously to form 3-P glycerate. High ATP concentrations inhibit the reaction so these must be carefully adjusted to optimum. The enzyme is usually assayed at maximal activities achieved by addition of ammonium sulfate or AMP (Korsrud and Baldwin, 1972a).

c. Comments and Discussion. Many metabolites interact with and alter the activity and kinetic properties of phosphofructokinase. Because of this, observations indicating that the phosphofructokinase reaction is rate limiting in many tissues *in vivo,* and the facts that phosphofructokinase is essentially irreversible and catalyzes a branch-point reaction, phosphofructokinase is considered an important determinant of glycolytic flux (Passonneau and Lowry, 1964). Positive effectors of the enzyme include AMP, ADP, cyclic AMP, fructose-1,6-diP and fructose-6-P while negative effectors include ATP, citrate, and alterations in the ATP/ADP ratio (Mansour, 1969). The general pattern of effector actions is consistent with high glycolytic flux when the energy status of a cell is low and low glycolytic flux when cellular energy status is high.

Mammary phosphofructokinase has not been studied very extensively. Even though available metabolite and some enzyme data indicate that the enzyme is far displaced from equilibrium and rate limiting *in vivo* (Table II) and unpublished data (Baldwin and Cheng) indicate that AMP and ATP are positive and negative effectors, respectively; a strong need for further study of mammary phosphofructokinase is suggested. An observation that may be of interest is that in most tissues citrate is a negative effector of phosphofructokinase. If this were true for the cow mammary enzyme, the extremely high citrate levels in this tissue (Table III) might be expected to severely depress phosphofructokinase activity. Until further studies of the mammary system have been reported, it seems appropriate, on the basis of data obtained in other tissues, to tentatively accept the view that mammary phosphofructokinase is a determinant of glycolytic flux in mammary tissue.

3. Fructose-1,6-diP aldolase (fructose-1,6-diphosphate:D-glyceraldehyde-3-phosphate-lyase; EC 4.1.2.13)

a. Reaction. Fructose-1,6-diP $\leftrightarrows$ dihydroxyacetone-P + D-glyceraldehyde-3-P

b. Assay. Couple with glyceraldehyde-3-P dehydrogenase or α-glycerol-P dehydrogenase as described above for phosphofructokinase (Baldwin and Milligan, 1966).

c. Comments and Discussion. The calculated mass action coefficients for the aldolase reaction are very close to K_{equil} for the rat and within approximately tenfold for the cow indicating that this reaction is close to equilibrium in both species (Table III). However, a major discrepancy is noted in comparing calculated forward velocities and net *in vivo* flux for this reaction (Table III). Forward velocities were calculated using the

K_m for fructose-1,6-diP of 3.2×10^{-4} M reported by Emery and Baldwin (1967) for the rat mammary enzyme. Only when the highest reported concentration of mammary fructose-1,6-diP (15.0 μmole/kg; Baldwin and Cheng, 1969) and lowest reported fructose-1,6-diP K_m for aldolase (1.4×10^{-5} M; rabbit muscle; Barman, 1969) are used is a calculated forward velocity (65 mmoles/day) comparable to net *in vivo* flux obtained for the aldolase reaction in rat mammary tissue. A similar relationship exists with the cow. In view of the complex kinetics of aldolase attributable to its interaction with triose-P isomerase as evaluated by Veech *et al.* (1969b) and noted below, and the apparent discrepancy noted above, further study of mammary aldolase is warranted before firm conclusions regarding its role and behavior *in vivo* are formulated.

4. Triose-P isomerase (D-glyceraldehyde-3-phosphate ketal-isomerase; EC 5.3.1.1.)

a. REACTION. D-Glyceraldehyde-3-P $\leftrightharpoons$ dehydroacetone-P

b. ASSAY. Using glyceraldehyde-3-P as substrate, measure rate of dihydroxyacetone-P formation by linking to α-glycerol-P dehydrogenase and NADH$_2$ (Beisenherz, 1955).

c. COMMENTS AND DISCUSSION. Despite the fact that triose-P isomerase activity and rates of interconversion of glyceraldehyde-3-P and dihydroxyacetone-P *in vivo* and *in vitro* are of critical concern in the interpretation of radioisotope tracer data (Wood *et al.*, 1958; Katz and Wood, 1963; Katz and Wals, 1972), very few data are available regarding the activity of this enzyme. In cow mammary gland, triose-P isomerase activity is very high such that the forward velocity computed for the *in vivo* state using a K_m for glyceraldehyde-3-P of 3.9×10^{-4} M (Barman, 1969) is more than 100 times *in vivo* net flux. With this observation suggesting rapid equilibration in mind, it is perhaps surprising to note that the mass action coefficient observed for the cow is almost 200 times greater than K_{equil}. This apparent discrepancy has been noted in several tissues and is apparently difficult to explain (Veech *et al.*, 1969b). This complication may produce the nonequilibration of isotope tracers in the triose-P isomerase reaction reported by Wood *et al.* (1958) and Katz and Wals (1972) and the lack of agreement between mass action coefficients and K_{equil} noted above. These results may be a good example of a case where an apparent large excess in enzymatic capacity is not expressed *in vivo*.

5. Glyceraldehyde-3-P dehydrogenase (D-glyceraldehyde-3-phosphate: NAD oxidoreductase [phosphorylating]; EC 1.2.1.12)

a. REACTION. D-Glyceraldehyde-3-P + NAD $\leftrightarrows$ 1,3-diP-D-glycerate + NADH$_2$

b. ASSAY. Glyceraldehyde-3-P + NAD + H$_2$O* $\xrightarrow{\text{ASO}_4}$ 3-P-glycerate + NADH$_2$

c. COMMENTS AND DISCUSSION. The data tabulated in Tables I and II are consistent with the view that enzyme capacity *in vivo* is in excess and with observations in other tissues, primarily liver, which suggest that the glyceraldehyde-3-P dehydrogenase, phosphoglycerate kinase and lactate dehydrogenase reactions *in vivo* are at close to equilibrium and responsive to changes in cellular redox (NAD/NADH$_2$) and energy (ATP/ADP·Pi) states (Stubbs *et al.*, 1972; Krebs and Veech, 1970). In rat mammary glands, changes in free NAD/NADH$_2$ ratios predicted by the lactic dehydrogenase couple and in (2 ATP + ADP)/2(ATP + ADP + AMP) ratios during lactation correspond closely with predicted liver patterns. These are presumed consistent with regulation of extent of carbon diversion via α-glycerol-P dehydrogenase to triglyceride synthesis and of glycolytic flux via glyceraldehyde-3-P dehydrogenase by cell redox and energy state (Baldwin and Cheng, 1969).

6. Other Glycolytic Enzymes

There are very few data available regarding the activities and regulatory functions in mammary of the remaining enzymes of glycolysis so only pyruvate kinase and lactic dehydrogenase will be discussed.

7. Pyruvate kinase (ATP:pyruvate phosphotransferase; EC 2.7.1.40)

a. REACTION. Phosphoenolpyruvate + ADP → ATP + pyruvate

b. ASSAY. Measure NADH$_2$ disappearance at 340 nm in the presence of lactic dehydrogenase to determine rate of pyruvate formation from phosphoenolpyruvate.

c. COMMENTS AND DISCUSSION. The occurrence of multiple forms of pyruvate kinase in various tissues and the kinetic properties of the enzyme were recently reviewed by Seubert and Schoner (1971). There appear to be two interconvertible forms of pyruvate kinase of which one (B)

---

* As noted in the description of the phosphofructokinase assay, rapid and spontaneous hydrolysis of 1-ASO$_4$-3-P-glycerate to 3-P-glycerate renders the reaction irreversible and enables assay by determination of NADH$_2$ production at 340 nm (Baldwin and Milligan, 1966).

exhibits sigmoidal kinetics and the other (A) normal Michaelis-Menten kinetics. Pyruvate kinase B is strongly activated by fructose-1,6-diP when phosphoenolpyruvate is low and is inhibited by ATP. In addition, fructose-1,6-diP causes conversion of the A form to the B form while ATP and citrate reverse this conversion. ATP and fructose diphosphate do not alter the kinetic characteristics of pyruvate kinase A. The characteristics of mammary pyruvate kinase in this regard are not known.

The K_{equil} for pyruvate kinase is 6500 while the mass action coefficients for rats and cows were 5.4 and 15.5, respectively, indicating a relative build-up of substrate and that pyruvate kinase is rate-limiting in mammary as has been observed in most tissues. Calculations of forward velocity in rats support this view (Table II).

8. Lactic dehydrogenase (L-lactate:NAD oxidoreductase; EC 1.1.1.27)

a. REACTION. L-Lactate + NAD $\leftrightarrows$ pyruvate + NADH$_2$

b. ASSAY. Pyruvate + NADH$_2$* $\rightarrow$ lactate + NAD

c. COMMENTS AND DISCUSSION. Lactic dehydrogenase consists of five isoenzymes, each a tetramer made up of two protein subunits—an "M" (muscle type) and "H" (heart type)—in combinations of HHHH (LDH1), HHHM(LDH2) . . . MMMM (LDH5). The "H" type isoenzymes have a higher apparent K_m for pyruvate and are more sensitive to inhibition by pyruvate than the "M" types. The kinetic properties of the isoenzymes appear to be of significant metabolic significance in that pyuruvate levels must become high before rapid conversion to lactate occurs in tissues rich in LDH1. This leads to more extensive oxidation of pyruvate. Tissues rich in LDH5, such as skeletal muscle, form lactate more readily at low pyruvate concentrations, a desirable trait supporting glycolytic flux under anaerobic conditions (Kaplan, 1966). This general thesis as to the metabolic significance of the LDH isoenzymes has been challenged based on results obtained while working with LDH at high concentrations (Wuntch *et al.*, 1970). However, a high correlation between the predominant molecular composition of LDH and relative amounts of oxygen uptake by cells of various types throughout the biological kingdom does exist and is of interest (Kaplan *et al.*, 1968).

Detailed studies by Karlsson and Carlsson (1968) and Simpson and Schmidt (1970) indicate that all five LDH isoenzymes exist in rat mammary tissue and that the proportion of LDH5, which is low in virgin and involuted glands, increases markedly during pregnancy and lactation.

---

* Measure NADH$_2$ disappearance at 340 nm.

If the above stated correlation between oxygen availability and/or uptake and the proportion of LDH5 is applicable to the mammary gland, it would seem that capacity for anaerobic metabolism increases during pregnancy and is maximal at peak lactation. The significance of these changes in LDH isoenzyme patterns during lactation is not completely clear. Karlsson and Carlsson (1968) suggested that the changes reflected changes in the proportions of the several mammary cell types favoring secretory cells during pregnancy and lactation while Simpson and Schmidt (1970) contended that the changes fit a binomial distribution at all stages and must occur in all cell types. *In vitro* studies with monkey heart cells (Goodfriend *et al.*, 1966), human lymphocytes (Hellung-Larsen and Andersen, 1968), and calf kidney cortex cells (Güttler and Clausen, 1969) indicate a tendency for low oxygen tensions to produce increases in the M-type isoenzymes. Estradiol administration to rats causes an increase in M-type isoenzymes in the immature uterus (Goodfriend and Kaplan, 1964; Kaplan, 1966). The possible role(s) or relationships of hormones and factors such as low oxygen tension to the observed increases in mammary LDH5 during lactation have not been evaluated.

E. Citric Acid Cycle and Related Functions

1. Acetyl-CoA synthetase (acetate:CoA ligase [AMP]; EC 6.2.1.1)

a. REACTION.   ATP + acetate + CoASH → AMP + PPi + acetyl-CoA

b. ASSAY.   Acetate + ATP + CoASH → Acetyl-CoA + AMP + PPi
   acetyl-CoA + NH_2OH → acetylhydroxamate[*] + CoASH

c. COMMENTS AND DISCUSSION.   Acetyl-CoA synthetase is distributed in the cytosol and mitochondria of mammary cells. Only total activities are presented in Tables I and II. As indicated in Figs. 1 and 2, this enzyme is very important in ruminant mammary glands in that it catalyzes the first reaction in acetate utilization for fatty acid synthesis and as an energy source. The reaction is much less important in rats. Available estimates of V_{max} are below estimates of *in vivo* flux (Table II) for the cow. On the

---

[*] Acetylhydroxamate formed is determined spectrophotometrically in acid ferric chloride solution at 540 nm (Berg, 1962). An alternate assay (Berg, 1962) is to determine acetyl-CoA formation by linking to citrate synthetase using malate as a precursor of oxalacetate for the citrate synthetase reaction. In the presence of NAD and excess malate dehydrogenase the rate of $NADH_2$ formation from malate is proportional (1:1) to the rate of acetyl-CoA formation (malate + NAD + acetyl-CoA → NADH + citrate + CoASH).

bases of observed sharp increases in cow mammary acetyl-CoA synthetase activity coincident with parturition and lactogenesis, of studies of inter-relationships between acetyl-CoA synthetase and a thiolase which hydro-lyzes acetyl-CoA forming acetate and CoASH (a pairing analogous to the opposing actions of phosphofructokinase and fructose-1,6 diphosphatase in liver), of observation of multiple forms of acetyl-CoA synthetase, and of the apparent rate limiting character of acetyl-CoA synthetase indicated by a low V_{max} to net *in vivo* flux ratio. Ponto *et al.* (1969), Marinez and Cook (1971), and Simon and Cook (1971) have suggested that the acetyl-CoA synthetase reaction is rate limiting and regulates acetate entry in ruminant mammary. Alternate, though not inconsistent, reason-ing might suggest that acetate availability limits the rate of this reaction. Consistent evidences are a high correlation between arterial acetate con-centrations and acetate uptake and activation (Baldwin and Smith, 1971) and the fact that physiological concentrations of acetate are in the same range as the acetyl-CoA synthetase K_m for acetate of 10^{-4} M (Barman, 1969).

2. Citrate synthetase (citrate oxalacetate-lyase [CoA-acetylating]; EC 4.1.3.7)

a. REACTION. Acetyl-CoA + oxalacetate + H_2O ⇆ citrate + CoASH

b. ASSAY. Malate + NAD ⇆ oxalacetate + $NADH_2$
   oxalacetate[*] + acetyl-CoA → citrate + CoASH

c. COMMENTS AND DISCUSSION. Citrate synthetase or condensing en-zyme is present in both the cytoplasmic and mitochondrial compartments of the mammary cell with about 75% of the total activity present in the mitochondrion (Table II). The mammary enzyme has not been studied. Although the *in vivo* status of this reaction is difficult to discern because of lack of data regarding intracellular distributions of oxalacetate, CoASH and acetyl-CoA, comparison of the V_{max} and net *in vivo* flux estimates in Table II suggests that the enzyme is present in considerable excess and, hence, that reaction rate *in vivo* is largely controlled by concentrations or availabilities of substrates.

3. Isocitrate dehydrogenase (*threo-D_S*-isocitrate : NADP oxidoreductase; EC 1.1.1.42)

a. REACTION. Isocitrate + NADP ⇆ 2-oxoglutarate + CO_2 + $NADPH_2$

---

[*] Excess malate dehydrogenase; determine $NADH_2$ formation at 340 nm (Ochoa, 1955).

b. ASSAY. Using isocitrate as substrate measure rate of NADPH$_2$ formation spectrophotometrically at 340 nm (Baldwin and Milligan, 1966).

c. COMMENTS AND DISCUSSION. Isocitrate dehydrogenase (NADP) activities are extremely high in cow mammary tissue (Table I) presumably reflecting its role in NADPH$_2$ formation for fat synthesis in this species (Bauman et al., 1970). In calculating free NADP/NADPH$_2$ ratios for cow mammary tissue (Table III) according to the methods and specifications of Veech et al. (1969a), the reaction is presumed to be in equilibrium in vivo. The facts that the concentrations of isocitrate and α-ketoglutarate (Table III) are close to their K_m's of 10^{-6} and 10^{-4} M, respectively, and that V_{max}/in vivo flux is very high suggest that net flux is dependent upon local redox state or NADP/NADPH$_2$ ratio (Tables II and III). The role of this enzyme in NADPH$_2$ generation for fatty acid synthesis is discussed in detail in Chapters 1 and 2, Vol. II.

The mitochondrial, NAD-linked isocitrate dehydrogenase which participates in the tricarboxylic acid cycle has not been studied in mammary tissue.

4. **Glutamate dehydrogenase (L-glutamate:NAD[P] oxidoreductase [deaminating]; EC 1.4.1.3)**

a. REACTION.   L-Glutamate + H$_2$O + NAD(P) $\leftrightarrows$ 2-oxoglutarate + NH$_3$ + NAD(P)H$_2$

b. ASSAY. In lysed mitochondria determine rate of NAD reduction at 340 nm using L-glutamate as substrate.

c. COMMENTS AND DISCUSSION. Glutamate dehydrogenase is found exclusively in the mitochondrion. V_{max} estimates for both the rat and cow are fairly high. From this, it might be presumed that the reaction in vivo is close to equilibrium since rates of either glutamate synthesis or degradation in mammary are probably small (Linzell, 1968) (Tables I and II). The enzyme of mammary tissue has not been well studied. Studies of the rate of [1-^{14}C]glutamate carbon incorporation into milk citrate in perfused goat mammary glands by Hardwick (1966) indicate a fairly rapid exchange of label between glutamate and α-ketoglutarate.

5. **Aspartate aminotransferase (L-aspartate:2-oxoglutarate aminotransferase; EC 2.6.1.1)**

a. REACTION.   L-Aspartate + 2-oxoglutarate $\leftrightarrows$ oxalacetate + L-glutamate

b. ASSAY. Determine rate of oxalacetate formation by linking with excess malate dehydrogenase to $NADH_2$ oxidation (Baldwin and Milligan, 1966).

c. COMMENTS AND DISCUSSION. Two isoenzymes of aspartate aminotransferase (GOT) have been reported for heart and liver in several species. Aspartate aminotransferase I (anodic) corresponds with the species found in cytoplasm while aspartate aminotransferase II (cathodic) originates from mitochondria. In addition to differing in electrophoretic mobilities, the two isoenzymes differ in amino acid composition (Martinez and Tiemeier, 1967), responses of pH changes and in K_m's for the several substrates (Boyd, 1961; Fleisher, 1960; Kaplan and Ciotti, 1961). The mitochondrial enzyme has a much greater affinity for aspartate while the cytoplasmic enzyme has a greater affinity for α-ketoglutarate (2-oxoglutarate).

Herzfeld and Greengard (1971) reported mammary aspartate aminotransferase activities were nil in the rat until late pregnancy when the activities of both the soluble and particulate enzymes rose sharply. After an initial increase in early lactation, activity of the particulate form remained constant through the remainder of lactation. The activity of the soluble enzyme rose steadily throughout lactation. The activities of both enzymes declined to virgin levels at involution. The activity of the soluble enzyme is higher than the particulate form in rat mammary (Herzfeld and Greengard, 1971) while activities of the two forms are similar in cow mammary (Baldwin and Cheng, unpublished).

The estimates of *in vivo* forward velocity presented in Table II were calculated based on α-ketoglutarate concentration because mammary aspartate levels are high (Table III) using the K_m reported for the cytoplasmic enzyme for α-ketoglutarate of 3.6×10^{-4} M (Boyd, 1961). Although the estimates of net *in vivo* flux for the aspartate aminotransferase reaction in Table II are most likely quite low due to lack of definitive data, it seems clear that enzyme capacity is in considerable excess *in vivo* and that the reaction is in equilibrium. It is suggested that advantage may be taken of this observation in estimating mammary oxalacetate concentrations. Oxalacetate is present at very low concentrations in all tissues (Greenbaum *et al.*, 1971) including mammary (Table III) and, hence, is very difficult to estimate directly. A better estimate may be obtainable by determining aspartate, glutamate, and α-ketoglutarate levels and calculating oxalacetate from these estimates and K_{equil}.

6. Succinate dehydrogenase (succinate:[acceptor] oxidoreductase; EC 1.3.99.1)

a. REACTION.   Succinate + acceptor ⇆ fumarate + reduced acceptor

b. ASSAY.   Usually determine rate of reduction of an artificial electron acceptor such as 2,6-dichlorophenol-indophenol or a tetrazolium dye spectrophotometrically in the presence of succinate (Baldwin and Milligan, 1966; Korsrud and Baldwin, 1972a).

c. COMMENTS AND DISCUSSION.   Succinic dehydrogenase is found mainly in mitochondria (Smith *et al.*, 1966). Estimates of activity based on assays with artificial acceptors are of limited value in evaluating metabolic parameters so these were not calculated (Table II).

7. Malate dehydrogenase (L-malate:NAD oxidoreductase; EC 1.1.1.37)

a. REACTION.   L-Malate + NAD ⇆ oxalacetate + $NADH_2$

b. ASSAY.   Oxalacetate + $NADH_2$[*] → malate + NAD

c. COMMENTS AND DISCUSSION.   Malate dehydrogenase (NAD) is one of the most active of the mammary enzymes. The enzyme is most often assayed in postmitochondrial supernatants so most estimates reflect only the activity of the cytosol enzyme. The mass action ratio (Table II) is very close to K_{equil} suggesting, when taken along with estimates of V_{max} and v_f far in excess of net *in vivo* flux, that the reaction is in equilibrium *in vivo*. Direction of reaction *in vivo* in the two cellular compartments and net flux are expected to depend greatly upon redox state in each intracellular location.

Mitochondrial malate dehydrogenase differs from the cytoplasmic enzyme in electrophoretic and kinetic properties. Grimm and Doherty (1961) characterized the enzymes from ox heart and found differing K_m and turnover numbers for malate and oxalacetate consistent with the view that the mitochondrial enzyme is better for malate oxidation while the cytoplasmic enzyme catalyzes the reverse reaction most efficiently. The mitochondrial enzyme is sensitive to oxalacetate inhibition while excess malate tends to inhibit the cytoplasmic enzyme. These characteristics appear to favor transport of reducing equivalent as malate from the cytosol to the mitochondrion.

Karlsson and Carlsson (1968) reported that the mitochondrial (cathodic) enzyme increased during pregnancy and lactation in rat mammary but was not observable in virgin glands or after involution. These changes may reflect increased mitochondrial numbers in active secretory cells.

---

[*] Determine $NADH_2$ oxidation at 340 nm. An alternate assay is to determine, at high pH to offset K_{equil}, $NADH_2$ formation from malate. In the latter assay, rates are 8 times lower and, generally, less reliable (Korsrud and Baldwin, 1972a).

In extensive studies, it has been noted that cytoplasmic malate dehydrogenase activities per secretory cell are quite constant and are not affected by changes in physiological and hormonal state (Korsrud and Baldwin, 1969, 1972a,b). For this reason and because mammary malate dehydrogenase levels are extremely high and easy to determine, malate dehydrogenase can be usefully employed as a reference enzyme to ascertain that changes in the activities of other secretory cell enzymes induced by hormones, endocrinectomies, or other experimental treatments, can be attributed to specific treatment effects and not artifacts such as general degeneration.

F. Fatty Acid Synthesis: Metabolism and Esterification

Most of the enzymes relevant to this section are discussed in some detail by Bauman and Davis (Chapters 1 and 2, Vol. II), and, hence, are considered only with reference to Tables I and II.

1. Malic enzyme (L-malate:NADP oxidoreductase [decarboxylating]; EC 1.1.1.40)

a. REACTION. L-Malate + NADP $\leftrightarrows$ pyruvate + CO_2 + $NADPH_2$

b. ASSAY. Measure $NADPH_2$ production at 340 mμ in presence of malate, NADP and enzyme (Korsrud and Baldwin, 1972a).

c. COMMENTS AND DISCUSSION. Malic enzyme fulfills an important role in $NADPH_2$ generation in rat mammary but not ruminant mammary tissue (Chapters 1 and 2, Vol. II). Malic enzyme levels are very low in the latter species (Table I). In computing free $NADP/NADPH_2$ ratios for rat mammary (Table III) it was found that estimates obtained using the NADP-linked isocitrate dehydrogenase and malic enzyme couples differed markedly (Baldwin and Cheng, 1969; Korsrud and Baldwin, 1972b). In discussion of this observation it was suggested that one or both of the two dehydrogenase reactions were not in equilibrium. The data in Table II tend to substantiate this suggestion for the malic enzyme. The calculated v_f is very close to net flux *in vivo* when a K_m for malate of 3.4×10^{-4} M (Barman, 1969) is used. Since, as discussed above, free NADP concentrations are likely quite low and rate limiting in mammary tissue and the v_f and *in vivo* flux estimates are very close, it is suggested that this reaction is not in equilibrium *in vivo* and that at physiological substrate concentrations, the activity of malic enzyme is rate limiting. This suggestion is consistent with a report by Katz and Wals (1972) that $NADPH_2$ generation by the malic enzyme in mammary tissue is proportionately less than in adipose tissue. It is suggested further that malic enzyme flux *in vivo* would be expected to be quite dependent on redox state or NADP availability.

2. Citrate cleavage enzyme (ATP:citrate oxalacetate-lyase [CoA acetylating and ATP-dephosphorylating]; EC 4.1.3.8)

a. REACTION. ATP + citrate + CoASH $\rightleftharpoons$ ADP + Pi + acetyl-CoA + oxalacetate

b. ASSAY. Determine rate of oxalacetate formation in presence of citrate, ATP and CoASH by linking to $NADH_2$ and malate dehydrogenase (Korsrud and Baldwin, 1972a).

c. COMMENTS AND DISCUSSION. Much attention has been directed at analyses of citrate cleavage enzyme function(s) in lipogenic tissues from simple stomached animals because of its essential role in the transfer of mitochondrial acetyl-CoA to the cytoplasm (Chapters 1 and 2, Vol. II). To accomplish this transfer, mitochondrial acetyl-CoA is incorporated into citrate (citrate synthetase) which diffuses from the mitochondrion and is cleaved to form oxalacetate and cytoplasmic acetyl-CoA by the citrate cleavage enzyme. The oxalacetate can re-enter the mitochondrion as malate after reduction with $NADH_2$, as aspartate after transamination or as pyruvate after conversion to malate and oxidation by the malic enzyme to form pyruvate and $NADPH_2$. Citrate cleavage enzyme activities are very high and in apparent excess in rats, sows and mice and very low in cows (Tables I and II). The low activity in the cow apparently reflects the fact that the primary source of cytoplasmic acetyl-CoA in this species is acetate and not mitochondrial acetyl-CoA (Hardwick, 1966).

3. Acetyl-CoA carboxylase (acetyl-CoA:carbon dioxide lyase [ADP]; EC 6.4.1.2)

a. REACTION. ATP + acetyl-CoA + CO_2 + H_2O → ADP + Pi + malonyl-CoA

b. ASSAY. Determine rate of $H^{14}CO_3{}^{2-}$ incorporation into malonyl-CoA (Miller and Levy, 1969).

c. COMMENTS AND DISCUSSION. Acetyl-CoA carboxylase catalyzes the first and, in most systems studied, rate-limiting reaction in the biosynthesis of fatty acids from acetyl-CoA. Purified preparations of acetyl-CoA carboxylase from various sources are activated by Mg^{2+}, fructose-1,6-diP, α-glycerol-P, glucose-6-P, palmityl carnitine, and related compounds.

Palmityl-CoA and other acyl-CoA thioesters are potent inhibitors of the enzyme (Miller and Levy, 1969). Rat mammary acetyl-CoA carboxylase is inhibited by certain nonesterified fatty acids in milk and has, hence, been implicated as the affected site accounting for the rapid decrease in mammary fatty acid synthesis at weaning (Howanitz and Levy, 1965; Levy, 1964).

Due to the complexity of acetyl-CoA carboxylase kinetics, computation of v_f was not considered useful, especially in view of the fact that reported V_{max} data are less than the *in vivo* flux estimates (Tables I and II). This may be due, in part, to association of the enzyme *in vivo* with membranes as discussed by Miller and Levy (1969).

4. Fatty acid synthetase

a. REACTION. Acetyl-CoA + n malonyl-CoA + $2n$ NADPH$_2$ → palmityl-CoA + $2n$ NADP + n CO$_2$

b. ASSAY. Determine NADPH$_2$ disappearance at 340 nm in presence of enzyme, acetyl-CoA, and malonyl-CoA.

c. COMMENTS AND DISCUSSION. Rat mammary fatty acid synthetase has been isolated and studied in great detail (Smith and Abraham, 1970, 1971b). The enzyme is subject to dissociation and inactivation in the cold and can be reassociated or activated by incubation at 30°. Unlike liver fatty acid synthetase, the activity of the mammary enzyme is not affected by malonyl-CoA and fructose-1,6-diP. Increasing concentrations of malonyl-CoA and high malonyl-CoA to acetyl-CoA ratios increase the chain length of fatty acids synthesized by cell free extracts and purified fatty acid synthetase (Carey and Dils, 1970; Hansen *et al.*, 1970; Smith and Abraham, 1971a). Interpretation of these data is complicated by the observation that butyryl-CoA is a better primer for fatty acid synthesis than acetyl-CoA (Smith and Abraham, 1971b; Lin and Kumar, 1971, 1972). In addition, mammary malonyl-CoA levels have not been reported so it is not known how this observation relates to the fact that milk fat fatty acids synthesized in the gland vary between C$_{12}$ and C$_{16}$ while palmitate is essentially the only fatty acid synthesized in other tissues. This difference in pattern of fatty acids synthesized is apparently not attributable to tissue differences in fatty acid synthetase (Lin and Kumar, 1972; Smith and Abraham, 1971a).

5. α-Glycerol-P dehydrogenase (L-glycerol-3-P:NAD oxidoreductase; EC 1.1.1.8)

a. REACTION.   L-Glycerol-3-P + NAD $\leftrightarrows$ dihydroxyacetone-P + NADH$_2$

b. ASSAY.   Determine NADH$_2$ production or formation in presence of α-glycerol-P or dihydroxyacetone-P, respectively.

c. COMMENTS AND DISCUSSION.   The role of α-glycerol-P dehydrogenase in the formation of α-glycerol-P required for milk triglyceride synthesis is essential and straightforward. The only alternate source of glycerol-P is formation from glycerol and ATP via the glycerol kinase reaction. Glycerol kinase is present in mammary tissue as evidenced by the fact that arterial glycerol is incorporated into lactose and other milk components (Wood et al., 1958; West et al., 1972). However, glycerol kinase levels in mammary tissue are very low (0.88 units/gm tissue; Baldwin and Milligan, 1966) and mammary A-V differences for glycerol are essentially zero (Linzell, 1969; West et al., 1972). Hence, a significant fraction of the α-glycerol-P required for esterification of fatty acids synthesized in the mammary gland must be formed via the α-glycerol-P dehydrogenase reaction. This holds whether or not one considers operation of a monoglyceride pathway and/or utilization of glycerol formed from blood lipoprotein triglycerides, since fatty acids synthesized in the gland must be esterified.

Comparisons of the K_{equil} and mass action ratios for the α-glycerol-P dehydrogenase reaction indicate that the reaction favors α-glycerol-P formation and is close to being in equilibrium in vivo under most conditions (Table II; Baldwin and Cheng, 1969). V_{max} and forward velocity estimates are high relative to net in vivo flux, further indicating excess enzymatic capacity and an equilibrium reaction. As was suggested above in discussion of the glyceraldehyde-3-P dehydrogenase reaction, it appears that net flux through the α-glycerol-P dehydrogenase reaction is determined primarily by the energy and redox (NAD/NADH$_2$) status of the cell and, perhaps, rate of triglyceride or fatty acid synthesis. In the latter regard it is important to note that a lack of α-glycerol-P can depress triglyceride synthesis, result in a build-up of fatty acyl-CoA and, as a result of fatty acyl-CoA feedback, depress fatty acid synthesis (Howard and Lowenstein, 1965).

G.   Other Enzymes

A number of additional mammary enzymes have been or should be investigated. Current available data were not considered sufficient to warrant discussion of these in detail; however, we felt that several should be discussed briefly. This is done in subsequent paragraphs.

Guinea pig, rat, and cow lipoprotein lipase(s) have been investigated relative to changes in activity with stage of lactation, the essential role of this enzyme in the hydrolysis of blood triglyceride prior to uptake by the mammary gland, characterization, and mechanisms of action (Benson *et al.*, 1969; Hamosh *et al.*, 1970; McBride and Korn, 1963; Robinson, 1963; Shirley *et al.*, 1971; Hamosh and Evans, 1972; Emery *et al.*, 1972). Since lipoprotein triglyceride hydrolysis is irreversible and is the first step in triglyceride fatty acid uptake, it seems reasonable to suggest that lipoprotein lipase is involved in regulation of lipoprotein triglyceride uptake by the mammary gland. There may be adequate provision for such regulation through activation of lipoprotein lipase and its substrate by serum and other factors and through variation in amount of lipoprotein lipase at the site of lipoprotein triglyceride hydrolysis. In addition, the possibility that availability (blood concentrations) of specific lipoprotein triglyceride fractions is a determinant of lipoprotein triglyceride uptake must be considered (Emery *et al.*, 1972). Due to the use of artificial substrates in the assay of lipoprotein lipase and uncertainty as to the proportion of total tissue lipoprotein lipase activity found at the site of triglyceride hydrolysis, interpretation of kinetic, V_{max}, and other data in relation to metabolism are difficult and tenuous. Further study is essential.

The enzymes of triglyceride synthesis in mammary tissue have not been investigated individually and, indeed, some questions still exist relative to their identity or what pathways are present (Benson *et al.*, 1969; Bickerstaffe and Annison, 1971). Benson *et al.* (1969) studied the effects of diet and stage of lactation on the activity of the triglyceride synthetase system (several enzymes). However, due to the complexity of the system and the assay used, it is difficult to relate the results obtained to *in vivo* flux or to evaluate the *in vivo* capacity of the system. Recently, the stearyl desaturase found in ruminant and pig mammary (Bickerstaffe and Annison, 1970; Kinsella, 1970) has been implicated as fulfilling an essential role in making critical amounts of oleate for optimal rates of triglyceride formation *in vivo* (Kinsella, 1972). Desaturase activities in rat, rabbit, sow, and goat mammary glands were 0.0, 0.0, 0.11, and 0.15 units/gm tissue, respectively (Lossow and Chaikoff, 1958; Bickerstaffe and Annison, 1970).

Two important enzymes involved in pyruvate metabolism and which fulfill essential roles in mammary energy metabolism and milk fat synthesis have received only minimal attention. These are pyruvate dehydrogenase and pyruvate carboxylase. Pyruvate dehydrogenase is a mitochondrial enzyme and has been implicated as a rate-limiting, regulatory site in several tissues (Wieland *et al.*, 1971; Coore, *et al.*, 1971). Important effectors of pyruvate dehydrogenase activity appear to be ATP and acetyl-CoA (Wieland and Siess, 1970). Greenbaum and Darby

(1964) reported data consistent with the view that the mammary pyruvate dehydrogenase reaction was depressed in adrenalectomized rats and that this depression is the cause of decreased fat synthesis from glucose in these animals. Pyruvate carboxylase catalyzes the conversion of pyruvate to oxalacetate with the uptake of carbon dioxide and expenditure of one ATP (Figs. 1 and 2). Regulation of the function of this enzyme has been reviewed in detail by Utter and Scrutton (1969). Pyruvate carboxylase is dependent upon the presence of acetyl-CoA for activity and in ruminant tissues is activated by butyryl-CoA (Ballard and Hanson, 1969). Pyruvate carboxylase was found in both mitochondrial and cytosol fractions prepared from rat mammary glands and mainly mitochondrial fractions from rabbit mammary glands (Gul and Dils, 1969). Pyruvate carboxylase activities in rat and rabbit tissues were 0.5 and 0.8 units/gm tissue, respectively.

β-Hydroxybutyrate dehydrogenase is an important mitochondrial enzyme in ruminant tissues in that it is required in β-hydroxybutyrate use as an energy source. The enzyme is of further interest because if its levels in mammary are sufficient to maintain the reaction in equilibrium, tissue levels of acetoacetate and β-hydroxybutyrate can be utilized along with the K_{equil} of the reaction to compute the ratio of free NAD to free $NADH_2$ in mammary mitochondria (Veech et al., 1969a). Rat and cow mammary β-hydroxybutyrate dehydrogenase levels were 25.0 and 2.73 units/gm tissue, respectively (Bauman et al., 1970).

Greenbaum and Greenwood (1954), Slater (1961), Slater et al. (1963), and Helminen and Ericsson (1970, 1971) studied the activities of a number of hydrolytic and degradative enzymes in mammary tissue. In general, the activities of these enzymes are low in lactating tissue and increase sharply at weaning. For example, acid phosphatase, aryl sulfatase, β-glucuronidase, and cathepsin D increase in total activity on the first day after weaning, reach peak values on the second and third day after weaning, and tend to decline thereafter (Helminen and Ericsson, 1970, 1971).

Very few data are available regarding the activities of specific enzymes involved in protein synthesis in mammary glands. Most aspects of mammary protein synthesis are reviewed by Denamur in Chapter 8 and Larson and Jorgenson in Chapter 4, Vol. II, and, hence, need not be discussed here. Bucovaz and Davis (1961) evaluated changes in amino acid activating enzyme activities in rat mammary gland and found dramatic changes in activity during pregnancy and lactation and maximum activities at midlactation. Since these workers used an exchange assay, it is not possible to relate their estimates to in vivo flux rates. Herrington and Hawtrey

(1970, 1971) have presented data which suggest that nonlactating cow mammary glands lack the enzyme which incorporates CTP and ATP into the 3′-terminus amino acid acceptor end of tRNA and thus makes tRNA which can accept amino acids. They reported further that a lack of specific proteins on ribosomes from nonlactating cow mammary glands renders these ribosomes incapable of protein synthesis. Formation of the tRNA nucleotide-incorporating enzyme and the missing ribosomal proteins is clearly essential for lactogenesis. These data suggest that just as is the case with enzymes of lactose and fat synthesis, several key enzymes involved in protein synthesis vary in activity in mammary glands and are possibly determinants of rates of protein synthesis.

Mammary activities of several additional enzymes not discussed herein were reviewed and discussed by Munford (1964) and Folley (1961).

III. REGULATION OF MAMMARY ENZYME ACTIVITIES

A. Changes in Enzyme Activities during Secretory Cell Development, Lactogenesis, Lactation, and Involution

1. General Patterns

The general pattern of changes in rat mammary enzyme activities during pregnancy, lactation, and involution is represented in Fig. 3. The mammary glands of virgin and early pregnant animals have very few secretory cells and, as might be expected from this, enzyme activities are low. Enzyme activity per gram tissue and per milligram DNA are low because enzyme activities in the adipose, connective, and other non-secretory elements which comprise the gland at this stage are low in comparison with enzyme activities in secretory cells. Total gland enzyme activities are low because the predominant cell types present are low in activity and because the gland is small. During mid-and late pregnancy, a major increase in DNA occurs (Fig. 3). This reflects the formation of secretory elements in the gland (Munford, 1963, 1964; Traurig, 1967). This increase in mainly secretory cells is followed closely by an increase in enzyme activities (Fig. 3). During this period, the activities of virtually all enzymes that have been studied increase. The increases are evident when enzyme data are expressed on a per gram tissue or per milligram DNA basis because the proportion of very active secretory to less active cell types such as adipose increases rapidly. Also, enzyme activities per milligram DNA increase because the increases in enzyme activities lag

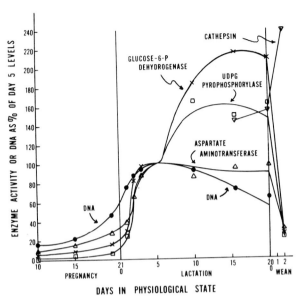

Fig. 3. Enzyme changes in rat mammary glands during lactation. Data plotted were derived from Greenbaum and Greenwood (1954) and Baldwin and Milligan (1966).

behind the increases in DNA. The changes in enzyme activities are, of course, most prominent when expressed on a total gland basis as in Fig. 3 because the gland is increasing in size. Since the activities of almost all enzymes increase during this period and the increases occur immediately after the formation of new secretory cells, it seems appropriate to conclude that the increases in enzyme activity which occur during this period reflect the development of newly formed secretory cells. These changes in enzyme activity have been reviewed and discussed by Munford (1964), Kuhn and Lowenstein (1967), and Baldwin (1968, 1969). Clear indications of the close relationship between secretory cell formation and general increases in enzyme activities illustrated in Fig. 3 for rats have also been reported for guinea pigs (Baldwin, 1966; Kuhn and Lowenstein, 1967), rabbits (Hartmann, 1969; Heitzman, 1967), and mice (Munford, 1963). A clear relationship has not been established for cows (Baldwin, 1966; Shirley et al., 1971, Mellenberger et al., 1972). This does not mean that such a relationship does not exist, but rather, that the conditions of experimentation were not sufficient to test for such a relationship. The primary limitation has been that, of necessity, biopsy techniques were used and as a result estimates of total gland DNA and enzyme activities were not obtained. Sampling frequency during the critical period of secretory cell formation and presumed development was also limited in these studies.

For the purposes of subsequent discussion, it is useful to consider the enzyme increases which occur during secretory cell development as including three possible groups of enzymes. The first group that might be considered would include constitutive enzymes whose activities are not hormone dependent or are hormone dependent in only the most general fashion in, for example, requiring only a hormonal environment consistent with secretory cell survival for their synthesis. A second group might include enzymes whose synthesis or levels are, in part, constitutive and, in part, hormone dependent. A third group would include enzymes whose synthesis is almost entirely subject to specific hormonal regulation. Although available data do not provide for clear definition of these suggested groups nor substantiate their existence, some distinctions can be made. These are discussed below with regard to possible relationships between changes in enzyme activities, lactogenesis, hormone actions and regulation of milk yields.

The general enzyme increases characteristic of mammary secretory cell development are, largely, complete by the third to fifth day of lactation in the rat (Fig. 3). This type of development may be completed earlier or later in other species or in different strains within a species (Munford, 1963; Baldwin, 1966; Hartmann, 1969) but is usually completed either late in pregnancy or early in lactation. The changes in enzyme activities which occur after general cell development is complete or during lactation, appear to be fairly specific in nature since not all enzymes are affected. Several not completely defensible but, nevertheless, useful generalizations can and have been made regarding changes in mammary enzyme activities during lactation (Baldwin, 1969; Emery and Baldwin, 1967; Korsrud and Baldwin, 1972a,b,c). The first generalization is that the activities of general metabolic or constitutive enzymes represented in Fig. 3 by aspartate aminotransferase do not change significantly after the fifth day of lactation while the activities of many enzymes involved in milk biosynthesis represented in Fig. 3 by glucose-6-P dehydrogenase and UDP-glucose pyrophosphorylase continue to increase reaching peak activities between the twelfth and nineteenth days of lactation (Baldwin, 1966). This generalization does not always hold true as can be seen from the ratios of day 11/day 5 enzyme activities presented in Table IV for several additional enzymes. A second suggestion is that the increases in enzyme activities which occur during this period can be attributed to specific increases in the rates of synthesis of the affected enzymes (Emery and

TABLE IV

SUMMARY EFFECTS OF ADRENALETOMY AND HYPOPHYSECTOMY AND HORMONE LEVELS
ON MAMMARY ENZYME LEVELS[a]

Enzyme	Day 11 activity/day 5 activity[b]			Basal level as % day 11[c]	Cortisol + prolactin required in hypophysectomy[d]
	Normal	AX	AXC		
Affected enzymes					
Glucose-6-P dehydrogenase	1.8	0.8	2.5	38	Yes
P-Glucomutase	1.3	1.3	1.6	39	Yes
UDPglucose pyrophosphorylase	1.5	0.7	2.3	42	Yes
UDPgalactose-4-epimerase	1.4	0.6	1.6	49	Yes
Lactose synthetase	—	—	—	54	—
Citrate cleavage enzyme	2.8	0.6	3.7	12	Yes
Malic enzyme	1.3	0.8	1.4	56	Yes
Fatty acid synthetase	—	—	—	12	Yes
Succinic dehydrogenase	1.3	0.9	1.4	—	—
Enzymes not affected					
Hexokinase	1.3	1.3	1.9	90	—
Phosphofructokinase	2.3	1.6	2.0	—	—
Fructose-1,6-diP aldolase	1.1	1.1	1.0	100	—
Pyruvate kinase	1.6	1.7	1.4	—	No
Aspartate aminotransferase	1.1	1.2	0.9	—	—
Isocitrate dehydrogenase (NADP)	1.0	0.9	1.0	0.8	No
Malate dehydrogenase (NAD)	0.8	0.9	0.8	—	No

[a] Summarized from Baldwin and Martin (1968) and Korsrud and Baldwin (1969, 1972a,b,c).

[b] Enzyme activities observed on day 11 in normal, adrenalectomized (AX), and adrenalectomized receiving cortisol (AXC) animals divided by enzyme activities on day 5 of lactation which was the day of adrenalectomy.

[c] Enzyme activity in mammary glands of rats 4 days after adrenalectomy on day 11 of lactation expressed as percentage of enzyme activities in normal day 11 rats. After adrenalectomy the activities of affected enzymes decrease rapidly and plateau at "basal" levels. A clear plateau is reached within 4 days and usually extends for 4–6 days. The ratio of plateau value per day 11 value is considered an index of basal (not glucocorticoid dependent) activity as a percentage of total activity at day 11 of lactation.

[d] Maintenance of normal activities per milligram DNA for several enzymes in hypophysectomized rat mammary glands requires administration of cortisol plus prolactin (in addition to oxytocin administered to facilitate milk removal). Enzymes requiring cortisol plus prolactin for normal activities are indicated by "yes." Enzymes whose activities per DNA are maintained without cortisol plus prolactin are indicated by "no."

Baldwin, 1967; Korsrud and Baldwin, 1972b,c). The third generalization is that these increases in enzyme activities are often hormone dependent (Korsrud and Baldwin, 1969, 1972a,b). These enzyme changes will be discussed in greater detail below in relation to specific hormone actions.

The final and, perhaps, most dramatic changes in mammary enzyme activities occur at weaning. Very soon after cessation of milk removal, a rapid decrease in mammary enzyme levels occurs (Fig. 3, Baldwin and Milligan, 1966; Jones, 1967). Also, after weaning a rapid increase in the activities of lysosomal enzymes occurs (Greenbaum and Greenwood, 1954; Slater, 1961; Helminen and Ericsson, 1970, 1971). This increase is represented by the cathepsin curve in Fig. 3. Helminen and Ericsson (1970) reported that total gland activities of four lysosomal enzymes (see previous section) increased markedly within a day of weaning, reached peak values on the second or third day of involution and declined slowly thereafter. Studies with cycloheximide indicated that the increases in lysosomal enzyme activities were due, at least in part, to new enzyme synthesis. Similar qualitative changes were produced when involution was induced by unilateral ligation of milk ducts in lactating rats, implying that hormone changes associated with weaning are not the cause of involution. Rather, it appears that accumulation of milk in the gland leading to feedback inhibition of milk synthesis (McLean, 1964; Levy, 1964), cell damage, ischemia induced by low blood flow rates through the distended gland, and possibly other local factors are the cause of involution (also see discussion of hypophysectomy below).

2. Enzyme Changes at Lactogenesis and during Lactation

Considerable thought, effort, and discussion have been directed at the hypothesis that the activities of a small group of key enzymes increase sharply at parturition in response to the hormone changes which occur at this time and that increases in the activities of these key enzymes are responsible for lactogenesis. In rats, guinea pigs, mice, and rabbits, it is almost impossible to address or test this hypothesis effectively because any specific or key enzyme changes that might lead to lactogenesis are thoroughly confounded with changes in cellularity and general enzyme increases associated with the development of newly formed secretory cells (Fig. 3). In the cow, on the other hand, secretory cell formation and development may be fairly complete a week or two prior to parturition (Baldwin, 1966; Mellenberger *et al.*, 1972) enabling identification and interpretation of key enzyme changes that might occur at parturition and cause lactogenesis. Several studies with cows have yielded data consistent with this hypothesis. The results reported imply that preferential (greater than increases in the activities of other enzymes) increases in the activities of lipoprotein lipase, lactose synthetase and acetyl-CoA carboxylase occur at lactogenesis. The NADP linked dehydrogenases and acetyl-CoA synthetase were implicated to a lesser extent (Shirley et al., 1971; Marinez and Cook, 1971; Mellenberger et al., 1972). The hypothesis is attractive and these supporting data are encouraging in terms of developing an explanation of lactogenesis. However, it must be noted that the data cited were reported as abstracts only and cannot be fully evaluated at this time in terms of experimental conditions and the real possibility that the reported changes reflect the development of newly formed secretory cells and are not a unique event responsible for lactogenesis. In the latter regard it should be noted that only the activities of enzymes highly associated with milk synthesis were reported. This makes the data difficult to interpret. The activities of constitutive enzymes should not increase at parturition if the required interpretive assumption that general cell development was complete when the prepartum samples were taken is to be accepted. Data on constitutive enzymes consistent with this assumption must be available before the hypothesis that lactogenesis is attributable to specific induction of the synthesis of a few key enzymes can be evaluated further and accepted.

The initiation and maintenance of lactation clearly requires the formation and maintenance of secretory cells, development within these cells of the enzymatic capacity for milk synthesis, the existence of mechanisms for regulating rates of milk component synthesis, an adequate supply of nutrients, and milk removal. In considering lactogenesis or lactation in a more general sense and with regard to these requirements, a number of critical and, largely, unresolved questions arise. One of these questions was treated briefly above with regard to the hypothesis that key enzyme changes are responsible for lactogenesis. A more general statement of the question is which, if any or all, of the above required processes are the "trigger(s)" for lactogenesis. In addition, it seems appropriate to determine which of these processes are regulated by hormones and in what fashion; and, further, to ask which of these processes are important determinants of milk yield. Various data discussed in other chapters and above with regard to cell proliferation and development during pregnancy and lactation clearly indicate that hormones regulate mammary secretory cell formation and development. Secretory cell formation and development are often coincident in time with lactogenesis but this is not always true as discussed above for the cow. In addition, one might suspect that in most species there are sufficient secretory cells present prepartum to support milk synthesis at some level prior to lactogenesis. These considerations suggest that secretory cell formation and general development are essential for lactation but are not likely the "trigger" event of lactogenesis.

The actions of hormones in the regulation of development within secretory cells of the enzymes required for milk synthesis as related to lactogenesis and regulation of milk yield are less clear. In *in vivo* and *in vitro* studies using milk component formation as a criterion, insulin, prolactin, glucocorticoids, and progesterone have been implicated as acting in the initiation and/or maintenance of milk synthesis (Topper and Oka, Chapter 6; Lyons *et al.*, 1958; Kuhn, 1969; Martin and Baldwin, 1971a; Korsrud and Baldwin, 1972a). The development of secretory cells after formation during pregnancy and early lactation is general in involving the formation of constitutive as well as biosynthetic enzymes as discussed above with regard to Fig. 3. Specific hormone actions regulating development of the enzymatic capacity for milk synthesis may or may not be reflected in these changes since in intact animals both inherent and hormone regulated development might occur simultaneously. Inherent development implies either no hormone actions or very general, permissive hormone actions while hormone dependent development implies specific homone actions involving enzyme synthesis. In both *in vitro* (Topper and Oka, Chapter 6) and *in vivo* (Martin and Baldwin, 1971a,b,c; Walters and McLean, 1968a,b) systems, the actions of insulin appear to be of the general or permissive type. Insulin insufficiency in diabetic animals or induced by administration of anti-insulin serum leads to almost immediate cessation of milk synthesis and within 36–48 hours to rapid losses in mammary secretory cells (Walters and McLean, 1968b; Martin and Baldwin, 1971a). The loss or death of secretory cells is accompanied by general decreases in enzyme activities as might be expected. However, the earlier effect of insulin insufficiency—cessation of milk synthesis—is not attributable to enzyme changes since none occur. This effect is due, rather, to a disruption in energy metabolism possibly involving electron transport (Martin and Baldwin, 1971b,c). These observations support the views that insulin acts in a permissive fashion in lactogenesis, does not induce the synthesis of specific mammary enzymes and, thereby, cause lactogenesis, and, that insulin, acting in a general fashion, regulates mammary metabolism and, hence, may contribute in the regulation of milk yield.

The studies with hypophysectomized and adrenalectomized rats (Korsrud and Baldwin, 1969, 1972a,b,c; Willmer and Foster, 1965) discussed in a later section of this chapter and *in vitro* studies summarized by Topper and Oka, in Chapter 6, indicate that prolactin and glucocorticoids may act in a specific fashion in regulating mammary enzyme synthesis and, thereby, possibly affect lactogenesis and rates of milk synthesis. Studies with hypophysectomized and adrenalectomized rats indicate that secretory cells have constitutive levels of several biosynthetic enzymes and that the activities of six to eight of these are increased by glucocorticoids and prolactin (Korsrud and Baldwin, 1969, 1972a). A clear requirement for glucocorticoids for the development and maintenance of normal mammary levels of several key mammary biosynthetic enzymes was demonstrated. The activities of other (constitutive) enzymes were not affected. Of the enzymes whose activities are affected by glucocorticoids, most are present in adrenalectomized animals at constitutive levels sufficient for maintenance of normal lactation according to the criteria of *in vivo* equilibrium, etc., discussed in the previous section (Korsrud and Baldwin, 1972b) and, hence, are not good candidates for consideration as "key" enzyme inductions responsible for lactogenesis. Further metabolic studies are required to determine which, if any, of the hormone dependent enzymes are good candidates to consider with regard to the regulation of lactogenesis and milk synthesis.

The case for prolactin is less clear. In *in vivo* studies, prolactin appears essential for secretory cell maintenance and survival (Folley, 1961; Jones, 1967; Korsrud and Baldwin, 1969) and cell losses complicate the interpretation of the enzyme data. In addition, prolactin has the effects of increasing the rates of synthesis of all RNA types, increasing tissue RNA levels, and increasing rates of protein (including casein) synthesis (Baldwin and Martin, 1968; Baldwin et al., 1969a). In hypophysectomized animals, both prolactin and a glucocorticoid must be administered to maintain the activities of a number of biosynthetic enzymes while the activities per milligram DNA of several other enzymes are maintained without therapy. Against this background of general prolactin actions and its interaction with glucocorticoids, it is difficult to evaluate apparent effects of prolactin upon the levels of specific enzymes. In *in vitro* systems the actions of prolactin have been evaluated in detail. It is interesting to speculate in comparing the results of *in vivo* and *in vitro* studies about the role of prolactin in lactogenesis and its specificity of action with regard to regulating of synthesis of specific enzymes, its general role in regulation of RNA and protein synthesis, and its interactions with glucocorticoids. Even so, further work directed at evaluation of the role of prolactin *in vivo* is required before specific actions of prolactin in the regulation of "key" enzyme synthesis and lactogenesis are proposed or accepted.

Ovariectomy and/or hysterectomy in late pregnancy results within 24–48 hours in a dramatic increase in mammary lactose levels indicating lactogenesis. This result can be prevented by administration of high levels of progesterone (Yokoyama *et al.*, 1969; Kuhn, 1969). In considering this observation along with data indicating that changes in plasma levels of several hormones, including glucocorticoids and prolactin, at lactogenesis are not sufficient to act as a lactogenic "trigger" or signal, Kuhn (1969) proposed that the dramatic decrease in progesterone prior to parturition is the lactogenic trigger. This view has several implications with regard to lactogenesis. One of these is that progesterone might act as a specific repressor and prevent the synthesis, prepartum, of key enzymes required for milk synthesis. The synthesis of these enzymes may or may not be regulated, in addition, by glucocorticoids and prolactin. Alternatively, progesterone might inhibit the function of key enzymes thereby preventing milk synthesis, or progesterone might be a general repressor of secretory cell proliferation and/or development. A number of additional possible implications can be drawn but these go beyond the current context. It is important to point out that even though it is convenient to consider specific hormone induction(s) of enzyme synthesis as a possible lactogenic trigger, a "depression" of enzyme synthesis or a release of enzyme inhibition would serve as well.

A reasonable summary view of possible relationships between the formation within secretory cells of the enzymatic capacity for milk synthesis and lactogenesis might be that secretory cells inherently form all or almost all of the enzymes required for milk synthesis; that the levels of a number of these enzymes are regulated in part by prolactin and glucocorticoids; and, that the synthesis of a few key biosynthetic enzymes at parturition resulting from decreases in progesterone levels and/or increases in prolactin and glucocorticoid actions might be a component of the lactogenic mechanism. Further evaluation of the latter possibility is required before acceptance of enzyme induction as the lactogenic "trigger" is appropriate.

It is easy to imply that enzyme changes induced by hormones at lactogenesis, during lactation or after endocrinectomy are essential to and/or responsible for changes in lactational performance. As has been emphasized in this chapter, establishing cause and effect relationships between changes in enzyme activities and metabolic activity or rate of milk synthesis requires application of additional data and in the case of mammary secretory cells, considerable additional study. For this reason, it must be emphasized that although hormonally regulated changes in mammary enzyme activity during pregnancy, lactogenesis, and lactation are correlated with changes in milk yield, cause and effect are not established. In view of this, several additional factors required for the initiation and maintenance of lactation and listed in a previous paragraph must be considered as participants in the regulation of mammary function. Several types of metabolic regulation not involving changes in enzyme activity may modulate mammary metabolism and act as determinants of lactogenesis and milk yield and composition. The action of insulin as evaluated in insulin insufficiency and noted above and in a subsequent section is a good example. In addition, factors such as feedback inhibition, allosteric effectors of enzyme functions, hormonal (or other) regulation of cyclic AMP, cellular energy and redox state, and nutrient supply have and should be considered. A number of these were discussed with regard to specific enzymes in a previous section. Unfortunately, effects of these factors in the regulation of mammary secretory cell metabolism, in the overall, have not been evaluated. Hence, beyond mention, further discussion is inappropriate. Milk removal is clearly a determinant of lactational performance. As was considered with regard to enzyme changes at involution, feedback of milk components, ischemia and, finally, a rapid loss of secretory cells accompany failure to remove milk. In the converse, simple removal of colostrum and possible inhibitors of milk biosynthesis may contribute to lactogenesis. Linzell (1969) considered the possibility that a sharp increase in blood flow to the mammary glands occurs at parturition and is responsible for lactogenesis. Whether or not the increased supply of nutrients resulting from increased blood flow at parturition is a component of the lactogenic trigger or not requires further evaluation. Baldwin and Cheng (1969) reported that mammary nutrient and metabolite levels were adequate in the rat or elevated relative to lactation in the prepartum cow and, hence, not the most limiting factor preventing milk synthesis prepartum. It is clear that mammary blood flow and supply of nutrients can limit milk yields during lactation (Barry, 1964; Kronfeld, 1969). High correlates between blood nutrient concentrations and mammary uptake have been reported (Baldwin and Smith, 1971) and the possibility that nutrient availability is a significant determinant of mammary metabolism and milk synthesis must be seriously considered. If nutrients are not provided, enzyme capacity cannot be expressed.

Interpretation of mammary enzyme changes at lactogenesis and during lactation are limited by a lack of several types of critical data and complexities introduced by the participation of multiple factors in the regulation of mammary function. This is especially true with regard to hypotheses that key enzyme changes at parturition initiate lactation and that increases in milk yields during lactation are a result of increases in mammary enzyme activities during this period. In this section an attempt was made to evaluate various possible interpretations of enzyme data with regard to secretory cell development, lactogenesis, lactation, and involution, to point out areas of uncertainty in interpretation and identify several types of experiments or data that might facilitate further interpretation.

B.   Hormones and the Regulation of Mammary Enzyme Activities

The effects upon mammary enzyme levels of adrenalectomy, adrenalectomy-ovariectomy, ovariectomy, thyroidectomy, hypophysectomy, alloxan diabetes and anti-insulin serum administration, and appropriate hormone therapies have been investigated in rats, to a lesser extent in mice and not at all or to a very limited extent in other species. The emphasis upon rats in subsequent discussion is forced by the available data. At the outset, it must be emphasized that studies with other species are so limited that great care in writing and reading must be taken to avoid unjustified extrapolations to other species. The same relationships may or may not hold. In addition, it is difficult to avoid the implications that when endocrinectomy results in reduced mammary enzyme levels and/or altered mammary metabolism and when these effects are reversed by appropriate hormone therapy, the action of the hormone was directly upon the mammary gland and, possibly, involved specific regulation of enzyme synthesis. This implication is often invalidated by general metabolic actions of hormones, by effects of one hormone upon the secretion of other hormones, by losses of secretory cells in endocrinectomized animals, or by general effects of hormones upon secretory cells which might indirectly affect enzyme synthesis. Most workers, of course, try to control or exclude these variables which preclude identification of specific hormone:enzyme relationships but, due to limitations imposed by the difficulties inherent in work with endocrinectomized, lactating animals, attempts at rigorous control are often frustrated. In the following discussions of the effects of insulin, ovarian hormones, adrenal glucocorticoids, pituitary hormones, and thyroxin, an attempt to remain cognizant of indirect effects was made but even further constraint in interpretation may be required.

1.   Insulin

Two important factors must be considered in evaluating effects of diabetes and/or insulin insufficiency upon mammary enzyme levels. The first is that alloxan treatments of lactating animals often result in mammary involution or do not induce diabetes (Korsrud and Baldwin, 1969). The second is that prolonged insulin insufficiency (2–3 days) leads to significant losses of mammary secretory cells and enzyme changes attributable to this. Recent studies wherein these variables were controlled indicate that insulin insufficiency does not affect the levels of enzymes other than hexokinase II (Walters and McLean, 1967a, 1968a,b; Korsrud and Baldwin, 1969; Martin and Baldwin, 1971a) as discussed earlier in this chapter. The determinant sites of insulin action in regulating mammary metabolism remain unclear but it is clear that insulin regulates the activities of the hexokinase isoenzymes, acts at other sites in an acute fashion, is required for secretory cell maintenance and does not regulate, in a specific fashion, the levels of enzymes other than hexokinase.

In vitro data regarding the actions of insulin upon enzymes in mammary explants are not clear. Green et al. (1971) reported that insulin induced glucose-6-P dehydrogenase and 6-P-gluconate dehydrogenase activities in mammary explants from late pregnant mice. This induction required DNA synthesis and could be mimicked by high glucose concentrations. The latter observation indicates that the effect might be nonspecific. Rivera and Cummins (1971a,b), on the other hand, found that insulin increased mammary explant glucose-6-P dehydrogenase, 6-P gluconate dehydrogenase, and 6-P-glucose isomerase activities and that this effect did not require DNA synthesis or mitosis. In considering these data along with in vivo data, one is tempted to suggest that insulin is acting in a general or permissive fashion in vitro and that the enzyme responses reported do not reflect specific enzyme inductions. However, the latter possibility cannot be discarded.

2. Ovarian Hormones

Ovariectomy during lactation does not appreciably affect mammary enzyme levels or lactational performance (Barker and Ludwick, 1967; Korsrud and Baldwin, 1969, 1972a,b). Administration of progesterone to ovariectomized rats decreased the activities of a few enzymes slightly while estrogen administration increased glucose-6-P dehydrogenase levels somewhat (Barker and Ludwick, 1967; Baldwin et al., 1969a; Korsrud and Baldwin, 1969). These data imply that the ovarian hormones may have some small effects upon mammary enzyme levels. However, it is difficult to ascribe these to specific actions on mammary tissue based on available data because of the possibilities for indirect actions, the small magnitudes of the responses noted, and the fact that ovariectomy had no effect on milk yield.

Ovariectomy in addition to adrenalectomy did not cause changes in enzyme levels in addition to those caused by adrenalectomy. 17β-Estradiol administration in low doses to adrenalectomized-ovariectomized rats caused a sharp depression in milk production, high pup mortality, and decreased the activities of several enzymes including hexokinase, glucose-6-P dehydrogenase, phosphofructokinase, and succinate dehydrogenase. These adverse effects were completely reversed by cortisol administration (Korsrud and Baldwin, 1972a,b). The reason(s) why estradiol has such adverse effects on milk production and mammary secretory cells in the absence of glucocorticoids is not clear.

3. Adrenal Glucocorticoids

The effects of adrenalectomy, hypophysectomy, and glucocorticoid replacement therapy upon lactating rat mammary enzyme levels have been investigated in some detail (Willmer, 1960; Willmer and Foster, 1965; Korsrud and Baldwin, 1969, 1972a,b,c). The pattern of results found with adrenalectomized rats and reported by these workers are presented in an idealized format for an affected enzyme (Table IV) in Fig. 4. Adrenalectomy on day 5 of lactation results in a leveling off of enzyme activity at a level comparable with that observed in normal animals on the fifth day of lactation indicating that the maintenance of normal day 5 enzyme levels during lactation is not glucocorticoid dependent (Fig. 4). In normal animals and adrenalectomized animals receiving glucocorticoid therapy enzyme activity continues to increase until midlactation and then tends to level off (Fig. 4). Daily administration of glucocorticoids to animals adrenalectomized on day 5 between the eighth and eleventh days of

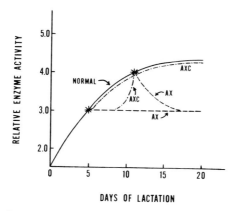

DAYS OF LACTATION

Fig. 4. Idealized representation of effects of adrenalectomy and glucocorticoid therapy upon levels of a glucocorticoid dependent enzyme in rat mammary glands. AX and (– – –) indicate adrenalectomy without replacement therapy; AXC and (– – – –) indicate adrenalectomized receiving glucocorticoid therapy; (–) indicates normal; and, (*) indicates times of adrenalectomy.

lactation results in achievement of normal day 11 enzyme levels. Adrenalectomy on day 11 of lactation results in a rapid decrease in enzyme activity to normal day 5 levels (Fig. 4). Glucocorticoid administration prevents this decrease. A simplistic interpretation of these observations might be that enzyme levels at day 5 are constitutive in the sense that glucocorticoids are not required for maintenance of these levels; and that increases above this level are hormone dependent. Several enzymes affected in this fashion are listed in Table IV along with some enzymes which are not effected by adrenalectomy. Also in Table IV are presented data regarding changes in enzyme activities in normal and adrenalectomized animals between days 5 and 11, estimates of the percentages of day 11 enzyme activities which are hormone dependent, and an assessment of correspondence between enzymes affected by adrenalectomy and hypophysectomy. The response pattern indicated in Fig. 4 and data summarized in Table IV, suggest that glucocorticoids determine, in some fashion, the activities of a number of biosynthetic mammary enzymes. Korsrud and Baldwin (1969, 1972a,b,c) discussed a number of data which support but do not rigorously establish the hypothesis that these glucocorticoid dependent changes in enzyme levels are due to differential increases in the rates of synthesis of the affected enzymes and may result from glucocorticoid mediated changes in patterns of nuclear RNA synthesis (Baldwin et al., 1969a). The extent of dependence upon glucocorticoids for the development and maintenance of normal, midlactation levels of glucocorticoid dependent enzymes listed in Table IV range from 40% for malic enzyme to 90% for citrate cleavage enzyme. It should be noted that the list of affected enzymes in Table IV may be incomplete since the possibility of effects upon several key proteins such as aceto-CoA carboxylase, triglyceride synthetase, α-lactalbumin, lipoprotein lipase, pyruvate dehydrogenase, and others have not been investigated. In addition, it has not been established that the specific site of glucocorticoid action is upon the secretory cell. The suggestion that this is true is strong but some reservation is still appropriate.

The bulk of the data cited above seems consistent with the views that glucocorticoids are intimately involved in the regulation of mammary enzyme levels; that the effects are specific; that the enzymes affected are primarily involved in milk synthesis; and, that the extent of dependence upon glucocorticoids for the development or maintenance of normal enzyme activities varies such that apparent enzyme inductions by glucocorticoids range from two- to tenfold (for malic enzyme and fatty acid synthetase, respectively).

The decreases in enzyme activities which occur after adrenalectomy are accompanied by decreases in pup growth rates which suggest decreases in milk production to levels of 40–60% of normal (Korsrud and Baldwin, 1972a,b,c). Some studies of effects of adrenalectomy upon mammary metabolism have been reported which indicate decreased rates of glucose and pyruvate utilization (Greenbaum and Darby, 1964) and some changes in tissue metabolite patterns (Korsrud and Baldwin, 1972b). Unfortunately, these data do not provide a sufficient basis for attempts to relate enzyme changes to metabolic changes in a cause and effect fashion. It is interesting to speculate, however, on the possibility that one or more of the glucocorticoid dependent enzymes becomes limiting after adrenalectomy and that this limitation results in decreased milk synthesis. Further studies based on this speculation might yield considerable insight relative to the role of enzymes in regulation of milk synthesis and relative to the discussions of enzymes presented in previous sections of this chapter.

Korsrud and Baldwin (1972c) took advantage of the observation that after adrenalectomy in midlactation, the levels of several mammary enzymes decrease in an exponential fashion until new steady state levels are attained to obtain estimates of the half-lives or turnover rates of several enzymes. The validity, theory, assumptions, and methods of obtaining half-life estimates based upon rates of change in enzyme activities during adaptation to a new physiological state were discussed by Segal and Kim (1963) and Szepesi and Freedland (1969). Based upon rates of decrease in the activities of citrate cleavage enzyme, malic enzyme, fatty acid synthetase, UDPglucose pyrophosphorylase, UDPglucose-4-epimerase, and glucose-6-P dehydrogenase in rat mammary glands after adrenalectomy on day 11 of lactation, estimates of half-lives for the enzymes of 28, 31, 28, 50, 20, and 24 hours, respectively, were obtained (Korsrud and Baldwin, 1972c). The half-life estimates for UDPglucose pyrophosphorylase and glucose-6-P dehydrogenase obtained in this manner compared favorably with previous estimates of 35 and 20 hours, respectively, obtained in normal rats using specific immunological techniques (Emery and Baldwin, 1967). Additional estimates of half-lives for mammary aldolase and α-glycerol-P dehydrogenase at midlactation of 19 and 18 hours, respectively, were also reported by the latter workers. It appears that the half-lives of many mammary enzymes are in the 20- to 40-hour range and further, that changes in mammary enzyme levels after adrenalectomy are attributable to decreases in rates of enzyme synthesis and not accelerated degradation as might be the case if involution were implicated.

4. Hypophysectomy: Prolactin

Hypophysectomy of lactating rats leads to dramatic decreases in milk production, in mammary enzyme levels, in mammary DNA levels and, essentially, to mammary involution (Jones, 1967; Korsrud and Baldwin,

1969). Replacement therapy with oxytocin (to provide for milk removal and prevent milk engorgement of gland), oxytocin plus a glucocorticoid, or oxytocin plus prolactin results in small improvements, but milk production falls far short of normal. Replacement therapy with oxytocin, cortisol, and prolactin results in restoration of milk production to almost normal levels (Baldwin and Martin, 1967, 1968; Korsrud and Baldwin, 1969). The response in milk production to administration of cortisol plus prolactin is much greater than the sum of the responses to each hormone administered alone, indicating an interaction between the hormones which produces a greater than additive response (Korsrud and Baldwin, 1969). Interpretations of enzyme data obtained with hypophysectomized animals are complicated by a similar interaction between cortisol and prolactin wherein responses in enzyme levels to administration of both hormones is much greater than responses to either hormone administered alone. Another complication is the loss of secretory cells which accompanies hypophysectomy. Expression of enzyme data on a units per milligram DNA basis helps prevent introduction of artifacts due to cell losses and differences in milk contents of glands from animals receiving different treatments but does not totally accomplish this objective since enzyme activities in dying cells might decrease faster than DNA content. Utilizing this method of expressing enzyme data, Baldwin and Martin (1967, 1968) and later Korsrud and Baldwin (1969) were able to demonstrate that the activities of "constitutive" enzymes per milligram DNA were not decreased by hypophysectomy or affected by the hormone treatments (this observation tends to alleviate the concern regarding relative rates of enzyme and DNA disappearance in dying cells expressed above) while the activities per milligram DNA of a number of (hormone dependent) biosynthetic enzymes were dramatically reduced by hypophysectomy. These activities were restored to almost normal levels by cortisol plus prolactin therapy but not by either hormone administered alone. "Constitutive" and "hormone dependent" enzymes identified in these studies are listed in Table IV and, as can be seen, correspond with those identified as being dependent or not dependent upon glucocorticoid therapy in adrenalectomized rats for maintenance of normal levels. If the implication discussed briefly in the adrenalectomy section that decreased synthesis of the "hormone dependent" enzymes is the reason for decreased enzyme activities after adrenalectomy is accepted, casein synthesis can be added to the hormone dependent list (Baldwin and Martin, 1967, 1968).

The nature of the interaction between cortisol and prolactin in regulating the activities of mammary biosynthetic enzymes and milk component synthesis has not as yet been evaluated in any detail. Baldwin and

Martin (1967, 1968) and later Baldwin *et al.* (1969a) presented data consistent with a hypothesis that the two hormones regulate nuclear RNA synthesis in an additive and complementary fashion. Prolactin appeared to increase rates of RNA synthesis in a general fashion and increased tissue RNA levels while cortisol appeared to act in a more specific fashion in increasing rates of synthesis of nonribosomal RNA. These *in vivo* observations appear to be consistent with results obtained in *in vitro* studies as discussed by Topper and Oka in Chapter 6. However, in the interpretation of *in vitro* studies emphasis has been placed upon specific actions of prolactin while the actions of glucocorticoids and interactions between prolactin and cortisol have received less attention. Since both prolactin and a glucocorticoid are clearly required for the maintenance of normal mammary secretory cell biosynthetic enzyme levels and normal rates of milk synthesis after endocrinectomy, the specific actions of each hormone and the nature of their interaction must be accommodated in explanations of lactogenesis, of the regulation of mammary biosynthetic enzyme levels and of the regulation of milk synthesis. Since these hormones are involved in several aspects of secretory cell formation, development, maintenance, and function, a few years may pass before adequate explanations can be formulated.

Jones (1967) studied rates of decrease in the activities of seven enzymes after hypophysectomy, hypophysectomy coupled with oxytocin therapy, and weaning in normal animals. The rates of decrease in enzyme activities were similar in the three treatments and were remarkably fast. The oxytocin treatment tended to exclude the possibility that the rapid decreases in enzyme activity after hypophysectomy and weaning are attributable to engorgement of the gland with milk. The weaning treatment and studies of unilateral weaning produced by ligating the nipples of some glands and allowing pups to continue nursing the remaining nipples (McLean, 1964) tend to exclude lack of hormones as a direct cause of the rapid decreases in enzyme activities after hypophysectomy. These observations suggest participation of an unknown, possibly local, factor in early decreases in enzyme activities induced by weaning and hypophysectomy (Jones, 1967). The data of Jones (1967) indicate decreases in enzyme activities per cell of 50% and more within periods of 8–12 hours. The studies of mammary enzyme turnover rates discussed briefly in the adrenalectomy section indicated enzyme half-lives of 20–40 hours. A half-life of 24 hours would indicate that if enzyme synthesis were stopped completely, 24 hours would pass before enzyme levels decreased to 50% of initial. If the turnover estimates are correct, it must be considered that cessation of enzyme synthesis after hypophysectomy or the onset of weaning does not fully explain the rapid decreases in enzyme activity observed by Jones (1967) and, hence, that rates of enzyme degradation must also increase. These implications, arising from the data of Jones (1967), must be seriously considered in the design and interpretation of studies with hypophysectomized animals and of weaning.

5. Thyroidectomy

Walters and McLean (1967b) evaluated the effects of thyroidectomy on pathways of glucose metabolism in lactating rat mammary glands using radioisotope tracer and enzymatic techniques. The treatment groups utilized were sham-operated, *ad libitum* fed controls, sham-operated, pair-fed controls, and thyroidectomized animals. The activities of hexokinase, glucose-6-P dehydrogenase, 6-P-gluconate dehydrogenase and NADP-linked isocitrate dehydrogenase were decreased in pair fed as compared to *ad libitum* fed controls and were decreased further in thyroidectomized animals indicating that both reduced food intake and thyroidectomy affect mammary enzyme levels. Based upon available data, it is not yet possible to determine whether the decreases in enzyme activities should be attributed to lack of a general or specific thyroxin action upon the mammary gland or a systemic effect. Similarly, as was discussed in a number of cases in this chapter, the changes in enzyme activities correlate well with the metabolic changes observed but it is not possible, based upon available data, to determine which, if any or all, of the enzyme changes are responsible for the metabolic changes.

IV. SUMMARY

In constructing this chapter, an attempt was made to describe a number of mammary enzymes in terms of their functions, their kinetic properties, their possible roles in regulation of lactogenesis and mammary metabolism and changes in their activities during pregnancy, lactation, and involution and after endocrinectomy. Emphasis was placed upon discussions of the application, value, and limitations of enzyme data in evaluations of mammary gland development, of hormone actions, of metabolism, and of metabolic regulation. In addition, some speculative hypotheses and reservations regarding relationships between enzyme changes and mammary development, lactogenesis, metabolic regulation, and specific hormone actions were introduced with a view toward identifying what the authors consider to be important aspects of mammary metabolism requiring further study and the careful application of enzymatic and other related techniques.

REFERENCES

Abraham, S., Cady, S. P., and Chaikoff, I. L. (1957). *J. Biol. Chem.* **224**, 995.
Aksamit, R. R., and Ebner, K. E. (1972). *Biochim. Biophys. Acta* **268**, 102.
Askew, E. W., Emery, R. S., and Thomas, J. W. (1970). *J. Dairy Sci.* **53**, 1415.
Baldwin, R. L. (1966). *J. Dairy Sci.* **49**, 1533.
Baldwin, R. L. (1968). *J. Dairy Sci.* **52**, 729.
Baldwin, R. L. (1969). In "Lactogenesis" (M. Reynolds and S. J. Folley, eds.), pp. 85–95. Univ. Pennsylvania Press, Philadelphia, Pennsylvania.
Baldwin, R. L., and Cheng, W. (1968). *J. Dairy Sci.* **52**, 523.
Baldwin, R. L., and Martin, R. J. (1967). *J. Dairy Sci.* **51**, 748.
Baldwin, R. L., and Martin, R. J. (1968). *Endocrinology* **82**, 1209.
Baldwin, R. L., and Milligan, L. P. (1966). *J. Biol. Chem.* **241**, 2058.
Baldwin, R. L., and Smith, N. E. (1971). *J. Dairy Sci.* **54**, 583.
Baldwin, R. L., Korsrud, G. O., Martin, R. J., Cheng, W., and Schober, N. A. (1969a). *Biol. Reprod.* **1**, 31.
Baldwin, R. L., Lin, H. J., Cheng, W., Cabrera, R., and Ronning, M. (1969b). *J. Dairy Sci.* **52**, 183.
Ballard, F. J., and Hanson, R. W. (1969). *Fed. Proc. Fed. Amer. Soc. Exp. Biol.* **28**, 218.
Barker, K. L., and Ludwick, T. W. (1967). *J. Dairy Sci.* **50**, 1978.
Barman, T. E. (1969). "Enzyme Handbook." Springer-Verlag, New York.
Bartley, J. C., Abraham, S., and Chaikoff, I. L. (1966). *Proc. Soc. Exp. Biol. Med.* **123**, 670.
Barry, J. M. (1964). *Biol. Rev.* **39**, 194.
Bauman, D. E., Brown, R. E., and Davis, C. L. (1970). *Arch. Biochem. Biophys.* **140**, 237.
Beisenherz, G. (1955). In "Methods in Enzymology" (S. P. Colowick and N. O. Kaplan, eds.), Vol. I, pp. 387–391. Academic Press, New York.
Benevenga, N. J., Stielau, W. J., and Freedland, R. A. (1964). *J. Nutr.* **84**, 345.
Benson, J. D., Askew, E. W., Emery, R. S., and Thomas, J. W. (1969). *Fed. Proc. Fed. Amer. Soc. Exp. Biol.* **28**, 623.
Berg, P. (1962). In "Methods in Enzymology" (S. P. Colowick and N. O. Kaplan, eds.), Vol. V, pp. 461–466. Academic Press, New York.
Bickerstaffe, R., and Annison, E. F. (1970). *Comp. Biochem. Physiol.* **35**, 653.
Bickerstaffe, R., and Annison, E. F. (1971). *Int. J. Biochem.* **2**, 153.
Boyd, J. W. (1961). *Biochem. J.* **81**, 434.
Bucovaz, E. T., and Davis, J. W. (1961). *J. Biol. Chem.* **236**, 2015.
Carey, E. M., and Dils, R. (1970). *Biochim. Biophys. Acta* **210**, 360.
Coore, H. G., Denton, R. M., Martin, B. R., and Randle, P. J. (1971). *Biochem. J.* **125**, 115.
Emery, R. S., and Baldwin, R. L. (1967). *Biochim. Biophys. Acta* **136**, 223.
Emery, R. S., Schurman, M., and Sidhu, K. S. (1972). *Fed. Proc. Fed. Amer. Soc. Exp. Biol.* **31**, 2634.

England, P. J., and Randle, P. J. (1967). *Biochem. J.* **105**, 907.
Fleisher, G. A. (1960). *Fed. Proc. Fed. Amer. Soc. Exp. Biol.* **19**, 6.
Folley, S. J. (1961). *Dairy Sci. Abstr.* **23**, 511.
Goodfriend, T. L., and Kaplan, N. O. (1964). *J. Biol. Chem.* **239**, 130.
Goodfriend, T. L., Sokol, D. M., and Kaplan, N. O. (1966). *J. Mol. Biol.* **15**, 18.
Green, C. D., Skarda, J., and Barry, J. M. (1971). *Biochim. Biophys. Acta* **244**, 377.
Greenbaum, A. L., and Darby, F. J. (1964). *Biochem. J.* **91**, 307.
Greenbaum, A. L., and Greenwood, F. C. (1954). *Biochem. J.* **56**, 625.
Greenbaum, A. L., and Slater, T. F. (1957). *Biochem. J.* **66**, 161.
Greenbaum, A. L., Gumaa, K. A., and McLean, P. (1971). *Arch. Biochem. Biophys.* **143**, 617.
Grimm, F. C., and Doherty, D. G. (1961). *J. Biol. Chem.* **236**, 1980.
Grossbard, L., and Schimke, R. T. (1966). *J. Biol. Chem.* **241**, 3546.
Gul, B., and Dils, R. (1969). *Biochem. J.* **111**, 263.
Güttler, F., and Clausen, J. (1969). *Biochem. J.* **114**, 831.
Hamosh, M., and Evans, A. J. (1972). *Fed. Proc. Fed. Amer. Soc. Exp. Biol.* **31**, 467.
Hamosh, M., Clary, T. R., Chernick, S. S., and Scow, R. O. (1970). *Biochim. Biophys. Acta* **210**, 473.
Hansen, H. J. M., Carey, E. M., and Dils, R. (1970). *Biochim. Biophys. Acta* **210**, 400.
Hansen, R., Pilkis, S. J., and Krahl, M. E. (1967a). *Fed. Proc. Fed. Amer. Soc. Exp. Biol.* **26**, 257.
Hansen, R., Pilkis, S. J., and Krahl, M. E. (1967b). *Endocrinology* **81**, 1397.
Hardwick, D. C. (1966). *Biochem. J.* **99**, 228.
Hartmann, P. E. (1969). In "Lactogenesis" (M. Reynolds and S. J. Folley, eds.), pp. 97–104. Univ. Pennsylvania Press, Philadelphia, Pennsylvania.
Hartmann, P. E., and Jones, E. A. (1970). *Biochem. J.* **116**, 657.
Heitzman, R. J. (1967). *Biochem. J.* **104**, 24.
Heitzman, R. J. (1969). *J. Dairy Res.* **36**, 47.
Hellung-Larsen, P., and Andersen, V. (1968). *Exp. Cell. Res.* **50**, 286.
Helminen, H. J., and Ericsson, J. L. E. (1970). *Exp. Cell. Res.* **60**, 419.
Helminen, H. J., and Ericsson, J. L. E. (1971). *Exp. Cell. Res.* **68**, 411.
Herrington, M. D., and Hawtrey, A. O. (1970). *Biochem. J.* **116**, 405.
Herrington, M. D., and Hawtrey, A. O. (1971). *Biochem. J.* **121**, 279.
Herzfeld, A., and Greengard, O. (1971). *Biochim. Biophys. Acta* **237**, 88.
Hines, M. C., and Wolfe, R. G. (1963). *Biochemistry* **2**, 770.
Holten, D. (1972). *Biochim. Biophys. Acta* **268**, 4.
Hori, S. H., and Matsui, S. (1967). *J. Histchem. Cytochem.* **15**, 530.
Howanitz, P. J., and Levy, H. R. (1965). *Biochim. Biophys. Acta* **106**, 430.
Howard, C. F., Jr., and Lowenstein, J. M. (1965). *J. Biol. Chem.* **240**, 4170.
Jones, E. A. (1967). *Biochem. J.* **103**, 420.
Jones, E. A. (1972). *Biochem. J.* **126**, 67.
Kaplan, N. O. (1966). *J. Cell. Comp. Physiol.* **66**, 1.
Kaplan, N. O., and Ciotti, M. M. (1961). *Ann. N. Y. Acad. Sci.* **94**, 701.
Kaplan, N. O., Everse, J., and Admiraal, J. (1968). *Ann. N. Y. Acad. Sci.* **151**, 400.
Karlsson, B. W., and Carlsson, E. I. (1968). *Comp. Biochem. Physiol.* **25**, 949.
Katz, J., and Wals, P. A. (1972). *Biochem. J.* **128**, 879.
Katz, J., and Wood, H. G. (1963). *J. Biol. Chem.* **238**, 517.
Katzen, H. M. (1967). *Adv. Enzyme Regulat.* **5**, 335.

Katzen, H. M., Soderman, D. D., and Wiley, C. E. (1970). *J. Biol. Chem.* **245**, 4081.

Kinsella, J. E. (1970). *J. Dairy Sci.* **53**, 1957.

Kinsella, J. E. (1972). *Lipids* **7**, 165.

Kirkman, H. N. (1962). *J. Biol. Chem.* **237**, 2364.

Korsrud, G. O., and Baldwin, R. L. (1969). *Biol. Reprod.* **1**, 21.

Korsrud, G. O., and Baldwin, R. L. (1972a). *Can. J. Biochem.* **50**, 366.

Korsrud, G. O., and Baldwin, R. L. (1972b). *Can. J. Biochem.* **50**, 377.

Korsrud, G. O., and Baldwin, R. L. (1972c). *Can. J. Biochem.* **50**, 386.

Krebs, H. A. (1969). *In* "Current Topics in Cellular Regulation" (B. L. Horecker and E. R. Stadtman, eds.), Vol. I, pp. 45–55. Academic Press, New York.

Krebs, H. A., and Veech, R. L. (1969). *Advan. Enzyme Regulat.* **7**, 397.

Krebs, H. A., and Veech, R. L. (1970). *In* "Pyridine Nucleotide-Dependent Dehydrogenases" (H. Sund, ed.), pp. 413–434. Springer-Verlag, New York.

Kronfeld, D. S. (1969). *In* "Lactogenesis" (M. Reynolds and S. J. Folley, eds.), pp. 109–120. Univ. Pennsylvania Press, Philadelphia, Pennsylvania.

Kuhn, N. J. (1968). *Biochem. J.* **106**, 743.

Kuhn, N. J. (1969). *J. Endocrinol.* **44**, 39.

Kuhn, N. J., and Lowenstein, J. M. (1967). *Biochem. J.* **105**, 995.

Levy, H. R. (1963). *J. Biol. Chem.* **238**, 775.

Levy, H. R. (1964). *Biochim. Biophys. Acta* **84**, 229.

Levy, H. R., Raineri, R. R., and Nevaldine, B. H. (1966). *J. Biol. Chem.* **241**, 2181.

Lin, C. Y., and Kumar, S. (1971). *J. Biol. Chem.* **246**, 3284.

Lin, C. Y., and Kumar, S. (1972). *J. Biol. Chem.* **247**, 604.

Linzell, J. L. (1968). *Proc. Nutr. Soc.* **27**, 44.

Linzell, J. L. (1969). *In* "Lactogenesis" (M. Reynolds and S. J. Folley, eds.), pp. 153–156. Univ. Pennsylvania Press, Philadelphia, Pennsylvania.

Lossow, W. J., and Chaikoff, I. L. (1958). *J. Biol. Chem.* **230**, 149.

Lyons, W. R., Li, C. H., and Johnson, R. E. (1958). *Recent Prog. Hormone Res.* **14**, 219.

Mahler, H. R., and Cordes, E. H. (1966). "Biological Chemistry." Harper, New York.

Malpress, F. H. (1961). *Biochem. J.* **78**, 527.

Mansour, T. E. (1969). *Advan. Enzyme Regulat.* **8**, 37.

Marinez, D. I., and Cook, R. M. (1971). *J. Dairy Sci.* **54**, 781.

Martin, R. J., and Baldwin, R. L. (1971a). *Endocrinology* **88**, 863.

Martin, R. J., and Baldwin, R. L. (1971b). *Endocrinology* **88**, 868.

Martin, R. J., and Baldwin, R. L. (1971c). *Endocrinology* **89**, 1263.

Martinez, C. M., and Tiemeier, D. (1967). *Biochemistry* **6**, 1715.

McBride, O. W., and Korn, E. D. (1963). *J. Lipid Res.* **4**, 17.

McKenzie, L., Fitzgerald, D. K., and Ebner, K. E. (1971). *Biochim. Biophys. Acta* **230**, 526.

McLean, P. (1958). *Biochim. Biophys. Acta* **30**, 303.

McLean, P. (1964). *Biochem. J.* **90**, 271.

Mellenberger, R. W., Bauman, D. E., and Nelson, D. R. (1972). *Fed. Proc. Fed. Amer. Soc. Exp. Biol.* **31**, 675.

Miller, A. L., and Levy, H. R. (1969). *J. Biol. Chem.* **244**, 2334.

Munford, R. E. (1963). *J. Endocrinol.* **28**, 1.

Munford, R. E. (1964). *Dairy Sci. Abstr.* **26**, 293.

Narayanan, R., and Ganguli, N. C. (1965). *Indian J. Biochem.* **2**, 240.

Ochoa, S. (1955). *In* "Methods in Enzymology" (S. P. Colowick and N. O. Kaplan, eds.), Vol. I, pp. 685–694. Academic Press, New York.

Opstvedt, J., Baldwin, R. L., and Ronning, M. (1967). *J. Dairy Sci.* **50**, 108.

Passonneau, J. V., and Lowry, O. H. (1964). *Advan. Enzyme Regulat.* **2**, 265–274.

Pilkis, S. J. (1970). *Biochim. Biophys. Acta* **215**, 461.

Ponto, K. H., Cook, R. M., and Thomas, J. W. (1969). *Fed. Proc. Fed. Amer. Soc. Exp. Biol.* **28**, 623.

Raineri, R. R., and Levy, H. R. (1970). *Biochemistry* **9**, 2233.

Ray, W. J., Jr., and Roscelli, G. A. (1964). *Biol. Chem.* **239**, 1228.

Rees, E. D., and Huggins, C. (1960). *Cancer Res.* **20**, 963.

Reiner, J. M. (1969). "Behavior of Enzyme Systems." Van Nostrand Reinhold, Princeton, New Jersey.

Richards, A. H., and Russell, H. (1971). *Fed. Proc. Fed. Amer. Soc. Exp. Biol.* **30**, 1172.

Rivera, E. M., and Cummins, E. P. (1971a). *J. Cell. Physiol.* **77**, 175.

Rivera, E. M., and Cummins, E. P. (1971b). *Gen. Comp. Endocrinol.* **17**, 319.

Robinson, D. S. (1963). *J. Lipid Res.* **4**, 21.

Saacke, R. G., and Heald, C. W. (1969). *J. Dairy Sci.* **52**, 917.

Saito, M., and Sato, S. (1971). *Biochim. Biophys. Acta* **227**, 344.

Segal, H. L., and Kim, Y. S. (1963). *Proc. Nat. Acad. Sci.* **50**, 912.

Seubert, W., and Schoner, W. (1971). *In* "Current Topics in Cellular Regulation" (B. L. Horecker and E. R. Stadtman, eds.), Vol. III, p. 237–267. Academic Press, New York.

Shatton, J. B., Gruenstein, M., Shay, H., and Weinhouse, S. (1965). *J. Biol. Chem.* **240**, 22.

Shirley, J. G., Emery, R. S., Convey, E. M., and Oxender, W. D. (1971). *J. Dairy Sci.* **54**, 780.

Simon, S., and Cook, R. M. (1971). *J. Dairy Sci.* **54**, 781.

Simpson, A. A., and Schmidt, G. H. (1970). *Exp. Biol. Med.* **133**, 897.

Slater, T. F. (1961). *Biochem. J.* **78**, 500.

Slater, T. F., Greenbaum, A. L., and Wang, D. Y. (1963). *In* "Lysosomes" (A. V. S. de Rebuck and M. P. Cameron, eds.), pp. 311–334. Little, Brown, Boston, Massachusetts.

Smith, S., and Abraham, S. (1970). *J. Biol. Chem.* **245**, 3209.

Smith, S., and Abraham, S. (1971a). *J. Biol. Chem.* **246**, 6428.

Smith, S., and Abraham, S. (1971b). *J. Biol. Chem.* **246**, 2537.

Smith, S., Easter, D. J., and Dils, R. (1966). *Biochim. Biophys. Acta* **125**, 445.

Smith, S., Gagne, H. T., Pitelka, D. R., and Abraham, S. (1969). *Biochem. J.* **115**, 807.

Spencer, A. F., and Lowenstein, J. M. (1966). *Biochem. J.* **99**, 760.

Stubbs, M., Veech, R. L., and Krebs, H. A. (1972). *Biochem. J.* **126**, 59.

Szepesi, B., and Freedland, R. A. (1969). *Arch. Biochem. Biophys.* **133**, 60.

Taketa, K., and Watanabe, A. (1971). *Biochem. Biophys. Acta* **235**, 19.

Traurig, H. H. (1967). *Anat. Record* **157**, 489.

Trujillo, J. M., Walden, B., O'Neil, P., and Anstall, H. B. (1965). *Science* **148**, 1603.

Tuttle, J. P., and Wilson, J. E. (1970). *Biochim. Biophys. Acta* **212**, 185.

Utter, M. F., and Scrutton, M. C. (1969). *In* "Current Topics in Cellular Regulation" (B. L. Horecker and E. R. Stadtman, eds.), Vol. I, pp. 253–297. Academic Press, New York.

Veech, R. L., Eggleston, L. V., and Krebs, H. A. (1969a). *Biochem. J.* **115**, 609.
Veech, R. L., Raijman, L., Dalziel, K., and Krebs, H. A. (1969b). *Biochem. J.* **115**, 837.
Walters, E., and McLean, P. (1967a). *Biochem. J.* **104**, 778.
Walters, E., and McLean, P. (1967b). *Biochem. J.* **105**, 615.
Walters, E., and McLean, P. (1968a). *Biochem. J.* **109**, 407.
Walters, E., and McLean, P. (1968b). *Biochem. J.* **109**, 737.
West, C. E., Bickerstaff, R., Annison, E. F., and Linzell, J. L. (1972). *Biochem. J.* **126**, 477.
Wieland, O., and Siess, E. (1970). *Proc. Nat. Acad. Sci.* **65**, 947.
Wieland, O., Siess, E., Schulze-Wethmar, F. H., Funcke, H. G., and Winton, B. (1971). *Arch. Biochem. Biophys.* **143**, 593.
Williamson, J. R. (1965). *J. Biol. Chem.* **240**, 2308.
Willmer, J. S. (1960). *Can. J. Biochem. Physiol.* **38**, 1265.
Willmer, J. S., and Foster, T. S. (1965). *J. Physiol. Pharm.* **43**, 905.
Wood, H. G., Jaffe, S., Gillespie, R., Hansen, R. G., and Hardenbrook, H. (1958). *J. Biol. Chem.* **233**, 1264.
Wuntch, T., Chen, R. F., and Vesell, E. S. (1970). *Science* **167**, 63.
Yokoyama, A., Shiada, Y., and Ota, K. (1969). *In* "Lactogenesis" (M. Reynolds and S. J. Folley, eds.), pp. 65–71. Univ. Pennsylvania Press, Philadelphia, Pennsylvania.
Young, W. J., Porter, J. E., and Childs, B. (1964). *Science* **143**, 140.

CHAPTER EIGHT

Ribonucleic Acids and Ribonucleoprotein Particles of the Mammary Gland

R. Denamur

I. Introduction 414
II. Ribonucleic Acids during Organogenesis and Secretory Differentiation of the Mammary Gland 415
  A. RNA Content of the Mammary Gland and RNA Synthesis during Mammary Growth not Associated with Secretory Activity 415
  B. Mammary RNA Content and Synthesis during Lactogenesis 417
  C. Mammary Content and Synthesis of RNA during Galactopoiesis 425
  D. Associated Pregnancy and Lactation 428
  E. RNA Content of the Mammary Glands and RNA Synthesis during the Involution of Mammary Structures .. 429
III. Nuclear RNA (nRNA) and Variations in DNA Transcription at the Moment of Functional Differentiation of the Mammary Gland 431
  A. Different Classes of nRNA Determined in the Mammary Gland 432
  B. Synthesis of the Different nRNA Classes 433
IV. RNP (Ribonucleoprotein) Particles and Ribosomal RNA .. 438
  A. General Properties of Mammary RNP Particles 438
  B. Degree of Aggregation and Intracellular Distribution of RNP during the Phase of Secretory Activity 442
  C. Variation in the Amount and Degree of Aggregation of RNP during the Functional Differentiation of the Mammary Gland 443
  D. Variations in the Synthetic Activity of RNP: Preferential Role during the Milk Protein Synthesis of the RNP's Bound to the Membranes of the Endoplasmic Reticulum 446
V. Transfer RNA of the Mammary Gland 447
  A. General Properties of Mammary Transfer RNA 447

B. Variations in the Mammary Content of tRNA and
    Their Rate of Synthesis 449
C. Do the tRNA's Control the Nature and Degree of Pro-
    tein Synthesis in the Mammary Gland? 450
References 454

I. INTRODUCTION

The mammary anlage, after having been differentiated during fetal life, progressively undergoes changes during the periods of postpuberty and first pregnancy leading to a canalicular arborization and full development of a lobulo-alveolar system (reviews of Mayer and Klein, 1961; Raynaud, 1970). These morphological transformations, which are chronologically controlled by well-defined hormonal balances (Lyons *et al.*, 1958; Nandi, 1959; Jacobsohn, 1961; Norgren, 1967 a,b,c,d,e), suppose the synthesis of numerous structural and enzymatic proteins. Lactogenesis, i.e., appearance of secretory activity at the level of the epithelial cells of the acini, takes place under the intervention of a hormonal combination that is different from that inducing growth of the mammary gland. Lactogenesis is characterized by general stimulation of protein synthesis and by induction of the synthesis of milk proteins which are species specific (caseins, α-lactalbumin, β-lactoglobulin). The continuation of secretory activity after parturition (galactopoiesis) is controlled by the hormonal secretions responsible for the appearance of this activity; however, the secretion level may be considerably modulated by other hormones (thyroxine, ovarian steroids).

Hormones and protein synthesis are thus closely bound together during all phases of mammary growth and secretion. Up until about 10 years ago it was still considered that the hormones acted on the nature and level of the protein synthesis by direct modification of enzymatic activity (Tepperman and Tepperman, 1960). At present, it has been proved that growth and secretion processes necessitate the de novo synthesis of specific proteins (Korner, 1965; Mueller, 1965; Williams-Ashman *et al.*, 1964; Tata, 1966, 1970). These considerations together with the very large number of experimental results showing the intervention of RNA's during the different phases of protein synthesis, have stimulated research on the RNA's in the mammary gland. These studies are mainly concerned with the content and degree of synthesis of the different RNA's in the mammary cells during the phases of growth and secretion as well as the effect of various hormones on these parameters. We shall try to summarize the present state of knowledge in this field, showing that the study of the mammary RNA's has allowed us to quantify the mammary response to hormonal stimuli and to analyze some of the cellular pathways used by the hormones to modify protein synthesis.

II.   RIBONUCLEIC ACIDS DURING ORGANOGENESIS AND SECRETORY DIFFERENTIATION OF THE MAMMARY GLAND

A.   RNA Content of the Mammary Gland and RNA Synthesis during Mammary Growth not Associated with Secretory Activity

In all species studied, the various classes of mammary ribonucleic acids are responsible for the synthesis of all structural proteins during mammary growth (not associated with any secretory activity). The RNA's are quantitatively limited and, on the average, undergo the same variations as mammary DNA.

1.   Fetal, Prepuberal, and Puberal Periods

a.   RNA CONTENT OF THE MAMMARY GLAND.   To my knowledge, fetal mammary RNA has not yet been studied biochemically. After birth, the mammary glands of the rat undergo allometric growth until puberty (Cowie, 1949; Sinha and Tucker, 1966) followed by isometric growth during the postpuberal period. This accelerated mammogenesis prior to puberty corresponds to an increase of total mammary RNA [Hackett and Tucker, 1969 (determinations on day 21, 35, or 49); Paape and Sinha, 1971 (determinations from day 30 to day 80)]. There is a positive correlation between the mammary RNA content or the RNA/DNA ratio on day 35 and on day 16 of lactation ($r = 0.55$ and 0.76) (Hackett and Tucker, 1969). Variations in the amount of RNA recorded during this phase of mammary organogenesis depend on ovarian secretions (Paape and Sinha, 1971). They are also under the control of prolactin, as shown by experiments on hypophysectomized-ovariectomized rats between day 26 and day 28 of life (Cole and Hopkins, 1962a). During the estrus cycle of the rat, variation of the mammary RNA content and of the RNA/DNA ratio parallels that of DNA content (increase between proestrus and estrus, and decrease between metaestrus and diestrus; Sinha and Tucker, 1969a). However, changes in mammary RNA are marked only during the first cycle following vaginal opening.

During the period prior to puberty, mammary growth of heifers (Sinha and Tucker, 1969b) is allometric, as is that of rats (Cowie, 1949; Sinha and Tucker, 1966) and mice (Flux, 1954). The increasing variations of mammary RNA content observed from birth to the age of 12 months correspond, however, to a decreasing RNA/DNA ratio. During the estrus cycle, changes in mammary RNA content and in the RNA/DNA ratio are comparable with changes in DNA content, the lowest values being attained on day 20 of the cycle and the highest on the day of estrus (Sinha and Tucker, 1969b). In the heifer, as in the rat, the metabolic activity of the mammary gland seems to be high during the estrogenic phase of the cycle.

b. RNA SYNTHESIS. ^{32}P incorporation into mammary RNA of virgin rats is increased by stilbestrol (Majumder and Ganguli, 1969a). At this physiological stage, progesterone alone or combined with estrogen does not affect the incorporation of ^{32}P into RNA. 17β-Estradiol also stimulates the incorporation of [^{14}C]formate into mammary RNA of ovariectomized virgin rats, whereas the action of testosterone is not significant (Libby and Dao, 1966). Lastly, the combination of estradiol and progesterone markedly stimulates [^{3}H]uridine incorporation into RNA, which occurs prior to the increase in [^{3}H]thymidine incorporation into mammary DNA in 3-4 week-old C_3H mice (Banerjee and Rogers, 1970).

2. Period of Pregnancy without Secretory Activity

a. RNA CONTENT. Variation in the mammary RNA content of the rabbit ($\bar{y} = 0.059\bar{x} + 0.96$, where $\bar{x}$ number of days of gestation; $P < 0.01$) is almost similar to that of the DNA content ($\bar{y} = 0.061\bar{x} + 1.6$; $P < 0.01$) for the first 19 days of pregnancy (Denamur, 1961, 1963a). During this phase of intense mitotic activity (Sod-Moriah and Schmidt, 1968), most of the newly formed cells contribute to the formation of the lobulo-alveolar system (Ancel and Bouin, 1909, 1911; Bouin and Ancel, 1909a,b). On the average, their RNA contents (RNA/DNA ratio) are not significantly different on day 6 (1.07), day 9 (0.89), day 14 (0.92), and day 19 (0.94). The RNA of these cells does not seem to be involved in the processes of secretion (Denamur and Gaye, 1967; Bousquet et al., 1969; Denamur and Delouis, 1972a).

The mammary RNA content of the rat increases throughout pregnancy. However, this increase is somewhat greater during the second half of this period (Shimizu, 1957; Tucker and Reece, 1963a; Denamur, 1965; Denamur and Gaye, 1967; Thibodeau and Thayer, 1967; Kelley and Pace, 1968; Paape and Sinha, 1971), which may be due to stimulation by placental secretions (Ray *et al.*, 1955; Wrenn *et al.*, 1966; Matthies, 1967, 1968; Desjardins *et al.*, 1968; Cohen and Gala, 1969; Kohmoto and Bern, 1970; Shani *et al.*, 1970). The RNA/DNA ratios increase as pregnancy progresses, but according to most authors they do not exceed unity (Tucker and Reece, 1963a; Kumaresan *et al.*, 1967a; Denamur and Gaye, 1967; Ferreri and Griffith, 1969). The relatively more limited mammary growth observed during pseudopregnancy in intact rats (Anderson and Turner, 1968; Desjardins *et al.*, 1968; Sinha and Schmidt, 1969) or hysterectomized rats (Anderson and Turner, 1968) as well as in rats with traumatic deciduomata (Anderson and Turner, 1968; Desjardins *et al.*, 1968) corresponds to a lower total mammary RNA than during pregnancy.

In the ewe, mammary growth is very slow during the first two-thirds of pregnancy (DNA content between 0 and 90 days: $\bar{y} = 0.023\bar{x} + 3.11$; $P < 0.01$) and the increase in RNA expressed per mammary gland ($\bar{y} = 0.032\bar{x} + 23.7$; $P < 0.01$) or per cell is small (RNA/DNA 0.56 on day 70) (Denamur, 1965; Denamur and Gaye, 1967).

Lastly, the higher milk yields in C_3H/HC mice correspond to greater mammary growth during pregnancy than in $C_{57}BC/6$ mice. The total quantities and cellular concentrations of RNA also differ significantly in these two strains and are greater in C_3H/HC mice on day 7 of pregnancy, at which time no secretory activity can be detected (Yanai and Nagasawa, 1971).

b. RNA SYNTHESIS. There is good chronological correlation between the activity of aspartate transcarbamylase, the first enzyme in the pathway of pyrimidine biosynthesis, and the amount of mammary RNA in pregnant rats (Thibodeau and Thayer, 1967).

B. Mammary RNA Content and Synthesis during Lactogenesis

The beginning of secretory phenomena generally corresponds to increases in cellular concentration (RNA/DNA) and in RNA synthesis (Denamur, 1969a). Moreover, *in vivo*, lactogenesis is associated with an important phase of cell proliferation, i.e., the continuation of mammogenesis (Denamur, 1965; see also reviews of Topper, 1968, 1970 and Denamur, 1969b, for a discussion of the role of mitosis in the functional differentiation of the mammary gland).

1. Induction of Secretory Phenomena in the Last Third of Pregnancy

a. RNA CONTENT OF THE MAMMARY GLAND. In the rabbit, there is a preferential increase in the content of mammary RNA ($\bar{y} = 1.509\bar{x} -$

31.6, where $\bar{x}$ = day of pregnancy; P < 0.01 between day 19 and day 30) compared to that of mammary DNA ($\bar{y}$ = 0.65$\bar{x}$ − 10.34; P < 0.01 after day 19 of pregnancy) (Denamur, 1963a; Denamur and Gaye, 1967). This acceleration slightly precedes the appearance of mammary lactose (detected by chromatography) between days 22 and 24 and corresponds to the beginning of [^{14}C]glucose incorporation into lactose (Denamur and Delouis, 1972a). The RNA/DNA ratio of 0.90 on day 19 increases to 0.95 by day 21 and to 1.29 by day 24. Although the mammary cells are proliferating (Sod-Moriah and Schmidt, 1968), there is also an increase in their RNA content in the period when lactose synthesis begins and a functional Golgi apparatus is formed (Bousquet *et al.*, 1969).

In the ewe, appearance of secretory phenomena about day 90 of pregnancy (judged by histological examination and by lactose content) is also concomitant with an increase in mammary RNA content ($\bar{y}$ = 0.98$\bar{x}$ + 206; P < 0.01, between days 90 and 145) even though there is greater cellular proliferation (DNA content $\bar{y}$ = 0.67$\bar{x}$ − 56; P < 0.01). The RNA/DNA ratio is 0.56 on day 70, and attains 0.85 on day 95, 1.03 on day 110, 1.25 on day 130, and 1.30 on day 145 (Denamur, 1965; Denamur and Gaye, 1967).

Lastly, the synthesis of milk proteins (caseins and α-lactalbumin) by the mammary glands of the mouse can be measured between days 12 and 15 pregnancy (Lockwood *et al.*, 1966; Palmiter, 1969a; McKenzie *et al.*, 1971). Concomitant with the appearance of secretory activity, an increase in the mammary RNA/DNA ratio is observed (Yanai and Nagasawa, 1971) as well as continuing cellular proliferation revealed by increases in mammary DNA (Lewin, 1957; Brookreson and Turner, 1959; Munford, 1963, 1964; Yanai and Nagasawa, 1971), higher incorporation of [^{3}H]thymidine into DNA (Traurig, 1967; Wang *et al.*, 1970), greater number of mitoses and decrease in the length of phase S (Banerjee and Walker, 1967).

b. RNA SYNTHESIS. In mice, synthesis of mammary RNA measured by the incorporation *in vivo* of [^{3}H]uridine is six times greater in mammary glands analyzed on day 15 of pregnancy than in mammary glands of virgin animals (strains C$_3$H and BALB/C; Banerjee *et al.*, 1971). Adrenalectomy on day 15 of pregnancy reduces by 20–30% the incorporation of [^{3}H]uridine into mammary RNA.

2. Induction of Secretory Phenomena a Little before or Immediately after Parturition

a. RNA CONTENT OF THE MAMMARY GLAND. Lactose (Shinde *et al.*, 1962, 1965; Denamur, 1965; Kuhn and Lowenstein, 1967; Kuhn, 1968) and α-lactalbumin (Kuhn, 1968; McKenzie *et al.*, 1971) appear in the mammary gland of the rat between days 19 and 20 of pregnancy. The increased activity of many enzymes (Glock and McLean, 1953; McLean, 1958; Malpress, 1961; Shatton *et al.*, 1965; Baldwin and Milligan, 1966; Kuhn and Lowenstein, 1967 and reviews of Munford, 1964; Folley and Jones, 1967) at parturition or immediately after can easily be related to the large increase in total quantities and cellular concentrations of RNA (Greenbaum and Slater, 1957; Tucker and Reece, 1963b; Denamur, 1965; Denamur and Gaye, 1967; Kuhn and Lowenstein, 1967) which takes place between day 20 of pregnancy and day 3 of lactation. On the other hand, it is known that amounts of mammary RNA similar to those existing on day 20 of normal pregnancy, as well as a level of enzyme activity as high as that of late pregnancy can be brought about in hypophysectomized-ovariectomized rats by a combination of the hormones estrone, progesterone, growth hormone, and prolactin for 14 days followed by prolactin, growth hormone, and cortisol for 3 days (Cole and Hopkins, 1962b). In the guinea pig, the period of lactogenesis, although not defined by biochemical criteria, seems to occur immediately after parturition according to histological data (Nagasawa, 1963). It is significant that the slow increase in the RNA/DNA ratio during the last 20 days of pregnancy (Nelson *et al.*, 1962) is followed by a considerable increase from the tenth hour after parturition (Nagasawa, 1963), and by the stimulation of many enzyme activities (Baldwin, 1966). In most of the other domestic animals (cow, goat, mare, sow) or laboratory animals (ferrets) the appearance in the mammary gland of a component characteristic for milk secretion cannot be related to the cellular RNA contents, since the latter have only been determined for a limited number of physiological stages (see review Denamur, 1965). However, it must be noted that in the mammary gland of pregnant hamsters, the total content and cellular concentration of RNA increase about sevenfold between days 5 and 15, while the DNA content is increased about 4 times (Sinha *et al.*, 1971).

b. RNA Synthesis. In the rat, Wang and Greenbaum (1962) have shown that RNA synthesis (incorporation of [2-^{14}C]glycine and [6-^{14}C]orotic acid for 24 hours) considerably increased between day 18 of pregnancy and the day following parturition.

3. Experimental Induction of Secretory Phenomena

a. *In vivo* Experiments. i. *RNA content of the mammary gland.* In the intact or hypophysectomized pseudopregnant rabbit all amounts of exogeneous prolactin that are lactogenic, judged by lactose synthesis, affect the amounts and cellular concentrations of mammary RNA (Denamur, 1965; Denamur and Gaye, 1967). There is a linear relationship between the logarithm of prolactin doses (between 2×6.25 IU and 2×100 IU/day injected from day 14 to day 19) and the resulting increase in RNA on day 19 (Denamur and Gaye, 1967). Moreover, variation in the mammary content of RNA occurring very rapidly after administration of the hormone, is significant 12 hours after the injection of prolactin (Gaye and Denamur, 1969) and shows considerable increase after 24 and 48 hours. Prolactin also causes marked cellular hyperplasia (Denamur and Gaye, 1967; Gaye and Denamur, 1969) (DNA $\times 2.7$ after 5 days of treatment), but the RNA/DNA ratio, which is 0.86 on day 14 of pseudopregnancy, attains 1.12, 1.25, and 1.5, respectively, 12, 24, and 48 hours after the beginning of the prolactin treatment (2×25 IU/day). Prolactin injected intraductally into pseudopregnant rabbits (Fiddler et al., 1970, 1971) induces milk secretion, synthesis of lactose (Chadwick, 1962), and stimulates the lipoprotein lipase activity (Falconer and Fiddler, 1970). Under similar experimental conditions (rabbits whose mammary glands have been developed by an estrogen–progesterone treatment), RNA cellular concentrations increase after intraductal injection of prolactin (Simpson and Schmidt, 1971). The mammary RNA enrichment caused by prolactin is reduced, especially in pseudopregnant-hypophysectomized-gonadectomized rabbits, by the estrogen–progesterone combinations that limit prolactin-induced milk secretion (Denamur et al., 1970).

In the rabbit, exogenous prolactin can also induce lactogenesis from the beginning of pregnancy (Denamur, 1963b). The increasing changes in total RNA, estimated after 5 days of hormonal treatment, are very large and an increase in the amount of RNA is even obtained by injecting prolactin into ovariectomized or hypophysectomized rabbits in which pregnancy is maintained by injections of progesterone (Denamur and Delouis, 1972a). Finally, cortisol administered to the rabbit during pregnancy (Talwalker et al., 1961; Meites et al., 1963; Denamur, 1965; Friesen, 1966; Denamur and Delouis, 1972b) induces more or less marked secretory phenomena according to the period of pregnancy. However, the increase in mammary RNA is only significant if the induced secretion attains some amplitude (Denamur, 1965; Denamur and Delouis, 1972b).

Ovariectomy performed in the rat during midpregnancy induces the secretory phenomena (Shinde et al., 1965; Liu and Davis, 1967). A significant increase in mammary RNA occurs 8–16 hours after operation on day 15 (Liu and Davis, 1967). The RNA content continues to increase after 16 hours and is doubled after 40 hours. The increase in total RNA precedes casein synthesis which is stimulated 24–32 hours after ovariectomy. Adrenalectomy (Davis and Liu, 1969) or injection of progesterone (Wickman and Davis, 1968) acts against the nucleic acid and secretory changes caused by ovariectomy. Administration of hydrocortisone or cortisone to pregnant ovariectomized and adrenalectomized rats reestablishes secretory phenomena of the same amplitude as those caused by ovariectomy of pregnant rats (Davis and Liu, 1969). Last, the lactogenic properties of cortisol showed in the pregnant rat by Talwalker *et al.* (1961) correspond to the increase in mammary RNA observed by Kumaresan *et al.* (1967a), and Ferreri and Griffith (1969). However, when cortisol is not lactogenic, as in the case of another strain of rats, it does not affect the RNA content of the mammary gland (Davis and Liu, 1969).

In the same way, the hormonal combination of prolactin (25 IU) and hydrocortisone (1 mg), administered for 5 days to rats whose milk secretion has ceased after hypophysectomy during lactation (day 5), leads to a higher mammary RNA content simultaneous with the reappearance of secretory phenomena. Larger amounts of prolactin (50 or 100 IU) or of hydrocortisone (2 mg) have no effect on either mammary RNA or milk secretion when they are administered separately (Denamur and Gaye, 1967; Denamur, unpublished). Finally, reinitiation of milk secretion in rats following the arrival of new litters 3, 5, and 9 days after forced total weaning corresponds to the preferential RNA enrichment of the mammary gland (Ota and Yokoyama, 1965).

ii. *RNA synthesis.* Incorporation of [^{3}H]uridine into RNA is greatly stimulated by intraductal injections of prolactin in pseudopregnant rabbits (Fiddler and Falconer, 1969), or in rabbits where the lobulo-alveolar structures have been developed by injections for 28 days of an estrogen-progesterone combination (Simpson and Schmidt, 1971). Stimulation of RNA synthesis precedes that of the proteins (Fiddler and Falconer, 1969) and also that of DNA (Simpson and Schmidt, 1971).

In the rat, incorporation of ^{32}P into cytoplasmic RNA is not stimulated when hydrocortisone does not induce milk secretion during pregnancy (Davis and Liu, 1969). In mice, incorporation of [^{3}H]uridine is even reduced after a cortisol treatment from day 7–8 till day 12–14 of pregnancy (Sirakov and Rychlik, 1968).

b. Experiments Using Organ Cultures of Mammary Gland Tissues. i. *RNA content of mammary explants.* (1) THE RNA CONTENT OF MAMMARY EXPLANTS IS INCREASED BY INSULIN AT THE BEGINNING OF CUL-

TURE. Total RNA of mammary explants of mice taken on day 11 and 13 of pregnancy and cultivated in medium 199 was increased by 26% in 24 hours under the influence of insulin (I) (El Darwish and Rivera, 1971). The addition of corticosterone (C_1), of prolactin (P), or of the lactogenic combination C_1P to the insulin medium has no positive effect in the first 24 hours of culture (El Darwish and Rivera, 1971; Mayne et al., 1968). In the absence of insulin, the RNA content decreases by 27% in 12 hours (Mayne and Barry, 1967) and by 20–40% in 5 days (El Darwish and Rivera, 1971).

(2) THE RNA CONTENT IS INCREASED AFTER 24 HOURS OF CULTURE BY THE ADDITION OF PROLACTIN OR PROLACTIN AND CORTICOSTERONE TO INSULIN. Between 24 and 48 hours the effect of prolactin or prolactin + corticosteroid added to insulin is positive. Thus, after 48 hours, the RNA content is increased by 53% when using the combination IP (El Darwish and Rivera, 1971) or by 37% (Mayne et al., 1968) with the lactogenic combination IC_1P. In the presence of the nonlactogenic hormonal component IC_1, however, the amount of RNA in mammary explants decreased by 23% in 48 hours (Mayne et al., 1968) and was not significantly different from that obtained with the insulin medium (El Darwish and Rivera, 1971). Thus, during the first 48 hours of culture, the mammary RNA increase results from synergic action between insulin and prolactin, whereas corticosterone only seems to intervene in order to maintain a rather high RNA level during lengthy (3–5 days) cultures (El Darwish and Rivera, 1971). Juergens et al. (1965) have shown that maximum synthesis of caseins by explants of mammary glands taken from midpregnant mice occurs 48 hours after beginning of the culture in the presence of insulin, cortisol (C_2), and prolactin. Consequently the synthesis of milk proteins closely parallels the amount of RNA in the tissue cultivated in presence of $I(^{C_1}_{C_2})P$. However, it is astonishing that the quantities of RNA in the mammary explants are not significantly different after 48 hours of culture in media IP or IC_1P (El Darwish and Rivera, 1971), whereas casein synthesis is possible only with the combination IC_1P. In addition, as cellular multiplication is very great (77%) when the culture starts (Stockdale et al., 1966) the mammary cells contain, on an average, half as much RNA after 48 hours of culture in the presence of $I(^{C_2}_{C_1})$, and the combination $I(^{C_1}_{C_2})P$ does not result in a higher RNA/DNA ratio in spite of the initiation of secretory phenomena.

ii. *RNA Synthesis.* Except for Turkington (1970a) who established that the specific radioactivity of UTP remains constant in the mammary cell whatever the hormonal balance of the culture medium, the other

authors who studied RNA synthesis did not measure the specific radioactivity of triphosphate nucleosides after addition of a radioactive precursor. Consequently the expression "RNA synthesis" used in this chapter
corresponds to the stimulation of radioactive adenine or uridine incorporation into RNA and does not necessarily signify the amount of RNA
elaborated.

(1) RNA SYNTHESIS DEPENDS MAINLY ON THE PRESENCE OF INSULIN AT THE
BEGINNING OF ORGAN CULTURE. At the beginning of the organ culture of
mammary glands from nonpregnant mice (from 0 to 24 hours), lactogenic
or nonlactogenic hormonal treatments bring about a very high stimulation or [^{3}H]- or [^{14}C]uridine incorporation into RNA [Palmiter, 1969b
(I = IPC$_2$); Stockdale *et al.*, 1966 (I = IC$_2$ = IP = IC$_2$P); Mayne and
Barry, 1970 (I = IC$_1$P); El Darwish and Rivera, 1971 (IC$_1$ = IP =
IC$_1$P)]. In the main, this represents the synthesis of the RNA needed for
the functioning of new cells resulting from the action of insulin (see
reviews Denamur, 1969b and Topper, 1968, 1970). This hormone very
quickly affects the mechanism inducing RNA synthesis. In fact, the rates
of incorporation of [^{3}H]uridine into RNA or of [^{3}H]thymidine into DNA
measured after 24 hours of culture are quantitatively rather similar
whether the insulin is continuously present or limited to the first 30 minutes of culture (Wang and Amor, 1971). Moreover, insulin stimulates
incorporation of [^{14}C]adenine into RNA after the first 3 hours (Mayne
et al., 1966), or first 12 hours (Mayne and Barry, 1967) of culture of
mammary explants from midpregnant mice. Incorporation of [^{14}C]adenine
6–9 hours after starting the culture is significantly higher in the presence
of IC$_1$P than with insulin, and this increase precedes the stimulation of
the [^{14}C]lysine incorporation (19%) into proteins (Mayne *et al.*, 1968).
So, the consequences of the nature of the hormonal environment on RNA
synthesis at the beginning of organ cultures are different if [^{14}C]adenine
is used as precursor instead of [^{3}H]- or [^{14}C]uridine. These differences
may partly be explained by the relative variations in the adenosine and
uridine pools, and consequently in the specific activities of adenosine and
uridine triphosphate nucleotides. A proportion of the incorporated [^{14}C]-
adenine may also correspond to the turnover of tRNA terminal adenosine
without any stimulation of RNA synthesis.

(2) RNA SYNTHESIS DEPENDS AFTER 24 HOURS OF CULTURE ON THE NATURE
OF THE HORMONES ADDED TO INSULIN. In fact, insulin seems to maintain
a high rate of RNA synthesis by itself (Mayne and Barry, 1970; El
Darwish and Rivera, 1971), contrary to the opinion previously expressed
by Stockdale *et al.* (1966). The action of insulin on RNA synthesis is

similar in timing to the activity of this hormone on DNA synthesis (El Darwish and Rivera, 1970, 1971; Wang and Amor, 1971). In spite of the continuation of some mitotic activity, 24 hours after beginning the culture of mouse mammary glands in the presence of IC_2, the addition of prolactin stimulates [^{3}H]uridine incorporation into RNA and increases at the same time total protein synthesis and especially that of α-lactalbumin and the A protein (Palmiter, 1969a). The combination IC_1P, acting from beginning of the culture, also induces a high rate of incorporation of [^{3}H]uridine on day 2 (Mayne and Barry, 1970), and even on day 5 (El Darwish and Rivera, 1971), in contrast to the combinations IC_1 and IP. Thus, corticosterone seems to have little effect on the amount of RNA synthesized at 48 hours of culture [it does not increase the incorporation rate of [^{3}H]uridine caused by insulin or by the combination IP (Mayne and Barry, 1970)], but, in the presence of IP, it brings about a higher rate of synthesis on day 5 (El Darwish and Rivera, 1971).

(3) SYNTHESIS OF RNA RELATED TO SECRETORY ACTIVITY. This RNA synthesis can more easily be studied if incorporation of a radioactive precursor into mammary RNA is observed after the mitotic phase of culture (see Topper, 1970). Thus, according to Green and Topper (1970), who used explants from midpregnant mice, after 96 hours of culture with insulin, the addition of hydrocortisone (C_2) reduces [^{3}H]uridine incorporation into mammary RNA, whereas prolactin stimulates this incorporation (+16 and +38%) or has no effect (Turkington, 1968). If C_2 is combined with insulin during the first 4 days of culture, prolactin added after 96 hours increases [^{3}H]uridine incorporation (Turkington, 1968; Green and Topper, 1970). Contrary to the results of Turkington (1970a), those of Green and Topper (1970) tend to show that RNA synthesis is independent of C_2 during the first 24 hours of prolactin action. Since the cells developed in the presence of IC_2 are only capable of producing caseins after the addition of prolactin, Green and Topper (1970) suppose that the nature of the RNA synthesized under the influence of prolactin is different in these two experimental situations (I or IC_2 for 96 hours, and then prolactin) or that a blocking in the translation of genetic messages occurs in the absence of cortisol [the membranes of the endoplasmic reticulum are only slightly developed in the absence of cortisol (Mills and Topper, 1969, 1970)].

Finally, simultaneous addition of progesterone and prolactin (after 96 hours in the presence of IC_2) reduces by more than 50% the [^{3}H]uridine incorporation into mammary RNA and produces a preferential inhibition of prolactin-induced α-lactalbumin synthesis (Turkington and Hill, 1969).

However, it seems impossible that such an important effect on RNA synthesis amounts only to an inhibition of the RNA coding for α-lactalbumin synthesis.

All these sometimes contradictory results show that the overall RNA synthesis responsible for secretory activity depends on the action of prolactin in the presence of insulin. The role of cortisol in the synthesis of specific RNA's has to be elucidated.

C. Mammary Content and Synthesis of RNA during Galactopoiesis

1. Increasing Phase of Lactation

A large increase in total quantities and cellular concentrations of RNA, corresponding to the stimulation of RNA synthesis, takes place from the beginning of galactopoiesis even in species where the number of secretory cells continues to increase after parturition.

a. RNA CONTENT OF THE MAMMARY GLAND. Shortly after parturition in the rat the RNA/DNA ratio is 1.9; it increases to 4.19 by day 16 of lactation (Denamur and Stoliaroff, 1966). Other authors have studied RNA variation during galactopoiesis in the rat and have found that even when the absolute quantities of RNA and the RNA/DNA ratios change at different rates (methods for determining them differ), the general conclusions that may be drawn are in favor of a close relationship between mammary RNA and milk secretion level. The RNA content and the RNA/DNA ratio reach a maximum on day 21 of lactation (Kirkham and Turner, 1953; Shimizu, 1957; Tucker and Reece, 1963b), on day 16 to day 20 (Tucker, 1966; Baldwin and Milligan, 1966), on day 18 (Greenbaum and Slater, 1957), or day 16 (Paape and Tucker, 1969a), whereas maximum milk secretion is obtained on day 18 (Kumaresan *et al.*, 1967b).

However, the RNA content of the mammary glands and the moment of lactation when they attain maximum values depend on many factors. Among these the most important is certainly the intensity of mammary suckling which, by stimulating the level of synthesis and excretion of hormones from the hypothalamo-hypophyseal complex, affects in the rat both the amount of milk secreted (Kumaresan *et al.*, 1967b; Moon, 1969), the mammary RNA content (Kumaresan *et al.*, 1967b; Tucker, 1964a, 1966; Tucker *et al.*, 1967a,b; Tucker and Thatcher, 1968; Smith and Convey, 1971), and the DNA content (Tucker, 1964a, 1966; Kumaresan *et al.*, 1967b; Tucker *et al.*, 1967b; Tucker and Thatcher, 1968; Smith and Convey, 1971). Thus, the correlation coefficient between the RNA content of the mammary glands and the milk secretion level attains 0.93

(P < 0.01; Tucker, 1966). Moreover, prolactin administered between day 7 and day 19 increases simultaneously both milk secretion and the RNA content of the mammary gland (Kumaresan et al., 1966). On the other hand, the mammary RNA content in rats on day 16 of lactation does not depend either on the age of the rats at the moment of conception (Pritchard and Tucker, 1970) or on the altitude at which they are kept (Kelley and Pace, 1968).

All these demonstrations of the close relationship between cellular RNA concentrations and secretory phenomena must, however, be contrasted with some experiments in which this interdependence has not been verified. Thus the reductions in milk secretion and in the amounts of lactose, caseins, and lipids synthesized after deprivation of insulin (alloxan-diabetic rats) do not correspond to changes in mammary RNA content and RNA/DNA ratio (Korsrud and Baldwin, 1969; Martin and Baldwin, 1971). In the same way, the fall in milk production after adrenalectomy is accompanied by great changes in certain enzyme activities (Willmer, 1960; Willmer and Foster, 1965; Korsrud and Baldwin, 1969), but not in the RNA content of the mammary glands (Korsrud and Baldwin, 1969). Lastly, in multiparous rats, the length of the dry period preceding parturition has an influence on the amount of milk secreted during the next lactation, but does not change the cellular RNA concentration on days 1, 8, or 16 of lactation; it acts on the magnitude of the secretory phenomena mainly by controlling the number of secretory cells (Paape and Tucker, 1969b).

As regards the other animal species, we generally notice that the period of galactopoiesis when cellular RNA concentrations are highest corresponds to maximum secretory activity. In the guinea pig, cellular RNA concentration and milk secretion rapidly increase to maximum values near day 6 (RNA/DNA, 4.2) (Nelson et al., 1962). The progressive increase in the RNA/DNA ratio at the beginning of galactopoiesis in the rabbit (Denamur, 1963a) and in the ewe (Denamur, 1965; Denamur and Gaye, 1967) coincides with the stimulation of numerous enzyme activities in the rabbit (Gul and Dils, 1969; Hartman and Jones, 1970), and with increasing milk production in the rabbit (Donovan and Van Der Werff Ten Bosch, 1957; Cowie, 1969; Hartman and Jones, 1970) and in the ewe (Ricordeau and Denamur, 1962). The periods of highest cellular RNA concentrations in the rabbit (RNA/DNA 4.1 on days 15–20, Denamur, 1963a), and in the ewe (RNA/DNA 2.7 on day 20, Denamur, 1965; Denamur and Gaye, 1967), can be correlated with maximum milk secretion in these species, and the correlation coefficient between the quantities of mammary RNA and the amounts of milk secreted is +0.91 in the ewe

(P < 0.01). Moreover, according to Yousef *et al.* (1969), the significantly higher mammary RNA/DNA ratios recorded in the lactating ewe, as compared with the lactating cow, can be related to the milk protein contents of these two species. As regards mice, there are no systematic studies of mammary RNA during lactation, but the RNA quantities as well as the RNA/DNA ratios are maximal on day 14 of galactopoiesis (Mizuno, 1961). The RNA content of the sow's mammary glands also increases during lactation, and attains higher levels during the second lactation, when secretion is more abundant, than in the course of the first lactation (Hacker, 1971).

b. RNA SYNTHESIS. i. *In vivo experiments.* Incorporation of [^{14}C]-orotic acid into mammary RNA is greatly increased between days 2 and 10 of lactation in the rat (Wang and Greenbaum, 1962), whereas acid or alkaline ribonuclease activities, expressed per unit of DNA, are not significantly changed (Slater, 1961). In C$_3$H and BALB/C mice, RNA synthesis measured by [^{3}H]uridine incorporation *in vivo* is 10 times higher on day 5 of lactation than in virgin animals (Banerjee *et al.*, 1971). Moreover, [^{3}H]uridine incorporation into mammary RNA of strain H mice is 4 times higher from day 12 to day 16 of lactation than on day 18 of pregnancy (Sirakov and Rychlik, 1968). Lastly, adrenalectomy during lactation in the mouse causes a 50% reduction of total protein synthesis and a total stoppage of casein synthesis. It reduces by more than 80% the [^{3}H]uridine incorporation into mammary RNA, whereas injection of cortisol into adrenalectomized mice reestablishes casein synthesis and induces a threefold increase in RNA synthesis measured 1–2 hours after administration of the hormone (Banerjee *et al.*, 1971).

ii. *In vitro experiments.* In the mouse (strain H), Sirakov and Rychlik (1968) found during incubation of mammary gland slices that [^{3}H]uridine incorporation is higher in mammary RNA of lactating animals (day 12–16) than of pregnant animals (day 18). In addition, 17β-estradiol dipropionate injected into lactating mice for 11 days reduces [^{3}H]uridine incorporation *in vitro* into mammary RNA.

2. Decreasing Phase of Lactation

In all species, this phase corresponds to a reduction in RNA content per cell. In the rabbit (Cowie, 1969) and the ewe (Ricordeau and Denamur, 1962) there is a stepwise decrease in level of milk secretion as lactation progresses. This reduction not only depends on the progressive slow disappearance of some mammary cells (fall in total DNA,

Denamur, 1965), but also on decrease in the RNA content and RNA/ DNA ratio (Denamur and Gaye, 1967), i.e., slowing down of the total synthetic activity.

In the rat, milk secretion decreases after day 20 of lactation; simultaneously, there is a rapid regression in the quantities of RNA and of the RNA/DNA ratio (Tucker, 1966). Prolongation of lactation beyond the normal duration (41 and 61 days, Tucker and Reece, 1963c; or 36 days, Thatcher and Tucker, 1968) leads to a significant reduction in ribonucleic acids (RNA/DNA 2.95 on day 21, 2.13 on day 41, 1.83 on day 61) as well as in the amount of milk secreted (fall on day 41 = 51.6% and on day 61 = 55.7%, Tucker and Reece, 1963c). Administration of cortisol-21 acetate (Thatcher and Tucker, 1970a) or of 9α-fluoroprednisolone acetate (Thatcher and Tucker, 1970b) delays the diminution in the milk production and maintains mammary RNA content when the suckling is prolonged from day 16 to day 32 (Thatcher and Tucker, 1970a). When 9α-fluoroprednisolone is injected from day 24 to day 32 (100 μg/day), both milk secretion and the amount of mammary RNA increase (Thatcher and Tucker, 1970b) and the effect of this steroid on the mammary RNA content exceeds that resulting from hypophyseal grafts under the capsule of the kidney (Thatcher and Tucker, 1970b). Finally, ingestion of "thyroactive" substance from the first day of galactopoiesis in rats reduces milk production as well as mammary RNA content (by 24–49% on day 15 and 20 of lactation), but does not affect either of these components differently since the RNA/DNA ratio is not changed (Sinha and Schmidt, 1970).

D. Associated Pregnancy and Lactation

In pregnant and lactating rats, Tucker and Reece (1964a) did not notice large changes in the RNA/DNA ratio on day 18 of lactation when the number of embryos was lower than 6. When this number exceeded 7, the authors observed a decrease in the amount of mammary RNA. The RNA content of the mammary glands and the amount of milk secreted by simultaneously suckling and pregnant rats are not significantly different from those of lactating rats on day 16 of lactation, but after day 20 pregnancy has a depressive effect on the amount of RNA and on milk secretion (Paape and Tucker, 1969a). Thus, between day 16 and day 24, the RNA/DNA ratio decreases by 13% in lactating animals and by 52% in rats both pregnant and lactating.

Last, suckling or suckling pregnant mice (fertilized at the postpartum estrus) show on day 19 of lactation identical mammary RNA contents and RNA/DNA ratios (Mizuno, 1961).

E. RNA Content of the Mammary Glands and RNA Synthesis during the Involution of Mammary Structures

Involution of the mammary gland is contemporaneous with the regression and then stoppage of milk secretion resulting from reduction in the frequency and intensity of suckling, or from the frequency of milking (domestic species). Cessation of secretory phenomena and involution of the mammary gland can also be obtained experimentally by early weaning, suppression of milking, or removal of various endocrine glands.

1. Mammary RNA Content after Bilateral Weaning

This is incomplete removal of the galactopoietic hormones, but without discharge of milk.

a. WEANING WITHOUT HORMONAL SUPPLEMENTATION. In the rabbit, total weaning carried out immediately postpartum or on day 5 of lactation (Denamur, 1962, 1965) leads to rapid decrease in the mammary RNA content (17% on day 1, 65% on day 3, 73% on day 5, 87% on day 10, if weaning starts on day 5) and a marked drop in the RNA/DNA ratios.

On the first day after weaning of lactating rats, the RNA/DNA ratio decreases by about 32% (Tucker and Reece, 1963d, weaning on day 21), 37% (Slater, 1962, weaning on day 16) or 18% (Darby *et al.*, 1964, weaning on day 16–18). The effects of weaning are very rapid, especially at the beginning of lactation. Thus, the removal of the litter for $12\frac{1}{2}$ hours on day 7 is sufficient to reduce the amount of RNA and the RNA/DNA ratio in the suckling rat (Smith and Convey, 1971), whereas on day 14 of lactation the regression of the RNA/DNA ratio can only be observed between 12 and 24 hours after weaning (Tucker and Reece, 1964b). When the intervals are longer, the losses of RNA, expressed as percentages of the preexisting quantities, are independent of the stage of lactation at which weaning is practiced (Paape and Tucker, 1969a). Decrease in the amount of RNA in the mammary gland occurs together with increase in the proportion of lysosomal hydrolyzing enzymes and, especially, acid ribonuclease (Slater *et al.*, 1963; Greenbaum *et al.*, 1965; review of Woessner, 1969).

The kinetics of the variation in the amount of RNA after total weaning in lactating mice are not known, whereas the quantities of DNA are greatly depressed as in other species (53.4% after 5 days, Anderson and Turner, 1963). The preferential reduction of RNA also takes place, presumably, after weaning in the mouse, since Wellings and deOme (1963) have described rapid and large modifications of the ergastoplasm in the mammary cells of mice weaned on day 15 of lactation.

b. WEANING WITH HORMONAL SUPPLEMENTATION. If the product of secretion is not ejected, the galactopoietic hormones, whatever the amount injected, maintain more easily the number of mammary cells than a high RNA content of these cells. Thus, in the rat, the decrease in the RNA/ DNA ratio after weaning may be reduced for 5–10 days by prolactin (2 × 25 IU/day). Cortisol (1 mg/day) or oxytocin (3 × 1 IU/day) (Denamur, 1965; Denamur and Stoliaroff, 1966) are less effective than prolactin, and these hormones maintain a great number of mammary cells (Ota *et al.*, 1962; Denamur and Stoliaroff, 1966). The effects of prolactin are still apparent after hypophysectomy, contrary to those of oxytocin (Denamur and Stoliaroff, 1966). In rabbits weaned on day 5 of lactation, results obtained after injection of cortisol, prolactin, or prolactin-cortisol (Denamur, 1962, 1965) are identical to those in rats. Oxytocin (Denamur, 1962), GH, and thyroxin (Denamur, 1965) do not delay the regression of the RNA/DNA ratio.

c. WEANING IN SUCKLING PREGNANT RATS. During the first days following weaning, pregnancy delays the reduction of mammary RNA content (Pappe and Tucker, 1969a). Thus, during the first 4 days of weaning the amount of RNA decreases by 60–77% in suckling-pregnant rats and by 83–87% in suckling animals.

2. Mammary RNA Content after Unilateral Weaning

Unilateral weaning is unilateral suppression of milk ejection ligature of the teats) in the presence of galactopoietic hormones. In rabbits (Denamur, 1965), rats (Tucker and Reece, 1963e; Tucker, 1966), and suckling mice (Mizuno, 1961) with unilateral ligature of the teats, a reduction of the RNA/DNA ratio is noted in the glands where the milk has not been removed, but in rabbits and rats this reduction is slower than after bilateral weaning. However, it cannot be prevented by increasing the suckling intensity between days 3 and 16 of lactation in the rat (Tucker, 1966) or, in the mouse, by injection of progesterone or prolactin or by pregnancy (Mizuno, 1961). Moreover in the rat (Tucker and Reece, 1963e; Tucker, 1966) and the mouse (Mizuno, 1961), the suckled contralateral mammary glands are more developed than those of intact animals (amounts of DNA and RNA), but this is not the case in rabbits (Denamur, 1965). It seems that a local factor associated with the non-ejection of milk from the mammary gland is the direct cause of changes in the enzyme activities (Jones, 1967) and cellular RNA concentrations.

3. Mammary RNA Content and Synthesis after Hypophysectomy

This is suppression of the galactopoietic hormones with or without induced milk ejection (injection of oxytocin). In all species, hypophysectomy leads to rapid cessation of secretory phenomena and involution of the mammary gland.

a. RNA CONTENT OF THE MAMMARY GLANDS. In the ewe, milk secretion is completely stopped 4–8 days after the operation (Denamur and Martinet, 1961; Denamur *et al.*, 1972). The decrease in milk secretion after 24–96 hours is partly due to the reduction in the number of mammary cells, but especially to the marked regression of the RNA content of these cells that occurs before the DNA content of the mammary gland decreases (Denamur *et al.*, 1972). Hypophysectomy of the lactating rat causes, prior to total cessation of secretory phenomena, changes in the respiratory metabolism (Bradley and Cowie, 1956), regression of many enzyme activities (Jones, 1967; Baldwin and Martin, 1968a,b; Korsrud and Baldwin, 1969), and decreased synthesis of mammary proteins (Baldwin and Martin, 1968b). If hypophysectomy is performed on the day of parturition (Baldwin and Martin, 1968a) or on day 5 of lactation (Denamur and Gaye, 1967), a very rapid reduction in mammary RNA content is noticed. Prolactin, and especially the prolactin-cortisol combination in the presence of oxytocin, maintains a large milk secretion and inhibits the regression of mammary RNA (Denamur and Stoliaroff, 1966; Baldwin and Martin, 1968a,b).

b. RNA SYNTHESIS AND METABOLISM. In ewes hypophysectomized during lactation, the regression of mammary RNA during the first 48 hours corresponds to a partial inhibition of RNA synthesis measured by [³H]uridine incorporation (Denamur *et al.*, 1972). Moreover, alkaline ribonuclease activity increases considerably after 48 hours (Denamur and Gaye, 1967; Denamur *et al.*, 1972), whereas the activity of ribonuclease inhibitor tends to disappear.

III. NUCLEAR RNA (nRNA) AND VARIATIONS IN DNA TRANSCRIPTION AT THE MOMENT OF FUNCTIONAL DIFFERENTIATION OF THE MAMMARY GLAND

Almost all RNA of the cell are synthesized in the nucleus; the amount of mitochondrial RNA being less and less as the species reach higher stages of evolution (Attardi *et al.*, 1970). nRNA represents a very complex population of evolved molecules or precursors of cytoplasmic RNA, whether bound to proteins or not, some of which have a very short life span (DNA-like RNA).

Moreover, the nuclear RNA content of the mammary gland undergoes quantitative variations; it is higher during galactopoiesis (22–23% of the DNA) than during pregnancy in the rabbit (14–16%) (Denamur, 1965; Simpson and Schmidt, 1969), and the mean nucleotide composition of these RNA is characterized by a high UMP–AMP content and a low GMP percentage (Denamur, 1965).

A. Different Classes of nRNA Determined in the Mammary Gland

Our knowledge of this topic remains limited. It proceeds from kinetic studies on [^{3}H]uridine incorporation into nuclear RNA in mouse mammary explants (Turkington, 1970a). After 20 hours of culture in an insulin medium and 5 minutes in the presence of [^{3}H]uridine, 98% of the incorporated radioactivity is localized in the nRNA with very heterogenous sedimentation constants (4–100 S). RNA 32 S and RNA 45 S, as well as heterodispersed RNA of high molecular weight (47–100 S), can be identified after 25 minutes of labeling. The RNA 18 S and 28 S appear after 4 hours, while a small amount of RNA 32 S and 45 S is still apparent. Finally, 24 hours after addition of [^{3}H]uridine, the radioactivity is mainly localized in the RNA 4 S, 18 S, and 28 S. The results of Turkington (1970a) are similar to those describing the kinetics of nRNA labeling in other tissues (reviews of Darnell, 1968; Tata, 1970; Grierson *et al.*, 1970; Penman *et al.*, 1970; Perry *et al.*, 1970; see also Gotoh *et al.*, 1971). The nuclear RNA 45 S of the mammary gland probably represent the rRNA precursors since they are converted into RNA 32 S and then 28 S and 18 S during a "chase" period in the presence of actinomycin D. In addition, the nucleotide composition established after ^{32}P incorporation shows that the RNA, 16–23 S, 24–40 S, and 40–47 S, isolated after sucrose gradient ultracentrifugation, show high GC contents, corresponding to those of rRNA. On the other hand, the heterodispersed RNA from 47 to 100 S have a DNA-like nucleotide composition. Little is known as yet about the role of the synthesis of rapidly turning over RNA that is restricted to the nucleus (Britten and Davidson, 1969). The metabolic instability of these RNA, their heterogenous sizes, and their rapid formation after hormonal stimulation signify that they could in part be precursors of messenger RNA (Penman *et al.*, 1970; Darnell *et al.*, 1970). However, further experiments would be necessary to confirm this. Moreover, it would be interesting to know if there is some relationship between these DNA-like RNA of mammary nuclei and the cytoplasmic RNA 15 S (Sirakov *et al.*, 1968; Sirakov and Richlik, 1969), or nuclear RNA 15–25 S (Baldwin *et al.*, 1969) to which was attributed, with insufficient proof, the role of messenger molecules.

B. Synthesis of the Different nRNA Classes

1. nRNA Synthesis Increases during the Phase of Mammary Secretion

The synthesis of the rapidly labeled nRNA is under strict hormonal control and it precedes that of the milk components. Insulin, free or bound to sepharose, causes in 1 hour a rapid stimulation of [^{3}H]uridine incorporation into nRNA, and maximum stimulation is attained in 24 hours (Turkington, 1970a,c). However, the addition of prolactin (free or bound to sepharose) to mouse mammary explants or mammary cells cultivated for 72 hours in the presence of IC_2 further increases the rate of nRNA synthesis in 30 minutes, attaining a maximum in 12 hours.

2. The Newly Synthesized RNA in the Nucleus is Necessary for Lactogenesis

This statement is based mainly on results using actinomycin D, which inhibits RNA synthesis governed by DNA (Reich *et al.*, 1962; and reviews of Gross, 1968; Waksman, 1968; Korner, 1969). In the mammary gland, RNA synthesis is almost entirely stopped if a sufficient quantity of actinomycin D is administered *in vivo* or added *in vitro* to the incubation medium or culture medium of mammary explants. Thus, during the incubation of the mouse mammary gland slices, 10 μg of actinomycin D per ml almost totally inhibits the insulin-induced increase in [^{14}C]adenine incorporation into RNA (Mayne *et al.*, 1966), and 5 μg/ml of actinomycin D reduces by 95% the [^{3}H]uridine incorporation induced by this hormone (Wang and Amor, 1971). The stimulation of RNA synthesis ([^{14}C]- or [^{3}H]uridine incorporation) by prolactin added after 24 hours (Mayne and Barry, 1970) or 96 hours (Turkington, 1968) of culture of mice mammary explants in IC_1 or IC_2 medium is reduced by 92% by 1 μg/ml of actinomycin D, and 5 μg of actinomycin D per ml completely inhibits the hormonal effect. Lastly, 80–90% of the polyribosomes of mice mammary adenocarcinoma are degraded by actinomycin D in 12 hours (Trakatellis *et al.*, 1965).

a. Actinomycin D Inhibition of the Synthesis of Milk Constituents Induced by Lactogenic Hormones. Actinomycin D used as described above reduces the casein synthesis in 8 hours by 20–45% when it is added after 20 or 40 hours of culture of mammary explants from midpregnant mice (medium IC_2P) (Stockdale *et al.*, 1966). It also inhibits the induction of synthesis of the different caseins and of α-lactalbumin by prolactin or HPL added after 96 hours of culture in IC_2 medium of mice mammary explants (Turkington, 1968; Turkington *et al.*, 1968). It is still active if introduced 16 hours after prolactin. Finally, actinomycin D (300 μg/kg) *in vivo* stops in the rabbit the induction of lactose synthesis caused by prolactin (Denamur and Gaye, 1967).

b. ACTINOMYCIN D INHIBITION OF THE STIMULATION OF SEVERAL ENZYME ACTIVITIES IN THE COURSE OF LACTOGENESIS. As mentioned above many enzyme activities are greatly increased when the initiation of secretory phenomena takes place; the enzymes include lipoprotein lipase, galactosyltransferase, glucose-6-phosphate dehydrogenase, and phosphogluconate dehydrogenase. The stimulation of lipoprotein lipase activity by prolactin is completely suppressed in the rabbit by injection of actinomycin D (0.1 μg/duct) at the same time as the hormone or 72 hours later (Falconer and Fiddler, 1968, 1970). The half-life of lipoprotein lipase being 2 hours after injection of actinomycin D, the authors think that the messenger RNA responsible for lipoprotein lipase synthesis has a short life span and that its synthesis is conditioned by prolactin. The increase in galactosyltransferase obtained by adding prolactin (after 96 hours) to the IC_2 culture medium of mouse mammary glands is also inhibited by actinomycin D (5 μg/ml) (Turkington *et al.*, 1968). Moreover, RNA synthesis is necessary during the first 4 hours of culture of pregnant mouse mammary glands to stimulate glucose-6-phosphate dehydrogenase and phosphogluconate dehydrogenase activities, determined by insulin or by high glucose, mannose, and fructose concentrations (Green *et al.*, 1971b). Contrary to its inhibitory activity during the first 4 hours of culture, actinomycin D added subsequently does not affect the increase in activity of these two enzymes (Leader and Barry, 1969; Green *et al.*, 1971b). This experiment is particularly interesting as it suggests the possibility in the mammary gland of regulating the genome (synthesis of the two enzymes) by varying the intracellular concentration of a metabolite common to mannose, fructose, and glucose, probably glucose-6-phosphate. However, the changes in glucose-6-phosphate dehydrogenase activity caused by actinomycin D are not always easy to explain, as shown by the observations made on virgin mice by Hilf *et al.* (1965). In fact, injections of estradiol do not lead to an increase in glucose-6-phosphate dehydrogenase activity; moreover, the activity is decreased by actinomycin D. However, if actinomycin D and estradiol are injected together, the glucose-6-phosphate dehydrogenase activity is stimulated. Whatever the interpretation of these results, a phenomenon of superinduction comparable with that described for tyrosine amino-transferase in HTC cells by Tomkins *et al.* (1969), and due to the addition of actinomycin D after prolactin, has not been demonstrated in the mammary gland as regards the synthesis of A and B proteins (Turkington *et al.*, 1968).

3. Is the Transcription of the Genome Quantitatively and Qualitatively Modified during the Phase of Mammany Secretion?

a. STIMULATION OF RNA POLYMERASE ACTIVITIES. The regulation of RNA synthesis independent of hormonal effects on precursor multiple pools can be demonstrated by a stimulated RNA polymerase activity in isolated nuclear preparation. The eukaryote nuclei contain multiple RNA polymerases that have been purified (Chambon *et al.*, 1970; Jacobs *et al.*, 1970; Kedinger *et al.*, 1970; Roeder and Rutter, 1970; Sethi, 1971; Smuckler and Tata, 1971) and play a specific role in rRNA synthesis (RNA polymerase α-amanitine insensitive, see Blatti *et al.*, 1970), or DNA-like RNA synthesis (RNA polymerase with multiple subunits). Such an analysis of the various RNA polymerases has not been made in the nuclei of mammary gland, but the RNA polymerase activity (nucleoside triphosphate: RNA nucleotidyltransferase, EC 2.7.7.6) has been measured at two ionic strengths. However, the significance of these determinations is limited as it is not possible to discern between the role played by the number of enzyme molecules, their activity (Stein and Hansen, 1970), and the "DNA template" length that can be transcribed. In spite of these difficulties of interpretation and of the existence of some artifacts (Dati and Maurer, 1971) it is interesting that the RNA polymerase activities are higher in the nuclei of lactating mammary glands than in those of pregnant mice and this is in agreement with the rate of RNA synthesis in these two physiological situations (Turkington and Ward, 1969). Moreover, the RNA polymerase activities are modified by the hormones in exactly the same way as they affect milk secretion or synthesis of ribonucleic acids. Thus, insulin definitely stimulates RNA polymerase activities from the eighth hour of culture of mouse mammary explants, whatever the molarity of the medium, and the enzyme activities increase up to 48 hours (the effect of insulin is independent of the rate of glucose penetration into the cell) (Turkington and Ward, 1969). The addition of hydrocortisone to insulin does not cause any change in RNA polymerase activities, but prolactin added 72 hours after the beginning of the culture IC_2 increases the activities by 100% in 10 hours and by 150–200% in 24 hours. In the same experimental conditions, the stimulation of [^{3}H]uridine incorporation into RNA caused by prolactin can be detected in the first 8 hours following its addition (Turkington, 1970a). Finally, the synthesis of new RNA polymerase molecules and perhaps of other proteins with a short life span precedes prolactin-induced RNA synthesis. In fact, cycloheximide or puromycin added at the same time as prolactin inhibit increases in RNA polymerase activities and RNA synthesis.

RNA polymerase activities have also been measured in the mammary gland nuclei of rats after different *in vivo* organectomies during lactation (adrenalectomy, ovariectomy, hypophysectomy) followed by the administration of various hormones (O-P, C-CP-I) (Baldwin *et al.*, 1969). The authors, by varying the molarity of the medium according to Widnell and Tata (1966) determined two RNA polymerase activities: RNA polymerase 1 [Mn^{2+} + $(NH_4)_2SO_4$] and RNA polymerase 2 ($MgSO_4$) whose reaction products are of the types DNA-like RNA and ribosomal RNA respectively. They have noted that the RNA polymerase 1 activity is much reduced after hypophysectomy or prolactin treatment of the hypophysectomized rats, whereas that of the RNA polymerase 2 is decreased by ovariectomy or hypophysectomy. Contrary to its effects on RNA polymerase 1, prolactin or prolactin-cortisol treatment administered to hypophysectomized rats increases the activity of RNA polymerase 2.

The dissociation of the behavior of the two RNA polymerase activities observed under certain hormonal conditions by Baldwin *et al.* (1969) does not perfectly agree with the results obtained by Turkington and Ward (1969). In addition, these two groups of authors have noted that the RNA polymerase activity of the mammary gland measured in the presence of a high [$(NH_4)_2SO_4$] molarity depends on the hormonal environment. The mammary enzyme therefore behaves like that of the hen's oviduct (McGuire and O'Malley, 1968), but differs from the liver RNA polymerase 1 that cannot be modified by GH (Pegg and Korner, 1965) or cortisone (Barnabei *et al.*, 1965), and from the RNA polymerase 1 of the prostate or seminal vesicles which are insensitive to testosterone (Liao *et al.*, 1965). In fact, it is difficult to interpret these experiments, since the ions may reveal the specificity of each RNA polymerase, or may have a selective action on the structure of the template chromatin.

b. VARIATIONS IN THE TEMPLATE CAPACITY OF DNA: EQUILIBRIUM AND RATE OF SYNTHESIS OF THE DIFFERENT CLASSES OF HISTONES. According to Stedman and Stedman (1950), Huang and Bonner (1962), Allfrey *et al.* (1963), Barr and Butler (1963), and Bonner *et al.* (1968), the selective expression of the genetic information contained in DNA could be controlled by the abundance and proportions of the different histones. This hypothesis seems to be interesting in the case of the mammary gland since DNA synthesis ([³H]thymidine incorporation) and that of the histones (lysine and arginine incorporation) (Hohmann and Cole, 1969; Marzluff *et al.*, 1969) are concomitant *in vivo* and *in vitro* (organ cultures). In addition, insulin that in 12 hours increases DNA and histone synthesis ([¹⁴C]lysine, [¹⁴C]arginine), but does not induce functional differentiation of mouse mammary cells *in vitro,* has no effect on the equilibrium of the different classes of histones (F₁, F₂b, F₂a + F₃b, F₂a 1) (Marzluff *et al.*, 1969). Lastly, although the proportions and the formation of the different histones are not modified between the phases of pregnancy and milk secretion in the rabbit or the rat (Stellwagen and Cole, 1968, 1969), the synthesis of various lysine-rich subfractions are representative of the secretory stage in the mouse (Hohmann and Cole, 1971).

However, the possibility of controlling the kind of nRNA synthesized by a specific interaction between histones and DNA is greatly limited by the fact that the number of histones is small (15–20, Fambrough and Bonner, 1969; Panyim and Chalkley, 1969; Bustin and Cole, 1969). A higher specificity could be obtained if the histones were subjected to rapid and temporary alterations of their charges following phosphorylation or acetylation of their peptide chains. It is, therefore, very important that the histones F₂a 1 and F₃ of the mammary nuclei are liable to be reversibly acetylated ([¹⁴C]acetate, Marzluff and McCarty, 1970) and that certain nuclear proteins, among which the histones (F₂a₂–F₂b), can be phosphorylated (Turkington and Riddle, 1969). Moreover, while phosphorylation of nuclear proteins is increased by insulin (in 8 hours; preformed histones, as the phosphorylation is only slightly inhibited by cycloheximide) at the same time as it stimulates synthesis of RNA and then of histones (12 hours), prolactin specifically increases the phosphorylation of certain classes of histones when inducing milk secretion. Thus, phosphorylation of the nuclear proteins and regulation of the expression of the genes responsible for secretory activity may be interrelated. Two phosphoprotein kinases (Majumder and Turkington, 1971a) (one of which is activated by a cyclic AMP binding protein—Majumder and Turkington, 1971b), would phosphorylate the nuclear proteins.

c. Characterization of nRNA Synthesized during the Secretory Phase. Synthesized nRNA has been characterized by two methods: analysis by sucrose gradient ultracentrifugation and competitive hybridization with DNA. The sedimentation profiles obtained by sucrose gradient ultracentrifugation of RNA, elaborated under the influence of insulin or prolactin, do not show the specific intervention of one hormone in the formation of different classes of nRNA. The formation of RNA 45 S, 32 S, and then 28 S and 18 S is equally strongly stimulated whatever the nature of the hormone, and after 4 hours of labeling, nRNA always constitutes the major part of the RNA synthesized in the nuclei (Turkington, 1970a). Nor can sucrose gradient ultracentrifugation reveal selective modifications, depending on the hormones present, of the rapidly labeled DNA-like RNA, even after incorporation of 5-bromo-2'-deoxythymidine into DNA (Turkington et al., 1971).

On the other hand, hybridization between nRNA and DNA and competitive hybridization between the rapidly labeled nRNA proceeding from mammary glands of virgin, pregnant, and lactating mice show that functional differentiation is associated with nuclear synthesis of nucleotide sequences that are absent or present in very small numbers in the mammary cells of virgin mice (Turkington, 1970b). There is also a slight difference between nRNA of pregnant mice and that of lactating animals (Turkington, 1970b). Similar modifications have been noticed in the rapidly labeled nRNA at the moment of the selective estrogen or progesterone induction of specific proteins in the oviduct of the hen (O'Malley and McGuire, 1968, 1969; O'Malley et al., 1968b, 1969; Hahn et al., 1968, 1969; Walker, 1969) and in the uterus of the rabbit (Church and McCarthy, 1970), as well as following hormonal stimulation of the liver by cortisol (Drews and Brawerman, 1967). Moreover, adenocarcinoma nuclei of C_3HBH mice or $R_{3230}AC$ carcinoma of rats synthesize polynucleotide molecules that are not formed by the mammary gland nuclei of C_3H/HcJ mice or those of normal lactating rats (Turkington and Self, 1970). The significance of Turkington's observations is, however, reduced by the fact that the nature of highly hybridizable RNA from the nucleus is still in doubt (Kennell, 1970; Tata, 1970) and also by the recent observation of Green et al. (1971a) showing that [3H]uridine incorporation into RNA of high molecular weight does not depend on the secretory stage, but on the presence of hydrocortisone.

IV. RNP (RIBONUCLEOPROTEIN) PARTICLES AND RIBOSOMAL RNA

A. General Properties of Mammary RNP Particles

All enzymatic and nucleic factors involved in the translation of the genetic message are assembled in a precise temporal and spatial sequence on a RNP support.

Mammary RNP's have been prepared by Denamur and Gaye (1967), Gaye and Denamur (1968, 1969, 1970), Baird and Herriman (1968), Herrington and Hawtrey (1969a, 1971), Turkington and Riddle (1970a), Herriman et al. (1971), and Gaye et al. (1972), by methods derived from Wettstein et al. (1963), Henshaw et al. (1963), and Blobel and Potter (1967). The monoribosomes have a sedimentation constant of 78 S measured by sucrose gradient ultracentrifugation, with 2 subunits of 40–60 S, whose presence is essential for the translation procedure. Each subunit proceeds from the interaction between ribosomal RNA and a great number of structural proteins. The monoribosomes are carriers of two specific sites, A and P, for the binding of aminoacyl-tRNA and peptidyl-tRNA.

Mammary RNP of lactating rabbits show absorbance maximum at 260 nm and a minimum at 235 nm. The absorbance ratios A 260/A 235 = 1.45 to 1.5 and A 260/A 280 = 1.8 to 1.9, as well as the RNA/protein ratio close to 1, allow us to conclude that they are only slightly contaminated by exogenous proteins (Gaye and Denamur, 1968). The RNP's isolated by ClCs gradient ultracentrifugation show a density of 1.55 gm/cm^3 (Houdebine, unpublished) identical to that determined for RNP of other organs (see Spirin, 1969; Scherrer et al., 1970). Lastly, mitochondrial ribosomes (55 S, Borst and Grivell, 1971) have not been studied in the mammary gland despite the considerable increase in the number of these organelles during the secretory phases (Howe et al., 1956).

1. Ribosomal RNA (rRNA): Physicochemical Properties

The extraction of the different constituent RNA's of mammary RNP has been accomplished by sodium dodecyl sulfate (SDS; 0.5%) (Gaye and Denamur, 1968), phenol (Herrington and Hawtrey, 1969a), or SDS-phenol treatment (Turkington and Riddle, 1970a; Green et al., 1971a). Sucrose gradient ultracentrifugation allows isolation of a small amount of material sedimenting toward 4–5 S, and two major peaks, 28 S and 18 S, corresponding to the ribosomal RNA of subunits 60 S and 40 S, respectively (Gaye and Denamur, 1968; Herrington and Hawtrey, 1969a; Turkington and Riddle, 1970a). Filtration on dextran gel (Sephadex G 200) or chromatography on methylated serum albumin columns according to Mandell and Hershey (1960) of the phenol-extracted rRNA enable tRNA not contaminated with RNA 5 S to be isolated (Gaye and Denamur, unpublished).

The molecular weights of the two main rRNA, estimated by polyacrylamide gel electrophoresis, are 1.8 and 0.73 × 10^6 (Green et al., 1971a). The nucleotide composition of the total ribosomal RNA of rabbit mam-

mary gland and of RNA 28 S, 18 S, and 5 S have been established after
alkaline hydrolysis and chromatography of the nucleotides 2′, 3′ on
Dowex 1 (Cl⁻ or formate) column. The nucleotide composition is as
follows in percent: rRNA total: Cp 29.4, Ap 17.3, Ψp 1.37, Up 16.7, Gp
34.4, GC 63.8—RNA 28 S: Cp 30.46, Ap 16.74, Ψp 1.34, Up 15.87, Gp
35.56, GC 66.9—RNA 18 S: Cp 28.06, Ap 20.21, Ψp 1.41, Up 18.14, Gp
32.17, GC 60.2 (Gaye and Denamur, unpublished). The high GC content
of mammary rRNA is characteristic for all ribosomal RNA of animal
origin (Wallace, 1961; Brown and Gurdon, 1964; Montagnier and Bellamy, 1964; Hirsch, 1966). This is particularly pronounced for RNA 28 S,
whereas the adenine and uridine contents of RNA 18 S are a little
greater. A similar difference between the nucleotide composition of the
two ribosomal RNA's has been determined for the RNA of chicken
embryo cells (Montagnier and Bellamy, 1964), of Hela cells (Zimmerman et al., 1963), of ascitic fluids (Lerner et al., 1963), of rat liver
(Munro, 1964), and rabbit liver (Hirsch, 1966). The significant proportion of Ψp (8% of Up) in the two rRNA's cannot be attributed to contamination of these RNA's by tRNA's. Finally, RNA 5 S, which is a
component of the subparticle 60 S, is characterized by a high Up content,
in accordance with the results of Rosset et al. (1964), Galibert et al.
(1965), and Knight and Darnell (1967). In accord with the hypothesis
put forward for bacteria (Erdmann et al., 1971; Jordan, 1971), mammary RNA 5 S could intervene in the specific fitting of tRNA on the
ribosomes through its CGAAC sequence that is complementary to the
GT ΨC/AG sequence present in all tRNA's.

The nucleotide composition of the microsomal RNA purified on a
methylated serum albumin column is similar to that of ribosomal RNA
isolated by ultracentrifugation. It remains unchanged during pregnancy
and lactation in the rabbit (Denamur, 1965). Baldwin and Martin
(1968a) have separated total mammary RNA of the rat according to a
method based on that of Greenman et al. (1965), Wicks et al. (1965), and
Tsanev et al. (1966). They obtained a fraction rich in ribosomal RNA or
precursors of these RNA (50–70% of total RNA) whose GC content
is high; however, its nucleotide composition determined after PEI cellulose thin-layer chromatography is very different from that of rabbit
mammary rRNA calculated after Dowex 1 chromatography (Gaye and
Denamur, unpublished). Wang et al. (1960), using rats, found no difference between the nucleotide composition of rRNA and that of tRNA's,
and Reich et al. (1963) found a high Up content and a low Cp percentage in the rRNA of goat, rabbit, and rat mammary glands; these
results seem clearly to show the influence of methods of rRNA prepara-

tions and analysis (time, $\theta°$, normality of alkali during the hydrolysis in mononucleotides) used by these authors.

2. Ribosomal Proteins

The ribosomal proteins in the mammary gland have been subjected to few investigations. Herrington and Hawtrey (1971) indicate that polyacrylamide gel electrophoresis allows the separation of at least 20 proteins from the mammary ribosomes of lactating cows (a much greater number of proteins have been identified in the particles 40 and 60 S of eukaryotes; Huynh-Vantan *et al.*, 1971; Schreiber, 1971; Warner, 1971). On the other hand, the mammary ribosomal proteins from nonlactating cows could not be separated by this method. Moreover, these authors have noticed that the ribosomes of nonsecretory mammary glands synthesize only a few proteins in a cell-free system, and that they differ from the ribosomes obtained from secreting glands in being unable to bind the poly U or tRNA aminoacyl complex. Herrington and Hawtrey (1971) speculate on the possibility that the deficiencies detected in the nonsecreting mammary RNP reflect the absence of a small number of ribosomal proteins that, without changing the sedimentation characteristics of the subunits, would inhibit the binding of the particle 40 S on the RNA messengers, the first stage in initiation of protein synthesis in the eukaryotes (Joklik and Becker, 1965; Heywood, 1970a,b; Huang and Baltimore, 1970; Pragnell and Arnstein, 1970; Burgess and Mach, 1971; Hoetz and McCarthy, 1971; Ilan and Ilan, 1971; Lebleu *et al.*, 1971; Pragnell *et al.*, 1971), as in the prokaryotes (Revel *et al.*, 1968, and reviews of Davis, 1971; Schreiber, 1971; Lucas-Lenard and Lipmann, 1971). In any case, three factors of ribosomal origin seem to be necessary in the cells of the eukaryotes [M_1, M_2, M_3—in the muscles and the reticulocytes or dissociation factor (DF) in yeast, liver, reticulocytes] (Fuhr *et al.*, 1969; Herzberg *et al.*, 1969; Heywood, 1970a,b; Petre, 1970; Pritchard *et al.*, 1970, 1971; Shafritz *et al.*, 1970, 1971a,b; Shafritz and Anderson, 1970a,b; Naora and Pritchard, 1971; Naora *et al.*, 1971; Crystal *et al.*, 1971; Lawford *et al.*, 1971; Lubsen and Davis, 1972), as well as in the prokaryotes (F_1, F_2, F_3), for initiating the synthesis of peptide chains. The peptidyl transferase enzyme responsible for the formation of the peptide bond is moreover a structural protein of the subunit 60 S. It is probably not responsible for the fact that the mammary microsomes have lost their capacity for elongating peptide chains in diabetic rats, as Wool *et al.* (1968) did not notice any difference in the number and the nature of ribosomal proteins of normal or diabetic rats.

Mammary ribosomes also bind a more or less large number of nonstructural proteins, among which are the nucleases that may affect the integrality of the RNA chains in the course of their preparation (Herrington and Hawtrey, 1969a). They are eliminated by washing (with 0.5 M NH$_4$Cl) the ribosomes (Herrington and Hawtrey, 1971).

B.   Degree of Aggregation and Intracellular Distribution of RNP during the Phase of Secretory Activity

In the eukaryotes, the active units in protein synthesis form structures called polyribosomes, consisting of messenger RNA, that are translated simultaneously by several ribosomes carrying tRNA and peptide chains in the process of construction. The ribosome-ribosomal subunit cycle has not been studied in the mammary gland during protein synthesis. However, we know that in eukaryote cells this cycle has the same essential characteristics as that of the bacteria (see reviews of Davis, 1971 and Schreiber, 1971), although the pool of ribosomes seems to equilibrate more slowly with that of the subunits (Howards et al., 1970; Jacobs-Lorena and Baglioni, 1970).

The total mammary ribosomes of lactating rabbits show a sucrose gradient sedimentation profile characterized by a prevalence of the hepta-, octa-, and nonamers (Denamur and Gaye, 1967; Gaye and Denamur, 1968; Herriman et al., 1971). The incubation of these polyribosomes, in the presence of ribonuclease, completely transforms the ribosomal aggregates into monomers (Gaye and Denamur, 1968; Herriman et al., 1971), but pronase does not change their sedimentation profile (Gaye and Denamur, 1968). EDTA, moreover, converts the polyribosomes into subunits 30 and 50 S (Gaye and Denamur, 1968) and into small RNP particles containing the rapidly labeled RNA (density in ClCs gradient, 1.46 gm/ml; Houdebine, unpublished).

The aggregation spectrum of the polyribosomes bound to the membranes of the endoplasmic reticulum is similar to that of total polyribosomes. On the other hand, free polyribosomes isolated according to Bloemendal et al. (1964) have a sedimentation profile different from that of polyribosomes bound to the membranes: the light forms and the monoribosomes are proportionally more abundant (Gaye and Denamur, 1968). The proportions of bound and free forms, determined by the method of Blobel and Potter (1967), are 80 and 20% respectively for lactating mammary glands of the rabbit (Gaye and Denamur, 1968) and the ewe (Gaye and Denamur, 1970). The sedimentation profiles characteristic for the bound and free polyribosomes of lactating rabbit mammary glands are the same as those for the bound and free ribosomal particles in the lactating ewe mammary gland (Gaye and Denamur, 1970) and lactating guinea pig mammary gland (Gaye and Denamur, unpublished).

C. Variation in the Amount and Degree of Aggregation of RNP during the Functional Differentiation of the Mammary Gland

1. RNP and RNA Content of the Mammary Gland

The amount of RNP is clearly more important in the mammary glands of lactating rabbits than in those of pseudopregnant (Denamur and Gaye, 1967; Gaye and Denamur, 1968, 1969) or pregnant females (Denamur and Gaye, 1967). This enrichment of the rabbit mammary gland during the secretory phase is in accordance with the preferential increase of ribosomal RNA between midpregnancy and maximum lactation noticed in this species by Deutsch and Norgren (1970) whatever the methods used to prepare the RNA (extraction by phenol-SDS or by phenol), or to analyze them (sucrose gradient centrifugation, polyacrylamide gel electrophoresis, selective precipitation). Ribosomal RNA's represent 70–85% of total RNA in the lactating rabbit mammary gland, whereas they do not exceed 60% of total RNA during pregnancy. Moreover, after unilateral ligature of the teats of lactating rabbits, resulting in a considerable regression of secretory activity, the rRNA decrease reaches 60–75%, whereas that of total RNA is limited to 40–50%. During pregnancy and lactation, the results obtained in the ewe (Gaye and Denamur, unpublished) are similar to those recorded for the rabbit, and hypophysectomy in the lactating ewe leads to a preferential reduction of the amount of polyribosomes (Denamur et al., 1972).

Induction of milk secretion corresponds, moreover, to an increase of the number of polyribosomes. Thus, the *in vivo* administration of prolactin to pseudopregnant rabbits stimulates the formation of polyribosomes, and after 4 days of treatment their number is close to that found in the mammary glands of lactating animals (Gaye and Denamur, 1969). The observations of Slater and Planterose (1958) also show that, in the rat, between the end of pregnancy (day 20) and day 3 of lactation, there is a definite increase in the proportion of ribosome-rich fractions. During the first 24 hours of culture of mammary explants from midpregnant mice, insulin increases the amount of polyribosomes (Turkington and Riddle, 1970a). Cortisol added to insulin has no positive effect, and the number of polyribosomes is even reduced between 24 and 72 hours of culture. The addition of prolactin after 72 hours of culture in the presence of insulin and cortisol considerably increases the amount of polyribosomes, inducing, at the same time, milk secretion. The stimulating action of prolactin requires the continued presence of insulin, and it does not occur if mitosis is inhibited by colchicine, or if mammary explants develop without a corticoid (Turkington and Riddle, 1970a). Increase in the amount of polyribosomes is significant 6 hours after addition of prolactin and coincides with the beginning of casein synthesis (^{32}P incorporation) (Turkington and Riddle, 1970a).

Finally, the abundance of RNP and rRNA, determined biochemically in actively secreting mammary glands, is confirmed by the ultrastructural features of these glands (see reviews of Bargman and Welsch, 1969; Hollmann, 1969; Hollmann and Verley, 1970; Wellings, 1969). The effect of prolactin on mammary RNP perfectly accords with that of the other morphogenic hormones on the amount and degree of aggregation of RNP in their receptor organs (see reviews of Tata, 1966, 1970).

2. Rate of rRNA Synthesis

The rate of rRNA synthesis is much stimulated during lactation or during the induction of milk secretion. Thus, ^{32}P incorporation into ribosomal RNA of rabbit mammary glands *in vivo* greatly increases during lactation (Majumder and Ganguli, 1969b). In the same way, intraductal injections of prolactin into pseudopregnant rabbits increase [^{3}H]uridine incorporation into microsomal RNA (Simpson and Schmidt, 1971). On the other hand, cortisol does not seem to be involved in the incorporation of ^{32}P into RNA of ribosomal type in the mammary glands of lactating hypophysectomized rats (Baldwin and Martin, 1968a,b). Injection of prolactin, however, and especially of the combination prolactin-cortisol, that reestablishes some secretory activity in the hypophysectomized rat, stimulates rRNA synthesis (Baldwin and Martin, 1968a,b). During the first 24 hours of mouse mammary culture, insulin increases *in vitro* the [^{3}H] uridine incorporation into monoribosomes and polyribosomes (Turkington and Riddle, 1970a). The addition of cortisol has no positive effect and rRNA synthesis even goes on decreasing until 72 hours of culture. The [^{3}H]uridine incorporation into monoribosomes and polyribosomes is stimulated by adding prolactin to the insulin-cortisol medium after 72–96 hours of culture. The period of labeling used by the authors (8–12 hours) localizes the radioactivity mainly in rRNA (Turkington, 1970a). Finally, Banerjee and Banerjee (1971), noticed a preferential increase in the binding of [^{3}H]uridine to the nucleolus (sites of rRNA synthesis, see reviews of Georgiev, 1967; Perry, 1967 and Perry *et al.*, 1970) between day 15 of pregnancy and day 5 of lactation in the mouse.

3. Variations in the Degree of Aggregation of RNP

During the phase of mammary growth in the pseudopregnant rabbit, a large amount of monoribosomes associated with a rather low percentage of very aggregated forms whose distinct separation generally does not exceed 5–6 ribosomal units can be detected (Gaye and Denamur, 1969). This distribution of ribosomal aggregates is also noticed during the second third of pregnancy, corresponding to a nonsecretory growth phase (Gaye and Denamur, unpublished). Thus, in the absence of secretion or when it begins (day 28 of pregnancy; Herriman *et al.*, 1971), total polyribosomes differ from those of lactation not in the size of the heaviest aggregates, but in a different distribution of the most numerous aggregates (Gaye and Denamur, 1969). In addition, on day 14 of pregnancy there are no great differences between the sedimentation profile for free polyribosomes, representing 75% of total ribosomes, and that for bound polyribosomes (Gaye and Denamur, 1969).

During the phase of mammary growth and secretion resulting from the administration of prolactin to pseudopregnant rabbits, a preferential increase in some aggregated forms occurs in 24 hours (Gaye and Denamur, 1969). After 48 hours, ribosomal aggregates of 7–8 units are the most abundant, and between 48 and 96 hours the sedimentation diagram for bound polyribosomes is similar to that existing during lactation. The aggregation degree of free polyribosomes is identical to that of bound polyribosomes 24–48 hours after starting prolactin treatment, but after 96 hours the sedimentation characteristics of free polyribosomes are identical to those of free mammary ribosomes obtained during lactation (Gaye and Denamur, 1969). Analysis of the distribution of free and bound polyribosomes in the mammary cell during prolactin treatment shows that the balance of free and bound forms progressively moves in favor of the latter. Lastly the secretory activity obtained in organ cultures of mouse mammary explants, influenced by IC_2P combinations, corresponds to the formation of polyribosomes with a large proportion of heavy aggregates (Turkington and Riddle, 1970a).

The changes in the sedimentation profiles of bound and free polyribosomes observed during the functional differentiation of the mammary gland are difficult to interpret. Schematically, these changes may be due to differences in the equilibrium between the peptide chain initiation, the chain elongations and release of peptide or to dissimilarities in the polyribosomes' contents of messenger RNA (Staehelin *et al.*, 1964).

D. Variations in the Synthetic Activity of RNP: Preferential Role during the Milk Protein Synthesis of the RNP's Bound to the Membranes of the Endoplasmic Reticulum

The synthetic activity (cpm of incorporated amino acids per unit RNA) of bound polyribosomes exceeds that of free polyribosomes during lactation in the rabbit or the ewe (Gaye and Denamur, 1968, 1970). Prolactin increases the capacity for synthesis of free and bound polyribosomes in the mammary glands of pseudopregnant rabbits (Gaye and Denamur, 1969) and alloxan diabetes reduces the synthetic activity of rat mammary microsomes (Martin and Baldwin, 1971). The stimulation produced by prolactin allows a partial interpretation of the growing changes in the synthetic capacity of the particle-containing fraction of mammary glands between the end of pregnancy and day 13 of lactation in the rabbit (Baird and Herriman, 1968). This stimulation seems to be associated with the degree of aggregation of the polyribosomes if the relationship, found in hepatic systems, between degree of aggregation and rate of protein synthesis (Noll *et al.*, 1963; Wettstein *et al.*, 1963) is also valid for the mammary gland.

The nature of the synthetic activity of polyribosomes differs in the pseudopregnant and the lactating rabbit and is subject to prolactin control. After injection of prolactin, there is a preferential stimulation of the quantities of proline (a major amino acid in caseins) incorporated into proteins by total polyribosomes (Gaye and Denamur, 1969). This modification in the nature of the polyribosomal activity is partly due to changes in the relative proportions of free and bound polyribosomes in association with the specificity of protein synthesis effected by these two classes of ribosomes. The free polyribosomes of lactating ewe mammary glands, although very active in protein synthesis, *in vitro* produce only negligible amounts of α-lactoglobulin, in contrast to the polyribosomes bound to the endoplasmic reticulum (Gaye and Denamur, 1970). On the other hand, in a cell-free system, bound polyribosomes synthesize α-lactalbumin and β-lactoglobulin. The latter has been identified by its chromatographic and electrophoretic behavior, its immunological properties, and by analysis of the peptide maps resulting from trypsin hydrolysis (Gaye and Denamur, 1970; Gaye *et al.*, 1972). The messenger RNA content of the two classes of RNP is therefore presumably different. Moreover, bound polyribosomes, representing 80% of total polyribosomes during the phases of active secretion, appear to be responsible *in vivo* for the almost total synthesis of these proteins. Our observations agree with those of Brew and Campbell (1967) showing α-lactalbumin synthesis by a microsomal fraction of guinea pig mammary gland, and with that of Beitz *et al.* (1969), who have synthesized chains immunologically identical to caseins from a microsomal cell-free system of bovine mammary gland. The functional difference in the mammary gland between bound and free polyribosomes has also been observed in the liver, where the synthesis of serum albumin takes place exclusively on polyribosomes bound to the membranes of the endoplasmic reticulum (Redman, 1968; Takagi and Ogata, 1968; Takagi *et al.*, 1969; Ganoza and Williams, 1969), whereas that of ferritin (structural protein) occurs mainly on the free forms (Redman, 1969; Hicks *et al.*, 1969). The mechanisms allowing separation, in the mammary cell, between the two categories of polyribosomes (free and bound) remain obscure. On the basis of our present understanding of this question it is difficult to say if the binding of ribosomes to the membranes reflects the presence of proteins peculiar to the 60 S particles of bound ribosomes [the subparticle 60 S could be the unit binding the ribosome to the endoplasmic reticulum (Sabatini and Blobel, 1970)], or if the nature of messenger RNA is the determining factor.

V. TRANSFER RNA OF THE MAMMARY GLAND

The role of tRNA in the genetic translation is essential and consists in specific binding of amino acids in the presence of aminoacyl-tRNA synthetase, followed by the formation of a ribosome-coding-triplet-aminoacyl-tRNA complex allowing insertion of amino acids into the peptide chain in positions determined by the sequence of messenger RNA codons (see review of Lengyel and Söll, 1969; Zachau, 1969). The nucleotide sequence of about 30 of these tRNA has been determined and their secondary structures are almost analogous (see Philipps, 1969, the so-called cloverleaf structure).

A. General Properties of Mammary Transfer RNA

1. Physicochemical Properties

The tRNA's of the mammary gland have been prepared from tissue homogenates (bovine mammary glands, Elska *et al.*, 1971), from the supernatant (105,000x *g*: ewe mammary glands, Petrissant, 1968, 1969), from the precipitate at pH 5 (bovine mammary glands, Herrington and Hawtrey 1969b), or from a postmitochondrial supernatant (ewe mammary glands, Petrissant, 1968). The proportions of molecules that are more or less degraded depend on the mammary material used for the extraction of tRNA as well as on other factors (addition of RNAse inhibitors, speed and duration of the mammary gland treatment, etc.; Petrissant, 1968, 1969). The method used in our laboratory by Petrissant (1968, 1969) can, for the early stages, be compared with that of Brunngraber (1962). The first part of the procedure is followed by selective isopropanol precipitation of impurities (Deutscher, 1967) and tRNA deacylation (Sarin and Zamecnik, 1964), a technique that is also used by Robison and Zimmerman (1970) to prepare large quantities of liver tRNA. In chromatography on methylated serum albumin column, the tRNA preparations obtained are homogeneous, but filtration on Sephadex G 100 indicates a 10% contamination by RNA 5 S. After elimination of which, the protein content of tRNA does not exceed 0.6%, the $\epsilon(P)$ is 7.4, the hyperchromicity expressed according to Klee and Staehelin (1962) attains 1.43 and their nucleotide composition expressed as a percentage of total nucleotides (Petrissant, 1968), is adenosine: 1.25, 5 Me Cp 0.94—Cp 28.2 —Ap 16.01—6 Me Ap 1.41—Ψp 3.41—Tp 0.71—Up 15.5—N_1 Me Gp 0.77—N_2 diMe Gp 0.98—Gp 30.04— Ip 0.23.

Supposing that the mean tRNA chain length is 80 nucleotides (75–87: Staehelin, 1971), there is consequently a terminal adenosine for each chain, which proves the structural integrity of the molecules. In addition, the proportion of Ψp (2.76) is in agreement with the amount of this nucleotide in most tRNA's of known structure (Staehelin, 1971; Ebel, 1971). On the other hand, the Tp (0.56 in 80 nucleotides) content established for all mammary tRNA of lactating ewes is lower than that determined by the same method in liver or yeast tRNA. Finally, 3 methylated guanines (N_1 Me Gp—N_2 Me Gp—N_2 diMe Gp) (Petrissant and Gaye, 1966) and 5 methylated bases (N_1 Me Gp—N_2 diMe Gp—6 Me Ap—Tp —5 Me Cp) (Petrissant, 1968) have been demonstrated in the tRNA of ewe mammary glands, whereas 6 have been detected in the tRNA of mouse mammary glands (Turkington, 1969) (N_2 diMe Gp—N_1 Me Gp —N_1 Me Ap—6 Me Ap—Tp—5 Me Cp). However, considering that about 50 modified nucleosides (the structure is known for 37 of them) have been isolated from the tRNA of various organisms (Söll, 1971), our knowledge concerning mammary tRNA seems still to be limited.

2. Acceptor Capacity of Transfer RNA in Lactating Mammary Glands

This capacity has been determined for mammary tRNA of lactating ewes and rabbits using aminoacyl-tRNA synthetases from ewe or rabbit mammary glands, from rabbit liver, or from *Escherichia coli,* and after studying the various parameters of the acylation reaction (pH, Mg/ATP ratio, etc.) (Petrissant, 1969).

The mammary tRNA of lactating ewes and those of rabbits may be distinguished by the amounts of acylated leucine and arginine. The acceptor activity of the tRNA in the ewe mammary gland, which attains 1389 pmoles per A 260, can be schematized in the following way: Ser > Leu > Ala > Arg ⩾ Val. It is also different from rabbit liver tRNA (Petrissant, 1969), whereas the acceptor capacity (for 4 amino acids) of mammary tRNA in lactating cows is characterized as follows: Glu > Leu > Phe > Gly (Elska *et al.*, 1971). Even if the number of amino acids studied is insufficient to draw conclusions, the acceptor capacity of the tRNA seems to be characteristic of the species for a given organ, and in the same species there seems to be an organ specificity, the expressions of which partly depend on the origin of the aminoacyl-tRNA synthetase used.

B. Variations in the Mammary Content of tRNA and Their Rate of Synthesis

The determination of the acceptor capacity of total RNA extracted by phenol-SDS from mouse mammary glands, as well as electrophoresis of these RNA on polyacrylamide gel, led Turkington (1969) to think that there is a preferential increase in tRNA concentrations during the phase of functional differentiation, between day 10 and day 20 of pregnancy. Together with the increase in the proportion of tRNA there is also, during this period of pregnancy, a stimulation of the tRNA methylase activities responsible for the achievement of the primary tRNA structure (Turkington, 1969). However, in spite of the continuation of mammary RNA enrichment during lactation in the mouse, the relative amounts of tRNA do not vary after pregnancy (between day 20 of pregnancy and day 10 of lactation) whatever the level of secretory activity (Turkington, 1969). Similar results have been obtained with organ cultures of mouse mammary tissue. Thus, insulin, a nonlactogenic hormone, stimulates RNA synthesis during the first 24 hours of culture but does not modify, either alone or in combination with hydrocortisone, the proportion of tRNA in total RNA (Turkington, 1969). On the other hand, the lactogenic combination IC_2P or IC_1P which increases the RNA content of mammary explants (Mayne *et al.*, 1968; El Darwish and Rivera, 1971) and stimulates RNA synthesis after 24 hours of culture brings about a preferential increase of tRNA and of the methylating enzyme activity (Turkington, 1969). However, these enzyme activities seem to be controlled by only two hormones: insulin and prolactin. Their stimulation corresponds to the synthesis of new enzyme proteins, as their increase is inhibited after injection *in vivo* or addition *in vitro* of actinomycin D or cycloheximide (Turkington, 1969). It would be interesting to know if the natural inhibitor of tRNA methylases which is present in certain tissues (Kerr, 1970, 1971) and whose activity in the uterus depends on estradiol (Sharma and Borek, 1970; Sharma *et al.*, 1971) is involved in the changes in tRNA methylase activities of the mammary gland. Whatever it may be, according to Turkington (1969) genetic translation at the moment of secretory differentiation of the mammary cells would only be possible by the intervention of larger amounts of tRNA. This opinion is in accordance with the results obtained in the chicken oviduct showing increase in the proportion of tRNA (Dingman *et al.*, 1969; O'Malley *et al.*, 1968a) and of tRNA methylases (Hacker, 1969) after estrogen induction of specific protein synthesis. In addition, the pH 5 fractions of pseudopregnant rabbit mammary glands contain about three times less tRNA than those of lactating rabbit mammary glands (Houdebine *et al.*, 1972). However, in this species the effect on tRNA does not seem to be selective as the amounts of rRNA and nRNA are also lower in the mammary cells of pseudopregnant animals. Moreover, an agreement has to be found between the observations of Turkington (1969) and those of Green *et al.* (1971a), who have shown, using cultures of mouse mammary explants, that the lactogenic combination IC_2P does not affect the distribution of rRNA, tRNA, or RNA 5 S and that [^{3}H]uridine incorporation into tRNA is not preferential.

C. Do the tRNA's Control the Nature and Degree of Protein Synthesis in the Mammary Gland?

It has been well established that for each amino acid there are several isoacceptor tRNA's (about 60 per 20 amino acids). The reasons for this multiplicity have not been elucidated yet, but it appears logical to suppose that it corresponds to the fact that the tRNA's act as regulators of genetic translation and of subsequent protein synthesis. This intervention could be of two kinds (see review of Sueoka and Kano Sueoka, 1970).

1. By allowing (presence of a new tRNA isoacceptor) or by inhibiting (disappearance of a tRNA isoacceptor) the translation of messenger RNA responsible for the synthesis of such and such a protein characteristic of a physiological stage (see reviews of Novelli, 1969; Sueoka and Kano Sueoka, 1970). In this case, the tRNA involved may consist of a polynucleotide chain synthesized on a newly derepressed gene or of a chain not proceeding from the intervention of a supplementary gene but under-

going variable degrees of methylation resulting or not in different properties of the anticodon (Peterkofsky *et al.*, 1966) (the neighboring bases of
the anticodon are often methylated). Attachment to the ribosomes could
also be effected (Capra and Peterkofsky, 1968; Gefter and Russell, 1969;
Stern *et al.*, 1970), but the changes according to the degree of methylation
in the interaction between tRNA and aminoacyl-tRNA synthetases described by Shugart *et al.* (1968a,b) have not been confirmed (Biekunski
et al., 1970). The formation in the liver of two new species of aspartic
tRNA after administration of growth hormone may illustrate the possibility of this type of regulation. However, the demonstration of this is still
not convincing (Jackson *et al.*, 1970).

2. By modulating the rate of translation of messenger RNA (Ames and
Hartman, 1963; Stent, 1964; Itano, 1966), after modification of the relative proportions of various tRNA isoacceptors, one of which is carrier of a
particular anticodon and becomes the limiting factor in the translation of
certain messenger RNA. This possibility has been verified experimentally
by Anderson (1969) for the artificial messenger, poly AG, whose translation rate depends on the amount of a tRNA arginine isoacceptor reacting
with the triplet AGA, and by Anderson and Gilbert (1969) for the rate
of synthesis of the α and β chains of globin. Alterations in balance of the
various tRNA isoacceptors have also been described in many experimental situations with microorganisms (see reviews of Sueoka and Kano
Sueoka, 1970), with cancer cells (Holland *et al.*, 1967; Taylor *et al.*,
1967, 1968; Axel *et al.*, 1967; Baliga *et al.*, 1969; Yang and Novelli,
1968a,b; Weinstein, 1968; Gallo, 1969; Goldman *et al.*, 1969; Mushinki and
Potter, 1969; Taylor, 1969, 1970; Gonano and Pirro, 1971a,b; Mittelman,
1971), and with normal cells under the influence of hormones (Maenpaa
and Bernfield, 1969, 1970; Beck *et al.*, 1970a; Sharma *et al.*, 1971—estradiol, tRNA Ser; Tonoue *et al.*, 1969—triiodothyronine, tRNA Leu; Yang
and Sanadi, 1969—thyroxine, tRNA Tyr).

Although some of the results obtained may correspond to artifacts
(Yang and Novelli, 1968a,b), the modulation of the translation phenomena by tRNA is a tempting hypothesis whose validity in the mammary
gland would be interesting to test. However, there are still too few experimental findings relative to the mammary gland, and we shall therefore
only rapidly mention the different experiments performed.

1. Is the Acceptor Capacity of Mammary tRNA Modified at Certain Physiological Periods?

For the Russian authors (Elska *et al.*, 1971) the acylation of glutamic
acid and leucine by total mammary tRNA of virgin or lactating cows
show an increase of 78 and 40% respectively for tRNA obtained during

lactation. On the other hand, the acylation of phenylalanine and glycine are lower (24 and 62%) in mammary tRNA of nonlactating cows. The increase in the amount of mammary glutamic tRNA is accompanied by growing variation of the glutamyl-tRNA synthetase activity. As already suggested (Fraser and Gutfreund, 1958; Elska and Matsuka, 1968a,b; Semonova et al., 1969) and concluded by Elska et al. (1971), the tRNA's acceptor capacity and the relative amounts of the various aminoacyl-tRNA synthetases are representative of the amino acid composition of the proteins synthesized at each physiological stage: secretory proteins during lactation or structural proteins during the growth periods [see also relative amount tRNA's in reticulocytes (Smith and McNamara, 1971), silk glands of silkworms (Garel et al., 1970), and fibroblasts of healing wounds (Lanks and Weinstein, 1970)]. However, the comparative studies in mammary glands are not conclusive enough because of the difficulty of interpreting the analysis of tRNA from virgin mammary glands that contain a small proportion of mammary parenchyma or from involuting mammary glands which contain many hydrolyzing enzymes.

2. Are the Levels and the Balances between the Various tRNA Iso-acceptors Indicative of the Synthetic Orientation of the Mammary Gland?

a. DEMONSTRATION AND PURIFICATION OF DIFFERENT tRNA ISOACCEP-TORS IN THE MAMMARY GLAND. The existence of several mammary tRNA isoacceptors for each amino acid has been demonstrated using different techniques of chromatography (Petrissant, 1970, 1971). The heterogeneity of alanine, leucine, arginine, valine, and serine tRNA of the ewe mammary gland has been revealed by chromatography on BD cellulose. As regards alanine, leucine, and valine, this heterogeneity was almost analogous to that of the corresponding yeast tRNA. On the other hand, the arginine tRNA's of the mammary gland seem to be more heterogenous, and serine tRNA's like those of yeast, show a heterogenous peak that is eluted late as well as another coinciding with that of methionine $Met \ II \atop GM$ tRNA. However, the author has not yet studied the chromatographic profile of these tRNA's in relation to the amount and the nature of the protein synthesized by the mammary gland. It is interesting that among mammary tRNA of lactating cows, two leucyl-tRNA's have been identified by chromatography on MAK column, whereas tRNA of involuting mammary glands have only one tRNA isoacceptor of this amino acid (Elska et al., 1971). Nevertheless, as five leucine isoacceptors have been isolated in the other organisms, it is still impossible to say if the isoacceptor, whose presence is localized during the secretory phase, is particular or identical to one of them.

In mammals, the number of isolated purified tRNA's is small and mainly of hepatic origin; tRNA serine (Staehelin *et al.*, 1968; Nishimura and Wettstein, 1969; Staehelin, 1971; Petrissant *et al.*, 1971); tRNA phenylalanine (Fink *et al.*, 1968; Petrissant *et al.*, 1971); tRNA tyrosine (Nishimura and Wettstein, 1969); tRNA's valine, tryptophan, Met I and II (Petrissant *et al.*, 1971). In the mammary gland, it is more particularly the heterogeneity of methionine tRNA that has been studied leading to the purification of two isoacceptors. Using several chromatographic techniques, Petrissant (1971) isolated the tRNA $^{\mathrm{Met\ I}}_{\mathrm{GM}}$ that can be acylated both by the homologous aminoacyl tRNA synthetase and by that of *E. coli* and whose activity exceeds 1200 pmoles of methionine per unit of absorption. Its terminal 3′ sequence differs from that of tRNA $^{\mathrm{Met\ f.}}_{E.\ coli}$; it can be formylated by the *E. coli* transformylase, responds to the codons AUG and GUG and leads to the formation of formylmethioninepuromycin. Consequently, the nonformylated tRNA $^{\mathrm{Met\ I}}_{\mathrm{GM}}$ is probably the tRNA initiating the synthesis of peptide chains in the mammary gland, in agreement with the role that has recently been allotted to tRNA Met I of mammals (Caskey *et al.*, 1967, 1968; Takeishi *et al.*, 1968; Gupta, 1968; Rajbhandary and Ghosh, 1969; Bhaduri *et al.*, 1970; Brown and Smith, 1970; Gupta *et al.*, 1970; Housman *et al.*, 1970; Jackson and Hunter, 1970; Smith and Marcker, 1970; Wilson and Dintzis, 1970; Anderson and Shafritz, 1971; Hunter and Jackson, 1971). The mammary tRNA $^{\mathrm{Met\ II}}_{\mathrm{GM}}$, that cannot be acylated by aminoacyl-tRNA synthetase of *E. coli,* has been obtained purified by the same system of successive chromatographies and phenoxyacetylation according to Gillam *et al.* (1968). Its specific activity exceeds 1200 pmoles of Met per unit of absorption. Its terminal 3′ sequence definitely differs from that of tRNA $^{\mathrm{Met\ m}}_{E.\ coli}$ (Petrissant, 1971).

b. Is the Structure of Certain tRNA Isoacceptors Modified as a Result of Variations in the Nature and Amount of Minor Nucleotides? i. *Degree of methylation.* The increase in the amount of methylating enzymes (guanine N^2N^2 dimethylase–guanine-N^1-methylase–amino purine-6-methylase–adenine-1-methylase–uridine-5-methylase–cytidine-5-methylase) is synchronous with that of the tRNA during mammary organogenesis, but the variations in these different enzyme activities are not strictly coordinated (Turkington, 1969). The author concludes, however, that there are no major changes in the tRNA methylation spectrum at the time of secretory differentiation in the mammary gland. In any case, the amount and number of methylating enzymes are more reduced in lactating mammary tissues than in mammary carcinoma containing in particular a guanine-7-methylase (Turkington and Riddle, 1970b). In fact, the abundance of methylating activities in cancer tissues seems to be a general phenomenon (see Turkington, 1971 and review of Craddock, 1970).

ii. *Amount of Ψp (pseudouridine phosphate)*. The tRNA's of lactating mammary glands contain more Ψp than those of nonsecretory mammary glands (Elska and Matsuka, 1968a).

Another form of alteration of the tRNA structure has been described by Herrington and Hawtrey (1969a,b; 1970a,b). These authors have shown that the tRNA extracted from the mammary glands of nonlactating cows have no terminal CCA sequence and cannot be acylated, contrary to the tRNA of lactating mammary glands. However, 30% of the tRNA extracted during the nonsecretory phase acquire the property of being acylated if they are prepared in the presence of RNAase inhibitors. As the loss of the triplet CCA, i.e., loss of the acceptor capacity in the main part of the tRNA, seems to be an artifact of the preparation, it cannot signify that tRNA regulate genetic translation in this way during the nonsecretory phases.

Lastly, the mitochondrial tRNA which, in the animal cells, are distinct from the cytoplasmic tRNA (Buck and Nass, 1968, 1969, 1970; Fournier and Simpson, 1968) have not been characterized in the mammary gland.

REFERENCES

Allfrey, V. G. Littau, V. C., and Mirsky, A. E. (1963). *Proc. Nat. Acad. Sci. U.S.* **49**, 414.

Ames, B. N., and Hartman, P. E. (1963). *Cold Spring Harbor Symp. Quant. Biol.* **28**, 349.

Ancel, P., and Bouin, P. (1909). *C. R. Soc. Biol.* **66**, 605.

Ancel, P., and Bouin, P. (1911). *C. R. Ass. Anat.* **1**,

Anderson, W. F. (1969). *Proc. Nat. Acad. Sci. U.S.* **62**, 566.

Anderson, W. F., and Gilbert, J. M. (1969). *Biochem. Biophys. Res. Commun.* **36**, 456.

Anderson, W. F., and Shafritz, D. A. (1971). *Cancer Res.* **31**, 701.

Anderson, R. R., and Turner, C. W. (1963). *Proc. Soc. Exp. Biol. Med.* **113**, 333.

Anderson, R. R., and Turner, C. W. (1968). *Proc. Soc. Exp. Biol. Med.* **128**, 210.

Attardi, G., Aloni, Y., Attardi, B., Ojala, D., Pica-Mattocia, L., Robberson, D. L., and Storrie, B. (1970). *Cold Spring. Harbor Symp. Quant. Biol.* **35**, 599.

Axel, R., Weinstein, I. B., and Farber, E. (1967). *Proc. Nat. Acad. Sci. U.S.* **58**, 1255.

Baird, G. D., and Herriman, I. D. (1968), *Biochim. Biophys. Acta* **166**, 162.

Baldwin, R. L. (1966). *J. Dairy Sci.* **49**, 1533.

Baldwin, R. L., and Martin, R. J. (1968a). *Endocrinology* **82**, 1209.
Baldwin, R. L., and Martin, R. J. (1968b). *J. Dairy Sci.* **51**, 748.
Baldwin, R. L., and Milligan, L. P. (1966). *J. Biol. Chem.* **241**, 2058.
Baldwin, R. L., Korsrud, G. O., Martin, R. J., Cheng, W., and Schober, N. A. (1969). *Biol. of Reprod.* **1**, 31.
Baliga, B. S., Borek, E., Weinstein, I. B., and Strinivasan, P. R. (1969). *Proc. Nat. Acad. Sci. U.S.* **62**, 899.
Banerjee, M. R., and Banerjee, D. N. (1971). *Exp. Cell. Res.* **64**, 307.
Banerjee, M. R., and Rogers, F. M. (1970). *J. Endocrinol.* **49**, 39.
Banerjee, M. R., and Walker, R. J. (1967). *J. Cell. Physiol.* **69**, 133.
Banerjee, M. R., Rogers, F. M., and Banerjee, D. N. (1971). *J. Endocrinol.* **50**, 281.
Bargmann, W., and Welsch, U. (1969). *In* "Lactogenesis" (M. Reynolds and S. J. Folley, eds.), p. 43. Univ. of Pennsylvania Press, Philadelphia, Pennsylvania.
Barnabei, O., Ramano, B., and Dibitanto, G. (1965). *Arch. Biochem. Biophys.* **109**, 226.
Barr, G. C., and Butler, J. A. V. (1963). *Nature (London)* **199**, 1170.
Beck, G., Hentzen, D., and Ebel, J. P. (1970a), *Biochim. Biophys, Acta* **213**, 55.
Beck, J. P., Stutinsky, F., Beck, G., Tambiah, R., and Ebel, J. P. (1970b). *Biochem. Biophys. Acta* **213**, 68.
Beitz, D. C., Mohren Weiser, H. W., Thomas, J. W., and Wood, W. A. (1969). *Arch. Biochem. Biophys.* **132**, 210.
Bhaduri, S., Chatterjee, N. K., Bose, K. K., and Gupta, N. K. (1970). *Biochem. Biophys. Res. Commun.* **40**, 402.
Biekunski, N., Giveon, D., and Littauer, U. Z. (1970). *Biochem. Biophys. Acta* **199**, 382.
Blatti, S. P., Ingles, C. J., Lindell, T. J., Morris, P. W., Weaver, R. F., Weinberg, F., and Rutter, W. J. (1970). *Cold Spring Harbor. Symp. Quant. Biol.* **35**, 649.
Blobel, G., and Potter, V. R. (1967). *J. Mol. Biol.* **26**, 279.
Bloemendal, H., Bont, W. S., and Benedetti, E. L. (1964). *Biochim. Biophys. Acta* **87**, 177.
Bonner, J., Dahmus, M. E., Fambrough, D., Huang, R. C., Marushige, K., and Tuan, D. Y. H. (1968). *Science* **159**, 47.
Borst, P., and Grivell, L. A. (1971). *FEBS Lett.* **13**, 73.
Bouin, P., and Ancel, P. (1909a). *C. R. Soc. Biol.* **67**, 466.
Bouin, P., and Ancel, P. (1909b). *C. R. Soc. Biol.* **66**, 689.
Bousquet, M., Fléchon, J., and Denamur, R. (1969). *Z. Zellforsch. Mikrosk. Anat.* **96**, 418.
Bradley, T.R., and Cowie, A.T. (1956). *J. Endocrinol.* **14**, 8.
Brew, K., and Campbell, P. N. (1967). *Biochem. J.* **102**, 265.
Britten, R. J., and Davidson, E. H. (1969). *Science* **165**, 349.
Brookreson, A. D., and Turner, C. W. (1959). *Proc. Soc. Exp. Biol. Rev.* **120**, 744.
Brown, D. D., and Gurdon, J. B. (1964). *Proc. Nat. Acad. Sci. U.S.* **51**, 139.
Brown, J. C., and Smith, A. E. (1970). *Nature (London)* **226**, 610.
Brunngraber, E. F. (1962). *Biochem. Biophys. Res. Commun.* **8**, 1.
Buck, C. A., and Nass, M. M. K. (1968). *Proc. Nat. Acad. Sci. U.S.* **60**, 1045.
Buck, C. A., and Nass, M. M. K. (1969). *J. Mol. Biol.* **41**, 67.
Buck, C. A., and Nass, M. M. K. (1970). *J. Mol. Biol.* **54**, 187.
Burgess, A. B., and Mach, B. (1971). *Nature (London) New Biol.* **223**, 209.
Bustin, M., and Cole, R. D. (1969). *J. Biol. Chem.* **244**, 5286.

Capra, J. D., and Peterkofsky, A. (1968). *J. Mol. Biol.* **33**, 591.

Caskey, C. T., Redfield, B., and Weisbach, H. (1967). *Arch. Biochem. Biophys.* **120**, 119.

Caskey, C. T., Beaudet, A., and Nirembert, M. (1968). *J. Mol. Biol.* **37**, 99.

Chadwick, A. (1962). *Biochem. J.* **85**, 554.

Chambon, R., Gissinger, F., Mandel, J. L., Kedinger, C., Gniazdowski, M., and Meihlac, M. (1970). *Cold Spring Harbor Symp. Quant. Biol.* **35**, 693.

Church, R. B., and McCarthy, B. J. (1970). *Biochim. Biophys. Acta.* **199**, 103.

Cohen, R. M., and Gala, R. R. (1969). *Proc. Soc. Exp. Biol. Med.* **132**, 683.

Cole, R. D., and Hopkins, T. R. (1962a). *Endocrinology* **71**, 395.

Cole, R. D., and Hopkins, T. R. (1962b). *Endocrinology* **70**, 375.

Cowie, A. T. (1949). *J. Endocrinol.* **6**, 145.

Cowie, A. T. (1969). *J. Endocrinol.* **44**, 437.

Craddock, V. M. (1970). *Nature (London)* **228**, 1264.

Crystal, R. G., Shafritz, D. A., Pritchard, P. M., and Anderson, W. F. (1971). *Proc. Nat. Acad. Sci. U.S.* **68**, 1810.

Darby, F. J., Wang, D. Y., and Greenbaum, A. L. (1964). *J. Endocrinol.* **28**, 329.

Darnell, J. E. (1968). *Bacteriol. Rev.* **32**, 262.

Darnell, J. E., Pagoulatos, G. N., Lindberg, U., and Balint, R. (1970). *Cold Spring Harbor Symp. Quant. Biol.* **35**, 555.

Dati, F. A., and Maurer, H. R. (1971). *Biochim. Biophys. Acta* **246**, 589.

Davis, B. D. (1971). *Nature (London)* **231**, 153.

Davis, J. W., and Liu, T. M. Y. (1969). *Endocrinology* **85**, 155.

Denamur, R. (1961). *Ann. Endocrinol.* **22**, 767.

Denamur, R. (1962). *C. R. Acad. Sci.* **255**, 1786.

Denamur, R. (1963a). *C. R. Acad. Sci.* **256**, 4748.

Denamur, R. (1963b). *C. R. Acad. Sci.* **257**, 1548.

Denamur, R. (1965). *Proc. Int. Congr. Endocrinol., 2nd Excerpta Medica.* **83**, 434.

Denamur, R. (1969a). *In* "Lactogenesis" (M. Reynolds and S. J. Folley, eds.), p. 53. Univ. of Pennsylvania Press, Philadelphia, Pennsylvania.

Denamur, R. (1969b). *Ann. Biol. Anim. Biochim. Biophys.* **9**, 287.

Denamur, R. (1969c). *Proc. Int. Congr. Endocrinol., 3rd, Mexico, 1968. Excerpta Med.* **184**, 959.

Denamur, R. (1971). *J. Dairy Res.* **38**, 237.

Denamur, R., and Delouis, C. (1972a). *Acta Endocrinol.* **70**, 603.

Denamur, R., and Delouis, C. (1972b). *C. R. Acad. Sci.* (accepted for publication).

Denamur, R., and Gaye, P. (1967). *Arch. Anat. Microsc. Morphol. Exp.* **56**, 596.

Denamur, R., and Martinet, J. (1961). *Ann. Endocrinol.* **22**, 759.

Denamur, R., and Stoliaroff, M. (1966). *Int. Pharmacolog. Congr., 3rd, Sao Paolo* p. 358.

Denamur, R., Delouis, C., and Gaye, P. (1970). *Arch. Int. Pharmacodyn. Thérap.* **186**, 182.

Denamur, R., Gaye, P., Houdebine, L., Bousquet, M., and Delouis, C. (1972). *Gen. Comp. Endocrinol.* **18**, 534.

Desjardins, C., Paape, M. J., and Tucker, H. A. (1968). *Endocrinology* **83**, 957.

Deutsch, A., and Norgren, A. (1970). *Acta Physiol. Scand.* **80**, 394.

Deutscher, M. P. (1967). *J. Biol. Chem.* **242**, 1123.

Dingman, C. W., Aronow, A., Bunting, S. L., Peacock, A. C., and O'Malley, B. W. (1969). *Biochemistry* **8**, 489.

Donovan, B. T., Van der Werff Ten Bosch (1957). *J. Physiol. London* **137**, 410.

Drews, J., and Brawerman, G. (1967). *J. Biol. Chem.* **242**, 801.

Ebel, J. P. (1971). *Symp. Soc. Chim. Biolog. Transfer Ribonucleic Acids: Structure, Biosynthesis, Function*, Strasbourg, December 9–11.

El Darwish, I., and Rivera, E. M. (1970). *J. Exp. Zool.* **173**, 285.

El Darwish, I., and Rivera, E. M. (1971). *J. Exp. Zool.* **177**, 295.

Elska, A., and Matsuka, G. (1968a). *Ukr. Biokhim. Zh.* **40**, 27.

Elska, A., and Matsuka, G. (1968b). *Ukr. Biokhim. Zh.* **40**, 120.

Elska, A., Matsuka, G., Matiash, U., Nasarenko, I., and Semenova, N. (1971). *Biochim. Biophys. Acta* **247**, 430.

Erdmann, V. A., Fahnestock, S., Higo, K., and Nomura, M. (1971). *Proc. Nat. Acad. Sci. U.S.* **68**, 2932.

Falconer, I. R., and Fiddler, T. J. (1968). *Biochem. J.* **110**, 56P.

Falconer, I. R., and Fiddler, T. J. (1970). *Biochem. Biophys. Acta* **218**, 508.

Fambrough, D. M., and Bonner, J. (1969). *Biochim. Biophys. Acta* **175**, 113.

Ferreri, L. F., and Griffith, D. R. (1969). *Proc. Soc. Exp. Biol. Med.* **130**, 1216.

Fiddler, T. J., and Falconer, I. R. (1969). *Biochem. J.* **115**, 58P.

Fiddler, T. J., Birkinshaw, M., and Falconer, I. R. (1970). *In* "Lactation" (I. R. Falconer, ed.), p. 147. Butterworths, London and Washington, D.C.

Fiddler, T. J., Birkinshaw, M., and Falconer, I. R. (1971). *J. Endocrinol.* **49**, 459.

Fink, L. M., Goto, T., Frankel, F., and Weinstein, I. B. (1968). *Biochem. Biophys. Res. Commun.* **32**, 963.

Flux, D. S. (1954). *J. Endocrinol.* **11**, 223.

Folley, S. J., and Jones, E. A. (1967). *Arch. Anat. Microsc. Morphol. Exp. Supp.* **56**, 584.

Fournier, M. S., and Simpson, M. V. (1968). *In* "Biochemical Aspects of the Biogenesis of Mitochondria" (E. C. Slater, J. M. Tager, S. Papa, and E. Quagheriello, eds.), p. 227. Adriatica Editrice.

Fraser, M. J., and Gutfreund, H. (1958). *Proc. Roy. Soc. London Ser. B* **149**, 392.

Friesen, H. G. (1966). *Endocrinology* **79**, 212.

Fuhr, J. E., London, I. M., and Graysel, A. I. (1969). *Proc. Nat. Acad. Sci. U.S.* **63**, 129.

Galibert, F., Larsen, C. J., Lelong, J. C., and Boiron, M. (1965). *Nature (London)* **207**, 1039.

Gallo, R. C. (1969). *J. Cell. Physiol. suppl. 1* **74**, 149.

Galper, J. B., and Darnell, J. E. (1969). *Biochem. Biophys. Res. Commun.* **34**, 205.

Ganoza, M. C., and Williams, C. A. (1969). *Proc. Nat. Acad. Sci. U.S.* **63**, 1370.

Garel, J. P., Mandel, P., Chavancy, G., and Daulie, J. (1970). *FEBS Lett.* **7**, 327.

Gaye, P., and Denamur, R. (1968). *Bull. Soc. Chim. Biol.* **50**, 1273.

Gaye, P., and Denamur, R. (1969). *Biochim. Biophys. Acta* **186**, 99.

Gaye, P., and Denamur, R. (1970). *Biochem. Biophys. Res. Commun.* **41**, 266.

Gaye, P., Viennot, N., and Denamur, R. (1972). *Biochim. Biophys. Acta* **262**, 371.

Gefter, M. L., and Russell, R. L. (1969). *J. Mol. Biol.* **39**, 145.

Georgiev, G. P. (1967). *Progr. Nucl. Acid Res. Mol. Biol.* **6**, 259.

Gillam, I., Blew, D., Warrington, R. C., Von Tigerstrom, M., and Jener, G. M. (1968). *Biochemistry* **7**, 3459.

Glock, G. E., and McLean, P. (1953). *Biochim. Biophys. Acta* **12**, 590.

Goldman, M., Johnston, W. M., and Griffin, A. C. (1969). *Cancer Res.* **29**, 1051.

Gonano, F., and Pirro, G. (1971a). *Biochem. Biophys. Res. Commun.* **45**, 984.

Gonano, F., and Pirro, G. (1971b). *Cancer Res.* **31**, 656.

Gotoh, S. Higashi, K., Matsuhisa, T., and Sakamoto, Y. (1971). *Biochim. Biophys. Acta* **254**, 265.

Green, M. R., and Topper, Y. J. (1970). *Biochim. Biophys. Acta* **204**, 441.

Green, M. R., Bunting, S. L., and Peacock, A. C. (1971a). *Biochemistry* **10**, 2366.

Green, C. D., Skarda, J., and Barry, J. M. (1971b). *Biochim. Biophys. Acta* **244**, 377.

Greenbaum, A. L., and Slater, T. F. (1957). *Biochem. J.* **66**, 155.

Greenbaum, A. L., Slater, T. F., and Wang, D. Y. (1965). *Biochem. J.* **97**, 518.

Greenman, D. L., Wicks, W. D., and Kenney, F. T. (1965). *J. Biol. Chem.* **240**, 4420.

Grierson, D., Rogers, M. E., Sartirana, M. L., and Loening, U. E. (1970). *Cold. Spring Harbor Symp. Quant. Biol.* **35**, 589.

Gross, P. R. (1968). *In* "Actinomycin" (S. A. Waksman, ed.), p. 87. Wiley (Interscience), New York.

Gul, B., and Dils, R. (1969). *Biochem. J.* **112**, 293.

Gupta, N. K. (1968). *J. Biol. Chem.* **243**, 4959.

Gupta, N. K., Chatterjee, N. K., Bose, K. K., Bhaduri, S., and Chung, A. (1970). *J. Mol. Biol.* **54**, 145.

Hacker, B. (1969). *Biochim. Biophys. Acta* **186**, 214.

Hacker, R. R. (1971). *Diss. Abst. Int. Sect. B* **31**, 4955.

Hackett, A. J., and Tucker, H. A. (1969). *J. Dairy Sci.* **52**, 1268.

Hahn, W. E., Church, R. B., Gorbman, A., and Wilmot, L. (1968). *Gen. Comp. Endocrinol.* **10**, 438.

Hahn, W. E., Schjeide, O. A., and Gorbman, A. (1969). *Proc. Nat. Acad. Sci. U.S.* **62**, 112.

Hartman, P. E., and Jones, E. A. (1970). *Biochem. J.* **116**, 657.

Henshaw, E. C., Bojarski, T. B., and Hiatt, H. H. (1963). *J. Mol. Biol.* **7**, 122.

Herriman, I. D., Baird, G. D., and Bruce, J. M. (1971). *J. Endocrinol.* **49**, 667.

Herrington, M. D., and Hawtrey, A. O. (1969a). *S. Agr. J. Med. Sci.* **34**, 49.

Herrington, M. D., and Hawtrey, A. O. (1969b). *Biochem. J.* **115**, 671.

Herrington, M. D., and Hawtrey, A. O. (1970a). *Biochem. J.* **119**, 323.

Herrington, M. D., and Hawtrey, A. O. (1970b). *Biochem. J.* **116**, 405.

Herrington, M. D., and Hawtrey, A. O. (1971). *Biochem. J.* **121**, 279.

Herzberg, M., Revel, M., and Danon, D. (1969). *Eur. J. Biochem.* **11**, 148.

Heywood, S. M. (1970a). *Proc. Nat. Acad. Sci. U.S.* **67**, 1782.

Heywood, S. M. (1970b). *Nature (London)* **225**, 696.

Hicks, S. J., Drysdale, J. W., and Munro, H. N. (1969). *Science* **164**, 584.

Hilf, R., Michel, I., Silverstein, G., and Bell, C. (1965). *Cancer Res.* **25**, 1854.

Hirsch, C. A. (1966). *Biochim. Biophys. Acta* **123**, 246.

Hoetz, W., and McCarty, K. S. (1971). *Biochim. Biophys. Acta* **228**, 526.

Hohmann, P., and Cole, R. D. (1969). *Nature (London)* **223**, 1064.

Hohmann, P., and Cole, R. D. (1971). *J. Mol. Biol.* **58**, 533.

Holland, J. J., Taylor, M. W., and Buck, A. (1967). *Proc. Nat. Acad. Sci. U.S.* **58**, 2437.

Hollmann, K. H. (1969). *In* "Lactogenesis" (M. Reynolds and S. J. Folley, eds.), p. 27. Univ. of Pennsylvania Press, Philadelphia, Pennsylvania.

Hollmann, K. H., and Verley, J. M. (1970). *In* "Lactation" (I. R. Falconer, ed.), p. 31. Butterworths, London and Washington, D.C.

Houdebine, L., Gaye, P., and Denamur, R. (1972). *Biochimie* (submitted for publication).

Housman, D., Jacobs Lorena, M., Rajbhandary, U. L., and Lodish, H. F. (1970). *Nature (London)* **227**, 913.

Howards, G. A., Adamson, S. D., and Herbert, E. (1970). *J. Biol. Chem.* **245**, 6237.

Howe, A., Richardson, K. C., and Birbeck, M. S. C. (1956). *Exp. Cell. Res.* **10**, 194.

Huang, A., and Baltimore, O. (1970). *J. Mol. Biol.* **47**, 275.

Huang, R. C., and Bonner, J. M. (1962). *Proc. Nat. Acad. Sci. U.S.* **48**, 1216.

Hunter, A. R., and Jackson, R. J. (1971). *Eur. J. Biochem.* **19**, 316.

Huynh-Van-Tan, Delaunay, J., and Schapira, G. (1971). *FEBS Lett.* **17**, 163.

Ilan, J., and Ilan, J. (1971). *Develop. Biol.* **25**, 280.

Itano, H. A. (1966). *J. Cell. Comp. Physiol. Suppl. 1* **27**, 65.

Jackson, R., and Hunter, T. (1970). *Nature (London)* **227**, 672.

Jackson, C. D., Irving C. C., and Sells, B. H. (1970). *Biochim. Biophys. Acta* **217**, 64.

Jacob, S. T., Sajdel, E. M., Muecke, W., and Munro, H. N. (1970). *Cold Spring Harbor Symp. Quant. Biol.* **35**, 681.

Jacobs-Lorena, M., and Baglioni, C. (1970). *Biochim. Biophys. Acta* **224**, 165.

Jacobsohn, D. (1961). *In* "Milk" (S. K. Kon and A. T. Cowie, eds.), Vol. 1, p. 127. Academic Press, New York.

Joklik, W., and Becker, Y. (1965). *J. Mol. Biol.* **13**, 496.

Jones, E. A. (1967). *Biochem. J.* **103**, 420.

Jordan, B. R. (1971). *J. Mol. Biol.* **55**, 423.

Juergens, W. G., Stockdale, F. E., Topper, Y. J., and Elias, J. J. (1965). *Proc. Nat. Acad. Sci. U.S.* **54**, 629.

Kedinger, C., Gniazdowski, M., Mandel, J. L., Gissinger, F., and Chambon, P. (1970). *Biochem. Biophys. Res. Commun.* **38**, 165.

Kelley, F. C., and Pace, N. (1968). *Amer. J. Physiol.* **214**, 1168.

Kennell, D. E. (1970). *Progr. Nucleic Acid Res.* **11**, 259.

Kerr, S. J. (1970). *Biochemistry* **9**, 690.

Kerr, S. J. (1971). *Proc. Nat. Acad. Sci.* **68**, 406.

Kirkham, W. R., and Turner, C. W. (1953). *Proc. Soc. Exp. Biol. Med.* **83**, 123.

Klee, C. B., and Staehelin, M. (1962). *Biochim. Biophys. Acta* **61**, 668.

Knight, E., and Darnell, J. E., Jr. (1967). *J. Mol. Biol.* **28**, 491.

Kohmoto, K., and Bern, H. A. (1970). *J. Endocrinol.* **48**, 99.

Korner, A. (1965). *Recent Progr. Horm. Res.* **21**, 205.

Korner, A. (1969). *In* "Inhibitors Tools in Cell Research" (Th. Bücher, H. Sies, eds.), p. 126. Springer-Verlag, Berlin.

Korsrud, G. O., and Baldwin, R. L. (1969). *Biol. Reprod.* **1**, 21.

Kuhn, N. J. (1968). *Biochem. J.* **106**, 743.

Kuhn, N. J., and Lowenstein, J. M. (1967). *Biochem. J.* **101**, 995.

Kumaresan, P., Anderson, R. R., and Turner, E. W. (1966). *Proc. Soc. Exp. Biol. Med.* **123**, 581.

Kumaresan, P., Anderson, R. R., and Turner, C. W. (1967a). *Endocrinology* **81**, 658.

Kumaresan, P., Anderson, R. R., and Turner, C. W. (1967b). *Proc. Soc. Exp. Biol. Med.* **126**, 41.

Lanks, K. W., and Weinstein, I. B. (1970). *Biochem. Biophys. Res. Commun.* **40**, 710.

Lawford, G. R., Kaiser, J., and Hey, W. C. (1971). *Fed. Proc. Fed. Amer. Soc. Exp. Biol.* **30**, 1311.

Leader, D. P., and Barry, J. M. (1969). *Biochem. J.* **113**, 175.

Lebleu, B., Marbaix, G., Huez, G., Temmerman, J., Burny, A., and Chantrenne, H. (1971). *Eur. J. Biochem.* **19**, 264.

Lengyel, P., and Söll, D. (1969). *Bact. Rev.* **33**, 264.

Lerner, A. M., Bell, E., and Darnell, J. E. (1963). *Science* **141**, 1187.

Lewin, I. (1957). *Proc. Roy. Soc. Med.* **50**, 563.

Liao, S., Leininger, K. R., Sagher, D., and Barton, R. W. (1965). *Endocrinology* **77**, 763.

Libby, P. R., and Dao, T. L. (1966). *Science* **153**, 303.

Liu, T. M. Y., and Davis, J. W. (1967). *Endocrinology* **80**, 1043.

Lockwood, D. H., Turkington, R. W., and Topper, Y. J. (1966). *Biochim. Biophys. Acta* **130**, 493.

Lubsen, N. H., and Davis, B. D. (1972). *Proc. Nat. Acad. Sci. U.S.* **69**, 353.

Lucas-Lenard, J., and Lipmann, F. (1971). *Amer. Rev. Biochem.* **40**, 409.

Lyons, W. R., Li, C. H., and Johnson, R. E. (1958). *Recent Progr. Horm. Res.* **14**, 219.

McGuire, W. L., and O'Malley, B. W. (1968). *Biochim. Biophys. Acta* **157**, 187.

McKenzie, L., Fitzgerald, D. K., and Ebner, K. E. (1971). *Biochim. Biophys. Acta* **230**, 526.

McLean, P. (1958). *Biochim. Biophys. Acta* **30**, 303.

Maenpaa, P. H., and Bernfield, M. R. (1969). *Biochemistry* **8**, 4926.

Maenpaa, P. H., and Bernfield, M. R. (1970). *Proc. Nat. Acad. Sci. U.S.* **67**, 688.

Majumder, G. C., and Ganguli, N. C. (1969a). *Indian J. Biochem.* **6**, 216.

Majumder, G. C., and Ganguli, N. C. (1969b). *Milchwissenschaft* **24**, 149.

Majumder, G. C., and Turkington, R. W. (1971a). *J. Biol. Chem.* **246**, 2650.

Majumder, G. C., and Turkington, R. W. (1971b). *J. Biol. Chem.* **246**, 5545.

Malpress, F. H. (1961). *Biochem. J.* **78**, 527.

Mandell, J. D., and Hershey, A. D. (1960). *Anal. Biochem.* **1**, 66.

Martin, R. J., and Baldwin, R. L. (1971). *Endocrinology* **88**, 863.

Marzluff, W. F., and McCarty, K. S. (1970). *J. Biol. Chem.* **245**, 5635.

Marzluff, W. F., McCarty, K. S., and Turkington, R. W. (1969). *Biochim. Biophys. Acta.* **190**, 517.

Matthies, D. (1967). *Anat. Rec.* **159**, 55.

Matthies, D. (1968). *Proc. Soc. Exp. Biol. Med.* **127**, 1126.

Mayer, G., and Klein, H. (1961). *In* "Milk" (S. K. Kon and A. T. Cowie, eds.), Vol. 1, p. 47. Academic Press, New York.

Mayne, R., and Barry, J. M. (1967). *Biochim. Biophys. Acta* **138**, 195.

Mayne, R., and Barry, J. M. (1970). *J. Endocrinol.* **46**, 61.

Mayne, R., Barry, J. M., and Rivera, E. M. (1966). *Biochem J.* **99**, 688.

Mayne, R., Forsyth, I. A., and Barry, J. M. (1968). *J. Endocrinol.* **41**, 247.

Meites, J., Hopkins, T. F., and Talwalker, P. K. (1963). *Endocrinology* **73**, 261.

Mills, E. S., and Topper, Y. J. (1969). *Science* **165**, 1127.

Mills, E. S., and Topper, Y. J. (1970). *J. Cell. Biol.* **44**, 310.

Mittelman, A. (1971). *Cancer Res.* **31**, 647.

Mizuno, H. (1961). *Endocrinol. Japan* **8**, 27.

Montagnier, L., and Bellamy, A. D. (1964). *Biochim. Biophys. Acta* **80**, 157.

Moon, R. C. (1969). *Proc. Soc. Exp. Biol. Med.* **130**, 1126.

Mueller, G. C. (1965). *In* "Mechanisms of Hormone Action" (P. Karlson, ed.), p. 228. Thieme Stuttgart.

Munford, R. E. (1963). *J. Endocrinol.* **28**, 17.

Munford, R. E. (1964). *Dairy Sci. Abstr.* **26**, 293.

Munro, A. J. (1964). *Biochem. J.* **91**, 22.

Mushinki, J. F., and Potter, M. P. (1969). *Biochemistry* **8**, 1684.

Nagasawa, H. (1963). *Jap. J. Zootech. Sci.* **34**, 181.

Nandi, S. (1959). *Univ. Calif. Publ. Zool.* **65**, 1.

Naora, H., and Pritchard, M. S. (1971). *Biochim. Biophys. Acta* **246**, 269.

Naora, H., Kodaira, K., and Pritchard, M. J. (1971). *Biochim. Biophys. Acta* **246**, 280.

Nelson, W. L., Heytler, P. G., and Ciaccio, E. I. (1962). *Proc. Soc. Exp. Biol. Med.* **109**, 373.

Nishimura, S., and Wettstein, I. B. (1969). *Biochemistry* **8**, 832.

Noll, H., Staehelin, T., and Wettstein, F. O. (1963). *Nature (London)* **198**, 632.

Norgren, A. (1967a). *Acta Univ. Lund. Sect. 2* **5**.

Norgren, A. (1967b). *Acta Univ. Lund. Sect. 2* **11**.

Norgren, A. (1967c). *Acta Univ. Lund. Sect. 2* **21**.

Norgren, A. (1967d). *Acta Univ. Lund. Sect. 2* **32**.

Norgren, A. (1967e). *Acta Univ. Lund. Sect. 2* **33**.

Novelli, G. D. (1969). *J. Cell. Physiol. Suppl. 1*, **74**, 121.

O'Malley, B. W., and McGuire, W. L. (1968). *Proc. Nat. Acad. Sci. U.S.* **60**, 1527.

O'Malley, B. W., and McGuire, W. L. (1969). *Endocrinology* **84**, 63.

O'Malley, B. W., Aronow, A., Peacock, A. C., and Dingman, C. W. (1968a). *Science* **162**, 567.

O'Malley, B. W., McGuire, W. L., and Middleton, P. (1968b). *Nature (London)* **218**, 1251.

O'Malley, B. W., McGuire, W. L., Kohler, P. O., and Korenman, S. G. (1969). *Recent Progr. Horm. Res.* **25**, 105.

Ota, K., and Yokoyama, A. (1965). *J. Endocrinol.* **33**, 185.

Ota, K., Yokoyama, A., and Shinde, Y. (1962). *Nature (London)* **1954**, 77.

Paape, M. J., and Sinha, Y. N. (1971). *J. Dairy Sci.* **54**, 1068.

Paape, M. J., and Tucker, H. A. (1969a). *J. Dairy Sci.* **52**, 380.

Paape, M. J., and Tucker, H. A. (1969b). *J. Dairy Sci.* **52**, 518.

Palmiter, R. D. (1969a). *Biochem. J.* **113**, 409.

Palmiter, R. D. (1969b). *Endocrinology* **85**, 747.

Panyim, S., and Chalkley, R. (1969). *Biochemistry* **8**, 3972.

Pegg, A. E., and Korner, A. (1965). *Nature (London)* **205**, 904.

Penman, S., Fan, H., Perlman, S., Rosbash, M., Weinberg, R., and Zylber, E. (1970). *Cold Spring Harbor Symp. Quant. Biol.* **35**, 561.

Perry, R. E. (1967). *Progr. Nucl. Acid Res. Mol. Biol.* **6**, 219.

Perry, R. P., Greenberg, J. R., and Tartof, K. D. (1970). *Cold Spring Harbor Symp. Quant. Biol.* **35**, 577.

Peterkofsky, A., Jesensky, C., and Capra, J. D. (1966). *Cold Spring Harbor Symp. Quant. Biol.* **31**, 515.

Petre, J., (1970). *Eur. J. Biochem.* **14**, 399.

Petrissant, G. (1968). *Bull. Soc. Chim. Biol.* **50**, 47.

Petrissant, G. (1969). *Bull. Soc. Chim. Biol.* **51**, 669.

Petrissant, G. (1970). *Ann. Biol. Anim. Biochim. Biophys.* **10**, 165.

Petrissant, G. (1971). *Biochimie* **53**, 523.

Petrissant, G., and Gaye, P. (1966). *Ann. Biol. Anim. Biochim. Biophys.* **6**, 333.

Petrissant, G., Boisnard, M., and Puissant, C. (1971). *Biochimie* **53**, 1105.

Philipps, G. R. (1969). *Nature (London)* **223**, 374.

Pragnell, I. B., and Arnstein, H. R. V. (1970). *FEBS Lett.* **9**, 331.

Pragnell, I. B., Marbaix, G., Arnstein, H. R. V., and Lebleu, B. (1971). *FEBS Lett.* **14**, 289.

462   R. *Denamur*

Pritchard, D. E., and Tucker, H. A. (1970). *Proc. Soc. Exp. Biol. Med.* **133**, 1318.
Pritchard, P. M., Gilbert, J. M., Shafritz, D. A., and Anderson, W. F. (1970). *Nature* (*London*) **226**, 511.
Pritchard, P. M., Picciano, D. J., Laycock, D. G., and Anderson, W. F. (1971). *Proc. Nat. Acad. Sci.* **68**, 2752.
Rajbhandary, U. L., and Ghosh, H. P. (1969). *J. Biol. Chem.* **244**, 1104.
Ray, E. W., Averill, S. C., Lyons, W. R., and Johnson, R. E. (1955). *Endocrinology* **56**, 359.
Raynaud, A. (1970). *In* "Lactation" (I. R. Falconer, ed.), p. 3. Butterworths, London and Washington, D.C.
Redman, C. M. (1968). *Biochem. Biophys. Res. Commun.* **31**, 845.
Redman, C. M. (1969). *J. Biol. Chem.* **244**, 4308.
Reich, E., Franklin, R. M., Shatkin, A. J., and Tatum, E. L., (1962). *Proc. Nat. Acad. Sci. U.S.* **48**, 1238.
Reich, E., Acs, G., Mach, B., and Tatum, E. L. (1963). *In* "Informational Macro-molécules" (H. J. Vogel, V. Bryson, and J. O. Lampen, eds.), p. 317. Academic Press, New York.
Revel, M., Brawerman, G., Lelong, J. C., and Gros, F. (1968). *Nature* (*London*) **219**, 1016.
Ricordeau, G., and Denamur, R. (1962). *Ann. Zootech.* **11**, 5.
Rivera, E. M., and Cummins, E. P. (1972). *J. Endocrinol* **52**, 205.
Robison, B., and Zimmerman, T. P. (1970). *Anal. Biochem.* **37**, 11.
Roeder, R. G., and Rutter, W. J. (1970). *Proc. Nat. Acad. Sci. U.S.* **65**, 675.
Rosset, R., Monier, R., and Julien, J. (1964). *Bull. Soc. Chim. Biol.* **46**, 87.
Sabatini, D. D., and Blobel, G. (1970). *J. Cell. Biol.* **45**, 146.
Sarin, P. C., and Zamecnik, P. C. (1964). *Biochim. Biophys. Acta* **91**, 653.
Scherrer, K., Spohr, G., Granboulan, N., Morel, C., Grosclaude, J., and Chezzi, C. (1970). *Cold Spring Harbor Quant. Biol.* p. 539.
Schreiber, G. (1971). *Angew. Chem. Int. Ed.* **10**, 638.
Semonova, N. O., Elska, A. V., and Matsuka, G. Kh. (1969). *Ukr. Biokhim. Zh.* **41**, 326.
Sethi, V. S. (1971), *Progr. Biophys. Mol. Biol.* **23**, 67.
Shafritz, D. A., and Anderson, W. F. (1970a). *Nature* (*London*) **227**, 918.
Shafritz, D. A., and Anderson, W. F. (1970b). *J. Biol. Chem.* **245**, 5553.
Shafritz, D. A., Pritchard, P. M., Gilbert, J. M., and Anderson, W. F. (1970). *Biochem. Biophys. Res. Commun.* **38**, 721.
Shafritz, D. A., Laycock, D. G., and Anderson, W. F. (1971a). *Proc. Nat. Acad. Sci. U.S.* **68**, 496.
Shafritz, D. A., Laycock, D. G., Crystal, R. G., and Anderson, W. F. (1971b). *Proc. Nat. Acad. Sci. U.S.* **68**, 2246.
Shani, J., Zanbelman, L., Khazen, K., and Sulman, F. G. (1970). *J. Endocrinol.* **46**, 15.
Sharma, O. K., and Borek, E. (1970). *Biochemistry* **9**, 2507.
Sharma, O. K., Kerr, S. J., Lipshitz-Wiesner, R., and Borek, E. (1971). *Fed. Proc. Fed. Amer. Soc. Exp. Biol* **30**, 167.
Shatton, J. B., Gruenstein, M., Shay, H., and Weinhouse, S. (1965). *J. Biol. Chem.* **240**, 22.
Shimizu, H. (1957). *Tohoku J. Agr. Res.* **7**, 339.
Shinde, Y., Ota, K., and Yokoyama, A. (1962). *J. Endocrinol.* **25**, 279.

Shinde, Y., Ota, K., and Yokoyama, A. (1965). *J. Endocrinol* **31**, 105.
Shugart, L., Chastain, B. H., Novelli, G. D., and Stulberg, M. P. (1968a). *Biochem. Biophys. Res. Commun.* **31**, 404.
Shugart, L., Novelli, G. D., and Stulberg, M. P. (1968b). *Biochim. Biophys. Acta* **157**, 83.
Simpson, A. A., and Schmidt, G. H. (1969). *Proc. Soc. Exp. Biol. Med.* **132**, 978.
Simpson, A. A., and Schmidt, G. H. (1971). *J. Endocrinol* **51**, 265.
Sinha, K. N., Anderson, R. R., and Turner, C. W. (1971). *Biol. Reprod.* **2**, 185.
Sinha, Y. N., and Schmidt, G. H. (1969). *Proc. Soc. Exp. Biol. Med.* **130**, 867.
Sinha, Y. N., and Schmidt, G. H. (1970). *J. Dairy Sci.* **53**, 1077.
Sinha, Y. N., and Tucker, H. A. (1966). *Amer. J. Physiol.* **210**, 601.
Sinha, Y. N., and Tucker, H. A. (1969a). *Proc. Soc. Exp. Biol. Med.* **131**, 908.
Sinha, Y. N., and Tucker, H. A. (1969b). *J. Dairy Sci.* **52**, 507.
Sirakov, L., and Rychlik, I. (1968). *Collect. Czech. Chem. Commun.* **33**, 637.
Sirakov, L., and Richlik, I. (1969). *Ann. Endocrinol.* **30**, 365.
Sirakov, L., Richlik, I., and Sorm, F. (1968). *Collect. Czech. Chem. Commun.* **33**, 951.
Slater, T. F. (1961). *Biochem. J.* **78**, 500.
Slater, T. F. (1962). *Arch. Int. Physiol. Biochem.* **70**, 167.
Slater, T. F., and Planterose, D. N. (1958). *Biochem. J.* **69**, 417.
Slater, T. F., Greenbaum, A. L., and Wang, D. Y. (1963). *Ciba Found. Symp. Lysosomes*, p. 311.
Smith, V. G., and Convey, E. M. (1971). *Proc. Soc. Exp. Biol. Med.* **136**, 588.
Smith, W. C., and McNamara, A. L. (1971). *Science* **171**, 577.
Smith, A. E., and Marcker, K. A. (1968). *J. Mol. Biol.* **38**, 241.
Smith, A. E., and Marcker, K. A. (1970). *Nature (London)* **226**, 607.
Smuckler, E. A., and Tata, J. R. (1971). *Nature (London)* **234**, 37.
Sod-Moriah, U. A., and Schmidt, G. H. (1968). *Exp. Cell. Res.* **49**, 584.
Söll, D. (1971). *Science* **173**, 293.
Spirin, A. S. (1969). *Eur. J. Biochem.* **10**, 20.
Staehelin, M. (1971). *Experentia* **27**, 1.
Staehelin, M., Rogg, H., Baguley, B. L., Ginsberg, T., and Wehrli, H. (1968). *Nature (London)* **219**, 1364.
Staehelin, T., Wettstein, F. O., Oura, M., and Noll, H. (1964). *Nature (London)* **201**, 264.
Stedman, E., and Stedman, E. (1950). *Nature (London)* **166**, 780.
Stein, H., and Hansen, P. (1970). *Cold Spring Harbor Symp. Quant. Biol.* **35**, 709.
Stellwagen, R. H., and Cole, R. D. (1968). *J. Biol. Chem.* **243**, 4456.
Stellwagen, R. H., and Cole, R. D. (1969). *J. Biol. Chem.* **244**, 4878.
Stent, G. S. (1964). *Science* **144**, 816.
Stern, R., Gonano, F., Fleissner, E., and Littauer, U. Z. (1970). *Biochemistry* **9**, 10.
Stockdale, F. E., Juergens, W. G., and Topper, Y. J. (1966). *Develop. Biol.* **13**, 266.
Sueoka, N., and Kano-Sueoka, T. (1970). *Progr. Nucl. Acid Res. Mol. Biol.*, pp. 10–23.
Takagi, M., and Ogata, K. (1968). *Biochem. Biophys. Res. Commun.* **33**, 55.
Takagi, M., Tanaka, J., and Ogata, K. (1969). *J. Biochem.* **65**, 651.
Takeishi, K., Ukita, T., and Nishimura, S. (1968). *J. Biol. Chem.* **243**, 5761.
Talwalker, P. K., Nicoll, C. S., and Meites, J. (1961). *Endocrinology* **69**, 802.
Tata, J. R. (1966). *Progr. Nucl. Acid Res. Mol. Biol.*, pp. 5–191.

Tata, J. R. (1970). *In* "Biochemical Action of Hormones" (G. Litwack, ed.), pp. 1–89. Academic Press, New York.

Taylor, N. W. (1969). *Cancer Res.* **29**, 1681.

Taylor, N. W. (1970). *Cancer Res.* **30**, 2463.

Taylor, N. W., Granger, G. A., Buck, C. A., and Holland, J. J. (1967). *Proc. Nat. Acad Sci. U.S.* **57**, 1712.

Taylor, N. W., Buck, C. A., Granger, G. A., and Holland, J. J. (1968). *J. Mol. Biol.* **33**, 809.

Tepperman, J., and Tepperman, H. M. (1960). *Pharmacol. Rev.* **12**, 301.

Thatcher, W. W., and Tucker, H. A. (1968). *Proc. Soc. Exp. Biol. Med.* **128**, 46.

Thatcher, W. W., and Tucker, H. A. (1970a). *Endocrinology* **86**, 237.

Thatcher, W. W., and Tucker, H. A. (1970b). *Proc. Soc. Exp. Biol. Med.* **134**, 705

Thibodeau, P. S., and Thayer, S. A. (1967). *Endocrinology* **80**, 505.

Tomkins, G. M., Gelehrter, T. D., Granner, D., Martin, D., Samuels H. H., and Thompson, E. B. (1969). *Science* **166**, 1474.

Tonoue, T., Eaton, J., and Frieden, E. (1969). *Biochem. Biophys. Res. Commun.* **37**, 81.

Topper, Y. J. (1968). *Trans. N.Y. Acad. Sci.* **30**, 869.

Topper, Y. J. (1970). *Recent Progr. Horm. Res.* **26**, 287.

Trakatellis, A. C., Montjar, M., and Axelrod, A. E. (1965). *Biochemistry* **4**, 1678.

Traurig, H. H. (1967). *Anat. Record* **157**, 489.

Tsanev, R. G., Markov, G. G., and Desser, G. N. (1966). *Biochem. J.* **100**, 204.

Tucker, H. A. (1964a). *Proc. Soc. Exp. Biol. Med.* **116**, 218.

Tucker, H. A. (1964b). *Proc. Soc. Exp. Biol. Med.* **112**, 1002.

Tucker, H. A. (1966). *Amer. J. Physiol.* **110**, 1209.

Tucker, H. A., Paape, M. J., and Sinha, Y. N. (1967a). *Amer. J. Physiol.* **213**, 262.

Tucker, H. A., Paape, M. J., Sinha, Y. N., Pritchard, D. E., and Thatcher, W. W. (1967b). *Proc. Soc. Exp. Biol. Med.* **126**, 100.

Tucker, H. A., and Reece, R. P. (1963a). *Proc. Soc. Exp. Biol. Med.* **112**, 370.

Tucker, H. A., and Reece, R. P. (1963b). *Proc. Soc. Exp. Biol. Med.* **112**, 409.

Tucker, H. A., and Reece, R. P. (1963c). *Proc. Soc. Exp. Biol. Med.* **112**, 688.

Tucker, H. A., and Reece, R. P. (1963d). *Proc. Soc. Exp. Biol. Med.* **112**, 1002.

Tucker, H. A., and Reece, R. P. (1963e). *Proc. Soc. Exp. Biol. Med.* **113**, 717.

Tucker, H. A., and Reece, R. P. (1964a). *Proc. Soc. Exp. Biol. Med.* **115**, 885.

Tucker, H. A., and Reece, R. P. (1964b). *Proc. Soc. Exp. Biol. Med.* **115**, 887.

Tucker, H. A., and Thatcher, W. W. (1968). *Proc. Soc. Exp. Biol Med.* **129**, 578.

Turkington, R. W. (1968). *Endocrinology* **82**, 575.

Turkington, R. W. (1969). *J. Biol. Chem.* **244**, 5140.

Turkington, R. W. (1970a). *J. Biol. Chem.* **245**, 6690.

Turkington, R. W. (1970b). *Biochim. Biophys. Acta* **213**, 484.

Turkington, R. W. (1970c). *Biochem. Biophys. Res. Commun.* **41**, 1362.

Turkington, R. W. (1971). *Cancer Res.* **31**, 644.

Turkington, R. W., Brew, K., Vanaman, T. C., and Hill, R. L. (1968). *J. Biol. Chem.* **243**, 3382.

Turkington, R. W., and Hill, R. L. (1969). *Science* **163**, 1458.

Turkington, R. W., and Riddle, M. (1969). *J. Biol. Chem.* **244**, 6040.

Turkington, R. W., and Riddle, M. (1970a). *J. Biol. Chem.* **245**, 5145.

Turkington, R. W., and Riddle, M. (1970b). *Cancer Res.* **30**, 650. ·

Turkington, R. W., and Self, D. J. (1970). *Cancer Res.* **30**, 1833.

Turkington, R. W., and Ward, O. T. (1969). *Biochim. Biophys. Acta* **174**, 291.

Turkington, R. W., Majumder, G. C., and Riddle, M. (1971). *J. Biol. Chem.* **246**, 1814.

Waksman, S. A. (1968). In "Actinomycin" (S. A. Waksman, ed.), p. 1. Wiley (Interscience), New York.

Walker, P. M. B. (1969). *Progr. Nucl. Acid Res. Mol. Biol.*, pp. 9–301.

Wallace, J. M. (1961). *Biochem. Biophys. Res. Commun.* **5**, 125.

Wang, D. Y., and Amor, V. (1971). *J. Endocrinol.* **50**, 241.

Wang, D. Y., Slater, T. F., and Greenbaum, A. C. (1960). *Nature (London)* **188**, 320.

Wang, D. Y., Amor, V., and Bulbrook, R. D. (1970). *J. Endocrinol.* **46**, 549.

Wang, D. Y., and Greenbaum, A. L. (1962). *Biochem. J.* **83**, 626.

Warner, J. R. (1971). *J. Biol. Chem.* **246**, 447.

Weinstein, I. B. (1968). *Cancer Res.* **28**, 1871.

Wellings, S. R. (1969). In "Lactogenesis" (M. Reynolds and S. J. Folley, eds.), p. 5. Univ. of Pennsylvania Press, Philadelphia, Pennsylvania.

Wellings, S. R., and de Ome, K. B. (1963). *J. Nat. Cancer Inst.* **30**, 241.

Wettstein, F. O., Staehelin, T., and Noll, H. (1963). *Nature (London)* **197**, 430.

Wickman, J., and Davis, S. W. (1968). *Fed. Proc. Fed. Amer. Soc. Exp. Biol.* **27**, 394.

Wicks, W. D., Greenman, D. L., and Kenney, F. T. (1965). *J. Biol. Chem.* **240**, 4414.

Widnell, L. L., and Tata, J. R. (1966). *Biochim. Biophys. Acta* **123**, 478.

Williams-Ashman, H. G., Liao, S., Hancock, R. L., Jurkovitz, L., and Silverman, D. A. (1964). *Recent Progr. Horm. Res.* **20**, 247.

Willmer, J. S. (1960). *Can. J. Biochem.* **38**, 1265.

Willmer, J. S., and Foster, T. S. (1965). *Can. J. Physiol. Pharmacol.* **43**, 905.

Wilson, D. B., and Dintzis, H. M. (1970). *Proc. Nat. Acad. Sci. U.S.* **66**, 1282.

Woessner, J. F. (1969). In "Lysosomes in Biology and Pathology" (J. T. Dingle and H. B. Fell, eds.), Chapter 11, p. 299.

Wool, I. G., Stirewalt, W. S., Kurihara, K., Low, R. B., Barley, P., and Oyer, D. (1968). *Recent Progr. Horm. Res.* **24**, 139.

Wrenn, T. R., Bitman, J., De Lauder, W. R., and Mench, M. L. (1966). *J. Dairy Sci.* **49**, 183.

Yanai, R., and Nagasawa, H. (1971). *J. Dairy Sci.* **54**, 906.

Yang, W. K., and Novelli, G. D. (1968a). *Proc. Nat. Acad. Sci. U.S.* **59**, 208.

Yang, W. K., and Novelli, G. D. (1968b). *Biochem. Biophys. Res. Commun.* **31**, 534.

Yang, S. S., and Sanadi, D. R. (1969). *J. Biol. Chem.* **244**, 5081.

Yousef, I. M., Emery, R. S., Askew, E. W., Benson, J., Thomas, J. W., and Huber, J. T. (1969). *J. Dairy Sci.* **52**, 1577.

Zachau, H. G. (1969). *Angew. Chem. Int. Ed.* **8**, 711.

Zimmerman, E. F., Heeter, M., and Darnell, J. E. (1963). *Virology* **19**, 400.

Author Index

Numbers in *italics* refer to the pages on which the complete references are listed.

A

Abad, A., 248, *273*
Abdallah, M., 314, *321*
Abdel Razek, S., 314, *321*
Abdou, I., 314, *322*
Abolins, J. A., 173, *220*
Abraham, S., 188, *220*, *224*, 334, *346*, 352, 354, 365, 385, *407*, *410*
Acs, G., 440, *462*
Adams, T. C., 288, 307, *321*
Adams, W. M., 288, *318*
Adamson, S. D., 442, *459*
Admiraal, J., 377, *408*
Ahmad, N., 300, *323*, 333, *347*
Ahren, K., 122, 127, 129, *135*
Akikusa, Y., 279, *321*
Aksamit, R. R., 368, *407*
Albert, T. F., 305, *318*
Albert-Recht, F., 288, *325*
Alcaraz, M., 233, 254, *269*
Allen, E., 118, 121, 122, *135*, *136*
Allen, M. S., 123, *138*
Allfrey, V. G., 436, *454*
Alloiteau, J. J., 262, *268*
Aloni, Y., 432, *454*
Amenomori, Y., 249, 250, 258, 259, *268*, *269*, 279, 285, 301, *318*, 332, *346*
Ames, B. N., 451, *454*
Ammar, R., 314, *322*
Amor, V., 418, 423, 424, 433, *465*
Anand, B. K., 250, *268*
Anastassiadis, P. A., 290, *324*
Ancel, P., 107, *135*, 416, *454*, *455*
Andersen, V., 378, *408*
Anderson, D. M., 196, *220*
Anderson, L. L., 109, *137*, 291, *321*
Anderson, M. S., 302, *326*
Anderson, R. R., 111, 114, 115, 117, 119, 120, 124, 125, 128, 129, 130, 134, *135*, *137*, *138*, *139*, 244, 262, 273, 287, 288, 298, 305, 310, *318*, *322*, 417, 419, 421, 425, 426, 429, *454*, *459*, *463*
Anderson, R. S., 190, *220*

Anderson, W. F., 441, 451, 453, *454*, *456*, *462*
Andersson, B., 233, *268*
Anguiano, G., 234, *274*
Annison, E. F., 144, 149, 151, 153, 170, 173, 178, 179, 183, 185, 186, 189, 191, 195, 196, 203, 205, 207, 208, 209, 210, 211, 212, 213, 214, 215, 216, 217, *220*, *223*, *225*, 386, 387, *407*, *411*
Anstall, H. B., 371, *410*
Antunes-Rodriguez, J., 246, 254, 258, *272*
Arai, Y., 285, *318*
Archer, F. L., 81, *91*
Arimura, A., 246, 258, *268*
Armstrong, D. T., 240, *269*, 282, *322*
Arndt, J. O., 172, *220*
Arnold, P. T. D., 155, 199, *220*
Arnstein, H. R. V., 441, *461*
Aronow, A., 450, *456*, *461*
Arvill, A., 127, *135*
Askew, E. W., 354, 387, *407*, 427, *465*
Astwood, E. B., 291, 310, *318*, *320*
Attardi, B., 432, *454*
Attardi, G., 432, *454*
Attramadal, A., 123, *139*
Atwood, B. L., 128, *137*
Aukland, K., 169, *220*
Aulsebrook, L. H., 239, *268*
Averill, R. L. W., 232, 248, 251, 254, *268*
Averill, S. C., 118, 128, *135*, *138*, 284, *324*, 417, *462*
Axel, R., 87, *94*, 451, *454*
Axelrod, A. E., 433, *464*
Axelrod, J., 315, *325*

B

Baba, N., 65, *93*
Baddeley, R. M., 233, 254, *270*
Bässler, R., 4, 33, 35, 69, 79, *91*, *94*
Baglioni, C., 442, *459*
Baguley, B. L., 453, *463*

Baird, G. D., 439, 442, 445, 446, *454*, *458*
Baker, B. L., 102, 127, *137*
Baker, D. W., 171, *225*
Baker, F. D., 107, *135*
Baker, R. D., 290, *324*
Baksi, S. N., 310, *318*
Baldwin, B. A., 148, *220*
Baldwin, R. L., 111, 117, 120, *135*, 298, 312, *318*, *323*, 419, 425, 426, 431, 433, 436, 440, 444, 446, *454*, *455*, *459*, *460*
Baldwin, R. L., 352, 353, 354, 360, 362, 363, 364, 365, 367, 368, 369, 370, 371, 372, 373, 374, 375, 376, 379, 380, 381, 382, 383, 384, 386, 390, 391, 382, 393, 395, 396, 398, 399, 400, 401, 402, 403, 404, 405, *407*, *409*, *410*
Baliga, B. S., 451, *455*
Balinsky, B. I., 98, *135*
Balint, R., 432, *456*
Ballantyne, B., 229, *268*
Ballard, F. J., 388, *407*
Baltimore, O., 441, *459*
Ban, T., 234, *268*
Banerjee, D. N., 342, *346*, 418, 427, 444, *455*
Banerjee, M. R., 342, *346*, 416, 418, 427, 444, *455*
Barcroft, J., 190, 194, *220*
Bárdos, V., 250, *271*
Bargmann, W., 4, 33, 37, 39, 43, 51, 61, 64, 65, 77, 79, *91*, 444, *455*
Barker, K. L., 400, *407*
Barley, P., 441, *465*
Barman, T. E., 359, 368, 375, 379, 383, *407*
Barnabei, O., 436, *455*
Barone, R., 155, 203, *220*
Barr, G. C., 436, *455*
Barraclough, C. A., 109, 126, *135*, *136*, 291, *320*
Barrett, M. A., 188, *221*
Barry, J. M., 151, 205, 209, 211, 213, 214, *220*, 329, 340, *347*, 398, 400, *407*, *408*, 422, 423, 424, 433, 434, 449, *458*, *459*, *460*
Barsantini, J. C., 313, *318*
Bartley, J. C., 334, *346*, 352, 354, *407*
Bartley, W., 213, 214, *220*

Barto, P. B., 300, *319*
Barton, R. W., 436, *460*
Bartoszewicz, W., 69, *91*
Baryshnikov, I. A., 231, 237, *268*
Bassett, J. M., 278, 285, 288, *318*
Bateman, V., 252, *268*
Bauer, A., 84, 85, *91*
Bauman, D. E., 352, 353, 354, 380, 383, 388, 390, 393, 394, *407*, *409*
Bauman, T. R., 309, *318*
Beard, R. W., 288, *320*
Beatty, J. F., 314, *324*
Beaudet, A., 453, *456*
Beck, G., 451, *455*
Beck, J. P., *455*
Beck, N., 118, *138*, 284, *323*
Becker, R. B., 153, 155, 199, *220*
Becker, Y., 441, *459*
Beisenherz, G., 375, *407*
Beitz, D. C., 447, *455*
Bell, C., 434, *458*
Bell, E., 440, *459*
Bell, F. R., 148, *220*
Bell, J. W., 194, *221*
Bell, P. H., 128, *136*
Bellamy, A. D., 440, *460*
Beller, T. K., 240, *268*
Ben-David, M., 287, 308, 314, *318*
Benedetti, E. L., 69, *91*, 442, *455*
Benevenga, N. J., 372, *407*
Benson, G. K., 124, *135*, 245, 255, *268*, *270*
Benson, J. D., 306, *320*, 387, *407*, 427, *465*
Benveniste, R., 287, *318*
Berg, P., 378, *407*
Bergman, A. J., 259, *274*
Bergman, E. N., 305, *318*
Berkow, S. G., 174, *220*
Berliner, R. W., 169, *220*
Bern, H. A., 85, *94*, 100, 101, 105, 128, 129, 131, 132, 133, *135*, *137*, *138*, *139*, 156, *225*, 246, *268*, 281, 282, 285, *323*, 417, *459*
Bernal, M., 230, *269*
Bernard, C., 191, *221*
Bernfield, M. R., 451, *460*
Bernhard, W., 41, 84, 85, *91*, 92

Beyer, C., 232, 233, 234, 235, 240, 244, 250, 251, 254, 255, 256, *268*, *269*, *274*
Bhaduri, S., 453, *455*, *458*
Bhatnagar, S., 314, *322*
Bialy, G., 314, *324*
Bickerstaffe, R., 144, 183, 185, 186, 189, 205, 207, 211, 212, 214, 216, 217, *220*, *223*, *225*, 386, 387, *407*, *411*
Biekunski, N., 451, *455*
Bintarningsih, 298, *318*
Birbeck, M. S. C., 439, *459*
Birk, S. A., 304, *325*
Birkinshaw, M., 4, 92, 420, *457*
Bishop, W., 315, *320*
Bisset, G. W., 232, 239, 240, 253, *269*, 305, *318*
Bitman, J., 102, 118, 119, *140*, 417, *465*
Bittner, J. J., 81, *91*
Black, A. L., 209, *220*
Blackwood, J. H., 147, 148, 192, 193, *220*
Blaha, G. C., 291, *322*
Blanchette, -Mackie, E. J., 214, *220*
Bland, K. P., 244, *269*
Blatherwick, N. H., 147, *223*
Blatti, S. P., 435, *455*
Blaxter, K. L., 244, *269*, 308, 309, *318*
Blecher, M., 330, *347*
Blew, D., 453, *457*
Blobel, G., 439, 442, 447, *455*, *462*
Bloemendal, H., 442, *455*
Bloor, C. M., 165, *224*
Bogdanove, E. M., 249, *269*
Bogden, A. E., 85, *91*
Boiron, M., 440, *457*
Boisnard, M., 453, *461*
Boivin, A., 101, *135*
Bojarski, T. B., 439, *458*
Bone, J. F., 194, *221*
Bonner, J., 436, 437, *455*, *457*, *459*
Bont, W. S., 442, *455*
Booker, D. E., 314, *318*
Boot, L. M., 262, *276*
Borek, E., 450, 451, *455*, *462*
Borglin, N. E., 314, *318*
Borst, P., 439, *455*
Borsuk, V. N., 231, *268*
Bose, K. K., 453, *455*, *458*
Bouckaert, J. H., 231, *274*

Bouin, P., 107, *135*, 416, *454*, *455*
Bousquet, M., 4, *91*, 416, 418, 431, 443, *455*, *456*
Bower, B. F., 169, *220*
Bowman, R. E., 288, *326*
Boycott, A. E., 194, *220*
Boyd, J. W., 381, *407*
Boyd, L. J., 314, *318*
Boyd, W. L., 191, *225*
Bradbury, J. T., 108, *135*, 243, *269*
Bradley, T. R., 431, *455*
Braun, R. K., 305, *318*
Brawerman, G., 438, 441, *457*, *462*
Brennan, M. J., 87, *93*
Bresciani, F., 124, *138*
Brethfeld, V., *91*
Breuer, C. B., 128, *136*
Brew, K., 328, 334, 338, 342, *346*, *348*, 434, 435, 446, *455*, *464*
Brewley, T. A., 282, *318*
Briley, M. S., 292, *322*
Britten, R. J., 432, *455*
Brodbeck, U., 334, *346*
Brody, S., 317, *324*
Bronson, F. H., 262, *269*, 332, *347*
Brookreson, A. D., 111, 115, 116, 120, 124, 125, *135*, 418, *455*
Brooks, C., Mc. C., 232, 239, *269*, 273
Brown, D., 101, *135*
Brown, D. D., 440, *455*
Brown, J. C., 453, *455*
Brown, L. D., 194, *221*
Brown, R. E., 352, 353, 354, 380, 388, *407*
Browning, H. C., 332, *346*
Bruce, H. M., 252, 262, *269*, 308, *318*
Bruce, J. M., 439, 442, 445, *458*
Bruce, J. O., 313, 314, *319*
Brumby, P. J., 301, *319*
Brunngraber, E. F., 448, *455*
Brush, M. G., 305, *319*
Bryant, G. D., 262, *269*, 285, 301, *319*
Buck, C. A., 451, 454, *455*, *458*, *464*
Bucovaz, E. T., 388, *407*
Buhi, W. C., 304, *325*
Bulbrook, R. D., 124, *136*, 418, *465*
Bullis, D. D., 300, *319*
Bunch, G. A., 229, *268*
Bunding, I., 305, *325*

Bunting, S. L., 343, *347*, 438, 439, 450, *456*, *458*
Burgess, A. B., 441, *455*
Burny, A., 441, *459*
Burrows, J. H., 87, *93*
Bush, L. J., 300, *319*
Bustin, M., 437, *455*
Butler, J. A. V., 436, *455*

C

Cabera, R., 352, 353, 354, 360, *407*
Cady, S. P., 365, *407*
Cahill, G. F., 193, *221*
Callahan, C. J., 290, 291, *320*, *321*
Campbell, I. L., 305, *319*
Campbell, P. N., 446, *455*
Capen, C. C., 310, *319*
Capra, J. D., 451, *456*, *461*
Carey, E. M., 385, *407*, *408*
Carlsson, E. I., 354, 377, 378, 382, *408*
Caro, L., 41, *93*
Carroll, E. J., 240, *269*
Carulo, E. V., 101, *135*
Cary, C. A., 147, *221*, *223*
Caskey, C. T., 453, *456*
Cathcart, E. P., 228, *269*
Catt, K. J., 284, *319*
Ceriani, R. L., 103, 105, 106, 130, 132, *135*
Cerruti, R. A., 118, *135*
Chadwick, A. 281, *319*, 420, *456*
Chaikoff, I. L., 334, *346*, 352, 354, 365, 387, *407*, *409*
Chalkley, G. R., 340, *347*, 437, *461*
Challis, J. R. G., 217, *221*
Chambon, P., 435, *459*
Chambon, R., 435, *456*
Chan, W. Y., 239, *269*
Chantrenne, H., 441, *459*
Charney, J., 84, 87, 88, *93*, *94*
Charton, A., 191, *221*
Chastain, B. H., 451, *463*
Chatterjee, N. K., 453, *455*, *458*
Chatterton, A. J., 124, *135*
Chatterton, R. J., Jr., 124, *135*
Chatterton, R. T., Jr., 124, *139*
Chatwin, A. L., *173*, 221
Chaudhury, M. R., 238, *269*

Chaudhury, R. R., 238, *269*
Chauveau, J. P. A., 193, *221*
Chavancy, G., 452, *457*
Chen, C. L., 248, 249, 250, 258, 259, 268, *269*, *274*, 279, 285, 289, 291, 301, 309, *318*, *319*, *323*, 332, *346*
Chen, R. F., 377, *411*
Cheng, W., 352, 353, 354, 360, 374, 375, 376, 381, 383, 386, 396, 398, 400, 402, 405, *407*, 433, 436, *455*
Chentsou, Y. S., 4, *91*
Chernick, S. S., 354, 387, *408*
Chezzi, C., 439, *462*
Childs, B., 371, *411*
Chopra, H. C., 85, 87, *91*
Chung, A., 453, *458*
Chung, A. C., 305, *325*
Chung, D., 119, 128, 131, *137*
Church, R. B., 438, *456*, *458*
Ciaccio, E. I., 101, 111, 117, 120, *138*, 419, 426, *461*
Ciotti, M. M., 381, *408*
Civen, M., 330, *348*
Clancy, D. P., 314, *319*
Clark, B. J., 239, 240, *269*, 305, *318*
Clark, E. R., 159, *221*
Clark, J. L., 131, *138*
Clary, T. R., 354, 387, *408*
Clausen, J., 378, *408*
Clemens, J. A., 248, *269*, 289, *323*
Cleverley, J. D., 237, *269*, 305, *319*
Clifton, K. H., 122, *135*
Cobo, E., 230, *269*
Cochrane, E. R., 241, *269*
Cocquyt, G., 186, 212, *224*, *225*
Coffey, R. G., 53, *91*
Cohen, H. A., 263, *276*
Cohen, R. M., 119, 128, *135*, 284, *319*, 417, *456*
Cole, H. A., 108, *135*
Cole, R. D., 415, 419, 437, *455*, *456*, *458*, *463*
Colgate, C. E., 122, *135*
Colley, V. B., 101, 105, *135*
Collias, N. E., 252, *269*
Collip, J. B., 118, *139*, 243, 253, 256, 257, *275*, 281, 297, *325*
Common, R. H., 290, *324*

Convey, E. M., 247, 258, *269*, 285, 286, 288, 293, 301, 302, 306, 309, 317, *319, 321, 322, 325,* 352, 353, 354, 390, 394, *410,* 425, 429, *463*
Cook, R. M., 353, 379, 394, *409, 410*
Cooper, R. A., 338, *348*
Coore, H. G., 387, *407*
Coppola, J., 128, *136*
Corbin, E. A., 183, *222*
Cordes, E. H., 363, *409*
Cotes, P. H., 299, 305, *319*
Coussens, R., 231, *275*
Cowie, A. T., 100, 107, 110, 124, *135, 136,* 186, 189, 213, 214, *222,* 244, 245, 255, 256, *268, 269, 270,* 278, 282, 294, 297, 298, 299, 300, 301, 305, 308, 311, 312, 313, *319,* 345, *347,* 415, 416, 426, 427, 431, *455, 456*
Cox, C. P., 124, *135,* 300, *319*
Craddock, V. M., 454, *456*
Crampton, E. W., 308, 309, *318*
Crichton, J. A., 299, 305, *319*
Crone, C., 182, *221*
Cross, B. A., 228, 229, 230, 231, 232, 233, 234, 236, 237, 238, 239, *270*
Crumpton, C. W., 196, *225*
Crystal, R. G., 441, *456, 462*
Cuatrecasas, P., 330, *347*
Cummins, E. P., 400, *410, 462*
Cupceancu, B., 104, *136*
Curtis, E. M., 315, *319*
Cuthbert, F. P., 312, *319*

D

Dabelow, A., 155, 156, 158, *221*
Dagg, C. D., 332, *347*
Daggs, R. G., 294, *319*
Dahmus, M. E., 436, *455*
Dalton, A. J., 41, *91*
Dalziel, K., 375, *411*
Damm, H. C., 127, *136*
Daniel, P. M., 255, *270*
Danon, A., 287, *318*
Danon, D., 441, *458*
Dao, T. L., 416, *460*
Darby, F. J., 387, 388, 403, *408,* 429, *456*
Darnell, J. E. Jr., 432, 440, *456, 457, 459, 465*

Darroch, R. A., 301, *324*
Das, M. R., 87, *91*
Dati, F. A., 435, *456*
Daulie, J., 452, *457*
Dauwalder, M., 53, *95*
Davey, A. W. F., 305, *319*
Davidson, E. H., 432, *455*
Davidson, J. N., 101, 111, *136*
Davis, B. D., 441, 442, *456, 460*
Davis, C. L., 352, 353, 354, 380, 383, 388, *407*
Davis, G. K., 193, 213, *223*
Davis, J. W., 286, 287, 291, 292, *319,* 388, *407,* 420, 421, *456, 460*
Davis, S. L., 285, *319*
Davis, S. W., 421, *465*
de Aberle, S. B., 108, *136*
Deanesley, R., 291, *321*
Debackere, M., 237, *270*
de Duve, Ch., 72, *91*
De Fremery, P., 281, *319*
Deis, R. P., 237, 238, 239, 240, 242, 249, 263, *270, 275, 276,* 291, *319*
De Lauder, W. R., 102, 118, 119, *140,* 417, *465*
Delaunay, J., 441, *459*
Delouis, C., 281, 285, *320,* 416, 418, 420, 431, 433, *456*
de Moor, A., 186, *224*
de Moss, W. R., 98, 107, 108, *140*
Dempsey, E. W., 310, *320*
Denamur, R., 4, 45, 57, *91, 92,* 111, 117, 120, *136,* 228, 232, 233, 235, 253, 255, *270, 275,* 280, 281, 285, 299, 300, 306, *320,* 416, 417, 418, 419, 420, 421, 423, 425, 426, 427, 428, 429, 430, 431, 432, 434, 439, 440, 442, 443, 445, 446, 450, *455, 456, 457, 458, 462*
Denenburg, V. H., 263, *276*
Denton, R. M., 387, *407*
Denton, W. L., 334, *346*
DeNuccio, D. J., 237, 239, 241, 242, *270, 272*
DeOme, K. B., 4, 6, 11, 15, 19, 21, 37, 51, 68, 69, 71, 72, 75, 77, 79, 85, *94, 95,* 100, 131, 132, *139,* 328, *348,* 430, *465*
de Robertis, E. D. P., 67, *94*

Desclin, J., 245, 249, 250, 253, *270*, 306, *320*

Desclin, L., 308, *320*

Deshpande, N., 124, *136*

Desjardins, C., 119, *136,* 306, *324,* 417, *456*

De Sombre, E. R., 329, 330, *347*

Desser, G. N., 440, *464*

Deutsch, A., 443, *456*

Deutscher, M. P., 448, *456*

De Vae, W. F., 250, *270*

Devita, J., 124, *139*

De Witt, G. W., 248, *273*

Dhariwal, A. P. S., 246, 247, 248, 249, 254, 255, 258, 261, 262, *272*

Dhondt, G., 165, 182, *221*

Dibitanto, G., 436, *455*

Dikstein, S., 287, 314, *318*

Dilley, W. G., 132, 133, 134, *136*

Dils, R., 352, 353, 354, 382, 385, 388, *407, 408, 410,* 426, *458*

Dingman, C. W., 450, *456, 461*

Dintzis, H. M., 453, *465*

Dion, A. S., 87, *91*

Dixon, J. S., 119, 128, 131, *137,* 282, *322*

Djojosoebagio, S., 295, 312, *320*

Dmochowski, L., 87, 88, *91, 92, 94*

Dodd, F. H., 316, *326*

Doe, R. P., 288, *325*

Doherty, D. G., 382, *408*

Doisy, E. A., 121, 122, *135*

Donker, J. D., 240, *270,* 294, *324*

Donné, A., 72, 75, 76, 77, *92*

Donoso, A. O., 315, *320*

Donovan, B. T., 128, 129, *136,* 244, 254, 269, *270,* 426, *457*

Downey, W. K., 316, *326*

Drews, J., 438, *457*

Dreyfus, Y., 88, *92*

Drost, M., 288, *320*

Drysdale, J. W., 447, *458*

Dugger, G. S., 245, *270*

Dunn, J. S., 194, *220*

Dutcher, R. M., 85, *92*

Dyusembin, Kh., 237, 241, *270, 276*

E

Easter, D. J., 352, 353, 354, 382, *410*

Eaton, J., 451, *464*

Eayrs, J. T., 232, 233, 254, 255, *270,* 315, *320*

Ebel, J. P., 448, 451, *455, 457*

Ebner, K. E., 188, *221,* 328, 334, 338, *346,* 347, 351, 352, 368, 369, *407, 409,* 418, 419, *460*

Eckles, N. E., 245, *270, 271*

Edgerton, L. A., 285, 286, 293, *324, 325*

Edgren, R. A., 314, *319*

Edwards, M. J., 186, 189, 213, 214, *222*

Edwardson, J. A., 229, 254, 255, *270,* 315, *320*

Eggleston, L. V., 359, 380, 388, *411*

Ehni, G., 245, *270, 271*

Ehrenbrand, E., 4, *92*

Ekman, L., 308, *320*

El-Darwish, I., 133, *136,* 422, 423, 424, 449, *457*

El Ganzoury, B., 314, *322*

Elger, W., 104, 127, *136, 138*

El Hagri, M. A. A. M., 155, 185, *221*

Elias, H., 53, *92*

Elias, J. J., 106, 129, *136,* 328, 339, *347,* 422, *459*

Elliott, J. R., 103, *136*

Ellis, F. G., 124, *136*

Ellis, G. H., 193, 213, *223*

Ellis, R. A., 79, 81, *92*

Ellis, S., 248, *274*

El Mahgoub, S., 314, *322*

Elska, A. V., 447, 449, 451, 452, 454, 457, *462*

Elsley, F. W. H., 196, *220*

Ely, F., 149, *221,* 236, 238, *271*

Emerson, K., 284, *326*

Emery, E. S., 194, *221*

Emery, R. S., 306, *320,* 352, 353, 354, 368, 370, 375, 387, 390, 391, 394, 403, *407, 410,* 427, *465*

Emmel, V. E., 241, *271*

Emmerson, M. A., 99, *136*

England, P. J., 366, *408*

Engle, G. C., 85, *92*

Erb, R. E., 290, 291, *320, 321*

Erdmann, V. A., 440, *457*

Ericsson, J. L. E., 4, 39, 61, 65, 68, 71, 72, 73, 79, *92,* 352, 388, 393, *408*

Eshchar, N., 315, *324*

Etienne, M., 129, *136*
Etta, K. M., 311, *320*
Evans, A. J., 387, *408*
Evans, H. M., 113, *137*
Evans, J. H., 340, *347*
Everett, J. W., 245, 246, 250, 253, *271*, 275
Everse, J., 377, *408*

F

Fahnestock, S., 440, *457*
Fajer, A. B., 109, *136*, 291, *320*
Falconer, I. R., 4, *92*, 278, *320*, 420, 421, 434, *457*
Fambrough, D. M., 436, 437, *455*, *457*
Fan, H., 432, *461*
Farber, E., 451, *454*
Farquhar, M. G., 19, 25, 26, 35, *92*, *94*
Faulkin, L. J., Jr., 101, *139*
Fawcett, C. P., 315, *320*
Faye, P., 191, *221*
Fazakerley, S., 210, 213, 214, 215, *220*, 223
Fegler, G., 166, 167, 173, 181, *221*
Feldman, D. G., 85, 88, *92*, *93*
Feldman, J. D., 4, 51, *92*, 101, *136*
Felig, P., 193, *221*
Felix, M. D., 41, *91*
Ferreri, L. F., 114, *136*, 286, *320*, 417, 421, *457*
Fick, A., 145, 216, *221*
Fiddler, T. J., 4, *92*, 420, 421, 434, *457*
Fiel, N. J., 134, *138*
Fikri, F., 314, *322*
Findlay, A. L. R., 228, 229, 230, 232, 237, 238, 239, 240, 252, 264, *270*, *271*, *272*
Fink, L. M., 453, *457*
Fiorindo, R. P., 246, 250, 258, *271*, *274*, 284, *324*
Fischer, J. E., 315, *325*
Fisher, E. W., 193, *221*
Fitzgerald, D. K., 328, 338, *347*, 352, *409*, 418, 419, *460*
Fitzpatrick, R. J., 237, *271*
Fitzpatrick, R. S., 305, *320*
Flamboe, E. E., 310, *320*
Flament-Durand, J., 250, *270*

Fléchon, J. E., 4, *91*, 416, 418, *455*
Fleet, I. R., 173, 182, 184, 189, 205, 217, 218, *222*, *223*
Fleischer, B., 334, *347*
Fleischer, S., 334, *347*
Fleischhauer, K., 4, 61, 64, 65, *91*
Fleisher, G. A., 381, *408*
Fleissner, E., 451, *463*
Flerkó, B., 250, *271*
Florini, J. R., 128, *136*
Flux, D. S., 100, *136*, 305, 313, *320*, 416, *457*
Foa, C., 146, 147, 189, 191, 209, *221*
Fohrman, M. H., 99, 100, 109, 110, *138*
Folley, S. J., 100, *136*, 148, 185, 188, 190, 192, 211, 212, 213, *221*, *224*, 237, 244, 245, 253, 256, *268*, *269*, *271*, 278, 280, 281, 294, 297, 299, 305, 308, 313, *319*, *320*, *324*, 345, *347*, 389, 396, *408*, 419, *457*
Forbes, A., 229, *271*
Forbes, A. P., 229, *271*
Forbes, D. A., 314, *318*
Forbes, T. R., 289, 292, *321*
Forsberg, J. G., 127, *136*
Forsyth, I. A., 188, *221*, 282, 284, *320*, 340, *347*, 422, 423, 449, *460*
Foster, T. S., 353, 395, 401, *411*, 426, *465*
Fournier, M. S., 454, *457*
Fowkes, F. M., 63, *93*
Fox, S., 240, *274*
Francis, B. F., 122, *135*
Frank, A. H., 100, *140*
Frank, R. T., 122, *136*
Frankel, F., 453, *457*
Franklin, D. L., 171, *221*
Franklin, R. M., 433, *462*
Frantz, A. G., 282, 302, *320*
Fraschini, F., 251, *274*
Fraser, M. J., 452, *457*
Fredrikson, H., 282, *320*
Freeland, R. A., 372, 403, *407*, *410*
Freinkel, N., 310, *321*
French, J. E., 214, *224*
French, T. H., 148, 188, 212, *221*, *224*
Friedberg, S. H., 132, *139*, 328, 329, 330, 334, 339, 340, *347*
Frieden, E., 451, *464*

Friedman, H. M., 250, *273*
Friedman, M., 288, *320*
Friedman, R. C., 134, *136*
Friesen, H. G., 282, 284, 285, 286, 302, *320, 321, 326,* 420, *457*
Fronek, A., 167, *221*
Fuchs, A. R., 237, *271*
Fürstenburg, M. H. F., 153, *221*
Fuhr, J. E., 441, *457*
Fujimoto, M., 102, 109, 110, 111, 116, *138*
Funcke, H. G., 387, *411*
Furth, J., 122, *135*

G

Gabel, A. A., 196, *221*
Gachev, E. P., 255, *271*
Gaddum, J. H., 165, *221*
Gagné, H. T., 188, *224,* 352, 354, *410*
Cairns, F. W., 228, *269*
Gaitan, E., 230, *269*
Gala, R. R., 119, 128, *135,* 284, 288, 289, 306, 307, 309, *319, 320,* 417, *456*
Gale, C. C., 255, *271*
Galibert, F., 440, *457*
Gallager, H. S., 87, *91, 94*
Gallo, R. C., 451, *457*
Galper, J. B., *457*
Ganguli, N. C., 352, 353, *409, 416,* 444, *460*
Ganoza, M. C., 447, *457*
Ganz, V., 167, *221*
Garcia, C., 314, *321*
Gardner, K. E., 101, *136*
Gardner, W. U., 100, 109, 118, 124, *136, 139, 140*
Garel, J. P., 452, *457*
Gartland, W. J., 131, *138*
Garven, H. S. D., 228, *269*
Garverick, H. A., 290, *321*
Gaunt, R., 281, *323*
Gaye, P., 45, 57, *91, 92,* 416, 417, 418, 419, 420, 421, 426, 428, 431, 434, 439, 440, 442, 443, 445, 446, 448, 450, *456, 457, 458, 461*
Gefter, M. L., 451, *457*
Gelehrter, T. D., 435, *464*
Gemzell, C. A., 289, *321*
Georgiev, G. P., 445, *457*

Geschwind, I. I., 249, *271*
Ghoneim, M., 314, *321*
Ghosh, H. P., 453, *462*
Giacometti, L., 228, *271*
Gibson, H. V., 122, *135*
Gilbert, J. M., 441, 451, *454, 462*
Gill, J. L., 302, *319*
Gillam, I., 453, *457*
Gillespie, R., 372, 375, 386, *411*
Ginsberg, T., 453, *463*
Giorgio, N. A., Jr., 330, *347*
Girardie, J., 4, 5, 8, 11, 23, 65, 69, 71, 75, 77, 79, 85, *92*
Gissinger, F., 435, *456, 459*
Giveon, D., 451, *455*
Glascock, R. F., 124, *136*
Glock, G. E., 419, *457*
Gniazdowski, M., 435, *456, 459*
Godman, G. C., 41, *93*
Goldman, M., 451, *457*
Goldzveig, S. A., 124, *135*
Gomez, E. T., 98, 100, 108, 125, *136, 137, 140,* 194, *222,* 281, *321*
Gonano, F., 451, *457, 463*
Goodfriend, T. L., 378, *408*
Gorbman, A., 438, *458*
Gorski, J., 307, *326*
Goss, D. A., 128, *137*
Gostev, A. V., 158, 174, *221*
Goto, T., 453, *457*
Gotoh, S., 432, *458*
Gowen, J. W., 99, *136*
Grachev, I. I., 229, 230, 237, 241, *271*
Graffi, A., 90, *93*
Graham, W. R., 148, 151, 167, 190, 193, 194, 202, 216, 218, *221, 222,* 308, *321*
Granboulan, N., 439, *462*
Granger, G. A., 451, *464*
Granner, D., 335, *347,* 435, *464*
Grant, G. A., 148, *222*
Gray, J., 312, *319*
Graysel, A. I., 441, *457*
Grazia, Y. R., 246, *275*
Green, C. D., 400, *408,* 434, *458*
Green, H. D., 165, *222*
Green, M. R., 342, 343, *347,* 424, 438, 439, 450, *458*
Greenbaum, A. C., 440, *465*

Greenbaum, A. L., 101, 111, *136*, 353, 359, 362, 381, 387, 388, 390, 393, 403, *408*, *410*, 419, 425, 427, 429, *456*, *458*, *463*, *465*
Greenberg, J. R., 432, 445, *461*
Greene, R. R., 243, *271*
Greengard, O., 353, 381, *408*
Greenhalgh, J. F. D., 101, *136*
Greenman, D. L., 440, *458*, *465*
Greenwood, F. C., 262, *269*, 285, 301, *319*, 353, 388, 390, 393, *408*
Greep, R. O., 282, 291, *318*, 322
Grégoire, C., 249, 253, *270*, 272
Grey, C. E., 88, *91*
Grierson, D., 432, *458*
Griffin, A. C., 451, *457*
Griffin, S. A., 310, *321*
Griffin, T. K., 240, *274*
Griffith, D. E., 114, *136*
Griffith, D. R., 102, 111, 114, 120, 124, 125, 127, 129, *136*, *138*, 258, *275*, 286, 313, *320*, *321*, *322*, 417, 421, *457*
Grimm, F. C., 382, *408*
Grivell, L. A., 439, *455*
Gros, C. M., 4, 75, 77, *92*
Gros, F., 441, *462*
Grosclaude, J., 439, *462*
Gross, L., 88, 89, *92*
Gross, P. R., 433, *458*
Grossbard, L., 364, *408*
Grossie, J., 134, *136*
Grosvenor, C. E., 232, 237, 238, 239, 240, 241, 242, 246, 247, 248, 249, 253, 254, 255, 257, 258, 259, 260, 261, 262, 263, 264, 265, *270*, *271*, *272*, *274*, 285, 292, 294, 295, 298, 300, 301, 303, 308, 310, 316, *321*
Grosz, H. J., 251, *272*
Gruenstein, M., 352, 368, *410*, 419, *462*
Grueter, F., 98, *139*, 281, *321*, *325*
Grumbach, M. M., 128, *137*, 284, *322*
Grunbaum, B. W., 4, 51, 85, *95*
Grynfeltt, J., 278, *321*
Guerin, M., 84, 85, *91*
Gueslin, M., 191, *221*
Güttler, F., 378, *408*
Guidry, A. J., 241, *274*
Gul, B., 388, *408*, 426, *458*

Gumaa, K. A., 359, 362, 381, *408*
Gupta, N. K., 453, *455*, *458*
Gurdon, J. B., 440, *455*
Gutfreund, H., 452, *457*
Guyda, H., 282, *320*, *321*

H

Hacker, B., 450, *458*
Hacker, R. R., 111, 117, 120, *136*, 427, *458*
Hackett, A. J., 415, *458*
Hafs, H. D., 279, 285, 286, 288, 293, 317, *321*, *324*, *325*
Hageman, E. C., 188, *221*
Haguenau, F., 41, 79, *92*
Hahn, D. W., 123, 126, 130, 131, *136*, 306, *321*
Hahn, W. E., 438, *458*
Haldar, J., 305, *318*
Hall, S. R., 134, *139*
Hamlin, R., 196, *221*
Hammond, J., 107, 108, 113, *137*, 278, *321*
Hamosh, M., 354, 387, *408*
Hamperl, H., 77, 79, *92*
Hancock, J., 301, *319*
Hancock, R. L., 414, *465*
Handwerger, S., 284, *325*
Hansel, W., 124, *139*, 309, *325*
Hansen, H. J. M., 385, *408*
Hansen, P., 435, *463*
Hansen, R., 365, *408*
Hansen, R. G., 372, 375, 386, *411*
Hanson, R. W., 388, *407*
Hanwell, A., 164, 173, 178, 181, 191, *222*
Hardenbrook, H., 372, 375, 386, *411*
Hardwick, D. C., 144, 149, 182, 183, 186, 189, 205, 209, 213, 214, *222*, 380, 384, *408*
Hardy, M. H., 101, 103, 131, 132, *137*
Harrington, R. B., 290, *321*
Harris, G. W., 236, *270*
Harrison, F. A., 288, *324*
Harrison, H. A., 190, *220*
Hart, P. G., 314, *323*
Hartman, P. E., 426, 451, *454*, *458*
Hartmann, P. E., 186, 189, 191, 194, 207, 213, 214, 216, 219, *222*, *270*, 298, *319*, 352, 353, 354, 390, 391, *408*

Hashimoto, I., 109, *137*, 291, *321*
Hassid, W. Z., 209, *225*, 334, *348*
Haug, H., 53, *92*
Haun, C. K., 249, *272*
Hawkins, R. A., 290, *326*
Hawtrey, A. O., 388, 389, *408*, 439, 441, 442, 447, 454, *458*
Heald, C. W., 353, *410*
Heap, R. B., 208, 217, *222*, 291, *321*
Hebb, C. O., 149, 151, 160, 161, 164, 181, 183, *222*, 229, 231, 239, *272*
Heeter, M., 440, *465*
Hefnawi, F., 314, *321*
Heitzman, R. J., 288, 307, *321*, 352, 353, 390, *408*
Hellman, L., 124, *135*
Hellung-Larsen, P., 378, *408*
Helminen, H. J., 4, 39, 61, 65, 68, 71, 72, 73, 79, *92*, 352, 388, 393, *408*
Henneman, H. A., 310, *321*
Hennig, A., 53, *92*
Henricks, D. M., 109, *137*, 291, *321*
Henshaw, E. C., 439, *458*
Hentzen, D., 451, *455*
Herbert, E., 442, *459*
Herrenkohl, L. R., 291, *321*
Herriman, I. D., 439, 442, 445, 446, *454*, *458*
Herrington, M. D., 388, 389, *408*, 439, 441, 442, 447, 454, *458*
Hershey, A. D., 439, *460*
Hervy, R., 191, *221*
Herzberg, M., 441, *458*
Herzfeld, A., 353, 381, *408*
Hesselberg, C., 11, *93*, 98, 108, *137*
Hey, W. C., 441, *459*
Heytler, P. G., 101, 111, 117, 120, *138*, 419, 426, *461*
Heywood, S. M., 441, *458*
Hiatt, H. H., 439, *458*
Hicks, S. J., 447, *458*
Higashi, K., 432, *458*
Higo, K., 440, *457*
Hilf, R., 434, *458*
Hill, R. L., 291, 293, *326*, 328, 334, 338, 342, 346, *346*, *348*, 424, 434, 435, *464*
Hillarp, N. A., 250, *272*
Hilliard, J., 249, *273*
Hills, F., 288, 289, *324*

Hilton, S. M., 184, *222*
Hindery, G. A., 110, *140*, 293, 308, *321*
Hines, M. C., 373, *408*
Hiromitsu, P., 85, *93*
Hirsch, C. A., 131, *138*, 440, *458*
Hjalmarson, A., 127, *135*
Hodson, A. Z., 193, 213, *223*
Hoeckstra, W. G., 124, *136*
Hoetz, W., 441, *458*
Hoffman, W., 289, 292, *321*
Hohmann, P., 437, *458*
Holbrook, D. J., Jr., 340, *347*
Holland, J. J., 451, *458*, *464*
Holland, R. C., 239, *268*
Hollander, V. P., 123, *138*
Hollmann, K. H., 4, 5, 6, 11, 12, 13, 14, 17, 21, 23, 25, 26, 33, 37, 39, 41, 43, 51, 53, 55, 57, 58, 59, 60, 68, 69, 71, 72, 73, 75, 76, 77, 79, 81, 84, 85, 87, 88, *92*, *93*, *94*, 338, *347*, 444, *458*
Holm, L. W., 288, *320*, *322*
Holst, V., 253, 256, *272*
Holten, D., 371, *408*
Holton, F. A., 184, *222*
Holton, P., 184, *222*
Holzbauer, M., 306, *321*
Holzman, G. B., 169, *222*
Hooker, C. W., 253, *272*
Hoover, C. R., 188, *221*ˈ
Hopkins, T. F., 285, 286, *323*, 420, *460*
Hopkins, T. R., 415, 419, *456*
Hori, S. H., 371, *408*
Horie, A., 85, *93*
Hoshino, K., 105, *137*
Houdebine, L., 431, 439, 442, 443, 450, *456*, *458*
Housman, D., 453, *458*
Houvenaghel, A., 165, 182, 184, *221*, *222*, 224, 239, *272*
Howanitz, P. J., 354, 385, *408*
Howard, C. F., Jr., 386, *408*
Howards, G. A., 442, *459*
Howe, A., 439, *459*
Hoyer, H., 159, *222*
Huang, A., 441, *459*
Huang, R. C., 436, *455*, *459*
Huber, J. T., 427, *465*
Huez, G., 441, *459*

Huggins, C., 352, 353, 354, *410*
Hughes, L. R., 314, *323*
Huhn, S., 79, *93*
Hunter, A. R., 453, *459*
Hunter, D. L., 290, *321*
Hunter, G. D., 288, 307, *321*
Hunter, T., 453, *459*
Huther, K. J., 288, *325*
Huynh-Van-Tan, Delaunay, J., 441, *459*
Hwang, P., 282, *321*

I

Ichinose, R. R., 106, 129, 131, 132, 133, *137*, 327, 345, *347*
Ieiri, T., 279, *321*
Iio, M., 169, *222*
Ilan, J., 441, *459*
Illingworth, D. V., 291, *321*
Illner, P., 251, 258, 259, *273*
Imai, T., 85, *93*
Ingalls, W. G., 285, 286, 288, 293, *321*
Ingbar, S. H., 310, *321*
Ingelbrecht, P., 253, 254, *272*
Ingles, C. J., 435, *455*
Ingraham, R. L., 101, *135*
Inskeep, E. K., 314, *325*
Irvin, J. L., 340, *347*
Irving, C. C., 451, *459*
Isaacs, B. L., 312, *319*
Isbister, C., 229, *272*
Ishikawa, T., 232, 239, *269*, *273*
Itano, H. A., 451, *459*
Ivy, A. C., 312, *319*
Iwahashi, H., 102, 109, 110, 111, 116, *138*

J

Jackson, C. D., 451, *459*
Jackson, R. J., 453, *459*
Jacob, S. T., 435, *459*
Jacobsen, M. S., 240, *269*
Jacobs Lorena, M., 442, 453, *458*, *459*
Jacobsohn, D., 99, 110, 122, 123, 127, 128, 129, *135*, *136*, *137*, 245, 254, *272*, 345, *347*, 414, *460*
Jacobsohn, I., 127, *136*
Jacobson, M. B., 174, *220*
Jaffe, S., 372, 375, 386, *411*

Jagenau, A. H. M., 165, *222*
Jamieson, J. D., 41, 45, 49, *93*
Jeffcott, L. B., 144, 183, 186, 189, 205, 211, 212, 216, 217, *223*
Jeffers, K. R., 279, *321*
Jener, G. M., 453, *457*
Jensen, E. M., 85, *91*
Jensen, E. V., 329, 330, *347*
Jesensky, C., 451, *461*
Jha, S. K., 194, *222*
Johke, T., 262, *273*, 301, 302, *321*
Johnson, C. B., 330, *347*
Johnson, R. E., 99, 118, 122, 123, 128, 131, *137*, *138*, 282, 284, 298, *318*, *323*, *324*, 333, *347*, 395, *409*, 414, 417, *460*, *462*
Johnson, R. M., 301, 306, *321*
Johnston, C. G., 122, *135*
Johnston, R. F., 194, *222*
Johnston, W. M., 451, *457*
Joklik, W., 441, *459*
Jones, E. A., 188, *221*, 352, 353, 354, 393, 396, 403, 405, 406, *408*, 419, 426, 431, *457*, *458*, *459*
Jones, T. S. G., 151, 216, 218, *221*
Jordan, B. R., 440, *459*
Joshi, U. M., 314, *321*
Josimovich, J. B., 128, *137*, 284, *321*
Juergens, W. G., 133, *139*, 334, 339, 340, 346, *347*, *348*, 422, 423, 434, *459*, *463*
Julien, J., 440, *462*
Jung, L., 148, 149, *222*
Jungblut, P. W., 329, 330, *347*
Jurkovitz, L., 414, *465*

K

Kahn, R. H., 102, 127, *137*, 246, *274*
Kaiser, J., 441, *459*
Kamal, I., 314, *321*
Kamberi, I. A., 246, *275*, 351, *321*
Kamoun, A., 288, 289, 306, *321*, *322*
Kand, S. S., 250, *268*
Kanematsu, S., 249, *273*
Kano-Sueoka, T., 450, 451, *463*
Kanzawa, F., 102, 109, 110, 111, 116, *138*
Kao, V. C. Y., 81, *91*
Kaplan, N. O., 377, 378, 381, *408*
Kaplan, S. L., 128, *137*, 284, *322*

Karg, H., 285, *324*
Karim, M., 314, *322*
Karlsson, B. W., 354, 377, 378, 382, *408*
Kasahara, M., 228, *274*
Kassouny, M., 240, *269*
Katz, J., 361, 372, 373, 375, 383, *408*
Katzen, H. M., 364, 365, 366, *408, 409*
Kaufmann, M., 146, 147, 192, 209, *222*
Kawashima, T., 329, 330, *347*
Kay, H. D., 148, 151, 185, 190, 193, 216, 218, *221, 222*
Kedinger, C., 435, *456, 459*
Keenan, T. W., 63, *93*
Kelley, F. C., 416, 426, *459*
Kennedy, P. C., 288, *322*
Kennell, D. E., 438, *459*
Kenney, F. T., 440, *458, 465*
Kephart, J. E., 53, *95*
Kerkof, P. R., 188, *220, 224*
Kerr, S. J., 450, 451, *459, 462*
Kety, S. S., 168, 169, *222*
Khazen, K., 308, *318*, 417, *462*
Kilpatrick, R., 282, *322*
Kim, Y. S., 403, *410*
King, S. F., 239, 241, 242, *272*
Kinsella, J. E., 188, *222*, 387, *409*
Kinzey, W. G., 119, *137*
Kirkham, W. R., 101, 110, 111, *137*, 425, *459*
Kirkman, H. N., 371, *409*
Kirschbaum, A., 245, *270*
Kistler, G. S., 53, *94*
Kjaersgaard, P., 168, 179, *222*
Klauske, J., 172, *220*
Klee, C. B., 448, *459*
Kleiber, M., 187, 213, *222, 224*
Klein, H., 414, *460*
Klein, M., 75, *93*, 100, *138*, 278, *323*
Kleinberg, D. L., 282, 302, *320*
Knaggs, G. S., 232, 233, 234, 235, 236, 237, 244, 251, 254, 255, *270, 271, 273*, 275, 289, 297, 315, *319, 325*
Knauer, E., 98, *137*
Knight, E., 440, *459*
Knodt, C. B., 305, *322*
Knook, H. L., 252, *273*
Knoop, A., 4, 33, 37, 51, 61, 64, 65, 79, *91*
Knopp, R., 289, *324*
Knox, F. S., 313, *322*

Kobayashi, Y., 65, *93*
Koch, B., 307, *322*
Koch, Y., 315, *322*
Kodaira, K., 441, *461*
Koelle, G. B., 239, *273*
Koen, P. F., 33, *94*
Kohler, P. O., 438, *461*
Kohmoto, K., 128, *137*, 417, *459*
Koivisto, E., 173, *225*
Koizumi, K., 232, 239, *269, 273*
Kokorina, E. P., 237, 241, *268, 273*
Kon, S. K., 313, *320*
Koprowski, J. A., 279, 301, 302, 303, 304, 306, 312, 313, *322*
Kora, S. J., 314, *322*
Korenman, S. G., 438, *461*
Korn, E. D., 354, 387, *409*
Korner, A., 414, 433, 436, *459, 461*
Korsrud, G. O., 352, 353, 354, 360, 364, 367, 369, 370, 372, 373, 382, 383, 384, 391, 392, 393, 395, 396, 399, 400, 401, 402, 403, 404, 405, *407, 409*, 426, 431, 433, 436, *455, 459*
Koshi, J. H., 240, *270*
Koulischer, L., 249, *270*
Kountz, W. B., 122, *135*
Kowalewski, K., 306, *322*
Kragt, C. L., 107, 122, 129, *135, 138*
Krahl, M. E., 365, *408*
Kramarsky, B., 87, *93*
Kratochwil, K., 345, *347*
Krebs, H. A., 359, 362, 375, 376, 380, 388, *409, 410, 411*
Kriesten, K., 11, 12, *93*
Krischke, W., 90, *93*
Kronfeld, D. S., 153, 169, 179, 180, 193, 194, 207, 208, 213, 215, 219, *222*, 312, *322*, 398, *409*
Krulich, L., 251, 253, 258, 259, *272, 273*, 303, 315, *320, 321*
Krulik, R., 289, 307, *322*
Krumholz, K. H., 240, *268*
Kühn, E. R., 240, 259, *273*
Kuhn, N. J., 53, *93*, 245, *273*, 288, 291, 292, *322*, 352, 354, 360, 369, 390, 395, 397, *409*, 418, 419, *459*
Kumar, S., 183, *222*, 385, *409*

Kumaresan, P., 114, 125, 126, 127, 129, 131, *137*, 295, 298, 304, 312, *322*, 417, 421, 425, 426, *459*
Kuramitsu, C., 313, *322*
Kuretani, K., 102, 109, 110, 111, 116, *138*
Kurihara, K., 441, *465*
Kurosumi, K., 65, 66, *93*
Kurotsu, T., 234, *268*
Kurz, M., 252, *273*

L

Lakshmanan, S., 183, *222*
Lane, N., 41, *93*
Langer, E., 79, *93*
Langford, P. L., 88, *92*
Lanks, K. W., 452, *459*
Lanner, M., 284, *325*
Lantos, C. P., 251, *273*
Larke, G. A., 332, *346*
Larsen, C. J., 440, *457*
Larson, B. L., 188, *221*, 225, 307, *326*
Lascelles, A. K., 77, *93*, 161, 186, 189, 194, 207, 213, 214, 216, 219, *222*, *223*
Lasfargues, E. Y., 85, 87, *93*, 101, 103, 131, 132, 133, *137*
Laslof, J. C., 310, *325*
Lassmann, G., 229, *273*
Laumas, K. R., 314, *322*
Laumas, V., 314, *322*
Lauritzen, C., 315, *322*
Lauryssens, M., 212, *225*
Law, L. W., 90, *93*
Lawford, G. R., 441, *459*
Lawson, E. C. M., 124, *137*
Laycock, D. G., 441, *462*
Layne, D. S., 314, *324*
Leader, D. P., 329, 340, *347*, 434, *459*
Leavitt, W. W., 291, *322*
Lebleu, B., 441, *459*, *461*
Leblond, C. P., 41, *93*
Lee, C. S., 161, *223*
Lee, T. H., 285, *318*
Le Gal, Y., 4, 75, 77, *92*
Lehrman, D. S., 252, *275*
Leininger, K. R., 436, *460*
Lelong, J. C., 440, 441, *457*, *462*
Leng, R. A., 213, 215, *223*
Lengyel, P., 447, *459*

Leon, M., 264, *274*
Leonard, S. L., 119, *137*
Lerner, A M., 440, *459*
Leslie, L., 101, 111, *136*
Levin, R., 264, *274*
Levitskaya, E. S., 231, *268*
Levy, H. R., 353, 354, 370, 371, 384, 385, 393, *408*, *409*, *410*
Lewin, I., 418, *460*
Lewis, A. A., 100, 113, *137*, *138*
Lewis, G. P., 239, 240, *269*
Lewis, U. J., 279, 282, *322*, *325*
Li, C. H., 99, 119, 122, 123, 128, 131, *137*, 282, 298, 300, *318*, *322*, *323*, 333, *347*, 395, *409*, 414, *460*
Liao, S., 414, 436, *460*, *465*
Libby, P. R., 416, *460*
Liebelt, A. G., 88, *92*
Liebelt, R. A., 88, *92*
Liggins, G. C., 288, *322*
Lin, C. Y., 385, *409*
Lin, H. J., 352, 353, 354, 360, *407*
Lind, J., 173, *225*
Lindberg, U., 432, *456*
Lindell, T. J., 435, *455*
Lindner, H. R., 288, 289, *322*
Linkie, D. M., 119, *137*, 333, *347*
Lintzel, W., 170, *223*
Linzell, J. L., 46, 47, 61, 65, 66, 77, *93*, 95, 99, 101, *137*, 144, 146, 148, 149, 150, 151, 152, 153, 155, 158, 159, 160, 161, 163, 164, 165, 166, 168, 169, 170, 173, 174, 177, 178, 179, 180, 181, 182, 183, 184, 185, 186, 187, 188, 189, 191, 192, 193, 194, 195, 196, 197, 198, 199, 200, 201, 202, 203, 205, 207, 208, 209, 210, 211, 212, 213, 214, 215, 216, 217, 218, 219, *220*, *221*, *222*, *223*, *224*, 225, 228, 229, 231, 236, 237, 239, 255, 262, *269*, *272*, *273*, 285, 292, 307, *319*, *322*, *324*, 380, 386, 398, *409*, *411*
Lipmann, F., 441, *460*
Lipshitz-Wiesner, R., 450, 451, *462*
Littau, V. C., 436, *454*
Littauer, U. Z., 451, *455*, *463*
Liu, T. M. Y., 286, 287, 291, 292, *319*, 420, 421, *456*, *460*
Liu, W. K., 282, *322*

Lo, T. B., 282, *322*
Lockwood, D. H., 328, 334, 338, 340, 341, 342, 343, *347*, *348*, 418, *460*
Lodish, H. F., 453, *458*
Loeb, L., 11, *93*, 98, 108, *137*, 313, *322*
Loening, U. E., 432, *458*
London, I. M., 441, *457*
Long, J. A., 113, 118, *137*, *138*
Longmire, D. B., 100, *139*
Lorscheider, F. L., 310, 311, *322*, *324*
Lossow, W. J., 387, *409*
Low, R. B., 441, *465*
Lowenstein, J. M., 354, 386, 390, *408*, *409*, *410*, 418, 419, *459*
Lowry, O. H., 374, *410*
Lu, F. C., 238, *269*
Lu, H. H., 232, *269*
Lu, K. H., 249, 250, 258, *269*, 315, *322*
Lubsen, N. H., 441, *460*
Lucas-Lenard, J., 441, *460*
Ludwick, T. M., 189, *224*
Ludwick, T. W., 400, *407*
Lugášová, J., 229, *273*
Luick, J. R., 187, 213, *222*, *224*
Lukáš, Z., 164, *223*, 229, *273*
Lukášová, J., 164, *223*
Lumb, W. V., 194, *222*
Lynch, J., 124, *140*
Lyons, W. R., 99, 118, 122, 123, 124, 125, 128, 131, *135*, *137*, *138*, *139*, 281, 282, 284, 298, 300, *318*, *322*, *323*, *324*, 333, *347*, 395, *409*, 414, 417, *460*, *462*

M

McAllister, H. C., 340, *347*
McBride, O. W., 354, 387, *409*
McCann, S. M., 240, 246, 247, 248, 249, 250, 253, 254, 255, 258, 259, 260, 261, 262, *270*, *272*, *273*, *275*, 303, 315, *320*, *321*
McCarthy, B. J., 438, *456*
McCarthy, R. D., 188, *222*
McCarty, K. S., 340, *347*, 437, 441, *458*, *460*
McCay, C. M., 193, 213, *223*
MacCleod, R. M., 248, *273*
McClymont, G. L., 213, 218, *223*

Macdonald, G. J., 100, 125, *137*, *138*, 300, *323*
McDowall, F. H., 305, *319*
McGinty, D. A., 124, 125, *137*
McGlone, J., 313, *323*
McGuire, W. L., 436, 438, *460*, *461*
Mach, B., 440, 441, *455*, *462*
Machlin, L. J., 300, *323*
McIntosh, R. A., 148, 190, 193, *221*
McKennee, C. T., 246, 250, 258, *274*
McKenzie, L., 328, 338, *347*, 352, *409*, 418, 419, *460*
MacLaren, J. A., 128, *137*, 284, *321*
McLaurin, W. D., 284, *325*
McLean, P., 352, 353, 354, 359, 362, 364, 365, 366, 370, 381, 393, 395, 400, 405, 406, *408*, *409*, *411*, 419, *457*, *460*
MacLeod, R. M., 123, *138*
McMurtry, J. P., 119, 134, *138*, 244, 262, *273*
McNabb, J. D., 33, *94*
McNamara, A. L., 452, *463*
Maenpaa, P. H., 451, *460*
Magne, H., 146, 147, 192, 209, *222*
Mahler, H. R., 363, *409*
Maiweg, H., 239, 241, 242, 246, 247, 248, 249, 255, 258, 261, 264, 272, *274*, 298, *321*
Majumder, G. C., 329, 331, 346, *347*, 416, 437, 438, 444, *460*, *465*
Malkani, P. K., 250, *268*, 314, *322*
Malpress, F. H., 244, *271*, 352, *409*, 419, *460*
Man, E. B., 310, *325*
Mandel, J. L., 435, *456*, *459*
Mandel, P., 452, *457*
Mandell, J. D., 439, *460*
Manente, B. A., 159, *223*
Mansour, T. E., 374, *409*
Marbaix, G., 441, *459*, *461*
Marcker, K. A., 453, *463*
Marey, E. J., 193, *221*
Marinez, D. I., 353, 379, 394, *409*
Markov, G. G., 440, *464*
Marliss, E., 193, *221*
Marshall, F. H. A., 107, *137*
Martin, B. R., 387, *407*
Martin, D., Jr., 335, *347*, 435, *464*

Martin, R. J., 298, 312, *318*, 323, 352, 353, 360, 365, 392, 395, 396, 400, 402, 404, 405, *407*, *409*, 426, 431, 433, 436, 440, 444, 446, *455*, *460*

Martinet, J., 233, 255, *270*, 299, 300, *320*, 431, *456*

Martinez, C. M., 381, *409*

Martini, L., 251, *274*

Martins, T., 252, *273*

Marushige, K., 436, *455*

Marzluff, W. F., Jr., 340 *347*, 437, *460*

Massart, L., 189, *224*

Masson, G. M. C., 313, *318*

Matiash, U., 447, 449, 451, 452, *457*

Matsuhisa, T., 432, *458*

Matsui, S., 371, *408*

Matsuka, G. Kh., 447, 449, 451, 452, 454, *457*, *462*

Matsumoto, A., 85, *93*

Matthews, C. A., 99, 100, 109, 110, *138*

Matthies, D. L., 119, 128, *138*, 284, *323*, 417, *460*

Maurer, H. R., 340, *347*, 435, *456*

Maximow, A., 147, *223*

Mayer, G. P., 75, *93*, 100, *138*, 278, 312, *322*, *323*, 414, *460*

Maynard, L. A., 193, 213, *223*

Mayne, R., 340, *347*, 422, 423, 424, 433, 449, *460*

Meigs, E. B., 147, 148, *223*

Meihlac, M., 435, *456*

Meites, J., 11, *93*, 102, 122, 123, 124, 129, 134, *138*, *139*, 244, 245, 246, 248, 249, 250, 252, 253, 254, 256, 257, 258, 259, *268*, *269*, *273*, *274*, *275*, *276*, 278, 279, 281, 285, 286, 287, 288, 289, 291, 292, 293, 295, 296, 298, 299, 300, 301, 306, 309, 310, 313, 314, 315, *318*, *319*, *321*, *322*, *323*, *325*, *326*, 332, *346*, 420, 421, *460*, *463*

Melampy, R. M., 109, *137*, 291, *321*

Mellenberger, R. W., 352, 353, 354, 390, 393, 394, *409*

Mena, F., 232, 233, 234, 235, 237, 238, 239, 240, 241, 242, 244, 246, 247, 248, 249, 250, 251, 253, 254, 255, 256, 257, 258, 259, 260, 261, 262, 263, 264, 265, *268*, *269*, *272*, *274*, 292, 298, 301, 316, *321*

Mench, M. L., 102, 118, 119, *140*, 417, *465*

Mepham, T. B., 182, 184, 186, 189, 191, 195, 196, 203, 205, 207, 208, 209, 211, 212, 213, 214, 216, 217, 218, *222*, *223*, *224*

Mess, B., 251, *274*

Metcalfe, J., 194, *221*

Mialhe-Voloss, C., 288, *322*

Mical, R. S., 315, *321*

Michel, I., 434, *458*

Middleton, P., 438, *461*

Midgley, A. R., Jr., 248, *274*

Milkovic, K., 288, 289, *323*

Milkovic, S., 288, 289, *323*

Miller, A. L., 384, 385, *409*

Miller, G. H., 314, *323*

Miller, M. R., 228, *274*

Miller, W. R., 127, *136*

Milligan, L. P., 352, 353, 354, 367, 368, 371, 374, 376, 380, 381, 382, 386, 390, 393, *407*, 419, 425, *455*

Mills, E. S., 57, *93*, 328, 338, 339, 341, 343, *347*, 424, *460*

Minaguchi, H., 248, *269*, 289, *323*

Mirsky, A. E., 101, *138*, 436, *454*

Mishkinsky, J., 315, *324*

Mittelman, A., 451, *460*

Mixner, J. P., 100, 113, *138*

Miyawaki, H., 85, *93*

Mizuno, H., 240, *274*, 315, *323*, 427, 430, *460*

Mochrie, R. D., 101, *135*

Moffat, B., 284, *319*

Moger, W. H., 129, *139*

Mohren Weiser, H. W., 447, *455*

Moloney, J. B., 90, *93*

Moltz, H., 264, *274*

Momongan, V. G., 237, *274*, 305, *323*

Monier, R., 440, *462*

Monnet, C., 155, 203, *220*

Montagna, W., 228, *271*

Montagnier, L., 440, *460*

Montjar, M., 433, *464*

Moon, R. C., 124, 125, 129, 131, *138*, 300, 308, *318*, *323*, 425, *460*

Moore, D. H., 84, 87, 88, 89, *91*, *93*, *94*

Moore, G., 33, *94*

Moore, L. A., 309, *323*

Morag, M., 240, *274*, 299, *323*
Morel, C., 439, *462*
Moriconi, A., 159, *224*
Morre, D. J., 63, *93*
Morris, B., 186, *223*
Morris, J. A., 313, *323*
Morris, L. J., 214, *220*
Morris, P. W., 435, *455*
Motta, M., 251, *274*
Mount, L. E., 153, *223*
Muecke, W., 435, *459*
Mueller, G. C., 414, *460*
Munford, R. E., 11, *93*, 100, 102, 110, *138*, 305, *319*, 389, 390, 391, *409*, 418, 419, *460*
Munro, A. J., 440, *460*
Munro, H. N., 435, 447, *458, 459*
Murad, T. M., 4, 75, *93*
Murray, M. R., 101, 103, 131, 132, 133, *137*
Mushinki, J. F., 451, *460*
Myers, B., 87, *91, 94*
Myers, J. A., 109, *138*

N

Nagasawa, H., 102, 109, 110, 111, 116, 117, 119, *138, 140*, 247, *276*, 284, 289, 299, 300, *323, 326*, 417, 418, 419, *460, 465*
Naito, M., 299, 300, *319, 323*
Nallar, R., 260, *272*
Nandi, S., 4, 6, 19, *93, 95*, 106, 129, 131, 132, 133, *137*, 281, 282, 285, *323, 327*, 345, *347*, 414, *461*
Naora, H., 441, *461*
Narayanan, R., 352, 353, *409*
Nasarenko, I., 447, 449, 451, 452, *457*
Nass, M. M. K., 454, *455*
Negro-Vilar, A., 248, 249, *276*
Neil, J. D., 279, *323*
Nelson, D. R., 352, 353, 354, 390, 393, 394, *409*
Nelson, W. L., 101, 111, 117, 120, *138*, 419, 426, *461*
Nelson, W. O., 281, *323*
Neumann, F., 104, 127, *136, 138*
Neutra, M., 41, *93*
Nevaldine, B. H., 370, 371, *409*
Newsome, J. F., 245, *270*

Newton, M., 238, *274*, 296, *323*
Newton, N. R., 238, *274*
Newton, W. H., 118, *138*, 284, *323*
Neyland, M., 229, *271*
Niall, H. D., 284, *319*
Nichols, B. W., 210, 214, *220*
Nichols, C. W., 284, *324*
Nicoll, C. S., 246, 248, 249, 250, 252, 254, 256, 257, 258, *268, 271, 273, 274*, 281, 284, 285, 296, 298, 299, 306, 309, *323, 324, 325*, 420, 421, *463*
Nicoll, C. W., 246, *274*
Niggli-Stokar, U., Von., 228, *274*
Nikitovitch-Winer, M., 245, 250, *271, 274*
Nir, I., 315, *324*
Nirembert, M., 453, *456*
Nisbet, A. M., 159, *224*
Nishimura, S., 453, *461, 463*
Nishinakagawa, H., 155, 156, 203, *224*
Nishizuka, Y., 85, *93*
Niswender, G. D., 119, *137*, 285, *319*, 333, *347*
Niswender, G. P., 248, *274*
Noel, G. L., 302, *320*
Noll, H., 439, 445, 446, *461, 463, 465*
Nomura, M., 440, *457*
Norgren, A., 414, 443, *456, 461*
Novelli, G. D., 450, 451, *461, 463, 465*
Novinski, W. W., 67, *94*

O

Oberling, C., 84, 85, *91*
Ochoa, S., 379, *410*
Ogata, K., 447, *463*
Ojala, D., 432, *454*
Oka, T., 132, *139*, 328, 329, 330, 331, 332, 333, 334, 338, 339, 340, 341, 342, 343, 344, 345, 346, *347, 348*
Olson, D. E., 63, *93*
O'Malley, B. W., 436, 438, 450, *456, 460, 461*
O'Neil, P., 371, *410*
Opstvedt, J., 352, 353, 354, *410*
Orahovats, D., 190, *220*
Orias, R., 253, *275*
Orrenius, S., 4, 72, 73, *92*
Osman, L. M., 288, *325*
Ota, K., 234, 252, 254, 255, *274, 276*,

291, 316, *324, 326,* 397, *411,* 418, 420, 421, *461, 462, 463*
Otero-Vilardebo, L. R., 41, *93*
Ott, I., 98, *138*
Oura, M., 445, *463*
Owen, E. C., 301, *324*
Owens, I. S., 328, 335, 336, 338, 343, 345, 346, *348*
Oxender, W. D., 285, *324,* 352, 353, 354, 390, 394, *410*
Oyaert, W., 231, *274, 275*
Oyer, D., 441, *465*
Ozawa, H., 334, *347*

P

Paape, M. J., 119, *136,* 241, 258, *274, 275,* 295, 301, 306, 313, 316, 317, *324, 326,* 415, 416, 417, 425, 426, 428, 429, 430, *456, 461, 464*
Pace, N., 416, 426, *459*
Pacheco, P., 233, 254, *269*
Padgett, F., 88, *91*
Paek, S., 35, *91*
Pagoulatos, G. N., 432, *456*
Pahl, I. R., 314, *318*
Palade, G. E., 19, 41, 45, 49, *92, 93*
Palic, D., 155, *224*
Palmiter, R. D., 328, 334, 338, 340, *348,* 418, 423, 424, *461*
Panda, J. N., 126, *138*
Paniagua, M., 314, *324*
Pankov, Y. A., 282, *322*
Panyim, S., 437, *461*
Pardue, F. E., 100, *139*
Parker, J. T., 194, *221*
Parkinson, R. D., 237, *276*
Parrot, D. M. V., 262, *269*
Parsons, J. A., 284, *324*
Parsons, J. T., 246, 250, 258, *274*
Passonneau, J. V., 374, *410*
Pasteels, J. L., 246, *274,* 282, *324*
Patel, M. D., 262, *274*
Paterson, J. Y. F., 217, *224,* 288, 289, 307, *324*
Patton, S., 63, *93*
Pavlov, E. F., 231, 237, *268, 276*
Pavlov, G. N., 231, *268*
Paymaster, J. C., 87, *93*

Peacock, A. C., 343, *347,* 438, 439, 450, *456, 458, 461*
Peaker, M., 61, 65, 66, *95,* 158, 182, 184, 188, 189, 205, 209, 217, 218, *223, 224*
Pearlman, W. H., 124, *137*
Peeters, G., 165, 182, 184, 186, 189, 207, 212, *221, 222,* 231, 237, *270, 274, 275*
Pegg, A. E., 436, *461*
Pencharz, R. I., 118, *138*
Penman, S., 432, *461*
Perlman, S., 432, *461*
Perrin, D. R., 237, *276*
Perry, J. S., 291, *321*
Perry, R. E., 445, *461*
Perry, R. P., 432, 445, *461*
Peskett, G. L., 148, 192, *221*
Peterkofsky, A., 451, *456, 461*
Peters, R. A., 194, *220*
Petersen, W. E., 67, *93,* 148, 149, 182, 184, 189, 191, 193, *221, 224, 225,* 236, 238, 240, 244, *270, 271, 275,* 305, 308, 309, *318, 322*
Petre, J., 441, *461*
Petrissant, G., 447, 448, 449, 452, 453, *461*
Pfeiffer, S. E., 335, *348*
Pharris, B. B., 291, *324*
Philp, J. R., 4, 39, 43, *95*
Phillips, G. R., 447, *461*
Pica-Mattocia, L., 432, *454*
Picciano, D. J., 441, *462*
Pickles, V. R., 173, 174, 183, *224*
Pilkis, S. J., 365, 366, *408, 410*
Pincus, G., 314, *321, 324*
Pirro, G., 451, *457*
Pitelka, D. R., 4, 6, 11, 15, 19, 21, 51, 69, 71, 72, 75, 77, 79, 85, *94, 95,* 101, 105, *135,* 188, *224,* 328, *348,* 352, 354, *410*
Plager, J. E., 289, *324*
Planterose, D. N., 443, *463*
Ponto, K. H., 353, 379, *410*
Popjak, G., 212, *224*
Popovici, D. G., 233, *275*
Porte, A., 4, 75, 77, *92*
Porter, J. C., 246, *275,* 315, *321*
Porter, J. E., 371, *411*
Posner, M., 131, *138*
Potter, M. P., 451, *460*

Potter, V. R., 439, 442, *455*
Poulton, B. R., 287, *324*
Powell, R. C., 191, *224*
Pozefsky, T., 193, *221*
Pragnell, I. B., 441, *461*
Price, S. M., 189, 209, *222*
Pritchard, D. E., 301, 316, *326*, 425, 426, *462, 464*
Pritchard, M. J., 441, *461*
Pritchard, M. L., 255, *270*
Pritchard, M. S., 441, *461*
Pritchard, P. M., 441, *456, 462*
Prop, F. J. A., 327, *348*
Puca, G. A., 124, *138*
Puget, E., 155, *224*
Puissant, C., 453, *461*
Purves, H. D., 251, *268*

Q

Quijada, M., 251, 258, *273*
Quinn, D. L., 250, *271, 275*
Quintero, C. A., 230, *269*

R

Rabinowitz, D., 169, *222*
Raggi, F., 153, 169, 179, 193, 194, 207, 208, 213, 219, *222*, 312, *322*
Ragsdale, A. C., 317, *324*
Raijman, L., 375, *411*
Raineri, R. R., 353, 354, 370, 371, *409, 410*
Rajbhandary, U. L., 453, *458, 462*
Ramano, B., 436, *455*
Ramberg, C. F., 153, 169, 179, 193, 194, 207, 208, 213, 219, *222*
Ramirez, V. D., 249, 250, *270, 275*, 314, *319*
Ramwell, P. W., 183, *224*
Ranadive, K., 6, *94*
Randel, R. D., 290, 291, *320, 321*
Randle, P. J., 366, 387, *407, 408*
Rao, S. S., 314, *321*
Rasmussen, F., 165, 168, 169, 177, 179, 182, 185, *224*
Ratner, A., 246, 250, 257, *275*
Ray, E. W., 118, 128, *135, 138*, 284, *324*, 417, *462*
Ray, W. J., Jr., 367, *410*

Raynaud, A., 103, 104, *138*, 414, *462*
Reddy, R. R., 294, *324*
Redfield, B., 453, *456*
Redman, C. M., 45, 94, 447, *462*
Reece, R. P., 11, *94*, 100, 101, 102, 111, 114, 120, 125, *137, 138, 139*, 247, 253, 256, 258, *269, 275*, 278, 279, 280, 281, 285, 286, 287, 292, 295, 296, 298, 300, 301, 309, 316, 317, *319, 323, 324, 326*, 416, 417, 419, 425, 428, 429, 430, *464*
Rees, E. D., 352, 353, 354, *410*
Reich, E., 433, 440, *462*
Reichert, L. E., 285, *319*
Reichlin, S., 134, *136*, 285, *324*
Rein, G., 98, *138*
Reineke, E. P., 191, *224*, 308, 309, 310, 311, *318, 320, 321, 322, 324, 325*
Reiner, J. M., 363, *410*
Reithel, F. J., 53, *91*
Relkin, R., 264, *275*
Rens, W., 165, *222*
Revel, M., 441, *458, 462*
Reynaert, H., 184, *224*
Reynolds, M., 165, 168, 174, 177, 181, 182, 186, *224*, 278, 280, *324*
Rice-Wray, E., 300, *323*, 333, *347*
Richard, P. H., 233, *275*
Richards, A. H., 371, *410*
Richards, M. P. M., 244, *275*
Richardson, K. C., 77, *94*, '100, *138*, 439, *459*
Richardson, R. C., 236, *275*
Richlik, I., 433, *463*
Richter, J., 313, *324*
Richterich, B., 101, 111, *139*
Ricordeau, G., 426, 427, *462*
Riddle, M., 340, *348*, 437, 438, 439, 443, 444, 445, 454, *464, 465*
Rigor, T. V., 67, *93*
Riis, P. M., 213, *224*
Ringler, I., 128, *136*
Ris, H., 101, *138*
Rivera, E. M., 101, 129, 131, 132, 133, *136, 138*, 338, 339, 340, *347, 348*, 400, *410*, 422, 423, 424, 433, 449, 457, *460, 462*
Riviere, M. R., 85, *92*
Robberson, D. L., 432, *454*
Roberts, J. S., 237, *275*

Robertson, J. M., 312, *322*
Robertson, L. L., 122, *135*
Robinson, D. S., 213, 214, *220*, 354, 387, *410*
Robinson, R., 290, *324*
Robison, B., 448, *462*
Roderig, H., 308, *318*
Roeder, R. G., 435, *462*
Rogers, E. B., 190, *220*
Rogers, F. M., 416, 418, 427, *455*
Rogers, M. E., 432, *458*
Rogg, H., 453, *463*
Rohr, H., 4, 43, 45, 56, *94*
Ronning, M., 352, 353, 354, 360, *407*, *410*
Rook, J. A. F., 191, 207, 212, *225*, 312, *324*
Rosbash, M., 432, *461*
Roscelli, G. A., 367, *410*
Rosenblatt, J. S., 134, *138*, 244, 252, 262, *275*
Rosenbloom, I., 122, *136*
Rosenthal, H. E., 288, *324*
Rosset, R., 440, *462*
Roth, L. L., 134, *138*, 244, 262, *275*
Rothballer, A. B., 251, *272*
Rothchild, I., 253, 255, *275*
Roussel, J. D., 314, *324*
Rowland, S. J., 305, *320*
Rushmer, R. D., 171, *221*
Rushmer, R. F., 171, *225*
Russell, H., 371, *410*
Russell, R. L., 451, *457*
Rutter, W. J., 435, *455*, *462*
Rychlik, I., 421, 427, *463*
Ryšánek, D., 164, *223*

S

Saacke, R. G., 353, *410*
Sabatini, D. D., 45, *94*, 447, *462*
Saez, F. A., 67, *94*
Sagher, D., 436, *460*
Saito, M., 246, 258, *268*, 365, *410*
Sajdel, E. M., 435, *459*
Sakamoto, Y., 432, *458*
Sakuma, M., 284, *324*
Samuels, H. H., 435, *464*
Sanadi, D. R., 451, *465*
Sandberg, A. A., 288, 289, *324*

Sandborn, E., 33, *94*
Sander, S., 123, *138*, *139*
Sandholm, L. E., 314, *318*
Sapirstein, L. A., 172, 173, 181, *224*
Sar, M., 248, 253, *269*, *275*, *276*, 288, 306, 310, *324*, *326*
Sarin, P. C., 448, *462*
Sarkar, N. H., 84, 87, 88, 89, *93*, *94*
Sartirana, M. L., 432, *458*
Sato, G., 131, *138*
Sato, S., 365, *410*
Satoh, K., 240, *274*
Saunders, F. J., 314, *324*
Sawyer, C. H., 232, 249, 254, *268*, *272*, 273
Schäfer, A., 4, *91*, *94*
Schaefgen, D. A., 246, 254, 257, 258, 260, 272
Schalch, D. S., 285, *324*
Schalm, O. W., 190, *225*
Schambye, P., 187, *225*
Schams, D., 285, *324*
Schanbacher, F. L., 294, *325*
Schaper, A., 165, *222*
Schapira, G., 441, *459*
Scharf, G., 125, *139*
Scherrer, K., 439, *462*
Scherle, W. F., 53, *94*
Schimke, R. T., 364, *408*
Schjeide, O. A., 438, *458*
Schlegel, W., 171, *221*
Schlein, P. A., 263, *276*
Schlom, J., 87, *94*
Schmalbeck, J., 4, 43, 45, 56, *94*
Schmidt, C. F., 168, 169, *222*
Schmidt, G. H., 102, 124, 129, *139*, 237, *274*, 305, 309, 312, *323*, *324*, *325*, 377, 378, *410*, 416, 417, 418, 420, 421, 428, 432, 444, *463*
Schmidt, K. D., 282, *322*
Schober, N. A., 360, 396, 400, 402, 405, *407*, 433, 436, *455*
Schoefl, G. I., 214, *224*
Scholz, H. R., 288, *325*
Schoner, W., 376, *410*
Schreiber, G., 441, 442, *462*
Schultze, A. B., 98, *140*
Schulze-Wethmar, F. H., 387, *411*
Schurman, M., 387, *407*

Schweizer, M., 281, *323*
Scott, J. C., 98, *137*
Scow, R. O., 214, *220*, 354, 387, *408*
Scrutton, M. C., 388, *410*
Seal, U. S., 288, *325*
Segal, H. L., 403, *410*
Seitter, U., 4, 43, 45, 56, *94*
Sekhri, K. K., 4, 6, 11, 15, 19, 21, 51, 69, 71, 72, 75, 77, *94*, 101, *139*, 328, *348*
Selby, F. W., 279, *325*
Seldinger, S. I., 193, 196, *224*
Selenkow, H. A., 284, *326*
Self, D. J., 438, *464*
Selinger, R. C. L., 330, *348*
Sells, B. H., 451, *459*
Selye, H., 118, *139*, 243, 253, 256, 257, 275, 281, 297, 313, *318*, *325*
Seman, G., 87, *91*, *94*
Semenova, N., 447, 449, 451, 452, *457*, *462*
Semm, K., 314, *325*
Sensui, N., 315, *323*
Setchell, B. P., 173, 181, 182, *221*, *224*
Sethi, V. S., 435, *462*
Seubert, W., 376, *410*
Shafritz, D. A., 441, 453, *454*, *456*, *462*
Sham, G. B., 165, *224*
Shani, J., 299, 315, *323*, *325*, 417, *462*
Share, L., 237, *275*
Sharma, O. K., 450, 451, *462*
Shatkin, A. J., 433, *462*
Shatton, J. B., 352, 368, *410*, 419, *462*
Shaw, G. H., 309, *325*
Shaw, J. C., 148, 183, 189, 191, 193, 213, *222*, *224*, *225*, 305, *325*
Shaw, J. E., 183, *224*
Shay, H., 352, 368, *410*, 419, *462*
Sheard, N. M., 252, *276*
Sherwood, L. M., 284, *325*
Shiada, Y., 397, *411*
Shiiba, N., 240, *274*
Shimizu, H., 101, 111, *139*, 416, 425, *462*
Shimizu, S., 234, *268*
Shinde, Y., 291, *326*, 418, 420, 430, *461*, *462*, *463*
Shirhama, S., 85, *92*
Shirley, J. G., 352, 353, 354, 390, 394, *410*
Shugart, L., 451, *463*

Sidhu, K. S., 387, *407*
Siess, E., 387, *411*
Silver, J. A., 13, *94*
Silverman, D. A., 414, *465*
Silverstein, G., 434, *458*
Simon, S., 379, *410*
Simpson, A. A., 102, *139*, 377, 378, *410*, 420, 421, 432, 444, *463*
Simpson, M. V., 454, *457*
Singh, D. V., 100, 129, 131, 132, 133, *139*
Singh, O. N., 310, *324*
Singh, R. N. P., 282, *322*
Sinha, K. N., 419, *463*
Sinha, Y. N., 107, 108, 109, 110, 111, 117, 120, *139*, 248, 258, 275, 278, 279, 282, 295, 301, 306, 313, 316, *322*, *325*, *326*, 415, 416, 417, 425, 428, *461*, *463*, *464*
Sirakov, L., 421, 427, 433, *463*
Sirsat, S. M., 87, *91*, *93*
Sitte, H., 53, *94*
Siu, P., 187, *225*
Sjöstrand, F. S., 63, *94*
Skarda, J., 400, *408*, 434, *458*
Slater, T. F., 101, 111, *136*, 353, 388, *408*, *410*, 419, 425, 427, 429, 440, 443, *458*, *463*, *465*
Slaunwhite, W. R., 288, 289, *324*
Sloviter, H. A., 308, *318*
Smith, A., 316, *326*
Smith, A. E., 453, *455*, *463*
Smith, C. R., 196, *221*
Smith, G. H., 85, *94*
Smith, K. L., 294, *325*
Smith, L. W., 314, *325*, *326*
Smith, N. E., 240, *269*, 362, 363, 379, 398, *407*
Smith, P. E., 98, *139*
Smith, R. E., 25, 26, 35, *94*
Smith, S., 188, *220*, *224*, 352, 353, 354, 382, 385, *410*
Smith, T. C., 101, 111, *139*
Smith, V. G., 286, 293, 302, 306, *319*, *325*, 425, 429, *463*
Smith, V. R., 67, *94*
Smith, W. C., 452, *463*
Smitt, M. C., 248, *273*
Smoller, C. G., 85, *94*
Smuckler, E. A., 435, *463*

Snedecor, G. W., 208, *225*
Snell, G. D., 332, *347*
Snyder, S. H., 315, *325*
Soderman, D. D., 364, 365, *409*
Sod-Moriah, U. A., 102, *139*, 416, 418, *463*
Soeldner, J. S., 284, *326*
Söll, D., 447, 448, *459*, *463*
Soemarwoto, I. N., 156, *225*
Sokol, D. M., 378, *408*
Sonksen, P. H., 284, *326*
Sorm, F., 433, *463*
Spellacy, W. N., 304, *325*
Spencer, A. F., 354, *410*
Spiegelman, S., 87, *94*
Spincer, J., 191, 207, 212, *225*
Spirin, A. S., 439, *463*
Spohr, G., 439, *462*
Srivastava, L. S., 126, 134, *139*, 312, *325*
Srukov, M. N., 155, *225*
Staehelin, M., 448, 453, *459*, *463*
Staehelin, T., 439, 445, 446, *461*, *463*, *465*
Stedman, E., 436, *463*
Stegall, R. F., 171, *225*
Stein, H., 435, *463*
Stein, O., 43, 51, *94*
Stein, Y., 43, 51, *94*
Stellwagen, R. H., 437, *463*
Stent, G. S., 451, *463*
Sterling, K., 310, *325*
Stern, R., 451, *463*
Stewart, C. P., 288, *325*
Stielau, W. J., 372, *407*
Stiles, E. P., 340, *347*
Stirewalt, W. S., 441, *465*
Stirling, J. D., 147, 192, 193, *220*
Stockdale, F. E., 132, 133, *139*, 328, 333, 335, 339, 340, 341, 343, 345, *347*, *348*, 422, 423, 434, *459*, *463*
Stocker, J. F., 290, *326*
Stockinger, L., 4, 65, *94*
Stoliaroff, M., 253, *270*, 306, *320*, 425, 430, 431, *456*
Stonecipher, W. D., 191, *224*
Storrie, B., 432, *454*
Storry, J. E., 312, *324*
Streicher, M. H., 241, *271*
Stricker, P., 98, *139*, 281, *325*

Strinivasan, P. R., 451, *455*
Strong, L. C., 109, *136*
Stubbs, M., 376, *410*
Stulberg, M. P., 451, *463*
Stumpf, W. E., 124, *139*, 329, 330, *347*
Stutinsky, F., 234, 235, *275*, 288, 289, *321*, *322*, *455*
Sud, S. C., 102, 124, *139*, 293, *325*
Sueoka, N., 450, 451, *463*
Sulman, F. G., 135, *139*, 287, 299, 308, 314, 315, *318*, *323*, *324*, 417, *462*
Sutter, N., 108, *139*
Suzuki, T., 329, 330, *347*
Svobodova, J., 289, 307, *322*
Swanson, E. W., 100, *139*, 311, *325*
Swanson, L. V., 279, *325*
Swett, W. W., 99, 100, 109, 110, *138*, *139*
Sykes, J. A., 88, *91*
Sykes, J. F., 134, *139*, 301, *326*
Szepesi, B., 403, *410*

T

Tabaschnik, I. I. A., 253, *275*
Takagi, M., 447, *463*
Takeishi, K., 453, *463*
Taketa, K., 371, *410*
Taleisnik, S., 238, 239, 253, *275*
Talwalker, P. K., 122, *139*, 246, *274*, 281, 285, 286, 298, 306, 315, *323*, *325*, 420, 421, *460*, *463*
Tambiah, R., *455*
Tanahashi, N., 334, *346*
Tanaka, J., 447, *463*
Tarten, M., 190, *225*
Tartof, K. D., 432, 445, *461*
Tata, J. R., 414, 432, 435, 436, 438, 444, *463*, *464*, *465*
Tatum, E. L., 433, 440, *462*
Tavenor, W. D., 196, *225*
Taylor, D. J., 87, *91*
Taylor, M. W., 451, *458*
Taylor, N. W., 451, *464*
Temmerman, J., 441, *459*
Tepperman, H. M., 414, *464*
Tepperman, J., 414, *464*
Terminn, Y., 234, 235, *275*

Thatcher, W. W., 296, 298, 299, 300, 301, 303, 304, 306, 307, 316, *325, 326,* 425, 428, *464*

Thayer, S. A., 416, 417, *464*

Thibodeau, P. S., 416, 417, *464*

Thomas, J. B., 104, *139*

Thomas, J. W., 302, 309, *319, 325,* 353, 354, 379, 387, *407, 410,* 427, 447, *455, 465*

Thompson, E. B., 435, *464*

Thomson, D. L., 118, *139,* 243, 253, 256, 257, *275,* 281, 297, *325*

Thorburn, G. D., 278, 285, 288, *318*

Tiemeier, D., 381, *409*

Tindal, J. S., 189, *225,* 232, 233, 234, 235, 236, 244, 245, 251, 254, 255, 256, *268, 270, 275,* 289, 297, 305, 315, *319, 325*

Tobey, E. R., 99, *136*

Tolbukhin, V. I., 231, *268*

Tomkins, G. M., 335, *347,* 435, *464*

Tomov, T., 300, *325*

Tonelli, G., 128, *136*

Tonoue, T., 451, *464*

Topper, Y. J., 57, *93,* 105, 106, 128, 132, 133, *139, 140,* 188, *225,* 280, 284, 292, *325, 326,* 328, 329, 330, 331, 332, 333, 334, 335, 336, 337, 338, 339, 340, 341, 342, 343, 344, 345, 346, *347, 348,* 417, 418, 422, 423, 424, 434, *458, 459, 460, 463, 464*

Toty, M., 155, *224*

Towers, K. G., 191, 207, 212, *225*

Trakatellis, A. C., 433, *464*

Tramezzani, H. J., 251, *273*

Traurig, H. H., 11, *94,* 389, *410,* 418, *464*

Trentin, J. J., 124, *139,* 253, *275*

Trujillo, J. M., 371, *410*

Tsakhaev, G. A., 183, *225,* 231, 233, 255, *268, 275, 276*

Tsanev, R. G., 440, *464*

Tuan, D. Y. H., 436, *455*

Tucker, H. A., 101, 102, 107, 108, 109, 110, 111, 114, 119, 120, 124, *136, 139,* 248, 258, 262, *275,* 278, 279, 280, 285, 287, 292, 293, 294, 295, 296, 298, 299, 300, 301, 302, 303, 304, 306, 307, 309, 313, 315, 316, 317, *319, 320,* 322, *324, 325, 326,* 415, 416, 417, 419, 425, 426,

428, 429, 430, *456, 458, 461, 462, 463, 464*

Turkington, R. W., 105, 128, 133, *139,* 188, *225,* 284, 291, 293, *326,* 328, 329, 330, 331, 334, 335, 338, 340, 341, 342, 343, 345, 346, *347, 348,* 418, 422, 424, 432, 433, 434, 435, 436, 437, 438, 439, 443, 444, 445, 448, 449, 450, 453, 454, *460, 464, 465*

Turner, C. W., 97, 98, 99, 100, 101, 102, 103, 104, 105, 107, 110, 111, 113, 114, 115, 116, 117, 119, 120, 122, 123, 124, 125, 126, 127, 128, 129, 130, 131, 134, *135, 136, 137, 138, 139, 140,* 191, 194, *222, 224,* 237, 244, 253, 256, 257, 258, 259, 260, *272, 273, 274, 275, 276,* 281, 285, 287, 288, 292, 293, 294, 295, 298, 300, 301, 304, 305, 306, 308, 309, 310, 311, 312, 313, 317, *318, 320, 321, 322, 323, 324, 325, 326,* 417, 418, 419, 421, 425, 429, *454, 455, 459, 463*

Turner, E. W., 426, *459*

Turner, G. D., 124, *140*

Turvey, A., 234, 235, 244, 251, 254, *270, 275,* 298, *319*

Tuttle, J. P., 365, *410*

Tuyttens, N., 237, *270*

Tverskoi, G. B., 231, 237, 254, 255, *268, 276*

Twarog, J. M., 188, *225*

Tyrrell, H. F., 309, *325*

Tyson, J. E., 302, *326*

U

Ukita, T., 453, *463*

Ulloa, A., 104, *136*

Urban, I., 233, *275*

Urquhart, J., 289, *326*

Utter, M. F., 388, *410*

V

Vaidya, A. B., 87, *91, 93*

Vanaman, T. C., 328, 334, 338, 342, *346, 348,* 434, 435, *464*

Van Der Hoeven, E., 4, 79, *94*

Vanderlaan, W. P., 279, 282, 322, *325*

Van der Lee, S., 262, *276*

van der Molen, H. J., 314, *323*

Van der Werff ten Bosch, J. J., 254, *270*, 426, *457*

Van Leersum, E. C., 194, *225*

van Rensburg, S. J., 288, *324*

van Tienhoven, A., 105, *140*

Van Wyk, J. J., 245, *270*

Varma, K., 284, *326*

Varma, S. K., 284, *326*

Veech, R. L., 359, 362, 375, 376, 380, 388, *409*, *410*, *411*

Vendrely, C., 101, *135*

Vendrely, R., 101, *135*

Verbeke, R., 184, 207, 212, *224*, 225

Verley, J. M., 4, 5, 12, 13, 14, 17, 21, 25, 37, 39, 41, 43, 55, 57, 58, 59, 60, 68, 69, 71, 72, 73, 75, 76, 77, 79, 84, 85, 87, 88, *92*, *93*, *94*, 444, *458*

Verschooten, F., 165, 182, *221*, 222

Vesell, E. S., 377, *411*

Viennot, N., 439, 446, *457*

Visscher, M. B., 189, *224*

Vladimirova, A. D., 155, 165, 173, *225*

von Berswordt-Wallrabe, R., 104, 127, 130, 131, *138*, *140*, 300, 308, 311, 312, *318*

Vonderhaar, B. K., 328, 335, 336, 337, 338, 342, 345, 346, *348*

von Haam, E., *93*

Von Tigerstrom, M., 453, *457*

Voogt, J. L., 248, 249, 250, 253, 258, *269*, 276, 288, 306, 326

Vorherr, H., 239, 240, *276*

Voytovich, A. E., 106, *140*, 331, 343, *348*

Vrbová, G., 184, *222*

Vuorenkoski, V., 173, *225*

W

Wada, H., 111, 116, 130, *140*

Wagner, G., 237, *271*

Wagner, H. N., 169, *222*

Wagner, W. C., 288, *318*

Wahl, H. M., 100, *140*, 155, *225*

Waites, G. M. H., 182, *224*

Wakabayashi, I., 246, 258, *268*

Waksman, S. A., 433, *465*

Walden, B., 371, *410*

Walker, P. M. B., 438, *465*

Walker, R. J., 418, *455*

Wallace, A. L. C., 285, *318*

Wallace, J. M., 440, *465*

Wals, P. A., 361, 375, 383, *408*

Walsh, J. P., 316, *326*

Walters, E., 352, 353, 354, 364, 365, 366, 370, 395, 400, 406, *411*

Wang, D. Y., 388, *410*, 418, 419, 423, 424, 427, 429, 433, 440, *456*, *458*, *463*, 465

Ward, O. T., 340, 342, 343, *348*, 435, 436, *465*

Warner, J. R., 441, *465*

Warner, R. G., 309, *325*

Warrington, R. C., 453, *457*

Wasz-Hockert, O., 173, *225*

Watanabe, A., 371, *410*

Watkins, W. M., 209, *225*, 334, *348*

Watson, P. S., 313, *326*

Watson, S. C., 282, *319*

Waugh, D. F., 4, 39, 79, *94*

Weatherford, H. L., 100, *140*, 241, *271*

Weaver, R. F., 435, *455*

Wehrli, H., 453, *463*

Weibel, E. R., 53, *94*

Weinberg, F., 435, *455*

Weinberg, R., 432, *461*

Weinhouse, S., 352, 368, *410*, 419, *462*

Weinstein, I. B., 451, 452, 453, *454*, *455*, *457*, *459*, *465*

Weirich, W. E., 196, *225*

Weisbach, H., 453, *456*

Weiss, R., 190, *220*

Weller, C. P., 287, *318*

Wellings, S. R., 4, 37, 39, 43, 51, 68, 71, 72, 75, 79, 85, *95*, 338, *348*, 430, *465*

Welsch, C. W., 248, 249, *276*

Welsch, U., 4, 33, 37, 39, 43, 65, 77, *91*, 444, *455*

West, C. E., 153, 174, 178, 185, 191, 195, 196, 203, 207, 208, 210, 211, 212, 213, 214, 215, 216, *220*, 223, *225*, 386, *411*

Westphal, U., 288, 289, 292, 306, 307, 309, *320*, *321*

Wettstein, F. O., 439, 445, 446, *461*, *463*, *465*

Wettstein, I. B., 453, *461*

Whaley, W. G., 53, *95*

Wheelock, J. V., 312, 316, *324*, *326*

White, F. C., 165, *224*

White, W. D., 332, *346*

Whitten, W. K., 262, 263, *276*

Whittlestone, W. G., 237, 238, *276*
Wickman, J., 421, *465*
Wicks, W. D., 440, *458, 465*
Widnell, L. L., 436, *465*
Wieland, O., 387, *411*
Wiesner, B. P., 252, *276*
Wiley, C. E., 364, 365, *409*
Will, J. A., 196, *225*
William, W. C., 87, *94*
Williams, C. A., 447, *457*
Williams, K. I. H., 314, *324*
Williams, R., 104, 110, 124, 127, *136, 140*
Williams, W. C., 88, *92*
Williams, W. F., 124, *140*
Williams, W. L., 253, 272, *276*
Williams-Ashman, H. G., 414, *465*
Williamson, J. R., 359, 362, *411*
Williamson, M. B., 191, *224*
Willmer, J. S., 353, 395, 401, *411*, 426, *465*
Wilmot, L., 438, *458*
Wilson, D. B., 453, *465*
Wilson, G. F., 305, *319*
Wilson, J. E., 365, *410*
Winton, B., 387, *411*
Witschi, E., 262, *276*
Woessner, J. F., 429, *465*
Wolf, R. C., 288, *326*
Wolfe, R. G., 373, *408*
Wood, H. G., 187, *225*, 372, 373, 375, *386, 408, 411*
Wood, W. A., 447, *455*
Wooding, F. B. P., 4, 51, 61, 63, 64, 65, 66, *95*
Wool, I. G., 441, *465*
Wrenn, T. R., 102, 118, 119, 134, *139, 140*, 301, *326*, 417, *465*
Wuntch, T., 377, *411*
Wymenga, H. G., 314, *323*
Wyngarden, L. J., 291, *324*

Y

Yagil, R., 299, *323*

Yamamoto, H., 124, 125, *140*
Yamamoto, L., 279, *321*
Yanai, R., 111, 116, 117, 119, *140*, 247, *276*, 284, 301, *326*, 417, 418, *465*
Yang, S. S., 451, *465*
Yang, W. K., 451, *465*
Yates, F. E., 289, *326*
Yokoyama, A., 234, 252, 254, 255, *274*, *276*, 291 316, *324*, *326*, 397, *411*, 418, 420, 421, 430, *461, 462, 463*
Yoshinaga, K., 290, *326*
Young, D. M., 310, *319*
Young, F. G., 299, 305, *319, 320*
Young, W. T., 371, *411*
Yousef, I. M., 427, *465*
Yunghans, W. N., 63, *93*

Z

Zachau, H. G., 447, *465*
Zaks, M. G., 231, 236, 237, *268, 276*
Zambrano, D., 249, *276*
Zamecnik, P. C., 448, *462*
Zanbelman, L., 417, *462*
Zanotti, D. B., 102, *137*
Zarrow, M. X., 263, *276*
Zarzicki, J., 4, 65, *94*
Zeilmaker, G. H., 67, *95*
Zelljadt, I., 85, *91*
Ziegler, H., 185, *225*
Zierler, K. L., 145, 169, 192, *222, 225*
Zietzschmann, O., 155, *225*
Zimbelman, R. G., 314, *326*
Zimmerman, E. F., 440, *465*
Zimmerman, T. P., 448, *462*
Zolman, J., 302, *319*
Zotikova, I. N., 231, *268*
Zuminiger, K., 240, *268*
Zweifach, B. W., 159, *225*
Zweig, M., 315, *325*
Zylber, E., 432, *461*

Subject Index

A

Abdominal mammary gland, 241
Acetate
    mammary use, 212–213
    precursor of milk fat, 213–216
Acetylcholine, effect on mammary blood
    flow, 183–184
Acetyl-CoA carboxylase
    amount in various species, 354
    characteristics, 384–385
    constants, 359
Acetyl-CoA synthetase
    amount in various species, 353
    characteristics, 378–379
    constants, 359
Acid phosphatase, 388
ACTH, see Adrenocorticotropic hormone
Actinomycin D
    inhibition of milk synthesis, 433–434
        of rRNA synthesis, 134, 432–433
        of tRNA synthesis, 450
Actomysin in myoepithelial cells, 81
Adenine incorporation into RNA, 423,
    433
Adenohypophysis, see also Pituitary gland
    anterior, 228
    function, effect of suckling, 253
    hormones (STH, TSH, ACTH)
        control of, species variation, 254–
        256
        in mammary growth, 113
        release in suckling, 253
    hypothalamic control of, 232
Adenosine and mammary vasodilatation,
    184
Adenosine monophosphate (AMP), 374,
    437
Adenosine triphosphate (ATP), 374,
    377, 384
Adrenal cortex
    activity in various species, 287, 288
    control of lactogenesis, 285–289
    maintenance of lactation, 305–308

Adrenal cortical extract, in lactogenesis,
    281, 282, 285, 286
Adrenal corticosterone, index of secretory
    activity, 306
Adrenal glands, 232, 241
    in lactogenesis, 281, 285–289
    in mammary development, 99, 132–
    133
Adrenal glucocorticoids, fetal, 278
Adrenal steroids, 245
    in mammary development, 129, 130
Adrenalectomy
    effect on mammary development, 122
        on mammary enzymes, 392, 401
        on mammary RNA synthesis, 418,
        421, 426, 427, 436
    impairment of milk secretion, 281, 282,
    305
    prevention of lactogenesis, 287
Adrenaline, see also Catecholamines,
    Epinephrine
    effect on mammary blood flow, 149,
    181, 182, 191
Adrenergic blocking agents, mammary
    effects, 239
Adrenocorticotropic hormone (ACTH),
    255
    in lactation, 297, 301, 306
    in lactogenesis, 281, 282
Aldolase, see Fructose-1,6-diphosphate
    aldolase
Aldosterone
    effect on mammary growth and differ-
    entiation, 105–107, 129
    in vitro studies, 132, 133
Alloxan diabetes, 128–129, 312, 426
Alveolar area index as measure of mam-
    mary development, 101
Alveolar cell development
    insulin, 339–341
        plus hydrocortisone, 341
    prolactin, 342–344
Alveolar structure
    blood vessels, 156, 158

insulin effects, 339
in lactation, 9, 17
lymphatics, 161, 163
in mammary regression, 13, 15, 16, 73, 74
in pregnancy, 7–9, 15, 17, 18
in regression, 13
in resting stage, 5–6
at weaning, 12, 13
Alveolar cell, synchrony of, 339–344
prolactin in, 345
Alveolar ultrastructure, *see also* Cell, mammary
hormonal effects on, 338–339, 342–343
Amino acids
arteriovenous differences, mammary, 147–149
as blood flow measurement, 171
precursors of milk proteins, 211–212
uptake (mammary) in various species, 211–212
Aminoacyl-tRNA, 439
Aminoacyl-tRNA synthetases, 447
heterogeneity of, 450–453
Amygdala in milk secretion, 251, 252
Anesthesia
avoidance of stress and, 191–192
effect on mammary blood flow and milk ejection reflex, 241, 242
on milk yield, 165
on prolactin release, 260
Androgens
inhibition of mammary growth and differentiation, 104–105, 335
role in mammary development, 127
Anlage (primordial structure), mammary, differentiation of, 102–104, 414
Antidiuretic hormone, effect on mammary blood flow, 182
Antipyrine, measure of blood flow, 169, 179
Apocrine secretion, 63–67
Arteries for blood sampling, 193–196
cow, 193–194
goat, 194
horse, 196
pig, 195, 196
sheep, 194

Arteriovenous difference of blood substances (a − v), 145
mammary blood flow measurements, 151
measurement *in vivo*, 190
minor milk components, 216–217
principles in measurement, 145, 146
Arteriovenous structures (mammary)
anastomoses, 159
bridges, 159
shunts (A-V), 159
Arylsulfatase, 388
Aspartate aminotransferase
amounts in various species, 353
characteristics, 380–381
isoenzymes, 381
constants, 358
Aspartate transcarbamylase, activity and mammary RNA content, 417
Auditory stimuli, lactation effects, 237, 263
Autophagocytosis in mammary regression, 71, 72
Autoradiographs
of milk protein synthesis, 43, 45
of milk fat synthesis, 51, 53

B

Baroceptors, cisternal, 233
Basement membrane
in lactating cells, 33
in mammary regression, 73
Binucleate cells in mammary gland, 11
Biogenic amines and milk yields, 315
Blood constituents as milk prescursors, 204–217
Blood flow of mammary gland, 143–219, 398
control of, 181–184
effect of anesthesia, 165
methods of measurement, 148–149, 165–174
rate of, 174–181
venous drainage, 153
Blood sampling
arterial, in various species, 191, 193–196
methods, 153
venous, 196–203

Blood supply, mammary gland, anatomy of, 154–163
Blood vessels, mammary gland
anatomy, 153
arteriovenous shunts, 158–161
large, 155
small, 155–158
teat, 159, 161
Bradykinin and mammary vasodilatation, 184
Brain stem
role in oxytocin release, 233, 239
in prolactin release, 233
Butyrophenones, mammogenic effects, 134

C

Calcium (Ca)
in blood, 309
mammary a − v differences, 151, 170
in milk, 216
Capillaries, in mammary gland, 155, 156, 158, 163
Capillary endothelium, triglyceride hydrolysis, 185, 214–216
Carbon dioxide pressure (pCO_2), effect on mammary blood flow, 183
Cardiac puncture, measure of cardiac output, 194
Carnitine in milk, 217
Casein synthesis
hormones in, 422
induced by hormones *in vitro*, 292, 293
mouse, 334
RNA levels in, 418, 421, 424, 427
nRNA in, 434
RNA-polyribosomes in, 444, 447
Cat
mammary blood flow, 180–183
mammary blood supply, 156
venous sampling, 196
Catecholamines, 240, *see also* Adrenaline, Epinephrine
effects on milk yields, 239, 315
histochemical identification, 231
neurotransmitters, 315
stimulation of prolactin-inhibiting factor, 315

Cathepsin D, 388
CBG, *see* Corticosteroid-binding globulin
Cell, mammary
culture of, identification of milk precursors, 188
cytoplasmic-nuclear ratios, 12
development
mitosis, critical, 335
in varying physiological states, 337–339
division, *see also* mitosis, 133, 417–418
enzyme levels and, 389–391
in gestation and early lactation, 292
induced by insulin and hydrocortisone *in vitro*, 292
in lactogenesis, 417–418
in mammary development, 111, 133
at parturition and lactogenesis, 393–395
hypophysectomy effects, 404–405
insulin effects, 399–400
in lactation, 334
membranes, insulin effects, 330
necrosis
Donné bodies and, 75–77
in mammary regression, 13, 71, 72
organelles, 17, *see also* Mitochondria, Ergastoplasm, Golgi apparatus
development and growth of, 53–60
in early pregnancy, 21, 23
in lactation, 30–36
in late pregnancy, 27
in mammary regression, 69–72
in milk stasis (weaning), 67, 68
at parturition, 29, 30
in resting stage, 19
secretion, 17
serum factor(s) effects, 331
structure
in lactation, 9
in various species, 3–5
ultrastructure (virgin mice), 328
wall, *see* Plasmalemma
Cell organelles of myoepithelium, 81
Cell wall, *see* Plasmalemma
Central nervous system
in lactation, 250–252

in milk ejection, 232–236, 239
prolactin release, 246
Cerebellum in oxytocin release, 239
Cerebral cortex
  effect on intramammary pressure, 241
  role in oxytocin release, 239
Chemoreceptors, 230
Cholinesterase, histochemical identification, 229, 231
Chorionic gonadotropin, 118, 128, 284
Chylomicra, uptake by mammary gland after hydrolysis, 213–216
Circulation of mammary gland, *see* Blood vessels, Lymphatics, Milk vein
Citrate cleavage enzyme
  amounts in various species, 354
  characteristics, 384
  constants, 359
Citrate synthetase
  amounts in various species, 353
  characteristics, 379
  constants, 358
Citric acid cycle enzymes, 378–383, *see also* specific enzymes
  amounts in various species, 353–354
  constants, 358
Colchicine, 134, 335
  effects on RNA-polyribosomes, 444
Colostrum, 244
Colostrum corpuscles, *see* Donné Bodies
Contractile tissue, mammary
  myoepithelium, 236
  smooth muscle (teat), 236
Contraction of mammary gland, mechanically induced, 238
Corpus luteum, 118, 128, 243
  prostaglandin inhibition, 291
  in pseudopregnancy, 113
  relaxin, 130
Corpuscles (nerve endings), Golgi-Mazzoni, Merkel's, Paccini, 228
Corticosteroid-binding globulin (CBG), 289
  levels in lactation (rat), 307
  progesterone binding, 291
  TSH in release, 309
Corticosteroids, 255
  binding of, serum, 289
  effects on RNA-polyribosomes, 444

fetal, species variations, 288–289
inhibition of milk yields (cow), 307
in lactogenesis, 244
in late pregnancy, 288
release of, ACTH in, 306
Corticosterone
  effect in lactation, 305–306
  maintenance of RNA levels, 421–422
  in mammary growth, 125, 129, 130
  response to exteroceptive stimuli, 263, 306
  in vitro studies, 133
Cortisol (17-hydroxycorticosterone)
  binding in bovine mammary cells, 307
  effect on casein synthesis, 427
    on DNA synthesis, 105
    in lactation, 306
    on mammary enzymes, 404–405
    on mammary growth, 125, 129, 130
    on mammary RNA synthesis, 419–421, 423–425, 427, 430, 431
      nRNA, 433
      RNA-polyribosomes, 443, 445
      rRNA, 444
      tRNA, 449–450
  enhancement of secretion, 103, 420
  in vitro studies, 133
Cortisone (11-dehydro-17-hydroxycorticosterone), 129
  effect in lactation, 306
  mammary RNA content and, 420, 421
  synergism with prolactin, 421
Cow
  amino acid uptake (mammary), 212
  arteries for blood sampling, 193–194
  induced lactation with estrogen and progesterone, 293
  intermediary metabolite levels, 360
  lipid uptake (mammary), 213
  mammary enzymes, 352–354, 357–359
  mammary growth in pregnancy, 112
  mammary RNA content, 419, 425
  prolactin effect in lactation, 299
  rate and duration of lactation (lactation curve), 295–296
  ribosomal proteins, 441
  udder blood flow, 179, 182
  veins for blood sampling, 199, 201, 202

Cycloheximide in RNA synthesis, 436
  tRNA, 450
Cyproterone, in mammary development, 104
Cytoplasmic crescents in milk, 65–66
Cytoplasmic vacuoles in milk protein secretion, 49
Cytosine arabinoside, 335–336

D

Deciduoma, 248, 264
Deciduomata in mammary growth, 114, 119
  RNA levels in, 417
Dense bodies
  in early pregnancy, 25, 26
  in late pregnancy, 27
  in mammary regression, 71
Deoxyribonucleic acid (DNA)
  mammary content
    in estrus cycle, 415–416
    measure of growth, 99, 101–102
    during pregnancy
      in rat, 111, 114
      in various species, 111, 116, 117
    in pseudopregnancy, 114
  synthesis, mammary cells
    insulin effects on, 330–332, 339–340, 437
    mitosis, 336
    prolactin in, 333
    varying physiological states, 330–332
  template, 435
    capacity, 436–437
  transcription in mammary gland, 431, 435, 436
Desmosome, 19, 37, *see also* Macula adhaerens
Dibenamine, adrenergic block, 231
Dibenzyline (phenoxybenzamine), adrenergic block, 240, 241
Diencephalon, periventricular, 234
Diestrus, 108, 415
  prolonged, 250
Differentiation of mammary gland
  cell division in, 111, 133
  early pregnancy, 6–9
  embryological, 98, 102

endocrine regulation, fetal, 102–107
  inhibition by androgens, 104–105
  late pregnancy, 8–10
  mammary lines, 98
  methods of measurement, 199–202
  postnatal, 107
  pregnancy and pseudopregnancy, 110–117
  puberty, 107
  in vitro, 131, 133
DNA, *see* Deoxyribonucleic acid
Dog
  mammary blood flow, 180, 181, 183
  mammary blood supply, 156
  venous sampling, 196
Donné bodies (colostrum corpuscles)
  cell necrosis and, 71, 72
  development of, 75–77
  in mammary regression, 13
  species variations, 76
Dopamine, effect on milk yields, 315
Dorsal root section (spinal)
  inhibition of milk ejection, 232–233
  intramammary pressure response, 242
DPN, *see* NAD
Draught reflex, 229
Drugs, mammary effects, 134
Duct system, mammary, 5–7, 14, 15, 21, 110–112, 240, 327
  differentiation of, 103, 106
Ductal resistance in milk ejection, 237, 238, 240, 242

E

Electromagnetic flowmeter, measure of blood flow, 165
Electron micrographs, mammary gland, 14–81, 101
Embden–Meyerhoff enzymes (glycolysis), 373–378
  amounts in various species, 353
  constants, 357
  fructose-1,6-diP aldolase, 374–375
  glyceraldehyde-3-P dehydrogenase, 375–376
  hexose-P-isomerase, 373
  lactic dehydrogenase, 377
  phosphofructokinase, 373–374

pyruvate kinase, 376
triose-P-isomerase, 375
Embryo
  differentiation from fetus in cow, human, and rat, 104
  hormonal control of mammary, 102
Emotional inhibition of milk ejection, 239
Endocrines, *see also* Hormones, Insulin, Prolactin
  regulation of mammary differentiation, 99–107
Endoplasmic reticulum, *see* Ribosomes, Ergastoplasm, Rough endoplasmic reticulum
Energy metabolism, insulin effects, 395, 397
Enzymes, mammary, 349–406, *see also* specific enzymes, Citric acid cycle, Embden–Meyerhoff enzymes
  activity
    in lactation, 391, 392
    in mid and late pregnancy, 389–391
    at parturition, 419
    and lactogenesis, 393–395
    virgin and early pregnancy, 389
    weaning, 392
  adrenalectomy effects, 392, 401
  constitutive, 391, 394–396, 402, 404
    hormone-dependent and, 391
  cortisol effects, 401
  demonstration of presence, 349–350
  equilibrium constants, 356–359
  estrogen effects, 400–401
  "feedback" inhibition of, 393
  glucocorticoid effects, 395–396, 401–403
  half-life estimates, 403
  hormonal regulation, 392, 395, 399–406
  hormone-dependent, 391, 395, 396, 404
  hypophysectomy effects, 392, 403–406
  inhibition by milk accumulation, 393
  insulin effects, 395, 397, 399, 400
  lipoprotein lipase, 387
  mass action coefficients, 356–359, 362
  maximum velocity, 356–359, 363

net flux, 356–359, 363
ovariectomy effects, 400–401
oxytocin effects, 392, 405
peak activities, 392
physiological state effects, 389–399
progesterone inhibition, 395–397
prolactin effects, 392, 395–397, 404–405
for protein synthesis, 388–389
regulation of, 389–406
RNA content and, 419
synthesis, actinomycin D in, 434
thyroidectomy effects, 406
units/gram of tissue, 352–355
velocity of reactions, 356–359, 363
weaning effects, 405
Epimerase, 372
Epinephrine, 231, *see also* Adrenaline, Catecholamines, Noradrenaline
  inhibition of milk ejection, 239
Ergastoplasm, *see also* Ribosomes, Polyribosomes
  in early pregnancy, 21
  hydrocortisone and, 57, 58
  in lactation, 30
  in late pregnancy, 27
  in mammary regression, 70
  in milk fat synthesis, 51
  in milk stasis, 68
  in polypeptide formation, 45
  polyribosome binding, 442
  prolactin effects, 57
  in protein formation, 39, 41
  in resting stage, 19
  volume of, in varying physiological states, 56–59
Estradiol
  effect on mammary development, 103, 127
    on LDH isoenzyme patterns, 378
    on tRNA synthesis, 450
  induction of lactation, 293–294
  in steer, 104
Estradiol-17β, 290
  effect on glucose-6-PO$_4$ dehydrogenase synthesis, 400, 434–435
    on RNA synthesis, 427
  mammary receptors, 329
  mammary uptake, 123–124

Estrogens
  concentration variations in stages of pregnancy, species variations, 289, 290
  effect on mammary development, 122, 345
    on mammary enzymes, 400–401, 434–435
    on mammary vascularity, 156
    on pituitary, 123, 291
  induction of milk secretion, 289
  inhibition of PIF, 246
  in vitro studies, 132
  to progesterone ratios
    induction of lactation, 293–294
    in lactogenesis, 245
    in mammary development, 124–125
  in RNA synthesis, 416, 420, 421
    nRNA, 438
  stimulation of hypothalamus, 249, 250
  synthetic, inhibition of lactation (human), 313
Estrone, 125, 419
Estrus
  continuous, 107
  cyclic, estrogenic phases, 278
  growth hormone in, 279, 301
  length of, species variations, 107–108
  luteal phase, 108, 278
  mammary gland in, 108, 328
  milk accumulation in, 278
  prolactin levels in, 278, 301, 332
  recurrence, mammary development in, 109–110
  variation in mammary RNA, 415–416
Ewe, mammary RNA content, 417, 418, 425, 427, 431
Exopinocytosis, 63, 67
Exteroceptive stimuli (ECS), litter to mother
  age of litters in, 264–266
  auditory, 263
  corticosterone release, 263
  development of responses, 263–266
  olfaction, 263
  pheromones, 263
  in prolactin secretion, 262–266
  spatial, 262, 264–266, 267
  visual, 263

F

F, *see* Hydrocortisone
Fasciculus, dorsal longitudinal (Bundle of Schultz), 233, 234
Fasting
  mammary blood flow in, 181
  metabolic effects, 219
Fat, effect of diets high in, 306
Fatty acid cycle enzymes, 383–389, *see also* specific enzymes
  amounts in various species, 354
  constants, 359
Fatty acid synthesis (mammary), 383–389, *see also* Milk fat, Lipids
Fatty acid synthetase
  amounts in various species, 354
  characteristics, 385
  constants, 359
Fatty acids
  free, *see* Free fatty acids
  uptake by mammary gland, 147
Fetal hormones, 278
Fetus, mammary development in, 104–107
Fick methods
  measure of blood flow, 168–171
  metabolic, 169–171
Fick principle, 144–145, 149, 151
Fistula, teat, 241
Fluorodeoxyuridine, 336
Forebrain bundle, medial
  in oxytocin release, 234
  in prolactin release, 252
Free fatty acids (FFA)
  arteriovenous differences in, mammary, 190
  milk fat synthesis, 214–215
Freemartin, cause and mammary development in, 105
Fructose-1,6-diphosphate aldolase
  amounts in various species, 353
  characteristics, 374–375
  constants, 357
Funiculus, dorsal and lateral, 233

G

Galactopoiesis
  definition of, 414
  hypothalamic influences, 245–252

neuroendocrine influences, 254–256
RNA content and synthesis (various species), 425–428
suckling influences, 245, 252–254
Galactopoietic hormones (TSH, STH, hydrocortisone, oxytocin), 261
Galactosyltransferase, 434
Genome transcription, 434–435
RNP in, 438
tRNA in, 447–450
heterogeneity of, 450–453
Glucocorticoids
effect on mammary enzymes, 392, 395, 397, 401–402
in lactogenesis, 281
in mammary development, 129, 130, 328–329, 346
in milk synthesis, 297, 334, 336
in RER formation, 342, 344
Glucose
mammary arteriovenous differences, 146, 147, 149, 151
as blood flow measurement, 170
precursor of lactose and other milk components, 146, 147, 209–211
Glucose activation enzyme (hexokinase), 364–366
Glucose-6-phosphate dehydrogenase
amounts in various species, 352
characteristics, 369–371
constants, 356
estradiol effects, 400, 434–435
inhibition by actinomycin D, 434–435
insulin effects on, 329, 337, 340, 400
isoenzymes, 371
β-Glucuronidase, 388
Glutamate dehydrogenase
amount in cow and rat, 353
characteristics, 380
constants, 358
Glyceraldehyde-3-phosphate dehydrogenase
amounts in various species, 353
characteristics, 375–376
constants, 357
α-Glycerol-phosphate dehydrogenase
amounts in various species, 354
characteristics, 385–386
constants, 359

Glycolysis enzymes, *see* Embden–Meyerhoff enzymes
Goat
arteries for blood sampling, 194
lipid uptake, mammary, 213, 214
mammary amino acid uptake, 211, 212
mammary blood supply, 156, 158
mammary RNA content, 419
rate and duration of lactation, 295
udder blood flow and milk yield, 174–179
venous blood sampling, 197–199, 203
Goitrogen, 308
Golgi apparatus
development, 59, 60
in early pregnancy, 21, 23
functions in milk secretion, 41, 43
in lactation, 30, 418
in lactose synthesis, 53
in late pregnancy, 9, 10, 27
in mammary regression, 71
in milk protein formation, 37, 39, 49, 63
in resting stage, 19
structure, 59
Gonadal steroids
in lactogenesis, 244
in mammary development, 122–123
Gonadectomy, 125
Gonadotropin
cyclic activity and mammary development, 107
pituitary, 244
Growth, mammary, *see also* Differentiation, mammary; Mammary development
allometric, 107, 415
animal models, 120–121
early pregnancy, 7, 8
estrous cycles, 108–110
experimental methods
in vitro, 131–133
in vivo, 120–131
fetal, 104–107
hormones in, 102–133
isometric, 107, 415
lactational, 9
species variations, 120
late pregnancy, 8, 9

mechanical stimulation of, 134
methods of measuring, 99–102
  biochemical, 101
  macroscopic, 99
  microscopic, 100
nutrition in, 133
pregnancy and pseudopregnancy, 110–117
puberty, 107–110
quantitation of, 110
Growth hormone (somatotropin, STH)
concentration
  at parturition, 285
  during pregnancy, 284
effect on mammary growth and differentiation, 103, 122, 125, 346
in estrous cycle, 279, 301
galactopoietic activities in various species, 300
human
  amino acid sequence, 283
  prolactin-like action, 282
  stimulation of lactation, 300
in lactation, 297
lactogenic properties, 282
levels in suckling, 303–304
in mammary RNA synthesis, 419
release and milk yields (cow), 302, 303
synergism with other hormones, 131
in vitro studies, 132
Growth stimulus, mechanical, 134
Guinea pig
mammary blood flow, 181
mammary DNA content, 117
mammary enzymes, 352–354
mammary RNA content, 419
venous sampling, 197

H

Hamster
mammary DNA content, 117
mammary RNA content, 419
Hematocrits in stressed and normal animals, 190
Heterophagocytosis, in mammary regression, 72, 76

Hexokinase
amounts in various species, 352, 366
characteristics, 364–367
constants, 356, 366
insulin effects on, 365, 400
isoenzymes, 364–365
Hexose monophosphate shunt, *see* Pentose cycle enzymes
Hexose-phosphate-isomerase (phosphoglucose isomerase)
amounts in various species, 353
characteristics, 372, 373
constants, 357
Histones
insulin effects on, 340
phosphorylation of, 437
synthesis of, 436–437
Hormonal control of mammary secretory activity
of lactogenesis, 243–245, 280–294, 414
before pregnancy, 278
during pregnancy, 279
of tRNA's in milk secretion, 451
Hormones, *see also* specific hormones
adenohypophyseal, 244
adrenal, 245
carriers for administration, 121
concentrations in various physiological states and species, 285
effect of actinomycin D, 433
fetal, 278
human placental, 118, 278, 284
induction of RNA synthesis, 419
inhibition of lactation, 291
in mammary development, 102–133
in mammary RNA synthesis, 419
mammary uptake, 217, 285
mammotropic, 132–133
  pituitary, 122
  placental, 128
    various species, 118–120, 284
  steroid, gonadal, 122–123
metabolic, 397–399
  in mammary development, 128–131
  pituitary, 131
  in vitro studies, 132–133
in mouse tumor virus growth, 85
pancreatic, *see* Insulin

regulation of mammary enzymes, 399–
406
release, methods of analysis, 254
replacement in hypophysectomy, 282,
297, 431
role in mammary growth, 113–119
serum levels at parturition, 293
synergism in RNA synthesis, *in vitro*,
422–425
treatment, means of administering, 121
Horse
arteries for blood sampling, 196
fatty acid uptake, mammary, 212
mammary RNA content, 419
sampling venous blood, 197, 203
Human(s)
chorionic gonadotropin, 118, 128
growth hormone, lactational effects,
300
mammary blood flow, 183
placental lactogen, 118, 128, 284
rate and duration of lactation, 296
Hydrocortisone (cortisol)
effects on ergastoplasm, 57, 58, 342
on RNA polymerase, 435–436
on RNA synthesis, 342, 421
on nRNA, 438
improvement of milk secretion, 255
in mammary development, 336
in milk secretion, 420–421
β-Hydroxybutyrate, mammary uptake,
213–216
β-Hydroxybutyrate dehydrogenase, 388
Hyperluteinization, 250
Hyperplasia, mammary, 111, 420
Hypertrophy, mammary, 111
Hypoglycemia, depressed milk yields,
312
Hypophysectomy
hormone therapy in, 255, 431
species variation, 256
during lactation
cessation of, 254, 297
hormone replacement, 282, 297, 431
during pregnancy
effect on lactogenesis, 281
on mammary development, 98–
99, 125–126
on mammary enzymes, 392; 403–
406

on mammary growth, 113
placental hormones in, 118
on mammary RNA synthesis, 419–
421, 431, 436, 443
rRNA, 444
Hypophysis, *see* Pituitary gland, Hypophysectomy
Hypothalamic extracts
growth hormone release, 284
prolactin release, 260, 282
Hypothalamo-adenohypophyseal system,
248, 425
Hypothalamus, 134
control of pituitary, 232
effect on galactopoietic hormones,
245–252
on prolactin secretion, 246, 247
estrogen stimulation of, 249, 250
in lactation (oxytocin release), 234–
235
lateral region, 234
prolactin secretion, 251
lesions and prolactin secretion controls,
250, 251
nuclei (neurosecretory neurons)
paraventricular, 232, 234, 239
supraoptic, 232, 239
periventricular diencephalic area in
milk ejection, 234
PIF and, 225, 248, 251
in prolactin secretion, 249–250
pituitary and, effects on milk secretion, 292
sites of actions, 251
tuberal region, prolactin secretion control, 249
Hypothyroidism, functional, in lactation,
310–311

I

I, *see* Insulin
Indicator dilution, measure of blood flow,
167, 168
Indicator fractionation, measure of blood
flow, 172–173
Innervation, mammary, 163–164
afferent, 232–236
efferent, 231–232
sensory nerve endings, 228–230

Insulin, 255
actions, dynamics of, 329
bound to sepharose, effect on virgin and pregnant mammary cells, 330–331
effects
on bovine milk production, 312–313
on DNA synthesis, 105, 330–332; 339, 437
on energy metabolism, 395, 397, 399, 400
on glucose-6-P dehydrogenase, 329, 337, 340, 400
on hexokinase, 365, 400
on histone synthesis, 340, 437
on mammary cell membranes, 330
on mammary cell proliferation, 292
on mammary development, 106–107, 128–129, 328, 329, 336
on mammary enzymes, 395, 397, 399–400
on mammary mitosis, 339
on mammary protein secretion, 334, 339–340
on milk yields, 312
on 6-P-gluconate dehydrogenase, 340, 400
on 6-P-glucose isomerase, 400
on ribosomes, 340, 341
on RNA content of mammary explants, 421–425
on RNA polymerases, 435–436
on RNA-polyribosomes, 443, 445
on RNA synthesis
nRNA, 433
rRNA, 444
tRNA, 449–450
on *in vitro* growth, mammary, 105
in combination with cortisol and prolactin in RNA synthesis, 423–425
synergism, with ovarian steroids, 122
with prolactin in RNA synthesis, 422
in vitro requirement, 132, 133
Insulin hypoglycemia, effect on mammary blood flow, 182
Insulin sensitivity, mammary
in involution, 332
prolactin effects on, 332–334

in varying physiological states, 328–344
Intramammary pressure response, 230, 231, 240, 242
Involution, mammary, *see also* Mammary regression, Weaning
effect of hormones, 430
retardation due to suckling, 252, 253
RNA content and synthesis in, 429–431
Iodine (I_2)
in mammary gland and milk, 310
in milk, 216
Isocitrate dehydrogenase (NADP)
amounts in various species, 353
characteristics, 379–380
constants, 358
Isotopes in milk precursor identification, 154, 186–188

J

Jugular vein, blood substances, 192–193
Junctional complexes
in lactating cells, 31, 35, 37
structure of, 19, 21

K

Kreb's cycle enzymes, *see* Citric acid cycle enzymes

L

α-Lactalbumin in mammary gland
RNA-polyribosomes in, 446
RNA synthesis and, 418–419, 424, 425
nRNA, 434
Lactation
adrenal hormones and, 129, 130, 305
cessation of, 266–268
concurrent pregnancy and, 316–317
RNA in, 428
early
cell division in, 292
growth during, 120
mammary RNA levels, 418–419
estrogen in, 313–314
exteroceptive stimuli in, 262–265
extrahypothalamic influences on, 245–252
hormonal requirements, 296–315

induced by hormones, 110, 126–127,
281, 293–294, 419–421
in vitro, 421–425
inhibition by high oxytocin levels, 240
initiation, hormonal control, 318, *see
also* Lactogenesis
prolactin and adrenal corticoids, 285
late, decline, 252
effects of hormones, 428
exteroceptive mechanism in, 265–
266
RNA levels in, 427–428, 443
maintenance
hormonal, 296–297, 318
suckling, 252–254, 296–297
mid-, 263
milk removal effects, 315–316
neuroendocrine control of, 228–268
ovarian steroids in, 313–315
period, in various species, 295, 296
progesterone in, 313–314
RNA and RNP in, 442–443
tRNA acceptor capacity in, 448–449
stage of
effect on blood flow, 174, 181
on exteroceptive mechanisms,
263–264
stimuli of, 262, 263
thyroid hormones, 308, 309
Lactation curves, 294–296
Lactational growth, endocrine control,
120
Lactic dehydrogenase
amounts in cow and rat mammary,
353
characteristics, 377
constants, 358
isoenzymes, 377, 378
Lactogen, *see also* Prolactin, Placental
hormones
placental and mammary development,
346
Lactogenesis
cell division in, 292, 417–418
characterization of, 414
circulating hormone levels, 244–245
criteria for, 286
experimental, farm animals, 293
hormonal control, 280–292, 414
sequences of, 292–293

hypothalamic lesions and, 251
increase of tRNA in, 449–450
inhibition by actinomycin D, 434
neuroendocrine mechanisms in, 243–
245
RNA synthesis in, 417–418
nRNA, 433
suckling effects, 244
Lactose
in mammary, during pregnancy, 418–
419
synthesis
effect of prolactin, 420
inhibition by actinomycin D, 434
in lactating cells, 53
RNA levels, 418–420
in mammary cell cultures, 188
Lactose synthesizing enzymes, 367–369,
see also specific enzymes
amounts in various species, 352
constants, 356
Lactose synthetase
amounts in various species, 352
characteristics, 368–369
constants, 356
hormonal effects on, 334
Langhans cells (placental), 118
Leukemia virus in mammary cells and
milk, 88–91
Lignocaine (Lidocaine, Xylocaine), 230,
238, 242
Lipoprotein lipase
actinomycin D inhibition, 434
amounts in various species, 354
characteristics, 387
effect on mammary lipid uptake, 214
effect of prolactin, 420
Litter size, effect on mammary mitotic
activity, 315
Litter weight, lactation index in rats,
294–295
Lobule-alveolar structure of mammary
gland, 110–112, 278, 415, 416
blood vessels, 158
differentiation of, 7, 8, 9, 414, 416
hormones in, 122
growth and lymphatics, 161, 163
Luteolysin, 243
Luteotropin (LTH), placental, 118, 119

Lymph flow, mammary, 184–186
  equilibration with blood, 185
Lymph nodes, mammary, 185, 186
Lymphatics, mammary, 161–163
Lymphocytes, decrease after milking, 241
Lysine incorporation into protein, 423
Lysosomes
  in early pregnancy, 25
  enzymes in weaning, 429
  in mammary regression, 71, 72

M

Macrophages in mammary regression, 72, 73
Macula adhaerens (desmosome), 19
Malate dehydrogenase (NAD)
  amount in various species, 353
  characteristics, 382–383
  constants, 359
  isoenzymes, 382–383
Malic enzyme
  amounts in various species, 354
  characteristics, 383
  constants, 359
Malphighian layer, source of mammary buds, 103
Mammary alveolus, *see* Alveolar structure
Mammary buds in male, 103
Mammary cell, *see* Cell, mammary
Mammary development, 414–415
  androgens in, 127
  biochemical methods of determining, 101
  embryonic and fetal, 98, 102–107
  enzyme levels in, 389–390
  estrogen effects, 327, 345
  estrogen:progesterone ratios in, 124–125
  estrous cycles, 107–110, 328
  extrauterine, 97–98, 107–131
  glucocorticoid effects, 328–329
  growth hormone, 103, 122, 125, 346
  hormonal effects, 327–346
    pregnant *vs.* virgin mice, 328–329
  insulin effects, 336, 339–340
  intrauterine, 97, 98, 102–107
  lactogen, placental, 118–120, 278, 284, 346

mechanical stimulation, 237–238
  mesenchymal cell in, 345
  methods of measurement, 99–102
  mitosis in, 111, 133, 292, 337, 417–418
  mouse, mature, 327–346
  nutrition, 133, 134, 219, 398
  postnatal, 107
  in pregnancy, 6–9, 110–117, 279, 416
  progesterone effects, 327, 345
  in puberty, 107–110, 327, 415–416
  RNA in, 414–429, 442–443
    tRNA in, 453
  RNP in, 443
  serum factor(s) affects, 328–329
  in varying physiological states, 237–246
  in vitro, 131–133
Mammary ductal system, 5–7, 14, 15, 21, 110, 112, 240, 327
Mammary end-buds, 5, 21, 110
Mammary enzymes, *see* Enzymes, mammary
Mammary gland, *see also* Cell, mammary, Lobule-alveolar structure of mammary gland
  abdominal, 241
  anatomic location, species variation, 154
  anlage, 102–104, 414
  binucleate cells in, 11
  blood flow, 143–219
    controlling factors, 181
    measurements, 148–149
  blood supply, species variation, 154
  cell division in gestation and early lactation, 292
  changes during estrous cycles, 108–110, 278, 328
  contractile tissue, 236–238, *see also* Myoepithelial cells
  differentiation, *see* Differentiation of mammary gland
  DNA content in pregnancy, 111–117
  ductal system, *see* Mammary ductal system
  embryonic, mouse, *in vitro*, 132
  end-buds, 5, 21, 110
  endocrinological control
    mammary development, 102–133

mature mouse, 327–346
  of milk secretion and ejection, 236–
    268
  of mammary enzymes, 389–406
  of mammary RNA and RNP, 414–
    454
  of mammary secretion, 277–317
explants, 132–133
glucocorticoid sensitivity, 328–329
growth, *see* Growth, mammary
inguinal, 104
inhibitory systems, activation of, 241–
    243
innervation
  afferent, 232–236
  efferent, 231–232
  sensory nerve endings, 228–230
insulin sensitivity, in varying physio-
    logical states, 328–334, 338
intermediary metabolite levels, 360
involution, *see also* Mammary gland,
    regression
  retardation due to suckling, 252,
    253, 429–430
  RNA levels in, 429–430
lymph flow, 184–185
maintenance of function, 245, 296–317
metabolism, feeding effects, 219, 398
in milk stasis (weaning), 12–14
mitosis in, 9, 11
morphology, *see also* Mammary gland,
    structure changes during dif-
    ferentiation, 102–107, 414
  lobule-alveolar, 110–112, 414, 416
  microscopic, 3–14, 100
mouse, in mid-pregnancy, 337, 338
  ovarian steroid effects, 125
neuroendocrine controls, 227–268
palpation of, inhibition of milk ejec-
    tion, 241–242
parenchyma of, 229
prolactin sensitization of, 332–334
protein synthesis, 336–338
rabbit, ovarian steroid effects, 125
regression
  of alveolus, 73
  macrophages in, 72–73
  processes in, 69–74
in resting stage, 5–6

RNA and RNP content, 414–454
serum factor(s) sensitivity, 328–334
structure, 5–13, 327
  electron micrographs, 14–81
  during lactation, 9
  during regression, 13, 15, 16
substrates for, 204–217
thoracic, 241
uptake of milk precursors
  fatty acids, 214–215
  isotope dilution, 154
  mechanism of, 218
venous drainage, species variation,
    196–203
whole organ perfusion, 147, 189
Mammary glandular tree, 5–6
Mammary involution, *see* Mammary
    gland, involution, regression
Mammary lines, 98
Mammary lobules, growth in early preg-
    nancy, 7, 8
Mammary regression, *see* Mammary
    gland, regression
Mammary secretion, *see also* Milk secre-
    tion
  lactation, 9, 296–317
  lactogenesis, 280–294
  metabolic regulation of, 397–398
  parturition, 29, 30, 280
  in pregnancy, 7, 8, 9, 23, 25, 27, 279
Mammary tissue
  effect of estrogen implants, 314
  uptake of hormones, 285
Mammillary peduncle, 234
Mammogenesis and hormones, 97–133
Mammotropic hormones, 122–128
  pituitary, 122
  placental, 128
    various species, 118–120, 284
  steroid, gonadal, 122–123
Mammotropin, *see* Prolactin
Maternal behavior, *see also* Nursing
  effect on milk secretion, 252, 253
Medial lemniscus, 233, 234
Medulla, oxytocin release, 233
Melanocyte-stimulating hormone (MSH),
    243
Melatonin, effect on milk yield, 315
Membranes of mammary cell, *see* Cell,

mammary, organelles; Plasma-lemma

Menstrual cycles, *see* Estrous cycles

Merocrine secretion of milk, 65–67

Mesencephalon
  dorsal, rostral and tegmentum
  in milk ejection, 233, 235
  prolactin release, 239

Mesenchymal cell factors in mammary development, 345

Messenger RNA, *see* Ribonucleic acid, messenger

Metabolic inhibitors, *see* specific substances

Metestrus, 108, 415

Methandrostenolone, 127

Methionine, heterogeneity of tRNA's for, 453

Methylase activity, tRNA, 449

Microbial fermentation, effect on milk fatty acids, 213

Microscopy, electron
  mammary gland, 14–81
  study of mammary innervation, 229

Microtubules of lactating cells, 33

Microvesicles
  in polypeptide transport, 49
  in protein formation, 41

Microvilli of lactating cells, 33

Midbrain in milk ejection, 233–235

Milk
  minor components, 216–217
  removal from mammary, *see also* Suckling, Nursing
    effect on enzymes, 393
    on milk secretion, 398
    mechanisms involved, 236–238
    inhibition of, 238–266

Milk ejection
  ductal resistance in, 237, 238, 240, 242
  frequency of stimulation, 237
  myoepithelium in, 237
  neuro-endocrine control, 236–243
  rate of, 237–238
  reflex, 236–238
    inhibition of, 238–243
    oxytocin in, 304–305

response to suckling, 230
stress effects, 238, 239, 242

Milk fat droplet (globule)
  in early pregnancy, 23
  growth of, 51, 53
  in lactation, 33
  in mammary regression, 71
  membrane (MFGM)
    formation of, 61, 63
    primary and secondary, 63
  in milk stasis, 68
  secretion from cell, 61

Milk fat, mammary a–v differences, 149

Milk fat synthesis
  cellular sites, 51
  in lactating cell, 49, 51
  sequence (autoradiographs), 51, 53

Milk fever (parturient paresis), 310

Milk precursors, 186–219
  in blood, 149, 204–217
  identification of, 143–219
  means of identification, 186–218
  mechanism of uptake, 218
  uptake by mammary, principles, 144–146

Milk production, as index of mammary development, 110

Milk protein, *see also* Casein, α-Lactalbumin
  granules (dense bodies, multivesicular bodies)
    in early pregnancy, 25
    in lactating cells, 37
    in milk stasis, 68
  hormones and RNA in, 424–425
  intracellular transport, 39, 41
  in lactating cells, 33
  secretion from cell, 63
  structure, 37, 39
  synthesis
    autoradiography, 43, 45
    during lactation, 37
    polypeptide formation, 45, 49
    during pregnancy, 25, 418
  vacuoles (cytoplasmic), 49

Milk reaccumulation, 262, 393

Milk secretion, *see also* Mammary secretion
  age of litters in, 421

apocrine *vs.* merocrine, 63–67
cessation of, 266–268
effect
of cortisol, 420–421
on mammary blood flow, 174
exteroceptive influences, 262–266
hormonal control, 296–315
hypophysectomy effects, 431
influence of suckling, 252–266
inhibition of, 260, 265–266
by milk accumulation, 393
interference with, species variations, 254–255
of lactating cells, 33
levels and suckling intervals, 261
in milk stasis, 69
neuroendocrine mechanisms
in galactopoeisis, 245–266
in lactogenesis, 243–245
onset, species variation, 5
ovariectomy effects, 420–421
before pregnancy, 278
in pregnancy, 7, 8, 9
RNA levels in, 424–425
RNA-polyribosomes in, 444
tRNA heterogeneity in, 452–453
stimulation of, 292
Milk stasis, 12–14, 67–69, *see also* Weaning
effect on mammary enzymes, 392
Milk synthesis
cessation after hypophysectomy, 297, 298
depressed, 260
inhibition by actinomycin D, 433–434
methods of study, 143–144
in milk stasis, 69
polyribosomes, bound *vs.* free in, 446–447
suckling effects, 316
Milk vein, 196–198, 202, 203
Milk yields
cow
corticosteroid in, 307
glucocorticoid inhibition, 305
growth hormone, 303–304
insulin effects, 312
serum prolactin and, 302–304
thyroid hormone in, 308

effects of anesthesia, 165
of oral contraceptives, 314–315
methods of measurement in various species, 294–295
oxytocin in, 305
Milking, *see also* Milk removal, Suckling, Nursing
insulin release in, 313
Mitochondria
in early pregnancy, 21
in lactation, 31
in late pregnancy, 27
in mammary regression, 71
in milk stasis, 68
in resting stage, 19
ribosomes of, 439
tRNA of, 454
volume of, in varying stages, 55, 56, 58
Mitogenic agents of mammary, 335, 339
Mitosis, mammary cells
critical
in cell development, 335, 424
DNA synthesis and, 335–336
hormonal effects, 335–337, 346
inhibition of, 335
in lactation and pregnancy, 11, 292
serum factor(s) in, 336
Monocytes in mammary regression, 76
Monoribosomes
characteristics, 439
hormonal effects, 444
in mammary development, 445
Morphology, *see* Mammary gland, morphology
Mouse
blood vessels, mammary, 155–156
embryonic mammary gland *in vitro*, 102–103
lactation curve, 296
mammary DNA content, 116, 117
mammary enzymes, 352–354
mammary RNA content, 417, 418, 427–430
mammary tumor virus, 81–85
prolactin levels, 301
Multivesicular bodies
in early pregnancy, 25, 26

in late pregnancy, 27
in mammary regression, 71
Myoepithelial cell, 17, 229, 239, 240
  actomysin in, 81
  calcium for contraction, 312
  lactation, 9, 10
  location of, 77, 236
  in mammary regression, 13, 73
  myofilaments in, 79, 81
  oxytocin effects, 236, 237
  ultrastructure, 78, 79

N

NAD/NADH$_2$, 376, 377, 380, 382, 386
NADH-cytochrome c reductase, insulin and hydrocortisone effects, 341–342
NADP (nicotinamide-adenine dinucleotide phosphate), 370, 371, 379, 380, 383, 385
Neonatal secretion of milk ("witches" milk), 278
Nerve endings, 228–230
  adrenergic, 239
  organs of Ruffini (receptor corpuscles), 229
  sensory receptors, 228, 237
Nerve fibers, myelinated and unmyelinated, 229
Nerves, mammary
  afferent, 228–230, 232–236
  cutaneous, 231
  external spermatic, 231, 232
  inguinal, 231
  segmental, 264
  supply of teat, 228
  sympathetic, 149, 163–164, 231, 232
  vasomotor, 163–165
Nervous system
  autonomic, 232
  central, *see* Central nervous system
  sympathetic, 231, 238
    control of mammary ducts, 240
    effect on mammary blood flow, 163–164
Neural pathways
  efferent, mammary, 231
  of milk ejection reflex, 232–236
  for prolactin release, 257

Neural refractoriness after suckling, to prolactin release, 260
Neuroendocrine control
  in galactopoiesis, 245–266
  in lactogenesis, 243–245
  in milk secretion and ejection, 236–243
Neurohypophyseal hormones (vasopressin, oxytocin) and suckling stimulus, 253
Neurohypophysis, 228, 239
  extrahypothalamic neural influences, 235
  hypothalamic control of, 232
Neurosecretory neurons of hypothalamus, 239
Neurotransmitters in prolactin release, 249
Neutrophils, decrease after milking, 241
Nitrous oxide, as measure of blood flow, 168
Noradrenaline, *see also* Adrenaline
  effect on mammary gland, 164
  inhibition of milk ejection, 239
Norepinephrine, *see* Noradrenaline
Norethisterone, mammogenic effects, 104
Nucleic acid, mammary content, 306
Nucleotide composition
  nRNA, 432
  rRNA, 440
  tRNA, 448
    methylation of, 453
    pseudouridine in, 454
Nucleus
  mammary cell
    in early pregnancy, 21, 23
    in lactation, 31
    in mammary regression, 69
    in milk stasis, 68
  parafascicular thalamic, 234
Nursing, *see also* Suckling
  behavior and intramammary pressure, 230, 231
  behavioral factors
    effect of litter's age, 252, 253
    stress in, 238
  effect on lactation, 315
  frequency, effect on mammary DNA and RNA content, 316

increase of pituitary prolactin, 301
  stimulus, effect on thyroid, 310
Nutrition, mammary effects, 133, 134,
  219, 398

O

Olfaction, effect on lactation, 263
Oral contraceptives, lactational effects,
  314–315
Organ culture, mammary
  embryonic and fetal mouse, 102–103
  identification of milk precursors, 188
  insulin and RNA synthesis in, 188,
    421–423
  mouse, RNA synthesis, 427
  prolactin and RNA synthesis, 422
  study of hormonal control, 99, 132–
    133, 327–334
  whole udder perfusion, 189, 230
Orotic acid incorporation into RNA, 419
  in early lactation, 427
Ovarian hormones
  carriers for administration, 121
  mammary uptake, 123–124
  naturally occurring, 123
  ratios for mammary growth, 124–125
  role in mammary development, 98, 99,
    107, 108, 113, 123
  stimulation of RNA synthesis, 415
Ovariectomy
  effects on lactation, 281, 282
    on lactation mitoses, 313
    on mammary enzymes, 400–401
    on mammary growth, 125
  in goat (lactogenesis effects), 244
  during lactation, effects on RNA, 436
  during pregnancy, effects on RNA,
    420–421
Ovary
  control in lactogenesis, 289–292
  maintenance of lactation, 313–315
Oxytocin, 228, 247, 254–255
  activation of teat receptors, 230
  effect on mammary enzymes, 392, 404
    on mammary gland, 236
      blood flow effects, 182
    on myoepithelium, 236, 237
  inhibitory effects (high levels), 240

in milk removal, 236, 297
  neuroendocrine control of, 236–238
  inhibition, 239
  release
    central nervous system in, 239
    neural pathways, 232
    response to auditory and visual
      stimuli, 237, 305
    to conditioned stimuli, 236, 237
    to suckling, 304
  in weaning, 430

P

P, *see* Prolactin
Pancreas (endocrine), lactation mainte-
  nance, 312–313
Parafascicular thalamic nucleus, 234
Parathyroid glands, in lactation, 311, 312
Parathyroid hormone
  maintenance of lactation, 297, 308,
    311–312
  mammary development, 130, 131
Paraventricular neurons (PV) of hypothalamus, 232, 234, 239
Parenchyma of mammary gland, 229
Parturient paresis syndrome (milk fe-
  ver), 310
Parturition
  mammary secretion in, 280
    RNA levels and, 418–419, 425
  premature, 288
Peduncle, mammillary, 234
Pentolinium (adrenergic block), 240, 241
Pentose cycle enzymes, 369–373, *see also*
  specific enzymes
  amounts in various species, 352
  constants, 356
Pentose phosphate-metabolizing enzymes,
  372 *see also* specific enzymes
  amounts in various species, 352
  constants, 357
Peptide chain formation, 441, 442, 445,
  447
Peptide transferase, 441
Peptidyl-tRNA, 439
Perfusion
  of fatty acids, 147
  whole udder, 189

Perphenazine, induced lactation, 287
Phenothiazine derivatives, mammotropic
    effects, 134
Phenoxybenzamine (Dibenzyline) adren-
    ergic block, 240
Pheromone, effect on prolactin release,
    263
Phosphate (PO_4),
    mammary vasodilation, 184
    in milk, 216
Phosphofructokinase
    amounts in various species, 353
    characteristics, 373–374
    constants, 357
Phosphoglucomutase
    amounts in various species, 352
    characteristics, 367
    constants, 356
6-Phosphogluconate dehydrogenase
    actinomycin D inhibition of, 434
    amounts in various species, 352
    characteristics, 371–372
    constants, 357
    insulin effects on, 340, 400
6-Phosphoglucose isomerase, glucose-in-
    sulin effects on, 400
Phospholipids, mammary a − v differ-
    ences, 147, 148
Phospho(P)-glucose isomerase, 353, 357
PIF, *see* Prolactin-inhibiting factor
Pig
    amino acid uptake (mammary), 212
    arteries for blood sampling, 195, 196
    fatty acid uptake, 212
    mammary DNA content, 117
    mammary enzymes, 352–354
    mammary RNA content, 419, 425
    sampling venous blood, 196, 203
Piloerection, oxytocin response, 240
Pineal gland, biogenic amines in lacta-
    tion, 315
Pinocytosis, 63, 67
Pituitary gland, *see also* Adenohypophy-
    sis, Neurohypophysis
    acidophils, prolactin secretion, 245,
        250
    anterior lobe
        control of lactogenesis, 281–285
        effect of estrogen implants, 314

    maintenance of lactation, 297–304
    autonomy
        hypothalamic influences, 258
        species differences, 249–250
        thyroid hormone effects, 309
    gonadotropin, 244
    hormones of, 243
        in mammogenesis, 122, 123
        in lactation, 227–268
        in mammary development and milk
            synthesis, 98–99, 131
    neuroendocrine mechanisms, 227–268
    posterior lobe, maintenance of lacta-
        tion, 304–305
    radioimmunoassay of prolactin, 254
    stalk transection
        effect on lactogenesis, 244
        milk secretion and, 254
        on prolactin release, 245
        replacement of hormones, 255
    transplants and autonomy of, 245–247,
        254, 299
    transplants and RNA, 428
Placental hormones
    human, 118, 128, 278, 284, 346
    in mammary development, species
        variations, 118–120, 128, 284,
        346
    in mammary RNA synthesis, 417
Placental lactogen, 118–120, 128, 244,
    278, 284, 346
Plasmalemma (cell wall)
    in MFGM formation, 61, 63
    regeneration, 63
Podophyllin, 134
Polyribosomes (ribonucleoprotein)
    bound to ER and free, 442
        functional differences in milk secre-
            tion, 446–447
        variation in physiological states, 445
    characteristics, 442–443
    development of, 443
    distribution of sizes in varying phys-
        iological states, 442, 443, 445
    effect of actinomycin D, 433
    hormonal effects, 443–444
    RNA (messenger), 442
Postpartum growth of mammary, 120
Potassium (K) in milk, 216

Pregnancy
    effect on lactation, 316
    late, corticosteroid concentration, 288
    mammary development during, 110–
        113, 279
    mammary RNA content during, 416–
        417
        concurrent lactation and, 428
        in weaning, 430
Prepartum hormone levels, 288
Pressure, intramammary, 240
Primary sprout, mammary growth and
    differentiation, 105–106
Primordial structure, *see* Anlage
Proestrus, 108, 279, 405
Progestagens, 128
Progesterone
    concentration variations in pregnancy
        species differences, 291, 292
    effect on lactogenesis, 245, 291, 395–
        397
        on mammary enzymes, 395–397
        on mammary growth and differen-
            tiation, 106, 107, 109, 122, 245,
            327, 345
        on mammary vascularity, 156
    to estrogen ratios
        induction of lactation, 293–294
        in lactogenesis, 245
        mammary development, 124–125
    inhibition
        of milk synthesis, 293, 346
        by prostaglandin, 291
    mammary gland spreading factor and,
        103
    metabolites of, 127, 292
    precursors, 127
    in RNA synthesis, 416, 419–421, 424,
        425
        nRNA, 438
    uptake by mammary gland, 124
    in vitro studies, 132
Progestins, lactational effects, 122, 314
Prolactin, 228
    in alveolar synchrony, 345
    in cellular hyperplasia, 420
    concentration
        circadian rhythms and, 301

    estrous cycles and, 278, 301, 332
    milk yields (cow) and, 302–303
    effect on adipose tissue, 103
        on mammary DNA synthesis, 105,
            333
        on mammary enzymes, 392, 404–
            405
        on mammary gland, local, 333
        on histones, 437
        on lactation, various species, 298–
            299
        on lipoprotein lipase, 420
        on mammary DNA synthesis, 105
        on mammary growth and differen-
            tiation, 103, 105–108, 132, 328,
            329, 333–334, 336
        on mammary protein secretion, 334,
            336
        on mammary RNA synthesis, 343,
            396, 404–405, 415, 419–422,
            425, 430, 431
        on milk yields, in various species,
            298–300
        on nRNA, 433–434
        on ribosomes, 343
        on RNA polymerase, 435–436
        on RNA-polyribosomes, 445
        on rRNA, 444
        on tRNA, 449–450
    in enzyme synthesis regulation, 392,
        395–397, 404–405
    in ergastoplasm development, 57, 446
    "feedback controls" of, 248, 249, 255
    human, growth hormone activity, 282
    inhibition of release, 248, 250, 257,
        258
    initiation and maintenance of lactation,
        281–284, 301–303
    levels in lactogenesis, 281, 282
        in pregnancy, 332–333
        in weaning, 266–268
    mechanism of secretion, 245–246
    in milk synthesis, 297
    neuroendocrine regulation of, 245–252
    pituitary
        concentration
            litter size and, 258, 259
            in pregnancy and at parturition,
                285

suckling intervals and, 257–261
  after suckling, 256, 257
  postpartum, 244
  radioimmunoassay of, 254, 301
placental, *see* Placental lactogen
release
  estrogen in, 289
  exteroceptive influences on, 262–266, 302
  neural pathways for, 232
  suckling, 247, 256–262
replacement in hypophysectomy, 255
sensitization of mammary cells to insulin and serum factor(s), 332–334
synergism
  with cortisone, 421
  with glucocorticoids, 285–286
  with insulin, 332–333
    in RNA synthesis, 422
  with ovarian steroids, 122
synonyms of, 113, 281
turnover rate, 246–247
Prolactin cell (acidophil)
  activities, 257, 258
  species variations, 250
Prolactin-inhibiting factor (PIF), 257, 258
  circulating prolactin levels and, 248, 250
  estrogen inhibition of, 246
  site of production, 251
Prolactin-releasing factor, 258
Propranolol (adrenergic block), 240
Prostaglandins
  effect on mammary blood flow, 183
  induction of lactogenesis, 291
Protein markers of mammary cells, 334
Protein secretion, mammary
  hormonal effects on, 334, 337, 339, 340
  RNA synthesis and, 422
Protein synthesis, mammary, 388, 389, *see also* Milk protein
  control by hormones, 328, 329, 334–338, 340, 342–346, 414, 415
  RNA-polyribosomes and, 444
  tRNA heterogeneity in, 452–453

rough endoplasmic reticulum and, 446–447
in varying physiological states, 334–338; 345–346
Pseudopregnancy, 250
  endocrine changes, 113
  mammary development in, 109, 113, 114, 118
  mammary RNA content, 417, 419, 420
  neural pathways of milk ejection, 235
Pseudouridine, 440, 454
Puberty
  endocrine changes, 107
  mammary growth in, 415
Puromycin, 134
  effects on RNA synthesis, 436
Pyruvate decarboxylase, 387–388
Pyruvate dehydrogenase, 387–388
Pyruvate kinase
  amount in rat mammary, 353
  characteristics, 376
  constants, 358
  isoenzymes, 376–377

Q

Quantitative measures of mammary growth, 101, 102, 110

R

Rabbit
  blood vessels, mammary, 155
  fatty acid uptake, mammary, 212
  mammary DNA content, 117
  mammary RNA content, 416–418, 427, 429, 430
  prolactin
    effect in lactation, 299
    induction of lactation, 282, 420
  venous blood sampling, 196
Radioactive isotopes, milk precursor identification, 154, 186–188
Radioimmunoassay of pituitary hormone content, 301
  of prolactin, 254
Rat
  blood vessels, mammary, 155, 156
  growth hormone in lactation, 300
  intermediary metabolite levels, 360

lactation
  age of litters in, 264–265, 421
  corticosterone levels, 306–307
  glucocorticoids in, 305–306
  lactation curve, 293, 296
  lactation index, 294, 295
  mammary blood flow, 181
  mammary DNA content in pregnancy,
      111, 114
  mammary enzymes, 352–354, 357–359
  mammary RNA content, 416, 417,
      419, 425, 427–431
  pituitary prolactin levels in suckling,
      301
  prolactin effect in lactation, 298–299
Receptors (nerve endings), mammary,
      228–230, 237
  adrenergic (α,β), 239
  stimulation by oxytocin, 230
Relaxin in mammary development, 130
Reserpine derivatives, mammogenic ef-
      fects, 134
  effects on polyribosomes, 442
  prolactin release and, 249, 250
  in weaning, 429
Ribonuclease, 427
Ribonucleic acid (RNA)
  DNA-like, 432, 433, 435, 438
  in enzyme synthesis, 434
  mammary content and synthesis of
      in concurrent pregnancy and lacta-
          tion, 428
      in estrus, 278, 415, 416
      fetal, 415
      in galactopoiesis, 295, 425–428
      in hypophysectomy, 431
      in involution, 427–428, 429–431
      in lactogenesis, 417–418
          induced *in vitro*, 421–425
          induced *in vivo*, 419–421
      in late pregnancy, 416–417
      at parturition, 286, 287, 418–419
      prepubertal, 414
      in pseudopregnancy, 417
      at puberty, 415–416
          species variations, 419
      suckling and, 425
  messenger (mRNA), 432–434, 442,
      445, 447

factors for binding rRNA, 441
  in genetic translation, 450
microsomal RNA
  hormonal effects, 444
  in milk protein formation, 446–447
  species variations, 440
nuclear (nRNA)
  actinomycin D effects, 432–433
  characterization of, 437–438
  classes of, 432, 437, 438
  in DNA transcription, 431
  hybridization with ribosomal RNA,
      438
  insulin effects, 432
  mammary content in galactopoiesis
      and pregnancy, 431
  nucleotide content, 432
  rRNA precursor, 432
  sedimentation profiles, 432, 437–
      438
  synthesis rate, 432
      hormonal control, 433, 438
      in lactogenesis, 433
  in protein synthesis, 414, 415, 424–
      425
ribosomal (rRNA)
  amounts in varying physiological
      states, 443
  characteristics of, 439–441
  hormonal effects on synthesis, 443–
      444
  nucleotide composition, species vari-
      ation, 440
  synthesis rate, 444
  synthesis in varying physiological
      states, 443
synthesis
  aspartate transcarbamylase in, 417
  cortisol in, 405, 423–425
  hormonal effects, 344, 427
  hormonal induction, 419
  hydrocortisone in, 342
  insulin effects, 330, 421–425
  prolactin effects, 343, 396, 405, 418–
      421, 423–425, 435
  protein secretion and, 422–423
  rough endoplasmic reticulum and,
      342
transfer (tRNA), 442

amino acid acceptor capacity
changes in physiological states, 448–450
heterogeneity of, 450–453
changes in physiological states, 451–452
minor nucleotides in, 453–454
species variations, 448–449
aminoacyl complex formation, 447
control of mammary protein synthesis, 450–451
in genetic translation, 447
hormonal effect on levels, 449–450
nucleotide content, 448
species variations, 440
physiochemistry, 447–448
variation in amounts and milk synthesis, 449–450
Ribonucleic acid polymerases
activity in lactation, 435–436
insulin effects, 340
Ribonucleoprotein (RNP)
aggregation of, 442
variation in physiological states, 443–445
amount, mammary, in varying physiological states, 442–443
characterization, 438–439
distribution in cell, 442–443
factors necessary for rRNA binding to mRNA, 441
hormonal effects on, 443–444
in milk protein synthesis, 446–447
monoribosomes, 439, 444
polyribosomes, 442–445
ribosomal proteins, 441
ribosomal RNA, 439–440
Ribosome-ribosomal subunits, 442
Ribosomes, *see also* Ribonucleic acid, ribosomal; Ergastoplasm
factors necessary for binding to mRNA, 441
free and bound in lactation, 442, 443
hydrocortisone effects, 341
insulin effects, 340–341
mammary
in resting stage, 19
secreting and nonsecreting cow, 441
in milk protein synthesis, 45, 446–447

nonstructural protein binding, 442
in peptide chain formation, 441
prolactin effects on, 343
RNA, *see* Ribonucleic acid
RNP, *see* Ribonucleoprotein
Rough endoplasmic reticulum (RER), 338, *see also* Ergastoplasm; Ribosomes
hydrocortisone effects on, 341, 342, 343
insulin effects, 340, 341, 343
polyribosomes, 442
prolactin effects, 343–344
protein synthesis (milk), 446–447
RNA synthesis, 342, 344
Ruminants
fatty acid uptakes (mammary), 212
growth hormone in lactation, 300
sampling of venous blood, 202–203

S

Self-licking (rat)
prolactin release, 262
role in mammary growth during pregnancy, 134, 244
Sensory stimuli from litter to mother, 262–266
auditory, 237, 263
olfactory, 263
optic, 237, 263
spatial, 264–266
Serotonin
effect on mammary blood flow, 149, 165, 182, 183
inhibition of oxytocin release, 315
Serum factor(s) sensitivity, mammary
effect on mammary development, 328–329
prolactin effects, 342–344
in varying physiological states, 328–334
Sheep, *see also* Ewe
arteries for blood sampling, 194
udder blood flow, 182, 184
Somatotropic activities, placental, 118
Somatotropin, 255, *see also* Growth hormone
Spinal cord, transection of
inhibition of milk ejection, 240

milk secretion effects, species variations, 254, 255
suckling effects in, 253
Spinal pathways for milk ejection, 232–233
Spinotectal tract, 233, 235
Spinothalamic tract in oxytocin release, 233, 235
Spiperone, stress avoidance, 191
Splanchnic nerves, 232
Stearyl desaturase, 387
Steer, mammary development in, 104
Steroids (gonadal, placental, corticoid), 244
    mammary uptake (gonadal), 123–125
STH, *see* Somatotropin, Growth hormone
Stilbestrol, 416
Stimulation of mammary gland
    mechanical, 134, 237–238
    oxytocin, 238
Stimuli of mammary gland
    conditional, auditory and visual in oxytocin release, 237, 263
    exteroceptive, 262–265
        corticosterone release, 263, 306
        of lactation, 262, 263
        tactile, 232, 264
Stress
    effect on arteriovenous measurements, 146, 148
        on blood flow, 149, 151, 164, 181, 190–192
        on milk ejection, 238, 242
Stressors, somatic and psychological, 238
Subthalamus, 234
Succinic dehydrogenase
    amounts in various species, 353
    characteristics, 381–382
Suckling, *see also* Nursing, Milk removal
    activation of nerves, 232
    effect
        of central nervous system, 232, 252
        on mammary RNA and DNA content, 425–426
        on maternal behavior, 252
        on prolactin release, 248, 252–256
    growth hormone release, 303–304
    initiation of lactation, 253–254

intervals
    effect on milk secretion, 261
    pituitary prolactin levels, 257–261
    neural refractoriness in, 260
    lactation stimulus, 292
    in lactogenesis, 244
    maintenance of secretion, 252–253, 316
    milk ejection response, 230
    pituitary secretions, 256
    prolactin release, 247, 256–262
    release of ACTH, 306
Suckling effects, methods of analysis, 254
Supraoptic neurons (SO) of hypothalamus, 232, 239
Sympathectomy, lumbar, mammary effects, 231
Sympathetic-adrenal system, inhibition milk ejection reflex, 239, 241
Sympathetic fibers, mammary, 231
Sympathetic nervous system, *see* Nervous system, sympathetic

T

Tactile stimuli, 232, 264
Teat
    blood supply, 159, 161
    nerve supply, 163, 229
Teat fistula, 241
Tegmentum, mesencephalic, 233
Telencephalon in prolactin secretion, 250, 251
Testosterone
    effect on DNA synthesis *in vitro*, 105
        on mammary bud, 104
        on mammary growth and differentiation, 105, 126
Thermodilution, measure of blood flow, 165–167; 179
Thermography, measure of blood flow, 173–174
Thermostromuhr, measure of blood flow, 151, 167
Thoracic mammary gland, 241
Thymidine, radioactive
    incorporation into DNA, 131
        into RNA, 418, 423
    uptake by organ cultures, 133

Thyrocalcitonin, 309, 310
Thyroidectomy
  effect on mammary enzymes, 406
  on milk yields, 308
Thyroid gland in lactation maintenance,
  308–311
Thyroid hormone (thyroxine), *see also*
  Triiodothyronine
  effect on mammary growth, 125–126
  in mammary development, 129
  in milk synthesis, 297
  in RNA synthesis, 428
  secretion rates, 310, 311
  site of action, 309
  stimulation of lactation, 308
  in vitro studies, 132–133
Thyroid-stimulating hormone (TSH),
  297
Thyroprotein
  feeding effects, 309
  in lactation, 301
  in prolactin release, 302
Thyroxine-binding globulin, 311
Tissue culture
  mammary
    cell division for lactogenesis, 292
    hormone sequences necessary for
      lactation, 292–293
    identification of milk precursors,
      187, 188
    induced casein synthesis with pro-
      lactin, 284
    insulin requirement, 129
    pituitary, 246–248
Tissue slices, *see also* Organ cultures
  mammary, identification of milk pre-
    cursors, 148, 187, 188
TPN, *see* NADP
Tract (central nervous system)
  spinotectal, 233, 235
  spinothalamic, 233
Transaldolase, 372
Transcortin and adrenal steroids, 245
Transketolase, 372
Triglyceride
  hydrolysis, capillary endothelium in,
    185, 214–216
  mammary uptake, 213, 215, 216

Triglyceride synthetases, 387
Triiodothyronine, *see also* Thyroid hormone
  mammary requirement after hypophy-
    sectomy, 255, 282
  stimulation of lactation, 308
TSH, *see* Thyroid-stimulating hormone
  (thyrotropin)
Triose-phosphate-isomerase
  amounts in cow, 353
  characteristics, 375
  constants, 357
Trophoblast in mammary development,
  119, 128
Tumor virus in mammary, 81–88

U

Udder, *see also* Mammary gland
  distension and denervation of, 241
UDP glucose-4-epimerase
  amounts in various species, 352
  characteristics, 368
  constants, 356
UDPG pyrophosphorylase
  amounts in various species, 352
  characteristics, 367–368
  constants, 356
Ultrasonic methods, measure of blood
  flow, 171, 172
Uridine incorporation into RNA, 416,
  418, 421, 423, 424, 427, 431
  into nRNA, 432–433
  into rRNA, 444
Uterus, lactogenic effects, 243, 244

V

Vasoconstriction, in mammary gland, 231
  blood flow effects, 181–182
Vasodilators, effect on mammary blood
  flow, 183–184
Vasomotor nerves, mammary, 163
Virus in mammary cells
  leukemia, 88–91
  tumor, 81–88
Vitamin D, substitution for parathyroid
  hormone, 312
Vitamins in milk, 217

W

Weaning, 266–268, *see also* Mammary
    regression, Milk stasis
  bilateral, RNA levels, 429–430
  effect on mammary enzymes, 405
  hormone effects, 430
  mammary RNA content and, 429–430

mammary structure and, 12–13, 67, 68
  myoepithelial cell and, 13
  unilateral, RNA in, 430, 431
"Witches milk," 278

Z

Zonula adhaerends, 19
Zonula occludentes, 17, 19